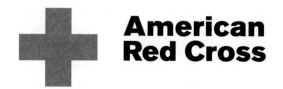

American
Red Cross

American Red Cross
Emergency Medical Response

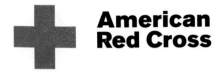
American Red Cross

This *Emergency Medical Response* textbook is part of the American Red Cross Emergency Medical Response program. By itself, it does not constitute complete and comprehensive training. Visit redcross.org to learn more about this program.

The emergency care procedures outlined in this book reflect the standard of knowledge and accepted emergency practices in the United States at the time this book was published. It is the reader's responsibility to stay informed of changes in emergency care procedures.

Published by StayWell Health & Safety Solutions

Printed in the United States of America
ISBN: 978-1-58480-327-0

Photo Credits

Select Photography: Barbara Proud and Steven Kovich

Chapter 2 Opener: Courtesy of Ted Crites

Chapter 5 Opener: Courtesy of Terry Georgia

Chapter 8 Opener: ©iStockphoto.com/Frances Twitty

Chapter 12 Opener: Image Copyright mangostock, 2010 Used under license from Shutterstock.com

Chapter 14 Opener: Image Copyright yamix, 2010 Used under license from Shutterstock.com

Chapter 18 Opener: Courtesy of Lake-Sumter Emergency Medical Services, Mount Dora, FL, Captain Phil Kleinberg, EMT-P

Chapter 21 Opener: Copyright Marina Bartel/ iStockphoto/Thinkstock

Chapter 23 Opener: Courtesy of Terry Georgia

Chapter 26 Opener: Image Copyright Phase4Photography, 2010 Used under license from Shutterstock.com

Chapter 28 Opener: ©iStockphoto.com/ Frances Twitty

Chapter 29 Opener: Image Copyright TFoxFoto, 2010 Used under license from Shutterstock.com

Chapter 30 Opener: Image Copyright Marlene DeGrood, 2010 Used under license from Shutterstock.com

Chapter 32 Opener: Image Copyright prism68, 2010 Used under license from Shutterstock.com

Many thanks to Capt. Jerome Williams, Battalion Chief Kenny Wolfrey, Capt. William Bailey and the Fairfax County, Virginia Fire and Rescue staff; and Executive Director Jim Judge, Capt. Deanna Chapman, Capt. Phil Kleinberg and the Lake-Sumter EMS staff, for opening their facilities to us and providing their expertise and assistance with our photography and video shoots.

Library of Congress Cataloging-in-Publication Data

American Red Cross emergency medical response.
    p. ; cm.
 Emergency medical response participant's manual
 Includes index.
 ISBN 978-1-58480-327-0
 1. Emergency medicine—Problems, exercise, etc. 2. Emergency medical services—Problems, exercises, etc. I. American Red Cross. II. Title: Emergency medical response participant's manual.
 [DNLM: 1. Emergency Treatment—methods—Problems and Exercises. 2. Emergencies—Problems and Exercises. 3. Emergency Medical Services—Problems and Exercises. WB 18.2]
 RC86.7.A476 2011
 616.02'5—dc22

                                                                    2011004133

Acknowledgments

This textbook is dedicated to the thousands of employees and volunteers of the American Red Cross who contribute their time and talent to supporting and teaching lifesaving skills worldwide and to the thousands of course participants and other readers who have decided to be prepared to take action when an emergency strikes.

Many individuals shared in the development and revision process in various supportive, technical and creative ways. The *Emergency Medical Response* textbook was developed through the dedication of both employees and volunteers. Their commitment to excellence made this textbook possible.

This training program and educational materials are consistent with the current Emergency Medical Services Educational Standards for Emergency Medical Responders. The care steps outlined within this product are consistent with the Guidelines 2010 for First Aid and the 2010 Consensus on Science for Cardiopulmonary Resuscitation and Emergency Cardiovascular Care. These treatment recommendations and related training guidelines have been reviewed by the American Red Cross Scientific Advisory Council.

The following members of the American Red Cross Scientific Advisory Council also provided guidance and review:

David Markenson, MD, FAAP, EMT-P
Chair, American Red Cross Scientific
Advisory Council
Chief, Pediatric Emergency Medicine
Maria Fareri Children's Hospital
Westchester Medical Center
Valhalla, New York

Jonathan L. Epstein, MEMS, NREMT-P
Vice Chair, American Red Cross Scientific
Advisory Council
Northeast EMS, Inc.
Wakefield, Massachusetts

David C. Berry, PhD, ATC, EMT-B
Member, American Red Cross Scientific
Advisory Council
Associate Professor of Kinesiology and Athletic
Training Education Program Director
Saginaw Valley State University
University Center, Michigan

Jim Judge, EMT-P, CEM
Member, American Red Cross Scientific
Advisory Council
Executive Director
Lake Sumter-EMS
Mount Dora, Florida

The **American Red Cross Scientific Advisory Council** is a panel of nationally recognized experts in the fields of emergency medicine, sports medicine, emergency medical services (EMS), emergency preparedness, disaster mobilization, and other public health and safety fields.

The Sounding Board for this edition included:

Craig C. Blaine, EMT-P
Health and Safety Instructor Trainer
Gastonia, North Carolina

Antonio E. Duran
Fire Captain, Safety Officer
Los Angeles County Fire Department
Temple City, California

Christina Fygetakes, MSEd, RRT, RPFT
Respiratory Therapist/Pulmonary Function
Technologist
Akron General Medical Center
Akron, Ohio

Donald Gregory, EMT-P
Health and Safety Instructor Trainer
UAW-GM Center for Human Resources
Montrose, Michigan

Elaine Kyte, LPN
Director, Health and Safety Services
Hazleton Chapter, American Red Cross
West Hazleton, Pennsylvania

Marlene Lugg, DrPH
Health and Safety Instructor Trainer
Glendale – Crescenta Valley Chapter,
American Red Cross
Senior Research Scientist
Southern California Kaiser Permanente
Adjunct Professor
West Coast University, Los Angeles
Winnetka, California

Lynne Osborne
Manager of Workplace Programs
Southeastern Michigan Chapter, American
Red Cross
Detroit, Michigan

Thomas Raines
Master Deputy Sheriff
Field Training Coordinator
Pensacola, Florida

Jonathan K. Rioch
Mechanical Engineer
Guardian Industries
Victor, New York

Paula Robinson, MA, EMT-B
Associate Professor
Parker College of Chiropractic
Dallas, Texas

The following individuals provided external guidance and review as Subject Matter Experts:

Paul B. Atkinson, MD
Neurologist
Ministry Health Care
Stevens Point, Wisconsin

Richard Ellis, BSOE, NREMT-Paramedic
Georgia Paramedic & EMS Level III Instructor
Chair, Paramedic Technology
Central Georgia Technical College
Treasurer, National Association of Emergency
Medical Technicians
Warner Robins, Georgia

Julie Gilchrist, MD
Centers for Disease Control and Prevention
Atlanta, Georgia

Jody Kakacek, M.A.
Program Manager, Special Projects
Quality of Life, Programs and Research
Epilepsy Foundation
Landover, Maryland

Jennifer Lugg
Aquatic Specialist
NAUI Open Water Certification
Health and Safety Instructor
American Red Cross of Greater Los Angeles
Glendale – Crescenta Valley Chapter,
American Red Cross
Winnetka, California

William Lugg, B.A., EMT
Firefighter, HAZMAT Specialist I
Los Angeles City Fire Department
Rescue 3 Swift Water Rescue I and NAUI
Rescue Diver
Health and Safety Instructor
American Red Cross of Greater Los Angeles
Glendale – Crescenta Valley Chapter,
American Red Cross
Los Angeles, California

Thomas J. McCarrier, NREMT-I
Professional Advisory Board Chair
Epilepsy Foundation Central/Northeast
Wisconsin
Stevens Point, Wisconsin
National Professional Advisory Board Member
Epilepsy Foundation
Landover, Maryland

Basim Uthman, MD
Neurologist
University of Florida
Gainesville, Florida
National Professional Advisory Board Member
Epilepsy Foundation
Landover, Maryland

The following organizations previewed the participant textbook and support the use of this program for training emergency medical responders:

Fairfax County Fire and Rescue Department
Fairfax County, Virginia

Fairfax County Police
Fairfax County, Virginia

International Association of Fire Chiefs
Fairfax, Virginia

International Association of Fire Fighters
Washington, D.C.

National Association of EMS Physicians®
Olathe, Kansas

National Athletic Trainers' Association
Dallas, Texas

The American Red Cross would also like to thank illustrators Annelisa Ochoa and Sara Krause; and Sherry Hinman and MaryAnn Foley, for their assistance in writing the textbook and supplementary materials.

In Memoriam
Donald Gregory was a valuable member of the American Red Cross Emergency Medical Response program team, a licensed paramedic, a First Aid/CPR/AED instructor trainer, an Authorized Provider and longtime First Aid Station Volunteer Coordinator for the Genesee-Lapeer Chapter in Flint, MI. He was also a policeman and firefighter. Don was very dedicated and passionate about safety and was respected by all who knew him.

Table of Contents

Detailed Table of Contents

UNIT 5: MEDICAL EMERGENCIES

UNIT 6: TRAUMA EMERGENCIES

UNIT 7: SPECIAL POPULATIONS

UNIT 8: EMS OPERATIONS

Key Features

The new American Red Cross Emergency Medical Response program represents the gold standard in training *emergency medical responders* (EMRs). This flexible, cutting-edge training solution is part of a comprehensive suite of high quality health and safety training programs offered by one of the most respected brands in the world.

This highly rated program has been completely revised to reflect the latest science in first aid, CPR and cardiovascular care. The course has also been redesigned to align with updated EMS Educational Standards.

Emergency Medical Response has also been revised with instructors' and students' needs in mind. The new affordable, user-friendly training materials enrich the learning experience for EMRs at every level. The new course includes—

- A more interactive course format featuring new rescue scenarios and hands-on exercises.
- Fully updated student materials, including a textbook and workbook.
- New ancillaries resources, such as an online learning companion.

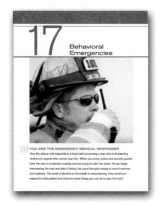

You Are the Emergency Medical Responder

At the start of each chapter, readers will find a unique, real-life scenario description that features an emergency involving different EMRs. Readers are asked to assess the situation and are prompted to think about what should be done. These scenarios help frame what will be discussed in the chapter, and encourage the student to start thinking about what to do and the proper sequence in a given emergency. A concluding scenario at the close of each chapter builds on the opening scenario and allows readers to apply the knowledge and skills gained to help answer the questions posed.

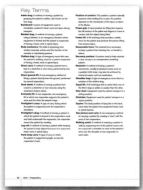

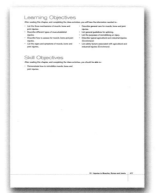

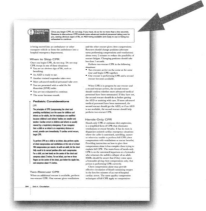

Key Terms

Each chapter defines the key terms used that all *emergency medical services* (EMS) personnel should know. A comprehensive glossary is also available.

Learning Objectives and Skills Objectives

These objectives represent the key material covered in the chapter, as well as the skills in which the students will be trained.

Critical Facts

Brief summaries of crucial parts of the chapter are called out for quick and easy reference.

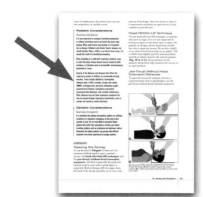

Pediatric Considerations and Geriatric Considerations

Focus on considerations in the pediatric and geriatric population EMRs should be aware of when responding to an emergency.

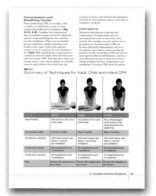

Tables

Clear, visual presentation of certain key information.

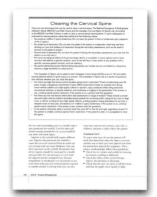

Sidebars

Supplementary information which enriches student knowledge and understanding of the chapter material.

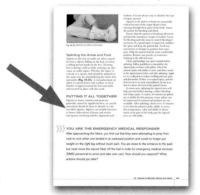

Putting It All Together

A wrap-up for each chapter, touching on the key objectives and points covered.

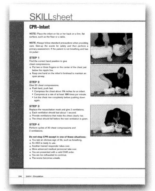

Skill Sheets

Step-by-step visual directions for performing specific skills that students will need to know in order to provide appropriate care for victims of an emergency.

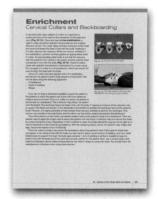

Enrichment

Areas of additional information and skills students will find valuable.

Student Resources

EMERGENCY MEDICAL RESPONSE WORKBOOK

This workbook is designed to accompany the *Emergency Medical Response* textbook. Specific workbook activities were created to help you review the most important material in the textbook, to help you practice making appropriate decisions about emergency care and to help you prepare for the skills and written evaluations. The material in each unit of this workbook reinforces key concepts and skills taught in the textbook and the course. This affords you the opportunity to build on learned material and apply your knowledge to emergency situations. Most of the workbook activities allow you to work at your own pace and evaluate your progress at various stages. The workbook includes learning activities, such as crossword puzzles, matching and labeling exercises, fill-in-the-blank and short answer questions; case studies; self-assessment; references to skill sheet pages; exams and more.

EMR INTERACTIVE

Enhance learning with EMR Interactive. This self-paced online tool supports traditional classroom training, allowing instructors to make more efficient use of class time and provide more hands on practice. Designed to appeal to a variety of learning styles, this interactive program is easy-to-navigate and filled with highly engaging content to improve learning results.

The program contains 14 modules that explore core concepts and skills. Appealing visuals, video clips, interactive activities and animations accompany the lessons. Key terms are also highlighted and defined within each module. A practice quiz and case scenarios are included in each module to help the participant apply knowledge and make decisions about care.

Health Precautions and Guidelines During Training

The American Red Cross has trained millions of people in first aid, CPR, and AED using manikins as training aids. The Red Cross follows widely accepted guidelines for cleaning and decontaminating training manikins. If these guidelines are adhered to, the risk of any kind of disease transmission during training is extremely low.

To help minimize the risk of disease transmission, you should follow some basic health precautions and guidelines while participating in training. You should take additional precautions if you have a condition that would increase your risk or other participants' risk of exposure to infections. Request a separate training manikin if you:

- Have an acute condition, such as a cold, sore throat or cuts or sores on your hands or around your mouth.
- Know that you are seropositive (have had a positive blood test) for hepatitis B surface antigen (HBsAg), which indicates that you are currently infected with the hepatitis B virus.*
- Know that you have a chronic infection as indicated by long-term seropositivity (long-term positive blood tests) for HBsAg* or a positive blood test for anti-HIV, that is, a positive test for antibodies to HIV, the virus that causes many severe infections, including AIDS.
- Have had a positive blood test for hepatitis C virus.
- Have a type of condition that makes you extremely likely to get an infection.

To obtain information about testing for individual health status, go to the Centers for Disease Control and Prevention website (cdc.gov).

After a person has had an acute hepatitis B infection, he or she will no longer test positive for HBsAg but will test positive for the hepatitis B antibody (anti-HBs). People who have been vaccinated against hepatitis B will also test positive for anti-HBs. A positive test for anti-HBs should not be confused with a positive test for HBsAg.

If you decide that you should have your own manikin, ask your instructor if he or she can provide one for you. You will not be asked to explain why you make this request. The manikin will not be used by anyone else until it has been cleaned according to the recommended end-of-class decontamination procedures. Because the number of manikins available for class use is limited, the more advance notice you give, the more likely it is that you can be provided a separate manikin.

GUIDELINES

In addition to taking the precautions regarding manikins, you can protect yourself and other participants from infection by following these guidelines:

- Wash your hands thoroughly before participating in class activities.
- Do not eat, drink, use tobacco products or chew gum during class when manikins are used.

---

*People with hepatitis B infection will test positive for HBsAg. Most people infected with hepatitis B virus will get better in time. However, some hepatitis B infections will become chronic and linger for much longer. People with these chronic infections will continue to test positive for HBsAg. Their decision to participate in CPR training should be guided by their physician.

- Clean the manikin properly before use.
- For some manikins, cleaning properly means vigorously wiping the manikin's face and the inside of its mouth with a clean gauze pad soaked with either a fresh solution of liquid chlorine bleach and water (¼ cup of sodium hypochlorite per gallon of tap water) or rubbing alcohol. The surfaces should remain wet for at least 1 minute before they are wiped dry with a second piece of clean, absorbent material.
- For other manikins, cleaning properly means changing the manikin's face. Your instructor will provide you with instructions for cleaning the type of manikin used in your class.
- Follow the guidelines provided by your instructor when practicing skills such as clearing a blocked airway with your finger.

PHYSICAL STRESS AND INJURY

Successful course completion requires full participation in classroom and skill sessions, as well as successful performance during skill and knowledge evaluations. Because of the nature of the skills in this course, you will participate in strenuous activities, such as performing CPR on the floor. If you have a medical condition or disability that will prevent you from taking part in the skill practice sessions, please tell your instructor so that accommodations can be made.

If you are unable to participate fully in the course, you may audit the course and participate as much as you can or desire but you will not be evaluated. To participate in the course in this way, you must tell the instructor before training begins. Be aware that you will not be eligible to receive a course completion certificate.

UNIT
1
PREPARATORY

1

The Emergency Medical Responder

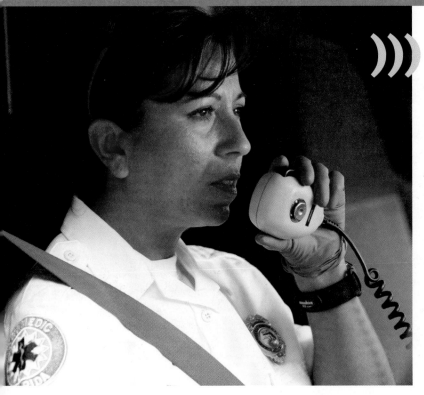

))) YOU ARE THE EMERGENCY MEDICAL RESPONDER

A terrified mother pulls her child from the bottom of a pool while a neighbor calls 9-1-1 for help. You are the first to arrive at the scene and see the neighbor trying to breathe air into the boy's limp body. The mother looks to you helplessly. How would you respond?

Key Terms

Advanced emergency medical technician (AEMT): A person trained in emergency care, with the additional training to allow insertion of IVs, administration of medications, performance of advanced airway procedures, and setting up and assessing of *electrocardiograms* (ECGs or EKGs); formerly referred to as EMT-Intermediate.

Certification: Credentialing at the local level; usually entails completing a probationary period and updating and/or recertification to cover changing knowledge and skills.

Direct medical control: A type of medical direction, also called "on-line," "base-station," "immediate" or "concurrent medical control"; under this type of medical direction, the physician speaks directly with emergency care providers at the scene of an emergency.

Emergency medical responder (EMR): A person trained in emergency medical care who may be called on to provide such care as a routine part of the job, paid or volunteer; often the first trained professional to respond to emergencies; formerly called "first responder."

Emergency medical services (EMS) system: A network of community resources and medical personnel that provides emergency medical care to people who are injured or suddenly fall ill.

Emergency medical technician (EMT): Someone who has successfully completed a state-approved EMT training program; EMTs take over care from EMRs and work on stabilizing and preparing the patient for transport; formerly referred to as EMT-Basic.

Indirect medical control: A type of medical direction, also called "off-line," "retrospective" or "prospective" medical control; this type of medical direction includes education, protocol review and quality improvement for emergency care providers.

Licensure: Required acknowledgment that the bearer has permission to practice in the licensing state; offers the highest level of public protection; may be revoked at the state level should the bearer no longer meet the required standards.

Local credentialing: Local requirements EMRs must meet in order to maintain employment or obtain certain protocols so that they may practice.

Medical direction: The monitoring of care provided by out-of-hospital providers to injured or ill persons, usually by a medical director.

Medical director: A physician who assumes responsibility for the care of injured or ill persons provided in out-of-hospital settings.

Paramedic: Someone with more in-depth training than AEMTs and who can perform all of the former's duties plus has additional knowledge of performing physical exams; may also perform more invasive procedures than any other prehospital care provider; formerly referred to as EMT-Paramedic.

Prehospital care: Emergency medical care provided before a patient arrives at a hospital or medical facility.

Protocols: Standardized procedures to be followed when providing care to injured or ill persons.

Scope of practice: The range of duties and skills that are allowed and expected to be performed when necessary, according to the professional's level of training, while using reasonable care and skill.

Standing orders: Protocols issued by the medical director allowing specific skills to be performed or specific medications to be administered in certain situations.

Learning Objectives

After reading this chapter, and completing the class activities, you will have the information needed to—

- Summarize the history and origins of the *emergency medical services* (EMS) system.
- Describe the components of an EMS system, and discuss factors related to "right to practice."
- Explain the different levels of EMS training.
- Discuss the continuity of care and the importance of working with other responders.
- Define who an *emergency medical responder* (EMR) is.
- List the roles and responsibilities of an EMR.
- Describe the personal characteristics and professional behavior expected of an EMR.
- Discuss medical oversight.
- Discuss factors related to the "right to practice."

INTRODUCTION

The ***emergency medical services* (EMS) system**, along with its front-line-trained ***emergency medical responders* (EMRs)**, plays a vital role in the health and safety of the population. By providing emergency services rapidly and effectively, EMRs save many lives and minimize many injuries.

The role of the EMR can vary, however, depending on the state and the location of practice. It is important for every EMR to understand the role of practice and any limitations, to be able to provide timely and skillful care.

As an EMR, you provide a link between the first actions of bystanders and more advanced care. An EMR is a person trained in emergency care, paid or volunteer, who is often summoned to provide initial care in an emergency (**Fig. 1-1**).

As the first trained professional on the scene, your actions are often critical. They may determine whether a seriously injured or ill person survives.

By taking this course, you will gain the knowledge, skills and confidence to provide appropriate care when you are called upon to help a person who has sustained an injury or sudden illness. You will learn how to assess a patient's condition and how to recognize and care for life-threatening emergencies. You will also learn how to minimize a patient's discomfort and prevent further complications until more advanced medical personnel take over.

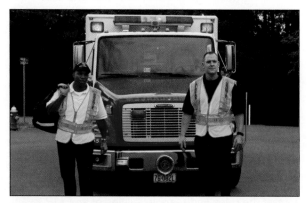

Fig. 1-1: As the first trained professional on the scene, an EMR's actions are often critical.

THE EMS SYSTEM
History and Origins

In the early 1960s in the United States, firefighters in some regions were taught how to perform CPR and basic first aid. There were two reasons for this. First, it prepared them to provide emergency care to colleagues injured in action. Second, because firefighters are based in communities all across the country, they were a practical choice to be available to answer emergency calls.

Although some firefighters received training in CPR and first aid, there was no organized EMS network in the early 1960s. This meant that there was no standardized or regulated training to ensure comparable emergency care education between the different regions.

This patchwork of resources resulted in response times and quality of care that differed between locations. Also, by not having a directed, formal EMS system, educational requirements differed by location.

In 1966, the *National Academy of Sciences/ National Research Council* (NAS/NRC) documented the problem in a white paper that found the quality of emergency care in the United States to be dismal.

Entitled "Accidental Death and Disability: The Neglected Disease of Modern Society," the white paper criticized both ambulance services and hospital emergency departments. In response to this white paper, in 1973, the U.S. Congress enacted the *Emergency Medical Services Act*, which created a multi-tiered, nationwide system of emergency health care. Among other things, the legislation called for standardized training within the EMS system.

The EMS System Today
Types of Systems

Today, there are several types of EMS services in the United States:

- Fire-based services: According to a survey by the *National Highway Traffic Safety Administration* (NHTSA), a division of the U.S. *Department of Transportation* (DOT), over half of all

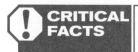

CRITICAL FACTS   As the first trained professional on the scene, your actions are often critical. They may determine whether a seriously injured or ill person survives.

communities in the United States depend on fire departments to provide emergency services. NHTSA found this was more common in urban areas.

- Third-party services: Third-party services are private companies that have been hired to perform EMS services. The NHTSA survey found that third-party services were more common in rural areas of the country.
- Hospital-based services: Hospital-based services are those that are backed up, monitored and run by a local hospital.
- Other systems: These include police and private systems.

At each of these levels, the delivery of care may be different, but the goal is always the same: to provide care according to community needs and resources.

Regulating Agencies

NHTSA's Office of Emergency Medical Services has been mandated to oversee the national EMS system. Its goal is to reduce death and disability by providing leadership and coordination to the EMS community. This is accomplished by assessing, planning, developing and promoting comprehensive, evidence-based EMS and 9-1-1 systems.

In addition to NHTSA's oversight of the EMS system, each state and territory has a lead EMS agency of its own. These can fall under the individual state health or public safety department. In some states, the agency is independent.

State EMS agencies are responsible for the overall planning, coordination and regulation of the EMS system within the state as well as licensing or certifying EMS providers.

Their responsibilities may include leading statewide trauma systems, developing and enforcing statewide **protocols** for EMS providers in addition to the national requirements, administering or coordinating regional EMS programs, operating or coordinating statewide communications systems, coordinating and distributing federal and state grants, and planning and coordinating disaster

and mass casualty responses, as well as homeland security medical initiatives.

Components of an EMS System
NHTSA Technical Assistance Program Assessment Standards

As a part of its mandate to oversee the national EMS system, NHTSA has designated 10 components that make up an effective EMS system, and has identified a method of assessing those areas. NHTSA's statewide EMS Technical Assistance Program allows states to request a team of outside experts, a *Technical Assistance Team* (TAT), to conduct a comprehensive assessment of each statewide EMS program. The assessment provides an overview of the current program in comparison to a set of standards. This evaluation outlines the program's strengths and weaknesses, as well as recommendations for improvement. Almost all states and territories have utilized this process and states may also request a reassessment by making joint requests to their state Highway Safety Office and NHTSA Regional Office. By measuring the progress of EMS systems against the standard set by NHTSA, states can ensure the EMS system is effective nationwide.

NHTSA's 10 components, also known as its *Technical Assistance Assessment Standards,* include—

1. Regulation and policy. State agencies have regulations and policies in place that govern their EMS systems. The regulations and policies regarding the EMS system vary among states. As an EMR, you are responsible for knowing and understanding the applicable regulations and policies in your state of practice.

2. Resource management. To ensure that all patients are able to receive the required care, all states must have central control of EMS resources. State EMS oversight includes ensuring that EMS personnel have adequate training and providing the equipment necessary to provide emergency care throughout the state. Equipment includes vehicles for transportation as well as tools and supplies necessary to provide care.

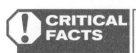

CRITICAL FACTS State EMS agencies are responsible for the overall planning, coordination and regulation of the EMS system within the state as well as licensing or certifying EMS providers.

Access to the EMS System

Mobile 9-1-1: Hundreds of Millions Served

The 9-1-1 service was created in the United States in 1968 as a nationwide telephone number for the public to use to report emergencies and request emergency assistance. It gives the public direct access to an emergency communications center called a *Public Service Answering Point* (PSAP), which is responsible for taking appropriate action.

The numbers 9-1-1 were chosen because they best fit the needs of the public and the telephone companies. They are easy to remember and dial, and they have never been used as an office, area or service code. Today, an estimated 200 million people call 9-1-1 each year. At least 99 percent of the population and 96 percent of the geographic United States is covered by some type of 9-1-1 service.

According to the *Federal Communications Commission* (FCC), over 50 million people now use mobile phones to call 9-1-1. That is more than double the number who used mobile phones to activate EMS services in 1995. However, because mobile phones are not associated with one fixed location or address, it can be difficult for dispatch to accurately determine the location of the caller or the emergency.

People who call 9-1-1 using a mobile phone should remember the following tips, to assist dispatch in finding their location:

- Callers should tell dispatch the location of the emergency right away.
- They should then give dispatch their mobile phone number so that dispatch can call back if the call gets disconnected. This is especially important if callers do not have a contract for service with a mobile phone service provider, because in these cases dispatch will have no way of obtaining their mobile phone number and will be unable to contact them.
- Callers should learn to use the designated number in their state for highway accidents or other non-life-threatening incidents, if there is one. States often reserve specific numbers for these types of incidents. For example, "#77" is the number used for highway accidents in Virginia. The number to call for non-life-threatening incidents in each state may be located in the front of the phone book.
- Callers should not program their mobile phone to automatically dial 9-1-1 when one button, such as the "9" key, is pressed. Mobile 9-1-1 calls often occur when autodial keys are pressed unintentionally. This causes problems for EMS call centers.
- Callers should turn off the autodial 9-1-1 feature if their mobile phone came preprogrammed with it already turned on. They can check their user manual to find out how.
- Callers should lock their keypad when they are not using their mobile phone. This action prevents accidental calls to 9-1-1.

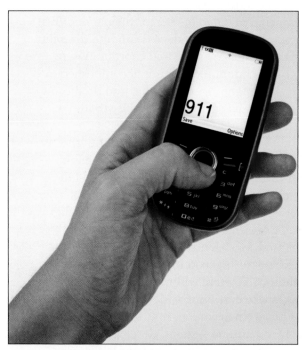

People who call 9-1-1 with a mobile phone should immediately tell dispatch the emergency location and the mobile phone number in case the call gets disconnected. *Courtesy of Michelle Lala Clark.*

3. Human resources and training. All EMS personnel must be trained to adequate levels, with the basic level being that of an EMR. Each state has its own rules and regulations regarding extra training or skills. For this, the agencies have to monitor training programs, and these programs must be re-evaluated on a regular basis.

4. Transportation. Safe and reliable transportation is needed for patients to reach

end destinations. This includes adequate and functioning transportation services for the area, which gives all citizens equal access to emergency care.

5. Facilities. EMS systems must have a range of appropriate receiving institutions available to meet the various and acute needs of injured or ill persons. Depending on the patient's age and condition, these can range from the hospital emergency department to specialty centers such as trauma, burn, stroke or pediatric centers.

6. Communications. EMS systems must have a designated communications number to be used by the public to get help and by members of the emergency response team to communicate effectively. Generally, 9-1-1 is used, although there are areas that must use a non-9-1-1 or seven- or 10-digit number.

7. Public information and education. The EMS system should offer information and education to the public on prevention of injury and illness and appropriate use of the EMS system.

8. **Medical direction** (also known as *"medical oversight"*). EMS systems are required to have a physician act as **medical director**, overseeing their operations.

9. Trauma systems. As part of the EMS system, each state is required to have a system that ensures timely and effective direction of patients to the appropriate receiving facilities, depending on the level of care required.

10. Evaluation. Improvement in care and assessment of the care provided are obtained through evaluation and upgrading of the EMS system, which is governed by each state.

Levels of EMS Training
National EMS Education Agenda for the Future: A Systems Approach

The need for standards in EMS care was identified back in the 1960s. At that time, the *National Standard Curricula* (NSC) were developed by the DOT and NHTSA, in response to a mandate by Congress. Between 1966 and 1973, NSC were developed for EMT-Basics, Intermediates and **Paramedics**. These curricula standardized aspects such as course

planning and structure, objectives, lessons, content and hours of instruction.

In 1996, the NHTSA and the *Health Resources and Services Administration* (HRSA) published a document entitled the *EMS Agenda for the Future* (the *Agenda*). The purpose of this document was to create a common vision for the future of EMS systems. The document was designed to be used by national, state and local governments, as well as by private organizations, in order to guide planning, decision making and policy around EMS care.

One of several areas addressed in the *Agenda* was the EMS education system. NHTSA, along with more than 30 EMS-related organizations, implemented steps to address the education section of the *Agenda*. The plan for this implementation was entitled the *National EMS Education and Practice Blueprint* (known as the *Blueprint*), and represents an important component of the EMS education system. The purpose of this document was to establish nationally recognized levels of EMS providers and scopes of practice, a framework for future curriculum development projects and a standardized way for states to handle legal recognition and reciprocity.

In 1998, a group under the NHTSA met to develop procedures to revise the *Blueprint* and developed a document entitled the *EMS Education Agenda for the Future: A Systems Approach* (the *Education Agenda*). The *Education Agenda* proposed an education system with five components:

1. National EMS Core Content
2. National EMS Scope of Practice Model
3. National EMS Education Standards
4. National EMS Education Program Accreditation
5. National EMS Certification

The main benefit of this systematic approach was the resulting consistency of instructional quality it would achieve through the system's three main components: the National EMS Education Standards, the National EMS Education Program Accreditation and the National EMS Certification.

The National EMS Education Standards replaced the NSC, and set minimum learning objectives for each level of practice. National EMS Certification now is available for all levels of providers and entails a standardized examination process, to ensure entry-level competence of EMS providers.

National Scope of Practice

The **scope of practice** of an EMR is defined as the range of duties and skills that the EMR is allowed and expected to perform when necessary, while using reasonable care and skill according to the EMR's level of training. While the scope of practice does not have regulatory authority, it does provide guidance to states. The EMR is governed by legal, ethical and medical standards. Since practices may differ by region, responders must be aware of the variations that exist for their level of training and licensing in their region.

Professional Levels of EMS Certification or Licensure

There are four nationally recognized levels of training for prehospital emergency care, including—

1. *Emergency medical responder* (EMR). EMRs have the basic knowledge and skills needed to provide emergency care to people who are injured or who have become ill. They are certified to provide care until a more highly trained professional—such as an EMT—takes over. This level of training used to be called *first responder*.
2. ***Emergency medical technician* (EMT).** EMTs have the next highest level of training. Their **certification** involves a minimum of 110 hours of training. EMTs take over the care from EMRs and work on stabilizing and preparing the patient for transport. This level of training used to be called *EMT-Basic*.
3. ***Advanced emergency medical technician* (AEMT).** AEMTs receive more training than EMTs, which allows them to insert IVs, administer medications, perform

advanced airway procedures, and set up and assess *electrocardiograms* (ECGs or EKGs). This level of care used to be called *EMT-Intermediate*.
4. Paramedic. Paramedics have more in-depth training than AEMTs, including more knowledge about performing physical exams. They may also perform more invasive procedures than any other **prehospital care** provider. This level of care used to be called *EMT-Paramedic*.

Working with Other Responders and Continuity of Care

Continuity of care in an emergency situation can be compared to a course of action. As an EMR, you are often the first on the scene and begin the course of action. While providing care, you will collect all the information you require to pass on to the next level of personnel when they arrive or to the receiving facility if you are providing transport. A smooth transition of care depends on the proper and thorough relay of information.

As an EMR, you will be working and communicating with other medical personnel including EMTs, AEMTs and paramedics as well as law enforcement personnel, emergency management, home health care providers and others.

EMERGENCY MEDICAL RESPONDER

Who Is an EMR?

An EMR is a person trained in emergency care who may be called on to provide such care as a routine part of his or her job, whether that job is voluntary or paid. EMRs have a duty to respond to the scene of a medical emergency and to provide emergency care to the injured or ill person. They are recognized and certified to provide emergency care to the general public until more advanced medical care takes over.

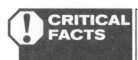 **CRITICAL FACTS** The scope of practice of an EMR is defined as the range of duties and skills that the EMR is allowed and expected to perform when necessary, while using reasonable care and skill according to the EMR's level of training.

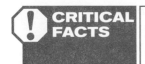
Some occupations, such as law enforcement and fire fighting, require personnel to respond to and assist at the scene of an emergency. These personnel are dispatched through an emergency number, such as 9-1-1, and often share common communications networks. When someone dials 9-1-1, this will contact police, fire or ambulance personnel. These are typically considered public safety personnel. However, EMRs do not necessarily work for public safety agencies. People in many occupations other than public safety are called to help in the event of an injury or sudden illness, such as—

- Athletic trainers.
- Camp leaders.
- Emergency management personnel.
- First aid station members.
- Industrial response teams.
- Lifeguards.
- Ski patrol members.

In an emergency, these people are often required to provide the same minimum standard of care as traditional EMRs. Their duty is to assess the patient's condition and provide necessary care, make sure that any necessary additional help has been summoned, assist other medical personnel at the scene and document their actions.

Responsibilities

To be an EMR means to accept certain responsibilities beyond providing care. Since you will often be the first trained professional to arrive at many emergencies, your primary responsibilities center on safety and early emergency care. Your major responsibilities are to—

- Ensure safety for yourself and any bystanders. Your first responsibility is not to make the situation worse by getting hurt or letting bystanders get hurt. By making sure the scene is safe as you approach it, you can avoid unnecessary injuries.

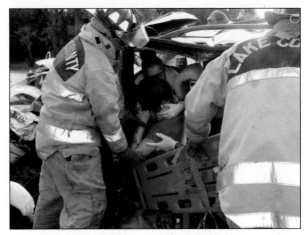

Fig. 1-2: One of an EMR's major responsibilities is gaining safe access to the patient.

- Gain access to the patient. Carefully approach the patient unless the scene is too dangerous for you to handle without help. Electrical or chemical hazards, unsafe structures and other dangers may make it difficult to reach the patient (**Fig. 1-2**). Recognize when a rescue requires specially trained emergency personnel.
- Determine any threats to the patient's life. Check first for immediate life-threatening conditions and care for any you find. Next, look for other conditions that could threaten the patient's life or health if not addressed.
- Summon more advanced medical personnel as needed. After you quickly assess the patient, notify more advanced EMS personnel of the situation, if someone has not done so already.
- Provide needed care for the patient. Remain with the patient and provide whatever care you can until more advanced medical personnel take over.
- Assist more advanced medical personnel. Transfer your information about the patient

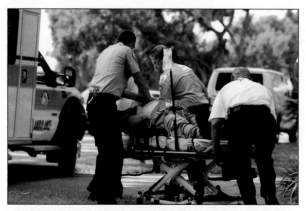

Fig. 1-3: The EMR assists more advanced medical personnel when they arrive at the scene. *Courtesy of Captain Phil Kleinberg, EMT-P, Lake-Sumter EMS.*

and the emergency to more advanced medical personnel (**Fig. 1-3**). Tell them what happened, how you found the patient, any problems you found and any care you provided. Assist them as needed within your level of training, and help with care for any other patients. When possible, try to anticipate the needs of those providing care.

In addition to these major responsibilities, you have secondary responsibilities that include—

- Summoning additional help when needed, such as special rescue teams, paramedic units or trauma alerts.
- Controlling or directing bystanders or asking them for help.
- Taking additional steps, if necessary, to protect bystanders from dangers, such as traffic or fire.
- Recording what you saw, heard and did at the scene.
- Reassuring the patient's family or friends.

Maintaining Certification

As an EMR, you have an obligation to remain up to date on the knowledge, skills and use of equipment needed for you to fulfill your role competently and effectively. Your employer should provide you with the requirements for your area. Some areas require a higher level of

knowledge for their EMRs, above and beyond the basic requirements.

Continuing Education

The field of health care, particularly emergency care, changes quickly as newer and better techniques and methods are discovered. EMRs must keep up to date on all of the new developments that affect them and the care they provide. As an EMR, you will be required to participate in various types of *continuing education* (CE) programs as outlined by the certifying body and your region.

Criminal Implications

Within the *National EMS Scope of Practice Model*, there are limitations placed on your scope of practice to ensure that what you do is in the interest of public protection and safety. Standards for EMR education, certification, **licensure** and credentialing are all mechanisms that set the parameters of practice. Criminal implications may arise for you if you perform procedures that are outside of what you are trained to do, what you are certified as competent to do, what you are legally licensed to do or what you have been *credentialed* (authorized by a medical director) to do.

EMRs must not be placed in situations in which they are expected to perform procedures they have not been sufficiently trained to do or for which they have insufficient experience. There are also criminal implications for falsification of care or training records, or for allowing your certification to lapse and continuing to practice.

Fees

One of your areas of responsibility is paying required fees. There is a fee to obtain licensure and recertification, and there may be fees for certain exams. You will also be required to obtain *continuing education units* (CEUs) to maintain your knowledge and skills. Fees vary widely

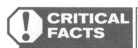 **CRITICAL FACTS**
As an EMR, you have an obligation to remain up to date on the knowledge, skills and use of equipment needed for you to fulfill your role competently and effectively.

from state to state and are usually your responsibility, though employers may sometimes assist with them.

Personal Characteristics and Professional Behavior

The responsibilities of EMRs require that they demonstrate certain characteristics. These include—

- Maintaining a caring and professional attitude. Injured or ill people are sometimes difficult to work with. Be compassionate; try to understand their concerns and fears (**Fig. 1-4**). Realize that anger shown by an injured or ill person often results from fear. A lay rescuer who helps at the emergency may also be afraid. Try to be reassuring. Even though citizen responders may not have done everything perfectly, be sure to thank them for taking action. Recognition and praise help to affirm their willingness to act. Also be careful about what you say. Do *not* volunteer distressing news about the emergency to the patient or to the patient's family or friends.
- Controlling your fears. Try not to reveal your anxieties to the patient or bystanders. The presence of blood, vomit, unpleasant odors, or torn or burned skin is disturbing to most people. You may need to compose yourself before acting. If you must, turn away for a moment and take a few deep breaths before providing care.
- Presenting a professional appearance. This helps ease a patient's fears and inspires confidence.
- Keeping your knowledge and skills up to date. Involve yourself in continuing education, professional reading and refresher training.
- Maintaining a safe and healthy lifestyle. Job stresses can adversely affect your health. As an EMR, it is important to maintain a safe and healthy lifestyle both on and off the job. Exercise, diet and common sense safety practices can help you manage physical, mental and emotional stress, and may help you be more effective as an EMR.

Medical Direction
Medical Director

Medical direction is the process by which a physician directs the care provided by out-of-hospital providers to injured or ill people. Usually this monitoring is done by a medical director, who assumes responsibility for the care provided. The physician also oversees training and the development of *protocols* (standardized procedures to be followed when providing care to injured or ill people).

Medical Control

Since it is impossible for the medical director to be present at every incident outside the hospital, the physician directs care through **standing orders**. Standing orders allow EMS personnel

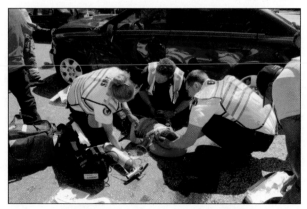

Fig. 1-4: An EMR should be compassionate and reassuring. *Courtesy of Captain Phil Kleinberg, EMT-P, Lake-Sumter EMS.*

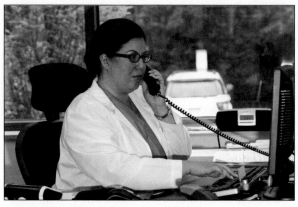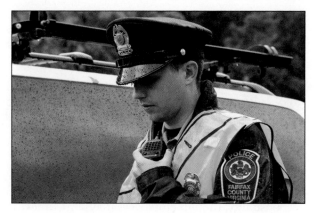

Fig. 1-5: Procedures that are not covered by standing orders require EMRs to speak directly with the physician. This is called direct medical control.

to provide certain types of care or treatment without speaking to the physician. This kind of medical direction is called **indirect medical control**. Indirect medical control, or "offline" medical direction, includes education, protocol review and quality improvement for emergency care providers.

Other procedures that are not covered by standing orders require EMRs to speak directly with the physician. This contact can be made via mobile phone, radio or telephone. This kind of medical direction is called **direct medical control**, or "online" medical direction (**Fig. 1-5**).

Right to Practice
Legislation and Scope of Practice

EMRs must follow state regulations that determine what they can and cannot do. Each state has very specific laws and rules governing how EMS personnel may practice in the out-of-hospital setting.

State EMS Office Oversight

EMRs must be licensed through the state EMS office, the licensing agency, before being allowed to work in that state. EMRs should be familiar with these laws and regulations. Typical legal concerns and issues are addressed in **Chapter 3**. For example, New York legislation does not allow certain individuals to assist with asthma medication.

Medical Direction

Medical direction is provided by the medical director, who assumes responsibility for care provided.

Levels of Credentialing

There are three aspects to credentialing of EMRs, all with the goal of protecting the public: certification, licensure and **local credentialing**.

Certification

Certification is achieved by obtaining and maintaining the National EMS Certification, by taking an approved EMS course as well as meeting other requirements. This does not grant you the right to practice as licensure does. EMS personnel generally need to recertify every 2 years, to ensure that they maintain a high degree of proficiency by upgrading their knowledge, skills and abilities.

Licensure

Licensure is an acknowledgement that the bearer has *permission* to practice in the licensing state. It is the highest level of public protection, which is granted at the state level. It is generally a requirement, with a few exceptions, for work on federal land or in the military. States often have requirements in addition to those required for certification, before they grant licensure. The state is the final authority for public protection; therefore, states can revoke state licensure if appropriate.

Local Credentialing

Often, EMS providers must meet local credentialing requirements in order to maintain employment or obtain certain protocols so that they may practice. Most employers also have additional requirements as part of an orientation program that would be similar to a local credentialing process.

Administrative Requirements

EMRs must follow any policies and procedures based on national, state, local or employer requirements. For example, the *Health Insurance Portability and Accountability Act* (HIPAA) is national; protocols can be state or local; and specifics of uniform (e.g., level of training and credentialing recognition) could be employer requirements.

Research

The field of emergency care and emergency medicine is constantly evolving. *Quality improvement* (QI), or *continuous quality improvement* (CQI), based on research, allows for continuing assessment and reassessment of all aspects of the EMS system. This includes viewing and evaluating the system internally, from the personnel's and administration's point of view, and also externally, from the public's point of view. It also entails keeping personnel and equipment up to date with the latest standards of care, ensuring that personnel are adequately trained and skilled in using new knowledge.

One example is the recent revamping of CPR procedures. As new recommendations came about and became the recognized standard, EMS systems across the country had to ensure that employees and volunteers were up to date and comfortable performing the new techniques.

The goal of an EMS system is to provide the highest quality of care possible throughout the country, equally accessible to all citizens. Through research, QI programs can assess whether that goal is being met.

PUTTING IT ALL TOGETHER

Since the EMS system was established in the United States, it has undergone significant changes as it has grown and adapted to citizens' needs. However, this growth needs to continue as the field of emergency and prehospital care continues to evolve.

The primary role of an EMR is to provide emergency care at the scene, while working with other services and health care personnel. It is important to understand that the role of the EMR does not stop at providing care. EMRs must continue to grow and learn along with the field. They must remain certified and retain their licensure in order to practice in their chosen state and, as such, must maintain the necessary standards as outlined by that state.

To be an effective EMR, you must not only be able to keep up the professional side of your work, but your personal side. EMRs have a responsibility to remain fit and healthy in order to perform their duties accordingly. This means maintaining a healthy lifestyle and being aware of your choices and how they would and could affect your performance on the job.

The size and scope of the EMS system in each state may vary according to population, needs and resources. However, all systems have some things in common: namely, their need for certification and licensure, and their goal of providing equal access to prehospital care to all citizens.

2 The Well-Being of the Emergency Medical Responder

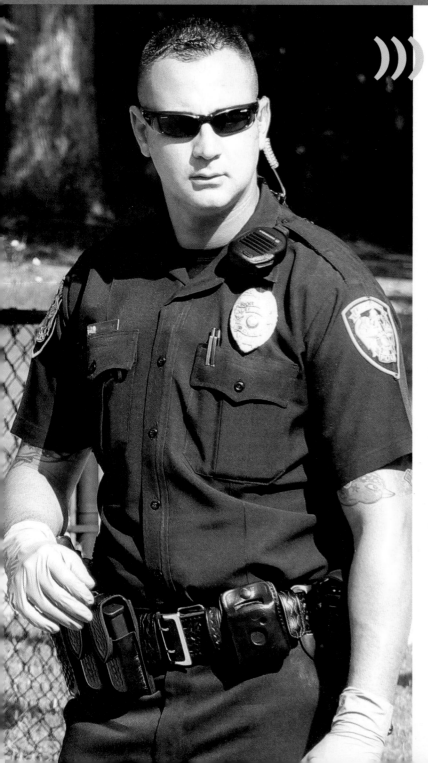

))) **YOU ARE THE EMERGENCY MEDICAL RESPONDER**

Your police unit responds to a call for a medical emergency involving a man who has collapsed in front of a school building. When you and your partner arrive, you see that the man is bleeding from the mouth and face. Vomit and blood are on the ground around him. "His face hit the ground when he fell," a bystander says. The victim does not appear to be breathing. How would you respond and what can you do to protect yourself from possible disease transmission?

Key Terms

Acute: Having a rapid and severe onset, then quickly subsiding.

Adaptive immunity: The type of protection from disease that the body develops throughout a lifetime as a person is exposed to diseases or immunized against them.

AIDS: A disease of the immune system caused by infection with HIV.

Antibodies: A type of protein found in blood or other bodily fluids; used by the immune system to identify and neutralize pathogens, such as bacteria and viruses.

Bacteria: One-celled organisms that can cause infection; a common type of pathogen.

Biohazard: A biological agent that presents a hazard to the health or well-being of those exposed.

Bloodborne: Used to describe a substance carried in the blood (e.g., bloodborne pathogens are pathogens carried through the blood).

Bloodborne pathogens: Germs that may be present in human blood or other body fluids that can cause disease in humans.

Body substance isolation (BSI) precautions: Protective measures to prevent exposure to communicable diseases; defines all body fluids and substances as infectious.

Chronic: Persistent over a long period of time.

Critical incident stress: Stress triggered by involvement in a serious or traumatic incident.

Debriefing: A method of helping people cope with exposure to serious or traumatic incidents by discussing the emotional impact of the event.

Defusing: Similar to a debriefing but shorter and less formal; a method of discussing a serious or traumatic event soon afterward; done to help people cope.

Direct contact: Mode of transmission of pathogens that occurs through directly touching infected blood or body fluid, or other agents such as chemicals, drugs or toxins.

Disease-causing agent: A pathogen or germ that can cause disease or illness (e.g., a bacterium or virus).

Droplet transmission: Mode of transmission of pathogens that occurs when a person inhales droplets from an infected person's cough or sneeze; also known as respiratory droplet transmission.

Engineering controls: Control measures that eliminate, isolate or remove a hazard from the workplace; things used in the workplace to help reduce the risk of an exposure.

Exposure: An instance in which someone is exposed to a pathogen or has contact with blood or body fluids or objects in the environment that contain disease-causing agents.

Exposure control plan: Plan in the workplace that outlines the employer's protective measures to eliminate or minimize employee exposure incidents.

Hepatitis: An inflammation of the liver most commonly caused by viral infection; there are several types including hepatitis A, B, C, D and E.

HIV: A virus that weakens the body's immune system, leading to life-threatening infections; causes AIDS.

Homeostasis: A constant state of balance or well-being of the body's internal systems that is continually and automatically adjusted.

Immune system: The body's complex group of body systems that is responsible for fighting disease.

Indirect contact: Mode of transmission of a disease caused by touching a contaminated object.

Infection: A condition caused by disease-producing microorganisms, called pathogens or germs, in the body.

Infectious disease: Disease caused by the invasion of the body by a pathogen, such as a bacterium, virus, fungus or parasite.

Innate immunity: The type of protection from disease with which humans are born.

Lividity: Purplish color in the lowest-lying parts of a recently dead body, caused by pooling of blood.

Meningitis: An inflammation of the meninges, the thin, protective coverings over the brain and spinal cord; caused by virus or bacteria.

Methicillin-resistant *Staphylococcus aureus* (MRSA): A Staph bacterium that can cause infection; difficult to treat because of its resistance to many antibiotics.

Multidrug-resistant tuberculosis (MDR TB): A type of *tuberculosis* (TB) that is resistant to some of the most effective anti-TB drugs.

Needlestick: A penetrating wound from a needle or other sharp object; may result in exposure to pathogens through contact with blood or other body fluids.

Occupational Safety and Health Administration (OSHA): Federal agency whose role is to promote the safety and health of American workers by setting and enforcing standards; providing training, outreach and education; establishing partnerships; and encouraging continual process improvement in workplace safety and health.

Opportunistic infections: Infections that strike people whose immune systems are weakened.

Pandemic influenza: A respiratory illness caused by virulent human influenza A virus; spreads easily and sustainably and can cause global outbreaks of serious illness in humans.

Passive immunity: The type of immunity gained from external sources such as from a mother's breast milk to an infant.

Pathogen: A term used to describe a germ; a disease-causing agent (e.g., bacterium or virus).

Personal protective equipment (PPE): All specialized clothing, equipment and supplies that keep the user from directly contacting infected materials; includes gloves, gowns, masks, shields and protective eyewear.

Severe acute respiratory syndrome (SARS): A viral respiratory illness caused by the *SARS-associated coronavirus* (SARS-CoV).

Standard precautions: Safety measures, including BSI and universal precautions, taken to prevent occupational-risk exposure to blood or other potentially infectious materials; assumes that all body fluids, secretions and excretions (except sweat) are potentially infective.

Stress: The body's normal response to any situation that changes a person's existing mental, physical or emotional balance.

Sudden death: An unexpected, natural death; usually used to describe a death from a sudden cardiac event.

Tuberculosis (TB): A bacterial infection that usually attacks the lungs.

Universal precautions: A set of precautions designed to prevent transmission of HIV, *hepatitis B virus* (HBV) and other bloodborne pathogens when providing care; considers blood and certain body fluids of all patients potentially infectious.

Vector-borne transmission: Transmission of a pathogen that occurs when an infectious source, such as an animal or insect bite or sting, penetrates the body's skin.

Virus: A common type of pathogen that depends on other organisms to live and reproduce; can be difficult to kill.

Work practice controls: Control measures that reduce the likelihood of exposure by changing the way a task is carried out.

Learning Objectives

After reading this chapter, and completing the class activities, you will have the information needed to—

- Describe how the immune system works.
- Identify ways in which diseases are transmitted and give an example of how each transmission can occur.
- Describe diseases that cause concern and how they are transmitted.
- Describe conditions that must be present for disease transmission.
- Explain the importance of standard precautions.
- Identify standard precautions to protect yourself against disease transmission.
- Describe the steps an *emergency medical responder* (EMR) should take for personal protection from bloodborne pathogens.
- Describe the procedure an EMR would use to disinfect equipment, work surfaces, clothing and leather items.
- Explain the importance of documenting an exposure incident and post-exposure follow-up care.
- Explain how the OSHA standard for bloodborne pathogens influences your actions as an EMR.
- Acknowledge the importance of knowing how various diseases are transmitted.
- Demonstrate the proper techniques for placing and removing *personal protective equipment* (PPE).

- Use appropriate PPE and properly remove and discard the protective garments, given a scenario in which potential exposure takes place.
- Identify the signs and symptoms of critical incident stress.
- Describe actions an EMR could take to reduce or alleviate stress.
- Describe reactions a person might have when confronted with the dying process or actual death of another individual.
- List possible emotional reactions an EMR may experience when faced with trauma, illness, death and dying.
- Explain the importance of understanding the response to death and dying and communicating effectively with the patient's family.
- Describe the steps an EMR might take when approaching the family of a dead or dying patient.
- Recognize possible reactions of the EMR's family to the responsibilities of an EMR.
- Communicate with empathy to patients and their family members and friends.

INTRODUCTION

The demands on an *emergency medical responder* (EMR) can be significant and are physical, emotional and mental in nature. To meet these demands, it is essential to take good care of yourself, by making healthy choices that promote your own physical, emotional and mental well-being. These choices will benefit not only you but also the patients and families you assist as you carry out your work each day.

Bloodborne pathogens, such as **bacteria** and **viruses**, may be present in blood and body fluids and can cause disease when certain conditions are present. Being aware of **disease-causing agents**, how they are spread and their signs and symptoms will help you prevent **exposure** to these illnesses and recognize them. It is also important for you to keep immunizations up to date to protect against vaccine-preventable diseases and wear proper *personal protective equipment* (PPE) while providing care (**Fig. 2-1**).

EMRs must also look after their mental and emotional health. A serious injury, sudden illness or death can have an emotional impact on everyone involved: patients, family, friends,

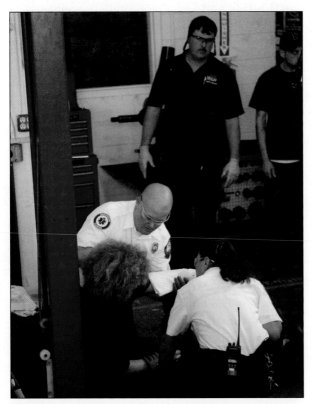

Fig. 2-1: Prevent exposure to bloodborne pathogens by wearing personal protective equipment, such as disposable gloves.

bystanders, EMRs and others. The degree of impact varies from person to person. The way one person responds to a stressful situation can differ substantially from the response of another person in a similar situation.

At times, you may encounter a patient who is experiencing an emotional crisis. Besides providing care for a specific injury or illness, you may also need to provide emotional support. Being able to understand some of what a patient feels when coping with an injury or illness is an important part of what you do as a responder.

PREVENTING DISEASE TRANSMISSION

To help prevent disease transmission, you need to understand how **infections** occur, how diseases spread from one person to another and what you as an EMR can do to protect yourself and others. **Infectious diseases** can be spread from infected people and from animals, insects or objects that have been in contact with them. EMRs must protect themselves and others from infectious diseases.

How Infection Occurs
Disease-Causing Agents

The disease process begins when a **pathogen** (germ) gets into the body. When pathogens enter the body, they sometimes can overpower the body's natural defense systems and cause illness. Bacteria and viruses cause most infectious diseases. Other disease-causing pathogens include fungi, protozoa, rickettsia, parasitic worms, prions and yeasts.

Bacteria are everywhere. They do not depend on other organisms for life and can live outside the human body. Most bacteria do not infect humans. Those that do may cause serious illness, such as bacterial **meningitis** and tetanus. The body may have difficulty fighting infection caused by bacteria. The body's ability to fight infection depends on its **immune system**. In people with healthy immune systems, a bacterial infection is often avoided. When an infection is present, health care providers may prescribe antibiotic medications that either kill the bacteria or weaken them enough for the body to get rid of them. Commonly used antibiotics include penicillin, erythromycin and tetracycline.

Table 2-1:
Pathogens and the Diseases and Conditions They Cause

PATHOGEN	DISEASES AND CONDITIONS
Viruses	Hepatitis, measles, mumps, chicken pox, meningitis, rubella, influenza, warts, colds, herpes, HIV (which causes AIDS), genital warts, smallpox, Avian flu
Bacteria	Tetanus, meningitis, scarlet fever, strep throat, tuberculosis, gonorrhea, syphilis, chlamydia, toxic shock syndrome, Legionnaires' disease, diphtheria, food poisoning, Lyme disease, anthrax
Fungi	Athlete's foot, ringworm, histoplasmosis
Protozoa	Malaria, dysentery, cyclospora, giardiasis
Rickettsia	Typhus, Rocky Mountain spotted fever
Parasitic Worms	Abdominal pain, anemia, lymphatic vessel blockage, lowered antibody response, respiratory and circulatory complications
Prions	*Creutzfeldt-Jakob disease* (CJD) or bovine spongiform encephalopathy (mad cow disease)
Yeasts	Candidiasis (also known as "thrush")

Unlike bacteria, viruses depend on other organisms to live and reproduce. Viruses cause many diseases, including the common cold (caused by the rhinovirus). Once in the body, viruses may be difficult to eliminate because very few medications are effective against viral infections. While there are some medications that kill or weaken viruses, the body's immune system is the main defense against them.

Some infections, such as measles, malaria, **HIV** and yellow fever, affect the entire body. Others affect only one organ or system of the body—for example, the virus that causes the common cold, which occurs in the upper respiratory tract. **Table 2-1** identifies some diseases and conditions caused by each of the types of pathogenic agents.

The Body's Natural Defenses

The body has a series of natural defenses that prevent germs from entering. The body depends on intact skin and mucous membranes in the mouth, nose and eyes to keep germs out. When the skin is damaged, germs can enter through openings, such as cuts or sores. Mucous membranes in the mouth, nose and eyes also work to protect the body from intruding germs, often by trapping them and forcing them out through a cough or sneeze. However, mucous membranes are less effective than skin at keeping bloodborne pathogens out of the body. If these barriers fail and a germ enters the body, the body's immune system begins working to fight the disease.

The immune system's basic tools are **antibodies** and white blood cells. Special white blood cells travel around the body and identify invading pathogens. Once they detect a pathogen, white blood cells gather around it and release antibodies that fight infection.

These antibodies attack the pathogens and weaken or destroy them. Antibodies usually can rid the body of pathogens. However, once inside the body, some pathogens can thrive and, under ideal conditions, multiply and overwhelm the immune system.

This combination of preventing pathogens from entering the body and destroying them once they enter is necessary for good health (**homeostasis**). Sometimes, however, the body cannot fight off infection. When this occurs, an invading pathogen can become established in the body, causing infection, which may range from mild to serious and brief (**acute**) to long-lasting (**chronic**). Fever and exhaustion often signal that the body is fighting off an infection. Other common signals include headache, nausea and vomiting.

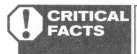 **CRITICAL FACTS** | Intact skin, as well as mucous membranes in the mouth, nose and eyes, are part of the body's natural defenses to help keep germs out.

There are three different types of human immunity: innate, adaptive and passive.

- **Innate immunity** is the type of protection with which we are born. The term "innate immunity" also refers to the natural barriers our bodies have, such as the skin and mucous membranes in the nose, throat and gastrointestinal tract, which prevent most diseases from entering our bodies.
- **Adaptive immunity** develops throughout our lives as we are exposed to diseases or are immunized against them.
- **Passive immunity** is immunity we gain from external sources such as from a mother's breast milk to an infant.

How Diseases Spread

Exposure to blood and other body fluids occurs across a wide variety of occupations. Health care workers, emergency response personnel, public safety personnel and other workers can be exposed to blood through injuries from needles and other sharps devices, as well as by **direct** and **indirect contact** with skin and mucous membranes.

For any disease to spread, including **bloodborne** diseases, all four of the following conditions must be met:

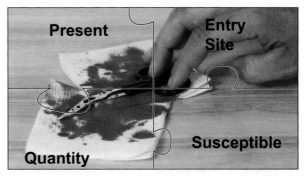

Fig. 2-2: To understand how infections occur, think of the four necessary conditions as pieces of a puzzle.

1. A pathogen must be present.
2. A sufficient quantity of the pathogen to cause disease must be present.
3. A person must be susceptible to the pathogen.
4. The pathogen must pass through the correct entry site (e.g., eyes, mouth and other mucous membranes or skin pierced or broken by **needlesticks**, bites, cuts, abrasions and other means).

To understand how infections occur, think of these four conditions as pieces of a puzzle **(Fig. 2-2)**. All of the pieces must be in place for the picture to be complete. If any one of the conditions is missing, an infection cannot occur.

Table 2-2:
How Bloodborne Pathogens Are Transmitted

DISEASE	SIGNS AND SYMPTOMS	MODE OF TRANSMISSION	INFECTIVE MATERIAL
Hepatitis B	Jaundice, fever, dark urine, clay-colored bowel movements, fatigue, abdominal pain, loss of appetite, nausea, vomiting, joint pain	Direct and indirect contact	Blood, semen
Hepatitis C	Jaundice, fever, fatigue, dark urine, clay-colored stool, abdominal pain, loss of appetite, nausea, vomiting, joint pain	Direct and indirect contact	Blood, semen
HIV	May or may not be signs and symptoms in early stage; late-contact stage symptoms may include fever, headache, fatigue, diarrhea, skin rashes, night sweats, loss of appetite, swollen lymph glands, significant weight loss, white spots in the mouth or vaginal discharge (signs of yeast infection) and memory or movement problems.	Direct and possibly indirect contact	Blood, semen, vaginal fluid

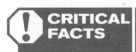 **CRITICAL FACTS**   For any disease to spread, pathogens must be present in sufficient quantity and pass through the broken skin or mucous membrane of a susceptible person.

Bloodborne pathogens, such as hepatitis B, hepatitis C and HIV, spread primarily through direct or indirect contact with infected blood or other body fluids (see **Table 2-2**). While these diseases can be spread by sexual contact through infected body fluids, such as vaginal secretions and semen, these body fluids are not usually involved in occupational transmission. Hepatitis B, hepatitis C and HIV are not spread by food or water or by casual contact such as hugging or shaking hands. The highest risk of occupational transmission is unprotected direct or indirect contact with infected blood.

Disease-causing germs can also cause infection through contaminated food or water. In this way, germs can spread to many people through a single source, such as sometimes occurs with *Escherichia coli (E. coli);* this type of infection is referred to as food poisoning.

Direct Contact

Direct contact transmission occurs when infected blood or body fluid from one person enters another person's body at a correct entry site (**Fig. 2-3**). For example, direct contact transmission can occur through infected blood splashing in the eye or from directly touching the body fluids of an infected person. The infected blood or other body fluid then enters the body through a correct entry site.

Indirect Contact

Some bloodborne pathogens are also transmitted by indirect contact (**Fig. 2-4**). Indirect contact transmission can occur when a person touches an object that contains the blood or other body fluid of an infected person, and that infected blood or other body fluid enters the body through a correct entry site. These objects include soiled

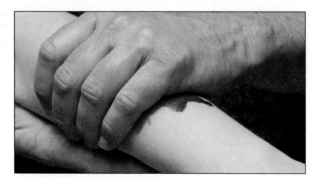

Fig. 2-3: Bloodborne pathogens can be transmitted by direct contact when an uninfected person directly touches the blood or body fluid of an infected person.

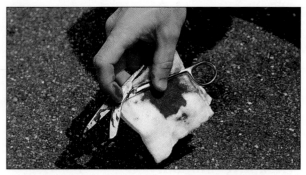

Fig. 2-4: Bloodborne pathogens can be transmitted by indirect contact when an uninfected person touches an object that contains the blood or other body fluid of an infected person.

dressings or equipment and work surfaces contaminated with an infected person's blood or other body fluid. For example, indirect contact can occur when a person picks up blood-soaked bandages with a bare hand and the pathogens enter through a break in the skin on the hand.

Respiratory Droplet and Vector-Borne Transmission

Other pathogens, such as the flu virus, can enter the body through **droplet transmission** (**Fig. 2-5**). This occurs when a person inhales droplets propelled from an infected person's cough or sneeze from within a few feet. A person can also become infected by touching a surface recently contaminated by infected droplets and then touching the eyes, mouth or

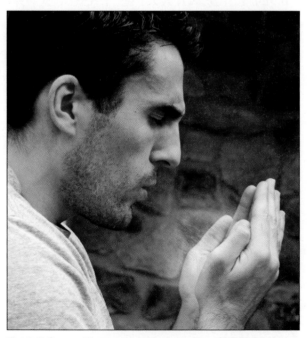

Fig. 2-5: Some pathogens enter the body through droplet transmission, when a person inhales droplets propelled from an infected person's cough or sneeze. *Courtesy of Michelle Lala Clark.*

nose with contaminated hands. **Vector-borne transmission** of diseases, such as malaria, rabies and West Nile virus, occurs when an infectious source, such as an animal or insect bite or a sting, penetrates the body's skin (**Fig. 2-6**).

Risk of Transmission

Infectious diseases have widely varying levels of risk of transmission. Hepatitis B, hepatitis C and HIV share a common mode of transmission—direct or indirect contact with infected blood or body fluids—but they differ in the risk of transmission. Workers who have received the hepatitis B vaccine and have developed immunity to the virus are at virtually no risk for infection by the *hepatitis B virus* (HBV). For an unvaccinated person, the risk for infection from a needlestick or cut exposure to hepatitis B-infected blood can be as high as 30 percent, depending on several factors. In contrast, the risk for infection after a needlestick or cut exposure to hepatitis C-infected blood is about 2 percent and the risk of infection after a needlestick or cut exposure to HIV-infected blood is less than 1 percent.

Diseases That Cause Concern
Hepatitis A, B, C, D and E

Hepatitis is a type of liver disease. Hepatitis A is caused by the *hepatitis A virus* (HAV). This disease is spread primarily through food or water that has been contaminated by stool from an infected person.

HAV is transmissible by—

- Eating food prepared by someone with HAV who did not wash hands after using the bathroom.
- Engaging in certain sexual activities, such as oral-anal contact with someone who has HAV.
- Changing a diaper and then not washing hands.
- Drinking water that has been contaminated.

HAV causes inflammation and swelling of the liver. The patient may feel ill, with flu-like symptoms, or may experience no symptoms at all. Symptoms of HAV usually disappear after several weeks. This disease rarely causes permanent damage or chronic illness.

HAV can be prevented with the hepatitis A vaccine, which is a series of two injections administered at least 6 months apart. The most effective prevention, though, is healthy habits. Always wash your hands thoroughly before preparing food, after using the toilet and after changing a diaper. International travelers should be careful about drinking tap water.

Hepatitis B is a liver infection caused by HBV. Hepatitis B may be severe or even fatal and it can be in the body for up to 6 months before symptoms appear. These may include flu-like symptoms such as fever, fatigue, abdominal pain, loss of appetite, nausea, vomiting and joint pain, as well as dark urine and clay-colored bowel movements. Later-stage symptoms include jaundice, which causes a yellowing of the skin and eyes (**Fig. 2-7**).

Medications are available to treat chronic hepatitis B infection, but they do not work for everyone. The most effective means of prevention is the hepatitis B vaccine. This vaccine, given in a series of three doses, provides immunity to the disease. Scientific data show that hepatitis B

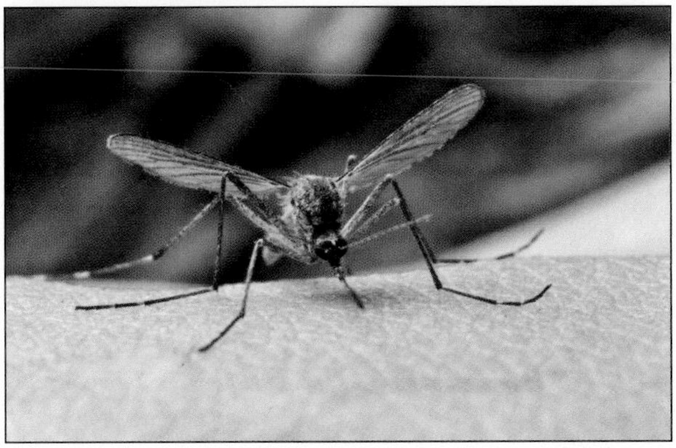

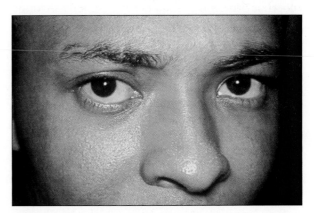

Fig. 2-6: Vector-borne transmission occurs when an insect bite or sting penetrates the body's skin. © *Shutterstock.com/Dmitrijs Bindemanis.*

Fig. 2-7: Later-stage symptoms of Hepatitis B include jaundice, which causes a yellowing of the skin and eyes. *Courtesy of CDC/Dr. Thomas F. Sellers, Emory University.*

vaccines are safe for adults, children and infants. There is no confirmed evidence indicating that the hepatitis B vaccine causes chronic illnesses.

The hepatitis B vaccination series must be made available to all employees who have occupational exposure, within 10 working days of initial assignment, after completing appropriate training. However, employees may decide not to have the vaccination. If an employee decides not to be vaccinated, the person must sign a form affirming this decision. However, if an employee who initially declines hepatitis B vaccination decides to accept the vaccination at a later date, the employer must make the hepatitis B vaccination available at that time, so long as the standard still covers the employee.

Hepatitis C is a liver disease caused by the *hepatitis C virus* (HCV). It is the most common chronic bloodborne infection in the United States. Its symptoms are similar to those of hepatitis B infection, including fever, fatigue, abdominal pain, loss of appetite, nausea, vomiting, dark urine, clay-colored stool, joint pain and jaundice. There is no vaccine against hepatitis C and no treatment available to prevent infection after exposure. For these reasons, hepatitis C is more serious than hepatitis B. Hepatitis C is the leading cause of liver transplants.

Hepatitis D is a serious liver disease caused by the *hepatitis D virus* (HDV) and relies on HBV to replicate. It is uncommon in the United States. It is transmitted through contact with infectious blood, similar to how HBV is spread. There is no vaccine for hepatitis D.

Hepatitis E is caused by the *hepatitis E virus* (HEV). It is commonly transmitted via the fecal-oral route and is associated with ingestion of drinking water contaminated with fecal material in countries with poor sanitation. It occurs primarily in adults. The potential for HEV transmission from contaminated food is still under investigation, and there is no evidence of transmission by percutaneous (through the skin) or sexual exposures. There is currently no FDA-approved vaccine for hepatitis E.

HIV/AIDS

HIV is the virus that causes **AIDS**. HIV attacks white blood cells and destroys the body's ability to fight infection. This weakens the body's immune system. Infections that strike people with weakened immune systems are called **opportunistic infections**. Some opportunistic infections that occur in patients with AIDS include severe pneumonia, *tuberculosis* (**TB**), Kaposi's sarcoma and other unusual cancers.

People infected with HIV may not feel or appear sick. A blood test, however, can detect the HIV antibody. When an infected person has a significant drop in a certain type of white blood cell or shows signs of having certain infections or cancers, the patient may be diagnosed as having AIDS. These infections can cause fever, fatigue, diarrhea, skin rashes, night sweats, loss of appetite, swollen lymph glands and significant weight loss. In the advanced stages, AIDS is a very serious condition. Patients with AIDS eventually develop life-threatening infections from which they can die. Currently, there is no vaccine against HIV.

Tuberculosis

TB is an infection caused by a bacterium called *Mycobacterium tuberculosis*. The bacteria usually attack the lungs, but they may also damage other parts of the body such as the brain, kidneys or spine. TB is spread through the air when an infected person coughs, sneezes or talks. Anyone exposed to TB should be tested. People with a weakened immune system are more likely to get TB.

Symptoms of TB in the lungs may include—
- A bad cough lasting 3 weeks or longer.
- A pain in the chest.
- Weight loss.
- Loss of appetite.
- Coughing up blood or bloody sputum (phlegm from inside the lungs).
- Weakness and/or fatigue.
- Fever and chills.
- Night sweats.

TB must be treated properly or it can lead to death. It can usually be cured with several medications over a long period of time. Patients with latent (asymptomatic) TB can take medicine to prevent development of active TB.

Multidrug-Resistant Tuberculosis

Multidrug-resistant tuberculosis (MDR TB) is TB that is resistant to at least two of the most effective anti-TB drugs, isoniazid and rifampicin. These drugs are the ones most widely used to treat TB. MDR TB is more likely to occur in patients who—

- Do not take their TB medicine regularly or who do not take all of the prescribed medication.
- Get active TB, after having taken medication to treat it in the past.
- Come from areas of the world where MDR TB is prevalent.
- Spend time with someone known to have MDR TB.

Meningitis

Meningitis is a contagious meningococcal infection that attacks the meninges, the protective coverings that surround the brain and spinal cord. Several different bacteria can cause meningitis, but a virus can also cause it. The bacteria are transmitted from person to person through droplets. Close and prolonged contact (e.g., kissing, sneezing or coughing on someone) and living in close quarters or dormitories (e.g., military or student housing) facilitates the spread of the disease. Meningitis can infect anyone but is more commonly found in those who have compromised immune systems and have trouble fighting infections.

The most common symptoms are stiff neck, high fever, light sensitivity, confusion, headache, nausea, sleepiness and vomiting. Bacterial meningitis is a serious infection; even when diagnosed early and properly treated, 5 to 10 percent of patients die, typically within 24–48 hours of the onset of symptoms. Bacterial meningitis may result in brain damage, hearing loss or learning disability in 10 to 20 percent of patients and sometimes death. *Viral* meningitis is less severe and usually resolves without specific treatment.

Bacterial meningitis is potentially fatal and is a medical emergency. Admission to a hospital or health center is necessary. There are vaccines available to prevent meningitis and antibiotics with which to treat it.

Community-Associated MRSA

***Methicillin-resistant* Staphylococcus aureus (MRSA)** is a type of bacterium. As one of the Staph bacteria, like other kinds of bacteria, it frequently lives on the skin and in the nose without causing any health problems. It only becomes a problem when it is a source of infection. These bacteria can be spread from one person to another through casual contact or contaminated objects. Infections with MRSA are more difficult to treat than ordinary Staph infections because they are resistant to many types of antibiotics, the medications used to treat bacterial infections. Infections can occur in wounds, burns and sites where tubes have been inserted into the body.

When MRSA occurs in groups of people who have not been recently hospitalized or have not had a medical procedure, this type of MRSA is referred to as *community-associated MRSA* (CA-MRSA). For example, it can occur among young people who have cuts or wounds and who are in close contact with one another, such as members of a sports team.

SARS

***Severe acute respiratory syndrome* (SARS)** is a viral respiratory illness caused by the *SARS-associated coronavirus* (SARS-CoV). It was first reported in Asia in February 2003. Over the following months, it spread to more than two dozen countries in North America, South America, Europe and Asia before the outbreak was contained.

SARS usually begins with a high fever (temperature greater than 100.4° F). Those infected may also experience headache, an overall feeling of discomfort and body aches. They may have mild respiratory symptoms at the outset. About 10 to 20 percent of those infected have diarrhea. After 2 to 7 days, SARS patients may develop a dry cough, and most develop pneumonia.

SARS spreads predominantly by close, person-to-person contact. The virus that causes SARS is thought to be transmitted most easily by respiratory droplets produced when an infected person coughs or sneezes and the droplets are deposited on the mucous membranes of the mouth, nose or eyes of people nearby. It can also spread when a person touches a surface or an object contaminated with infectious droplets and then touches the mouth, nose or eyes.

Influenza

Seasonal influenza is a respiratory illness caused by both human influenza A and human influenza B viruses, which can be transmitted from person to person. Most people have some immunity to influenza and there is a vaccine available.

Seasonal influenza usually has a sudden onset, with symptoms of fever (usually high), headache, extreme tiredness, dry cough, sore throat, runny or stuffy nose and muscle aches. Abdominal symptoms such as nausea, vomiting and diarrhea may also be present, but these symptoms occur more often in children than in adults.

Influenza is transmitted from person to person via large virus-laden droplets from coughing or sneezing. These large droplets settle on the mucosal surfaces of the upper respiratory tracts of susceptible persons who are within 3 feet of infected people. Transmission can also occur through direct contact or indirect contact with respiratory secretions—for example, when touching surfaces contaminated with influenza virus and then touching the mouth, nose or eyes.

Pandemic influenza (or pandemic flu) is a virulent human influenza A virus. The term "pandemic" refers to a worldwide epidemic occurring over a wide geographic area that affects a large number of people. Pandemic flu causes a global outbreak, or pandemic, of serious illness in humans. Because there is little natural immunity, the disease spreads easily from person to person.

Although we do not know for sure when the next pandemic influenza will strike or that it would present in the same way as seasonal influenza, it is helpful to be aware of the symptoms of seasonal influenza in order to plan for a pandemic flu. The best defense is to take steps to prevent disease transmission, such as frequent hand washing.

Protecting Yourself From Disease Transmission

There are many other illnesses, viruses and infections to which an EMR may be exposed. Keep immunizations current, have regular physical checkups and be knowledgeable about other pathogens. For more information on infectious diseases and illnesses of concern, contact the *Centers for Disease Control and Prevention*

(CDC) at (800) 342-2437 or visit the website at *www.cdc.gov*. You may also refer to your organization's exposure control officer.

Exposure Control Plan

Federal *Occupational Safety and Health Administration* (**OSHA**) regulations require employers to have an **exposure control plan**. The exposure control plan is a written program outlining the protective measures the employer will take to eliminate or minimize employee exposure incidents. The exposure control plan should include exposure determination, methods for implementing other parts of the OSHA standard (e.g., ways of meeting the requirements and recordkeeping) and procedures for evaluating details of an exposure incident. The exposure control plan guidelines should be available to employees and should specifically explain what they need to do to prevent the spread of infectious diseases.

Immunizations

Before working as an EMR, you should have a physical examination to determine your baseline health status. Your immunizations should be current while practicing in health care and should include protection against—

- Tetanus, diphtheria, pertussis.
- Hepatitis B.
- Measles/mumps/rubella (*German measles*).
- Chicken pox (*varicella*).
- Influenza.
- Meningococcal.

In addition to immunizations, it is recommended that you be screened for TB and have an annual tuberculin test.

Standard Precautions

Standard precautions are safety measures taken to prevent occupational-risk exposure to blood or other potentially infectious materials such as body fluids containing visible

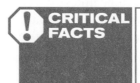

CRITICAL FACTS Exposure control plans, as required by OSHA, contain policies and procedures that help employers eliminate, minimize and properly report employee exposure incidents.

Standard precautions are safety measures to prevent occupational-risk exposure to blood or other potentially infectious materials. It assumes all body fluids may be infective.

Table 2-3:

Recommended Protective Equipment Against Hepatitis B, Hepatitis C and HIV Transmission in Prehospital Settings[1]

TASK OR ACTIVITY	DISPOSABLE GLOVES	GOWN	MASK	PROTECTIVE EYEWEAR
Bleeding control with spurting blood	Yes	Yes	Yes	Yes
Bleeding control with minimal bleeding	Yes	No	No	No
Emergency childbirth	Yes	Yes	Yes	Yes
Oral/nasal suctioning manually clearing airway	Yes	No	No, unless splashing is likely	No, unless splashing is likely
Handling and cleaning contaminated equipment and clothing	Yes	No, unless soiling is likely	No	No

[1]Department of Health and Human Services, Public Health Services: *A curriculum guide for public safety and emergency response workers prevention of transmission of immunodeficiency virus and hepatitis B virus,* Atlanta, Georgia, February 1989, Department of Health and Human Services, Centers for Disease Control. With modifications from Nixon, Robert G., *Communicable Diseases and Infection Control for EMS,* Prentice Hall, 2000.

blood. Standard precautions combine ***body substance isolation* (BSI)** and **universal precautions** and assume that all body fluids may be infective.

Universal precautions are OSHA-required practices of control to protect employees from exposure to blood and certain body fluids. These precautions require that all human blood and certain body substances be treated as if known to be infectious for hepatitis B, hepatitis C, HIV or other bloodborne pathogens.

BSI precautions are a group of measures to prevent exposure to pathogens. This approach to infection control can be applied through the use of—

- PPE.
- Good hand hygiene.
- **Engineering controls**.
- **Work practice controls**.
- Proper equipment cleaning.
- Spill cleanup procedures.

Personal Protective Equipment

PPE is equipment that is appropriate for your job duties and should be available in your workplace and identified in the exposure control plan. PPE includes all specialized clothing, equipment and

supplies that keep you from directly contacting infected materials. These include, but are not limited to, CPR breathing barriers, disposable (single-use) gloves, gowns, masks, shields and protective eyewear (**Table 2-3**, **Fig. 2-8**).

Disposable Gloves

Wear disposable gloves for all patient contact when providing care to injured or ill people. Disposable gloves are made of materials such as latex, vinyl and nitrile. There are gloves that are powder-free as well as other nonlatex disposable gloves. For information on glove removal, refer to the Removing Disposable Gloves Skill Sheet on page 37.

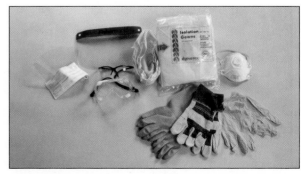

Fig. 2-8: Personal protective equipment

The History of Isolation Precautions

Isolation precautions have evolved over the last few decades, in response to the expansion of health care delivery from a mostly primary care hospital setting to a wide range of settings, as well as our understanding of new pathogens and how they spread.

While isolation precautions were already in place in the early 1980s, new guidelines, called *universal precautions,* were developed in the mid-1980s in response to the HIV/AIDS epidemic. These precautions dictated the application of blood and body fluid precautions to all patients, whether or not they were known to be infected. These precautions included such measures as hand washing immediately following glove removal, handling of needles and other sharps devices and PPE to protect health care personnel from mucous membrane exposures.

In 1987, new precautions were developed, called *BSI precautions,* which shared some features with universal precautions but emphasized the need to avoid contact with all moist and potentially infectious body substances, even if blood was not present. Another difference from universal precautions was that BSI precautions did not specify hand washing after glove removal unless there was visible soiling.

Most recently, in 1996, the *Healthcare Infection Control Practices Advisory Committee* (HICPAC) blended the major features of universal and BSI precautions in a broader guideline referred to as *standard precautions,* directing health care workers to apply these precautions to all patients at all times. Standard precautions address some gaps in the earlier guidelines, by including three transmission-based categories of precautions: airborne, droplet and contact.

Today, standard precautions constitute the primary strategy to prevent health care-associated infection among patients and health care personnel.

Eye Protection

Safety glasses with side shields may be worn for eye protection. Use goggles or a full-face shield if there is a risk of splash or spray of body fluids. These reduce the risk of contamination of the mouth, nose or eyes. Examples of when these are necessary are when a patient is bleeding profusely, when delivering a baby, when suctioning and when providing ventilatory support (e.g., *bag-valve-mask resuscitator* [BVM] or resuscitation mask).

CPR Breathing Barriers

CPR breathing barriers include resuscitation masks, face shields and BVMs. CPR breathing barriers help protect you against disease transmission when performing CPR or giving ventilations to a patient.

Masks

A mask is a personal protective device worn on the face that covers at least the nose and mouth, and reduces the wearer's risk of inhaling hazardous airborne particles (including dust particles and infectious agents such as TB), gases or vapors. A *high-efficiency particulate air* (HEPA) or N95 mask filters out at least 95 percent of airborne particles, and is therefore given a "95" rating. Respirators that filter out at least 99 percent receive a "99" rating. Those that filter at least 99.97 percent (essentially 100 percent) receive a "100" rating. Remember that masks must be fit-tested to be effective. Place a surgical mask on the patient if you suspect an airborne disease.

Gowns

Wear a disposable gown in situations with large amounts of blood or body fluids. If your clothing becomes contaminated, remove it and shower as soon as possible. Wash the clothes in a separate load, preferably at work.

Hand Hygiene

Hand washing is the most effective measure to prevent the spread of infection. By washing your hands often, you physically remove disease-causing germs you may have picked up from other people, animals or contaminated surfaces. In addition, jewelry, including rings, should not be worn where the potential for risk of exposure exists.

Wash your hands frequently. When practical, wash your hands before providing care and always after providing care—whether or not gloves are worn (**Fig. 2-9**). Local protocols may vary and should be followed.

Wash your hands with soap and running water, and dry your hands thoroughly. Wash your hands and other exposed skin immediately

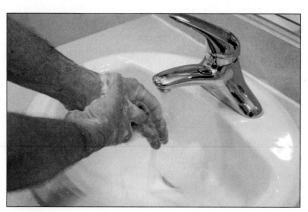

Fig. 2-9: Hand washing is the most effective way to prevent the spread of infection.

if exposed to contaminants, such as blood and body fluids. Always wash hands after using the restroom and before and after handling food. Use alcohol-based hand sanitizers when soap and running water are not available.

Hand Washing Tips

To ensure you wash your hands correctly, follow these steps:

- Wet hands with warm water.
- Apply soap to hands.
- Rub hands vigorously for at least 15 seconds, covering all surfaces of the hands and fingers. Use soap and warm running water. Scrub nails by rubbing them against the palms.
- Rinse hands with water.
- Dry hands thoroughly with a paper towel.
- Turn off the faucet using the paper towel.

In addition to washing your hands frequently, keep your fingernails less than one-quarter of an inch long and avoid wearing artificial nails.

Hand Sanitizer and Hand Washing Stations

At some outdoor events or workplaces, for example on a farm or at a fair, the only source of clean water may be a portable hand wash station. These stations consist of a supply of soap and potable water, and a bucket, cooler or other container with a turn-spout that allows the water to run over your hands to rinse soap away. The stations also include

a catch bucket to catch the wastewater, and an ample supply of paper towels.

Alcohol-based hand sanitizers allow you to cleanse your hands when soap and water are not readily available and your hands are not visibly soiled. If your hands contain visible matter, you should use soap and water instead. When using an alcohol-based hand sanitizer—

- Apply the product to the palm of one hand.
- Rub hands together.
- Rub the product over all surfaces of the hands and fingers until hands are dry.
- Wash your hands with anti-bacterial hand soap and water as soon as it is available.

Engineering and Work Practice Controls

Engineering controls are control measures that isolate or remove a hazard from the workplace. In other words, engineering controls are objects used in the workplace to help reduce the risk of an exposure incident. Examples of engineering controls include—

- Sharps disposal containers (**Fig. 2-10**).
- Self-sheathing needles.
- Safer medical devices, such as sharps with engineered sharps injury protections or needleless systems.
- Use of **biohazard** containers and labels, and posting of signs at entrances to areas where infectious materials may be present.
- PPE.

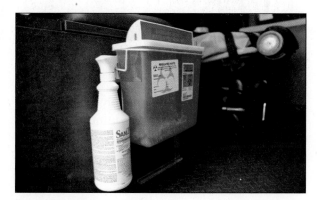

Fig. 2-10: Biohazard containers are one type of engineering control.

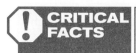 **CRITICAL FACTS** Engineering controls, such as biohazard containers and PPE, are control measures that isolate or remove a hazard from the workplace.

Biohazard containers are marked with a biohazard symbol—a three-sided design in bright, fluorescent orange or orange-red, or predominantly so with lettering or symbols in a contrasting color. This symbol warns of potential infection hazards. The origin of the biohazard symbol dates back to the 1960s. It was created out of a need for a standardized, unique symbol to use as a warning symbol in response to accidental infections that occurred as a result of biomedical research. These unfortunate incidents were viewed as preventable. The symbol's development was spearheaded by Charles Baldwin, an environmental health engineer at Dow Chemical Corporation. The symbol that was eventually chosen best met the criteria that were tested in development of the symbol. It is easy to recognize, has three sides so it can be identified from any angle, and can be easily stenciled for labeling purposes. The symbol was soon adopted by the National Institutes of Health, the CDC and OSHA.

Work practice controls reduce the likelihood of exposure by changing the way a task is carried out. These are the methods of working that help reduce the risk of an exposure incident. Examples of work practice controls include—

- Placing sharps items (e.g., needles, scalpel blades) in puncture-resistant, leak-proof and labeled containers, and having the containers at the point of use.
- Avoiding splashing, spraying and splattering droplets of blood or other potentially infectious materials when performing all procedures.
- Removing and disposing of soiled protective clothing as soon as possible.
- Cleaning and disinfecting all equipment and work surfaces possibly soiled by blood or other body fluids.
- Washing your hands thoroughly with soap and water immediately after providing care, using a utility or restroom sink (not one in a food preparation area).
- Not eating, drinking, smoking, applying cosmetics or lip balm, handling contact lenses or touching your mouth, nose or eyes when you are in an area where you may be exposed to infectious materials.

- Using alcohol-based sanitizers where hand-washing facilities are not available.

Vehicle and Equipment Cleaning and Disinfecting

After providing care, the equipment and surfaces you used should always be cleaned and disinfected or properly disposed of **(Fig. 2-11)**. Handle all soiled equipment, supplies and other materials with care until it is properly cleaned and disinfected. Place all used disposable or single-use items in labeled biohazard containers. Place all soiled clothing in marked plastic bags for disposal or washing.

Take the following steps to clean up spills:
- Wear disposable gloves and other PPE when cleaning spills.
- Clean up spills immediately or as soon as possible after the spill occurs.
- If the spill is mixed with sharp objects, such as broken glass and needles, do not pick these up with your hands. Use tongs, a broom and dustpan or other similar items.
- Dispose of the absorbent material used to collect the spill in a labeled biohazard container.
- Flood the area with a fresh disinfectant solution. Use a commonly accepted disinfectant of approximately $1\frac{1}{2}$ cups of liquid chlorine bleach to 1 gallon of water (1 part bleach per 9 parts water, or about a 10% solution), and allow it to stand for at least 10 minutes. Other commercial disinfectant/antimicrobial solutions are available and may have different set times. Follow local protocols and manufacturer's instructions.
- Use appropriate material to absorb the solution, and dispose of it in a labeled biohazard container.
- Scrub soiled boots, leather shoes and other leather goods such as belts with soap, a brush and hot water. If you wear a uniform to work, wash and dry it according to the manufacturer's instructions.

Clean and disinfect the vehicle according to standard procedures. Wear appropriate PPE (disposable gown and gloves) during the cleaning process and discard after use.

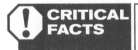

CRITICAL FACTS Work practice controls reduce the likelihood of exposure by changing the way tasks, such as disposal of sharps items or soiled clothing, are carried out.

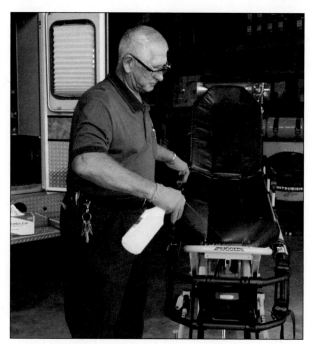

Fig. 2-11: Always clean and disinfect the equipment you use after providing care. *Courtesy of Terry Georgia.*

Thoroughly clean and disinfect all surfaces that may have come in contact with the patient or materials that may have become contaminated while providing care for the patient (e.g., stretcher, rails, control panels, floors, walls, work surfaces). Use an *Environmental Protection Agency* (EPA)-registered hospital disinfectant and use according to manufacturer's recommendations.

If an Exposure Occurs

Exposure incidents involve contact with blood or body fluids—for example, a patient's blood gets into a cut on your hand, you are stuck with a needle used on a patient or bloody saliva splashes into your mouth or eyes. You may also be exposed when in unprotected, close contact with someone who has an airborne disease involving exposure to aerosolized, respiratory droplets (e.g., coughing, sneezing), such as with a patient infected with influenza (including pandemic flu), TB or MDR TB.

What to Do If You Are Exposed

If you are exposed, take the following steps immediately:

- Clean the contaminated area thoroughly with soap and water. Wash needlestick injuries, cuts and exposed skin with soap and water.
- Flush splashes of blood or other potentially infectious materials to the mouth and nose with water.
- If the eyes are involved, irrigate with clean water, saline or sterile irrigants for 20 minutes.
- Seek immediate follow-up care as identified in your department exposure control plan.

Reporting Exposures

Following any exposure incident—

- Report the exposure incident to the appropriate person identified in your employer's exposure control plan immediately and to the *emergency medical services* (EMS) providers who take over care of the patient. This step can be critical to the success of post-exposure treatment.
- Write down what happened. Include the time and date of the exposure as well as the circumstances of the exposure, any actions taken after the exposure and any other information required by your employer.

OSHA Regulations

OSHA has issued regulations about on-the-job exposure to bloodborne pathogens. OSHA determined that employees are at risk when exposed to blood or other body fluids. OSHA therefore requires employers to reduce or remove hazards from the workplace that may place employees in contact with infectious materials.

OSHA regulations and guidelines apply to employees who may come into contact with blood or other body substances that could cause an infection. These regulations apply to you as an EMR because you are expected to provide emergency care as part of your job. In 2001, in response to passage of the federal Needlestick

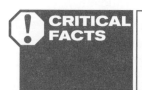
CRITICAL FACTS

If you are exposed to blood or other potentially infectious materials, immediately take the appropriate steps, such as cleaning contaminated areas, as part of a proper exposure control plan.

Per OSHA regulations, employers are required to remove items that might put employees in contact with infectious materials.

Safety and Prevention Act, OSHA revised the Bloodborne Pathogens Standard 29 CFR 1910.1030. These guidelines may help you and your employer meet the OSHA bloodborne pathogens standard to prevent transmission of serious diseases. (For additional information on the Bloodborne Pathogens Standard 29 CFR 1910.1030, visit OSHA's website at *www.osha.gov/SLTC/bloodbornepathogens/standards.html.*)

OSHA regulations regarding bloodborne pathogens have placed specific responsibilities on employers for protection of employees, including—

- Identifying positions or tasks covered by the standard.
- Creating an exposure control plan to minimize the possibility of exposure and making the plan easily accessible to employees.
- Developing and putting into action a written schedule for cleaning and decontaminating at the workplace.
- Creating a system for easy identification of soiled material and its proper disposal.
- Developing a system of annual training for all covered employees.
- Offering the opportunity for employees to get the hepatitis B vaccination at no cost.
- Establishing clear procedures to follow for reporting an exposure.
- Creating a system of recordkeeping.
- In workplaces where there is potential exposure to injuries from contaminated sharps, soliciting input from non-managerial employees with potential exposure regarding the identification, evaluation and selection of effective engineering and work practice controls.
- If a needlestick injury occurs, recording the appropriate information in the sharps injury log, including—
  - The type and brand of device involved in the incident.
  - The location of the incident.
  - A description of the incident.
- Maintaining a sharps injury log in such a way that protects the privacy of employees.
- Ensuring confidentiality of employees' medical records and exposure incidents.

Needlestick Safety and Prevention Act

Blood and other potentially infectious materials have long been recognized as potential threats to the health of employees who are exposed to these materials through penetration of the skin. Injuries from contaminated needles and other sharps have been associated with an increased risk of disease from more than 20 infectious agents. The most serious pathogens are hepatitis B, hepatitis C and HIV. Needlestick and other sharps injuries resulting in exposure to blood or other potentially infectious materials are a concern because they happen frequently and can have serious health effects.

In 2001, OSHA revised the Bloodborne Pathogens Standard 29 CFR 1910.1030. The revised standard clarifies the need for employers to select safer needle devices and to involve employees in identifying and choosing these devices. Needleless systems are one option to reduce the possibility of accidental needlestick injuries and possible infection. The updated standard also requires employers to maintain a log of injuries from contaminated sharps. (For additional information on the Needlestick Safety and Prevention Act, visit OSHA's website at *www.osha.gov/SLTC/bloodbornepathogens/standards.html.*)

Also, be aware of any areas, equipment or containers that may be contaminated. Biohazard warning labels are required on any container holding contaminated materials, such as used gloves, bandages or trauma dressings. Post signs at entrances to work areas where infectious materials may be present.

EMOTIONAL ASPECTS OF EMERGENCY CARE
Stressful Situations

EMRs experience an extraordinary number of stressful situations beyond what others may encounter. Some of the more powerful situations include—

- Dangerous situations. Fires, scenes of violent crime, agricultural accidents and other

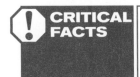

CRITICAL FACTS OSHA regulations regarding bloodborne pathogens have placed specific responsibilities on employers for protection of employees. These include creating exposure control plans, scheduling decontamination and cleaning of the workplace, training on OSHA regulations and free hepatitis B vaccinations.

emergency scenes all involve a certain measure of danger.

- Physical and psychological demands. Some rescues, such as extrications, may place substantial physical burdens on the EMR; others, such as rescuing an abused child, may involve extraordinary psychological demands.
- Critically injured or ill people. Responding to a call to help someone who is critically injured or ill can be highly stressful because of the possibility of not being able to save the patient.
- Death and dying patients. Death is disturbing to most people, but the feelings of powerlessness at not being able to save someone's life may also bring about tremendous guilt and grief.
- Overpowering sights, smells and sounds. Disturbing sights, strong smells and sounds that are upsetting to the EMR may accompany scenes of illness and accidents, especially those that are severe.
- Multiple-patient situations. All of the above situations can occur when a single person is injured or ill, but the effects are magnified in a multiple-casualty incident, which can be truly overwhelming.
- Angry or upset patients, family and bystanders. In an emotionally charged situation, tempers may flare, adding to the intensity of the situation.

During stressful situations, cooperate with other personnel responding to the situation. It is important that you handle the situation in a professional manner when dealing with law enforcement, other EMS providers, the patient and the family.

Death and Dying

Experiencing the dying process is difficult for most people. The following measures may help the patient and family deal with the dying process:

- Recognize that the patient's and the family's needs include dignity, respect, sharing, communication, privacy and control.
- Allow the patient and the family to express rage, anger and despair.

- Listen empathetically and remain calm and non-judgmental.
- Do not falsely reassure.
- Use a gentle tone of voice.
- Let the patient and the family know that everything that can be done to help will be done.
- Use a reassuring touch, if it is appropriate.
- Comfort the patient and the family.

Resuscitation

You may be summoned to an emergency in which one or more people have died or are dying. The cause could be natural, accidental or intentional. Though your responses will vary according to the situation, you must recognize that death will have an emotional impact on you, as well as on others involved.

You may be in a situation in which you think a person has been dead for a while and you are unsure whether you should attempt to resuscitate that person. The general rule is to always attempt to resuscitate a patient without a pulse or breathing except in the following situations:

- A valid *Do Not Resuscitate* (DNR) order that meets local guidelines is present at the scene.
- Obvious signs of death are present in the patient. These signs include tissue decay (putrefaction); rigor mortis (stiffening of joints that occurs after death; assess two or more joints, such as the fingers and jaw, to verify); obvious mortal wounds (injuries clearly not compatible with life, such as decapitation); or dependent **lividity** (purplish color in the lowest-lying parts of a recently dead body, due to pooling of blood).
- The situation is so dangerous (such as a gunman on the scene) that attempting to resuscitate the patient would endanger your life.

To determine that a person is dead, the patient is often placed on a heart monitor and vital signs are assessed. When it is determined that the patient has no electrical activity of the heart and no respirations and blood pressure, the person may be declared dead. This may occur after prolonged resuscitation attempts, or it may occur immediately if one of the above conditions is present.

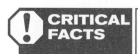 **CRITICAL FACTS** Measures such as listening empathetically, speaking gently and allowing anger or despair to be expressed may help the patient and family cope with the dying process.

Some patients may have advance directives or DNR orders, written legal documents saying that they do not wish to be resuscitated or kept alive by mechanical means. In most instances, you should honor the wishes of the patient if they are expressed in writing. However, since state and local laws about these situations vary, you should summon more advanced medical personnel immediately to provide care. If you are in doubt about the validity of the advance directives, attempt to resuscitate the patient. (For more information on advance directives and DNR orders, refer to **Chapter 3**.)

Individual Responses to Death

Dying is part of the living process. Death affects everyone, and the way we respond varies widely. Be prepared to handle your feelings and the feelings of others. Remember that reactions to death and dying range from anxiety to acceptance. How well you and others handle the situation will depend on both personal feelings about death and the nature of the incident.

One of the most disturbing emergency situations is **sudden death**. Sudden death generally refers to an unexpected, natural death. It is commonly used to describe death resulting from an abrupt cardiac event, but it also describes a death that occurs within a few hours after an abrupt onset of symptoms in an otherwise healthy person. Sudden death of an infant can be especially disturbing to new parents, though it is difficult for anyone involved. EMRs can never fully prepare themselves for an emergency involving sudden death.

Stages of Grief

There will be times you are called to assist grieving patients or family members. There are some predictable responses to grief, though people do not always experience them in any particular order. Keep in mind that everyone's reactions to death and dying is unique and not everyone will experience every stage of grief, nor will everyone experience grief in the same order.

Remain non-judgmental throughout the grieving process. The stages of grieving include—

- Denial. The patient or family member denies the seriousness of the situation in order to buffer the pain of the event.
- Anger. The patient or family member projects feelings of anger toward other people, especially those closest to the individual. Do not take anger personally, even though it may seem to be directed toward you. Be alert to anger that may become physical and endanger you or others.
- Bargaining. The patient or family member may attempt to negotiate with a spiritual higher being or even with EMS providers in an effort to extend life.
- Depression. The patient or family member exhibits sadness and grief, is usually withdrawn and may cry continually. Allow the affected person to express these feelings, and help the patient or family member to understand that these are normal feelings associated with death.
- Acceptance. The patient or family member ultimately accepts the situation and incorporates the experience into the activities of daily living, in an effort to survive or to support a loved one. Use good listening skills in this phase.

Helping the Patient and the Family

The care EMRs provide to patients often focuses on the patient's physical needs, but care must also include supporting patients and their families through the emotions they may experience when someone is injured or ill. In these situations, be calm, supportive and non-judgmental. Allow the patient or family member to safely vent feelings.

STRESS MANAGEMENT
What Is Stress?

Stress is the body's normal response to any situation that changes a person's existing mental, physical or emotional balance. Stress can result from positive experiences, such as a wedding, or more difficult situations, such as responding to a life-threatening emergency.

Stress can arise from any situation or thought that brings about feelings of frustration, anger or

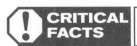 **CRITICAL FACTS** Denial, anger, bargaining, depression and acceptance are the five stages of grief.

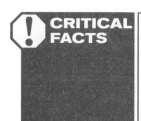
anxiety. Stress is unique to the individual; what is stressful to one person may not be so to another. Stress is a normal part of life. In small quantities, it can be positive, motivating people and helping them to be more productive. Too much stress or a strong response to stress, however, can be harmful, contributing to illnesses such as heart disease or depression.

An event like a serious injury, illness or death may produce great stress in patients, family members and EMRs. By learning how stress builds up, how to identify its signs and symptoms and how to manage stress, you can help yourself and others cope with the stressful impact of an emergency situation.

While providing care, you may encounter angry, scared or violent patients and family members, especially when the patient is seriously injured or ill. Personal feelings triggered by these situations can affect you. Learn what to expect and how to assist patients, their families, yourself and others in dealing with this stress.

Those involved in a serious injury, sudden illness or death may face an emotional crisis. Their reactions to the crisis will depend on a number of factors and will differ from person to person. Often, reactions will come during or immediately following the event, but in some cases they may be delayed for hours, days or even longer.

Warning Signs of Personal Stress

As an EMR, be sure to note if you or those around you are exhibiting any signs of personal stress during or following a response. When interacting with patients and their families during an emergency, you may hear them talk about or exhibit certain signs of stress. Warning signs of stress include—

- Difficulty sleeping and nightmares.
- Irritability with co-workers, family and friends.
- Feelings of sadness, anxiety or guilt.
- Indecisiveness.
- Loss of appetite.
- Loss of interest in sexual activity.
- Isolation.
- Loss of interest in work.
- Feelings of hopelessness.
- Alcohol or drug misuse or abuse.
- Inability to concentrate.

INCIDENT STRESS MANAGEMENT

An EMR's job can be highly stressful, often involving "critical incidents." These emergencies involve a serious injury or death. Critical incidents are especially stressful if you feel you did something wrong or failed to do something even after responding exactly as you were trained. A particular type of stress, called **critical incident stress**, can result from such a situation. It is important to understand the powerful impact this stress can have on you.

The stress of the emergency can cause distress or disruption in a person's mental or emotional balance. It can cause sleeplessness, anxiety, depression, exhaustion, restlessness, nausea, nightmares and other problems. Some effects may appear right away and others only after days, weeks or even months have passed. People suffering from critical incident stress might not be able to do their job well.

Closely monitor your performance and watch for the following signs of critical incident stress reactions:
- Confusion
- Shortened attention span
- Poor concentration
- Denial
- Guilt
- Depression
- Anger
- Change in interactions with others
- Increased or decreased eating

- Uncharacteristic, excessive humor or silence
- Any other unusual behavior

EMS Incidents Likely to Produce Stress

Events that trigger critical incident stress are often powerful and traumatic, and are usually outside of the range of what we consider normal human experiences on the job. This might include the death or serious injury of a co-worker, the death of a child or a multiple-casualty event.

Preincident Education

To help EMRs cope with job-related stress before it occurs, employers sometimes offer stress-management classes and crisis mitigation training. This preparation helps responders set expectations and improve their ability to cope with stress.

It is also a good idea to create a self-care plan that lays out how you will take care of your own well-being while involved in emergency work. This should include mental health considerations. For example, your employer may offer prearranged professional counseling to help you cope with work-related stress.

Finally, an EMR's job often requires long hours, including weekends and evenings. To lower your stress level, it is a good idea to arrange in advance for personal responsibilities such as care for children and elderly parents.

Stress Management During an Emergency

Pay attention to your own stress responses during an emergency, through continual self-monitoring. In monitoring your stress, consider factors such as stamina, expectations, prior traumatic experiences and eating habits. Partner with a colleague so that you can help monitor each other's stress levels to determine when relief is necessary. If you feel your stress level rising to a concerning level, you may need a second to step back from a situation, recollect your thoughts and then continue with care.

Post-Incident Stress Management

To relieve stress, the following steps can help:
- Use quick relaxation techniques, such as deep, slow breathing.
- Eat a good meal and avoid beverages with caffeine.

- Avoid alcohol or drugs.
- Review the event and clear up any uncertainties.
- Get enough rest.
- Get involved in some type of physical exercise or activity, either alone or in a group.

Two techniques are commonly used to help deal with an incident stress situation: **debriefing** and **defusing**. These processes bring you together with peer counselors and mental health professionals trained in techniques to help accelerate the recovery process after a critical incident.

Staff Debriefing

Debriefing usually takes place in a group setting and should be conducted in a controlled environment by a trained professional. The team talks about what happened before, during and after the emergency. It is important to avoid assigning blame or criticizing anyone's actions. Team leaders and mental health professionals evaluate the information and offer suggestions on overcoming stress. The goals of a debriefing are to reduce the impact of the traumatic event, accelerate the normal recovery process from a traumatic event, normalize the stress response for emergency workers in traumatic events and provide education in stress management and coping techniques. All information shared at these meetings is confidential.

Debriefings are not just for those incidents involving death or major disasters. Any incident, such as a dramatic, lifesaving rescue, is a potential source of emotional stress. It is important that responders involved in any incident involving significant stress be debriefed.

Defusing

A defusing is much shorter than a debriefing. It is less formal and less structured. Defusings are effective in the first few hours after the event and usually last 30 to 45 minutes. One advantage of a defusing is that it allows for immediate, initial venting, and may even eliminate the need for a formal debriefing. Also, if the choice is made to have a formal debriefing meeting, discussions shared in the defusing may enhance the subsequent meeting. Defusings are often done on a one-on-one basis between the responder and a peer counselor.

Follow-Up

EMRs sometimes do not recognize how much the stress of what they do can affect their family and friends. They sometimes complain that their loved ones show a lack of understanding for what they do. Family members can experience frustration because of an EMR's unwillingness to share information and feelings about an incident. EMRs do not always realize that family members and friends suffer fear of separation and are afraid of being ignored for something "more exciting." An EMS career can be cut short by the invisible dangers of unmanaged stress. By taking a serious look at your life and making necessary adjustments, you can ensure a healthy balance in all the things you choose to do.

If you begin to exhibit signs and symptoms of critical incident stress that do not seem to be going away after an emergency, work with your supervisor to arrange for professional counseling by a licensed mental health professional.

When to Access Professional Help

If you or another colleague show signs of critical incident stress, work with your employer as soon as possible to arrange for professional counseling by a licensed mental health professional. Do not wait until after an emergency to figure out where you should go if you begin to exhibit signs and symptoms of critical incident stress.

Incidents that could lead to a necessity to access professional counseling by a licensed mental health professional include—
- Line-of-duty death or serious injury.
- Multiple-casualty incidents.
- Suicide of an emergency worker.
- Serious injury or death of children.
- Events with excessive media attention.
- Victims known to EMS personnel.
- Events that have unusual impact on EMS personnel.
- Any disaster.

Activation protocols vary from area to area. Your employer should be able to supply you with information on how to access this service in your community.

Some people think that participating in counseling is an admission of weakness. Quite the contrary is true. Counseling should be—and in many areas is—a routine part of any overwhelming incident, such as an airline disaster. Counseling can help in any situation, regardless of how minor you may think the event was. The most important thing you can do to minimize the effects of any emergency is to express your feelings and thoughts after the incident.

PUTTING IT ALL TOGETHER

In order to provide emergency care to others, it is important first to look after yourself. This includes physical, emotional and mental health concerns.

One of the ways EMRs must look after themselves is by preventing illness. Bloodborne pathogens—most commonly bacteria and viruses—are present in blood and body fluids and can cause disease in humans. The bloodborne pathogens of primary concern to EMRs are hepatitis B, hepatitis C and HIV. These pathogens spread primarily through direct or indirect contact with infected blood or other body fluids.

To prevent the spread of bloodborne pathogens and other diseases, EMRs should follow standard precautions. These precautions require that all blood and other body fluids be treated as if known to be infectious. Apply these precautions by using PPE, frequently washing your hands, using engineering controls, following work practice controls, properly cleaning and disinfecting equipment, cleaning up after spills and properly disposing of used disposable or single-use equipment.

If exposed to blood or other potentially infectious materials, you should immediately wash, flush or irrigate the exposed area of your body and report the incident to your supervisor.

It is equally important that you attend to mental and emotional health concerns in yourself and the patients and families you are helping. An emotional crisis often results from an unexpected, shocking and undesired event, such as the sudden loss of a loved one. Although people react differently in different situations, everyone experiences some or all of the stages of grief. By considering the nature of the incident, you can begin to prepare yourself to deal with its emotional aspects.

Regardless of the nature of the event, the care you provide to patients in any emotional crisis is very similar. Your care involves both verbal and nonverbal communication. It also requires you to understand that in some cases death is inevitable. In some situations, you may be overcome by emotion. Remember, that self-help involves sharing your feelings with others.

))) YOU ARE THE EMERGENCY MEDICAL RESPONDER

After EMS personnel assumed the care of your patient, you note that, in addition to the blood and vomit on the ground, there is some blood on your disposable gloves and the mask of your BVM. What steps would you follow to avoid coming in contact with the blood and other body fluids? How should the area be decontaminated?

SKILLsheet

Removing Disposable Gloves

NOTE: To remove gloves without spreading germs, never touch your bare skin with the outside of either glove.

STEP 1

◆ Pinch the palm side of one glove near your wrist.
◆ Carefully pull the glove off so that it is inside out.

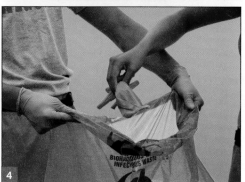

STEP 2

◆ Hold the glove in the palm of your gloved hand.
◆ Slip two fingers under the glove at the wrist of the remaining gloved hand.

STEP 3

◆ Pull the glove until it comes off, inside out.
◆ The first glove should end up inside the glove you just removed.

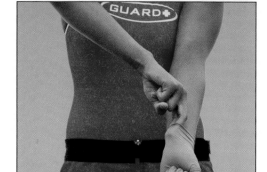

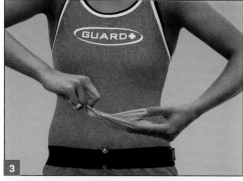

STEP 4

◆ Always wash your hands after removing gloves.

NOTE: Always dispose of gloves and other PPE in a proper biohazard container.

Wash hands thoroughly with soap and running water, if available. Otherwise rub hands thoroughly with an alcohol based hand sanitizer if hands are not visibly soiled.

Enrichment
Health of the Emergency Medical Responder

Being an EMR is a rewarding experience, but it also can be physically, emotionally and mentally challenging. Making healthy lifestyle choices benefits not only yourself, but also the patients who will rely on you in their moments of need.

PHYSICAL WELL-BEING

Taking care of your body is a must for an EMR. There are situations you may face where physical strength and stamina will be key components in successfully caring for patients or assisting other responders. There are many factors to obtaining good physical well-being, and you should consider it your responsibility to address all of them as part of a healthy lifestyle. Physical activity not only helps you keep fit but also is an effective way to reduce stress.

Physical Fitness

Your physical well-being is one of the most important assets you hold to ensure that you are able to effectively perform your job as an EMR **(Fig. 2-12)**. Maintaining your own physical fitness is necessary for having the stamina and strength to respond at the level required.

One of the key aspects of physical fitness is cardiovascular endurance. Be sure to get regular cardiovascular training. According to the American College of Sports Medicine, 30 minutes of physical activity per day can help lower blood pressure and cholesterol and help you maintain a healthy weight. The more you exercise, the better your endurance—resulting in better health, strength and stamina.

Muscle strength and flexibility are also important assets for EMRs to assist in day-to-day tasks. Strength training develops

Fig. 2-12: Strength training develops strong bones, increases bone density and controls body fat.

strong bones, increases bone density and controls body fat. Strength training will also reduce your risk of injury, as muscle protects your joints and helps you maintain flexibility and balance.

Stretching on a regular basis is the best way to maintain flexibility. Therefore, in tandem with your aerobic and strength training, make sure to incorporate stretching as part of your daily workout routine.

Nutrition

Following basic nutrition strategies will help keep you fit, reduce stress and assist in maintaining your stamina throughout the day. Try to cut down on foods that are high in sugar and caffeine and follow the Food Guide Pyramid for a healthy diet *(www.mypyramid.gov)*.

Sleep

Sleep deprivation is one of the most potentially dangerous challenges EMRs may face, as it affects your ability to think clearly and can decrease your eye-hand coordination. This means you are less productive and may make mistakes that can lead to injury or negatively affect the patients you treat. If you find yourself consistently feeling drowsy, adjust your sleep schedule to ensure you are getting enough rest. Speak to your health care provider if you are experiencing sleeplessness.

Disease Prevention

Emergency care personnel must take precautions against disease transmission by potentially infectious substances. Make sure to protect yourself against disease transmission by following standard precautions and using recommended PPE. Remember, hand washing is the most important way to prevent the spread of infection, even if you were wearing gloves when possibly exposed.

Controlling risk factors for heart disease is the best way to minimize your chance of cardiovascular disease. Taking steps to maintain a healthy lifestyle by quitting smoking, becoming more active, lowering stress in your life and eating a healthy diet will dramatically reduce your risks.

Injury Prevention

As mentioned, strength training is a good start to helping prevent injury on the job. As an EMR, it is challenging to keep your own safety in mind, especially when your patient is in a life-threatening situation. Trying to remain aware of your surroundings, using proper lifting techniques and following proper procedures and protocols, however, will help ensure your safety and that of your patient.

Sun Safety

According to the American Academy of Dermatology, 1 in 5 Americans will develop some form of skin cancer during their lifetime. Remember when exposed to the sun to drink plenty of fluids and dress appropriately, such as in long-sleeved shirts, pants, hats and sunglasses. Wear sunscreen with a *sun protection factor* (SPF) of at least 15, one that provides broad-spectrum protection from *ultraviolet A* (UVA) and *ultraviolet B* (UVB) rays. Reapply sunscreen every 2 hours, even on cloudy days, and especially when sweating.

MENTAL WELL-BEING

There is no doubt that being an EMR is stressful **(Fig. 2-13)**. The sense of responsibility for other people's lives can be overwhelming. Mental well-being, like physical well-being, is important to allow you to stay focused and be prepared to deal with the day-to-day stress of your job.

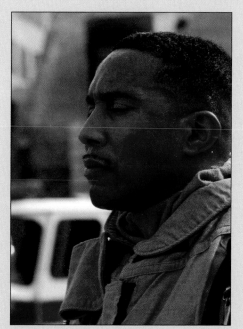

Fig. 2-13: Being an EMR can be overwhelming. Mental well-being is important to help prepare for the everyday stress of the job.

Reducing Stress

If you find yourself feeling overwhelmed or indifferent toward your job, irritable, angry, sarcastic or quick to argue, chances are you are not coping well with the stress in your life. It is important to find ways to help relieve your feelings of stress before they begin to affect your job performance.

There are three types of stress reactions common to EMRs: acute, delayed and cumulative. Recognizing the warning signs of stress is imperative, as the earlier they are identified, the easier they are to address. The warning signs include—

- Irritability.
- Lack of concentration.
- Difficulty sleeping and nightmares.
- Anxiety.
- Indecisiveness.
- Guilt or shame.
- Loss of appetite and sexual desire.
- Isolation.
- Loss of interest in work.

If you feel stress affecting your life, it is important to get it under control. These stress management techniques may be helpful:
- Reprioritize work goals and tasks.
- Perform physical activity every day.
- Make sure you eat at every meal and avoid fast food.
- Share household chores with family members.
- Practice relaxed breathing or muscle relaxation.
- Put a positive spin on negative thoughts.

Continued on next page

Enrichment
Health of the Emergency Medical Responder (continued)

Personal Relationships

Finding work-life balance is always challenging, and must be managed properly so you can enjoy a rewarding personal life. Too much focus on work can place stress on your relationships. Often, when faced with difficulties in your personal life, concentrating on your job can be difficult. This can lead to mistakes or injuries. Some people throw themselves into work as a way to avoid dealing with relationship problems at home, which can lead to burnout.

Discovering you are having difficulty coping with problems at home can be overwhelming. Counseling can help you cope with conflict in your personal relationships and be better prepared to focus while on the job. Family therapy and marriage counseling can help mend strained relationships, teach new coping skills and improve how you interact with family and partners. Counseling gives families the tools to communicate better, negotiate differences, problem solve and even argue in a healthier way.

Alcohol and Drug Problems

High levels of stress, anxiety or emotional pain can lead some people to drink alcohol to excess or use drugs. In actuality, this increases stress.

Addiction is a complex problem, including both psychological and physical aspects. If you are addicted to a drug, you will experience intense cravings for it, sometimes many times throughout the day. Your cravings for the substance will persist in spite of the physical, psychological and social consequences it brings. You may find yourself repeatedly trying to stop taking the drug but being unable to do so because of the unpleasant reactions to stopping, such as insomnia, anxiety and tremors. You may also find yourself rationalizing the need to do things you would not normally do, such as stealing or lying, to continue drug use. Or, you may try to convince yourself that you need the drug in order to cope with your problems. If you show any of the signs of addiction, seek help immediately through addiction services in your community.

If you are a smoker, deciding to quit smoking will be one of the best and most responsible decisions you make in your life. It will also be one of the most challenging. Speak to your health care provider for advice on quitting, and remember the health benefits as a way to stay focused on your goal.

HEALTH RISKS AND ASSESSMENTS

Your employer may offer wellness tools, such as online health profiles, to help you identify health risks and develop wellness goals through personalized health assessments. Take advantage of these and other tools that may be offered to you in an effort to lead a healthier lifestyle.

3 Medical, Legal and Ethical Issues

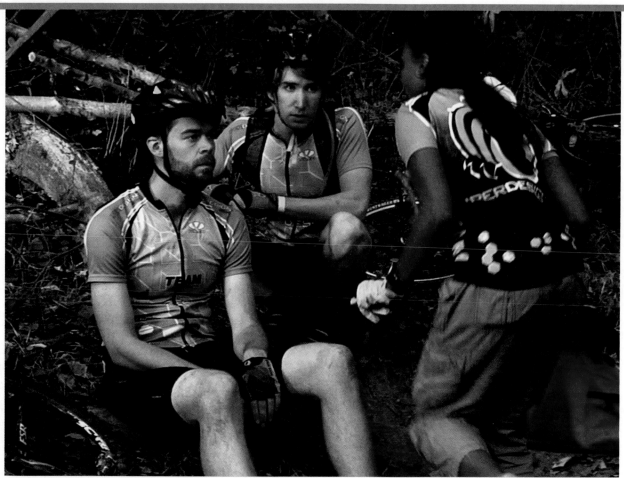

)))) YOU ARE THE EMERGENCY MEDICAL RESPONDER

A 20-year-old cyclist on a mountain bike team was temporarily unconscious after falling off his bike during practice. As the athletic trainer for the team, you respond to the incident. The injured cyclist is awake but complaining of dizziness and nausea. After assessing and taking a history and baseline vital signs, you tell the cyclist to go home and rest. Was this an appropriate response? Why or why not?

Key Terms

Abandonment: Ending the care of an injured or ill person without obtaining that patient's consent or without ensuring that someone with equal or greater training will continue care.

Advance directive: A written instruction, signed by the patient and a physician, which documents a patient's wishes if the patient is unable to communicate his or her wishes.

Applied ethics: The use of ethics in decision making; applying ethical values.

Assault: A crime that occurs when a person tries to physically harm another in a way that makes the person under attack feel immediately threatened.

Battery: A crime that occurs when there is unlawful touching of a person without the person's consent.

Competence: The patient's ability to understand the *emergency medical responder's* (EMR's) questions and the implications of decisions made.

Confidentiality: Protection of a patient's privacy by not revealing any personal patient information except to law enforcement personnel or *emergency medical services* (EMS) personnel caring for the patient.

Consent: Permission to provide care; given by an injured or ill person to a responder.

Do no harm: The principle that people who intervene to help others must do their best to ensure their actions will do no harm to the patient.

Do not resuscitate (DNR) order: A type of advance directive that protects a patient's right to refuse efforts for resuscitation; also known as a *do not attempt resuscitation* (DNAR) order.

Durable power of attorney for health care: A legal document that expresses a patient's specific wishes regarding his or her health care; also empowers an individual, usually a relative or friend, to speak on behalf of the patient should he or she become seriously injured or ill and unable to speak for him- or herself.

Duty to act: A legal responsibility of some individuals to provide a reasonable standard of emergency care.

Ethics: A branch of philosophy concerned with the set of moral principles a person holds about what is right and wrong.

Expressed consent: Permission to receive emergency care granted by a competent adult verbally, nonverbally or through gestures.

Good Samaritan laws: Laws that apply in some circumstances to protect people who provide emergency care without accepting anything in return.

Health care proxy: A person named in a health-care directive, or durable power of attorney for health care, who can make medical decisions on someone else's behalf.

Implied consent: Legal concepts that assume a patient would consent to receive emergency care if he or she were physically able or old enough to do so.

In good faith: Acting in such a way that the goal is only to help the patient and that all actions are for that purpose.

Legal obligation: Obligation to act in a particular way in accordance with the law.

Living will: A type of advance directive that outlines the patient's wishes about certain kinds of medical treatments and procedures that prolong life.

Malpractice: A situation in which a professional fails to provide a reasonable quality of care, resulting in harm to a patient.

Medical futility: A situation in which a patient has a medical or traumatic condition that is scientifically accepted to be futile should resuscitation be attempted and, therefore, the patient should be considered dead on arrival.

Moral obligation: Obligation to act in a particular way in accordance with what is considered morally right.

Morals: Principles relating to issues of right and wrong and how individual people should behave.

Negligence: The failure to provide the level of care a person of similar training would provide, thereby causing injury or damage to another.

Next of kin: The closest relatives, as defined by state law, of a deceased person; usually the spouse and nearest blood relatives.

Patient's best interest: A fundamental ethical principle that refers to the provision of competent care, with compassion and respect for human dignity.

Refusal of care: The declining of care by a competent patient; a patient has the right to refuse the care of anyone who responds to an emergency scene.

Standard of care: The criterion established for the extent and quality of an EMR's care.

Surrogate decision maker: A third party with the legal right to make decisions for another person regarding medical and health issues through a durable power of attorney for health care.

Learning Objectives

After reading this chapter, and completing the class activities, you will have the information needed to—

- Define the legal duties of an *emergency medical responder* (EMR), including scope of practice and the standard of care.
- Define and discuss the ethical responsibilities of an EMR.
- Describe the various forms of consent and explain the methods of obtaining consent.
- Explain the difference between expressed consent and implied consent.
- Have a basic understanding of Good Samaritan laws.
- Describe the ethical responsibilities of an EMR.
- Discuss the implications of and steps to follow if a patient refuses care.
- Discuss advance directives and explain their implications on emergency medical care.

- Explain other legal issues including assault and battery, abandonment and negligence.
- Explain the importance, necessity and legality of maintaining confidentiality about the condition, circumstances and care of the patient.
- Discuss the *Health Insurance Portability and Accountability Act* (HIPAA) Privacy Rule, including instances where disclosure of information is permitted.
- Describe the signs of obvious death.
- Understand the importance of and need for crime scene/evidence preservation.
- Understand the circumstances and general requirements of mandated reporting.

INTRODUCTION

Many emergency medical care providers are concerned about the possibility of a lawsuit resulting from their actions while providing emergency care. While there is nothing to stop a patient or a patient's family from filing a lawsuit against those who provide care at the scene of an emergency, there are often defenses and immunities that can be asserted. By becoming aware of some basic legal principles involved in providing emergency assistance, you may be able to reduce the chances of a successful lawsuit.

This chapter addresses, in general terms, some medical and legal principles and a few ethical responsibilities that relate to emergency care. Because laws vary from state to state, your instructor will need to inform you on the laws in your state that apply to you or tell you where you can find such information.

LEGAL DUTIES
Scope of Practice

The *emergency medical responder's* (EMR's) scope of practice is defined as the range of duties and skills an EMR is allowed and expected to perform as appropriate. The scope of practice also defines boundaries and distinctions within the health care system, ensuring that each level of provider operates within a legally accepted range of duties and skills. Scope of practice also draws a distinction between these professionals and the layperson.

The EMR, like other out-of-hospital care providers, is governed by legal, ethical and medical guidelines. Since practice may differ from state to state or in regions of the same state, you must be aware of variations existing for your level of training in your state or area. The term scope of practice also refers to the authority to practice, given by the state to individuals licensed to practice in that state.

Standard of Care

The public expects a certain **standard of care** from personnel summoned to provide emergency care. The standard of care is the criterion established for the extent and quality of EMR care.

When providing emergency care, EMRs are expected to perform to at least the minimum standard set forth by their training. State laws and other authorities, such as national organizations, may govern the actions of EMRs. If your actions do not meet the set standards, and harm another person, you may be successfully sued for **negligence** or **malpractice**.

Duty to Act

While on duty, an EMR has an obligation to respond to an emergency and provide care at the scene. This obligation is called a **duty to act (Fig. 3-1)**. It applies to public safety officers, certain government employees,

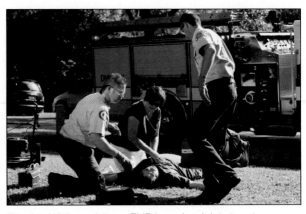

Fig. 3-1: While on duty, an EMR has a legal duty to act.

CRITICAL FACTS

The EMR's scope of practice is defined as the range of duties and skills an EMR is allowed and expected to perform as appropriate.

The public expects a certain standard of care from personnel summoned to provide emergency care. The standard of care is the criterion established for the extent and quality of EMR care.

While on duty, an EMR has an obligation to respond to an emergency and provide care at the scene. This obligation is called a duty to act.

licensed and certified professionals and medical paraprofessionals while on duty. For instance, members of a volunteer fire department have a duty to act based on participation in the fire department. An athletic trainer has a duty to provide care to an injured athlete. Failure to fulfill these duties could result in legal action.

As an EMR, if you see a motor-vehicle crash while driving to work, in most states, you have a **moral obligation**, as opposed to a **legal obligation**, to stop. However, once you have begun to provide care, you are legally obligated to continue until the patient is turned over to someone with an equal or a higher level of training.

Competence

Competence refers to the patient's ability to understand the EMR's questions and the implications of decisions made. EMRs must obtain permission from competent patients before beginning any care. To receive **consent** or **refusal of care**, the EMR should determine competence. In certain cases, such as those involving intoxication, drug abuse or cognitive impairment such as dementia or Alzheimer's disease, the patient is not considered competent. Some individuals, such as minors, are not competent to make decisions about their care as a matter of law. In such cases, call more advanced medical care and law enforcement personnel or send someone to call.

Good Samaritan Laws

EMRs who act in a reasonable and prudent way consistent with the standard of care should prevail if a negligence claim is asserted. Furthermore, **Good Samaritan laws** and other laws for EMRs may provide protection from negligence claims if the EMR acts **in good faith** and is not willful or reckless.

In addition, the vast majority of states and the District of Columbia have Good Samaritan laws that protect people against claims of negligence when they provide emergency care in good faith

without accepting anything in return. These laws, which differ from state to state, may apply when an EMR volunteers to assist in an emergency when not on duty. Although professional rescuers such as EMRs are not usually considered Good Samaritans when on the job, many states have other laws that protect EMRs from negligence claims arising out of job activities in some situations.

When a responder's actions are willful or reckless, however, these liability protections most likely will not apply.

Along with the lay public, Good Samaritan laws may protect off-duty EMRs who are providing emergency care in good faith. The laws do not protect individuals from acts deemed to have been grossly negligent or who provided care significantly below the standard of care.

Good Samaritan laws vary from state to state. For more information, check your local and state laws or consult with a legal professional to see if Good Samaritan laws protect you.

Ethical Responsibilities

As an EMR, you have an ethical obligation to carry out your duties and responsibilities in a professional manner. This includes showing compassion when dealing with a patient's physical and emotional needs, and communicating sensitively and willingly at all times. Try to avoid becoming satisfied with meeting minimum training requirements and instead strive to develop your professional skills to surpass the standards for your area. Doing so includes not only practicing and mastering the skills taught in this course but seeking out further training and information, such as through workshops, conferences and supplemental or advanced educational programs. Your instructor may be able to provide ideas and information about opportunities in your area for further education and professional development.

In addition to being the best you can be in providing care, be honest in reporting your actions and the events that occurred when you respond to an emergency. Make it a personal goal to be a person whom others trust and can

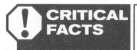 **CRITICAL FACTS** If a responder acts in a reasonable and prudent way consistent with the standard of care, a negligence claim against the responder will likely fail.

depend on to give accurate reports and provide effective care.

Address your responsibilities to the patient at every emergency. Periodically, carry out a self-review of your performance (e.g., patient care, communication, documentation) to help improve any areas of potential weakness or opportunities for professional growth.

Ethical responsibilities include the following concepts:

- **Morals:** Morals are a set of principles relating to issues of right and wrong and how individual people should behave. To understand the morals of a society, you have to know what that society believes.
- **Ethics:** Ethics is a branch of philosophy that deals with the set of moral principles a person holds about what is right and wrong.
- **Applied ethics:** The term "applied ethics" refers to the application of ethical values in decision making.

Decision-Making Models

A decision-making model is a tool or technique to assist you in making decisions. The term can also refer to a set of principles which, when applied, lead to the desired decision. Some of those principles include the following:

- **Do No Harm:** The phrase "do no harm" is attributed to Hippocrates and first appeared in his treatise, Of the Epidemics. The treatise states "Practice two things in your dealings with disease: either help or do not harm the patient." "Do no harm" has been brought into several trained and professional health care practices. In essence, it means that people who intervene to help others must do their best to ensure their actions will do no harm to the patient or patients. (For more information on the National Association of Emergency Medical Technicians' Code of Ethics, see *www. naemt.org/aboutNAEMT/EMTCodeOfEthics.htm*).
- **Act in Good Faith:** To act in good faith means to act in such a way that the goal is only

to help the patient and that all actions are for that purpose.
- **Patient's Best Interest:** To act in the patient's best interest is a fundamental ethical principle that refers to providing competent care with compassion and respect for human dignity. This implies that the care one provides serves the integrity of the patient's physical well-being while at the same time respecting the patient's choices and self-determination.

PATIENT CONSENT AND REFUSAL OF CARE

Individuals have a basic right to decide what can and cannot be done to their bodies; they have the legal right to accept or refuse care. Therefore, to provide care to an injured or ill person, you must first obtain the patient's consent. Usually, the patient needs to tell you clearly that you have permission to provide care.

To obtain consent, you must—
- Identify yourself to the patient.
- Give your level of training.
- Ask the patient whether you may help.
- Explain what you observe.
- Explain what you plan to do.

Forms of Consent

Consent may be either directly expressed or implied. There are also some special situations in which exceptions or alternate means of providing consent may apply.

Expressed Consent

After you have provided the required information, the patient can give **expressed consent** either verbally or through a gesture. If the patient is a minor, the law requires that an EMR obtain consent from a parent or guardian, if one is available. The patient has the right to withdraw consent for care at any time. If this should occur, step back and call for more advanced medical personnel. In some

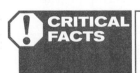
CRITICAL FACTS

Ethical responsibilities include morals, ethics and applied ethics.

Individuals have the legal right to refuse or accept care. To obtain consent, you must identify yourself, give your level of training, ask the patient whether you may help, explain what you observe and what you plan to do.

circumstances, you may be asked to explain why the person needs your care.

To give expressed consent, a patient must be competent. This means the patient must be able to understand the EMR's questions as well as the implications of accepting or refusing any care that the EMR has proposed. The EMR should ensure that the patient understands the condition and both the risks and benefits of the proposed treatment.

Implied Consent

Certain patients may not be able to give expressed consent. This includes patients who are unconscious, confused, mentally impaired, seriously injured or seriously ill. In these cases, the law assumes that the patient would give informed consent for care if he or she were able to do so. This legal concept is called **implied consent**.

Implied Consent and Minors

Remember, when the patient is a minor, an EMR is required by law to obtain permission to provide care from a parent or guardian, if one is available. However, if the condition is life threatening and a parent or guardian is not present, consent is implied. A minor is usually considered anyone under the age of 18, but this varies by state.

If you encounter a parent who refuses to allow you to provide care, try to explain the consequences of not caring for the patient. Use terms the parent or guardian will understand. If a law enforcement officer is not present, send someone to call or find one. If necessary, do so yourself. Do not argue with the parent or guardian. Doing so can create a potentially unsafe situation.

Emancipated minors are minors who have been granted the legal rights to make their own decisions, such as consent for emergency or medical care. Examples include a minor who is married, pregnant, a parent, a member of the armed forces or financially independent and living away from home.

Special Situations

In certain cases, such as those involving intoxication and drug abuse, patients may not be considered competent and therefore are unable to make rational decisions or give expressed consent. In such cases, call more advanced medical care and law enforcement personnel or send someone to call. If possible, attempt to provide care, but do not endanger your personal safety. Always maintain a safe distance from potentially violent or hostile patients.

If a patient appears to be mentally incompetent, the EMR should verify if there is a guardian present with the legal right to consent to treatment. A mentally incompetent patient who is seriously injured or ill falls under implied consent when a parent or guardian is not present.

If an adult is legally incompetent—that is, determined by a court to be unable to handle personal or financial affairs, and under a legal guardian's care—you must also get that guardian's consent to provide care. Summon a law enforcement officer if necessary.

Refusal of Care

Some injured or ill people may refuse care, even those who may desperately need it. Even though patients may be seriously injured or ill, you should honor their refusal of care. Patients with decision-making capacity who are of legal age have a right to refuse care. If this occurs, you must ensure that the person is competent and is able to make rational, informed decisions.

Refusal of care does not have to be all or nothing. Patients can agree to receive part of the care that an EMR has suggested, but refuse another part. For example, a patient could choose to be assessed at the scene but refuse transport to the hospital, or agree to be transported to the hospital but not to be treated at the scene.

If a patient refuses care, be sure to—

- Follow local policies related to refusal of care.
- Tell the patient what treatment is needed and why. Explain the benefits of receiving treatment as well as the risks of refusing treatment, and mention any reasonable alternative treatments that fall within the parameters of care.
- Try again to convince the patient that the care is needed or that the patient should consider going to the hospital instead, but do not argue. If possible, have a witness listen to and document the refusal, to make it clear that you did not abandon the patient.
- Remind injured or ill persons that they can call *emergency medical services* (EMS) personnel again if the situation changes or if they change their mind and decide to accept care before you leave the scene.

- Notify local EMS personnel about the situation.
- Notify medical direction, if required by your local protocols.

- Document the patient's refusal, according to local policy. If the patient continues to refuse care, document any assessment you performed and have the patient sign the

Lake-Sumter Emergency Medical Services
INFORMED REFUSAL RELEASE FORM
FORMA INFORMADA DEL LANZAMIENTO DE LA DENEGACIÓN

Date (Fecha): _____   **RUN #:** _____

Name (Nombre): _____   **Street Address** (Direccion de Calle): _____

City (Ciudad): _____   **State** (Estado): _____   **Zip:** _____   **Age** (Edad): _____   **Sex** (Sexo):   M   F

Phone # (Numero de Telefono):   (   ) _____   **Date of Birth** (Fecha de Nacimiento): _____

Refusal of Care (Negación del cuidado)

I (the patient or patient's guardian) have been informed of:
Yo (el paciente o guardian del paciente) he estado informado de:

☒ **The reason I (the patient) should go to a hospital for further medical care; and**
La razon qua yo (el paciente) debo de ir al hospital para mas tratamiento; y

☒ **The evaluation and/or treatment that will/may occur when I (the patient) arrive(s) at the hospital; and**
De la evaluacion y/o tratamiento que va/o puede ocurrir quando yo (el paciente) llegue al hospital; y

☒ **The potential consequences and/or complications that may result in my (or patient guardian's) refusal to go to the hospital for further emergency care; and**
De las consecuencias potenciales y/o complicaciones qua pueden resultar de mi (o guardian del paciente) rechazamiento de ir al hospital para tratamiento de emergencia; y

As a competent adult, I understand the above and I am responsible for making a rational decision on my (the patient's) behalf, and have been advised that emergency medical care is necessary, and that refusal of recommended care and transport to a hospital may result in death or imperil my (the patient's) health by increasing the opportunity for morbidity. Understanding the above, I (patient guardian) refuse to accept emergency medical care and/or transport to a hospital facility, assume all risks and consequences resulting from my (patient guardian's) decision, and release Lake-Sumter EMS from any and all liability resulting from my (patient guardian's) refusal. The patient(s) was/were advised that Lake-Sumter EMS stands ready to return at any time and can be reached by dialing 911.

Como un adulto competente, yo comprendo antedicho y estoy capaz de hacer una decision racional en mi (el paciente) enteres, y estoy avisado que el tratamiento de emergencia as necesario, y que mi rachazamlento para cuidame y transportaclon al hospital puede resultar en muerte o poner an pellgro mi (el paciente) salud para aumentar la oportunidad de morbosidad. Comprendiendo lo antedicho, yo (guardian del paciente) me niego a aceptar tratamiento de emergencia o transporte al hospital, asumi todos los peligros y consecuencias que resultan de mi (guardian del paciente) decision, y suelto a Lake-Sumter EMS de algunas y todas obligaciones resultando de mi (guardian del paciente) rechazamiento. El paciente eralfue avisado que Lake-Sumter EMS esta listo para volver al cualquier hora y puede alcanzarlos marcando 911.

Notice of Privacy Practices(Aviso de las prácticas de la aislamiento)

I hereby acknowledge that I have received a copy of the LSEMS Notice of Privacy Practices as required by Federal Law.
Reconozco por este medio que he recibido una copia del aviso de LSEMS de las prácticas de la aislamiento según los requisitos de ley federal.

Patient Initials(Iniciales):_____(required)

A copy of the LSEMS Notice of Privacy Practices was given to: ☐ Patient   ☐ Authorized Representative

Patient Signature
(Firma del Paciente):   **X** _____   Date(Fecha):_____

Print Name (Imprenta su Nombre): _____

Print Patient(s) under care of Guardian(Imprenta el paciente que esta al cuidado del guardian)

Name (Nombre): _____   **Age** (Edad): _____   **Name** (Nombre): _____   **Age** (Edad): _____

Name (Nombre): _____   **Age** (Edad): _____   **Name** (Nombre): _____   **Age** (Edad): _____

Signature of Guardian (Firma del Guardian):   **X** _____

Print Guardian's Name (Imprenta el nombre del guardian del paciente): _____

WITNESS
(TESTIFICAR)

Signature (Firma): _____   **Print Name** (Imprenta Nombre): _____   ID: _____

Signature (Firma): _____   **Print Name** (Imprenta Nombre): _____   ID: _____

Effective: June 2003

Fig. 3-2: Refusal of care form. *Courtesy of Lake-Sumter EMS.*

refusal documentation (**Fig. 3-2**). If the patient refuses to sign the form, have a family member, police officer or bystander sign the form, verifying the patient refused to sign. Also, have a family member, police officer or bystander sign the form as a witness. A law enforcement officer is preferable, if available.

- Try one more time to persuade the patient to go to a hospital before leaving the scene.

Advance Directives

An **advance directive** is a set of written instructions that describes a person's wishes about medical care. These instructions, signed by the patient and a physician, make a person's intentions known while he or she is still capable of doing so and are used when the patient can no longer make his or her own health care decisions.

Do Not Resuscitate Orders and Medical Futility

One type of advance directive, a ***Do Not Resuscitate* (DNR) order**, also called a *Do Not Attempt Resuscitation* (DNAR) order, protects a patient's right to refuse efforts for resuscitation (**Fig. 3-3**). These orders are usually written for people who have a terminal illness. They differ from state to state. You must be aware of your state and local legislation and protocols relative to these orders. Your state EMS office is a good source of this information.

There must be written proof of a DNR order unless your state is one of the few that accepts verbal verification. If there is no proof of a DNR order, you must act and provide care as you would in any similar situation where a DNR order does not exist. The exception to this is in cases of **medical futility** or obvious death.

The term medical futility is used to describe situations where emergency medical interventions, such as CPR, would not provide any likely benefit to the patient. Be familiar with and follow local protocols and medical control for these situations. If there is any doubt as to whether medical futility exists, treatment should be provided.

Living Wills

A **living will**, another kind of advance directive, is a legal document that outlines a patient's wishes about certain kinds of medical treatments and procedures that prolong life. In the event that the patient cannot communicate health care decisions, this document takes effect.

As an EMR, you must assess the validity of a living will before agreeing to its terms. If in doubt, you must provide care until the matter has been clarified. More general than a DNR order, which refers only to the act of resuscitation, living wills can go further into dictating what may and may not be done to a patient.

When assessing an advance directive, check for written doctor's instructions that most often accompany the directive. The phrasing must be clear and understandable, with no room for interpretation. It is vital that you review your particular state's laws to see if advance directives and/or living wills are permitted in your area of practice. Also, clarify whether they require more than one health care provider to verify the patient's condition, which is the case in some states.

Surrogate Decision Making

A **surrogate decision maker** is a third party who has been given the legal right to make decisions regarding medical and health issues on another person's behalf through a **durable power of attorney for health care**. A person

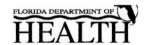

FLORIDA DEPARTMENT OF

HEALTH

State of Florida
DO NOT RESUSCITATE ORDER

(please use ink)

Patient's Full Legal Name: _____Date:_____

(Print or Type Name)

PATIENT'S STATEMENT

Based upon informed consent, I, the undersigned, hereby direct that CPR be withheld or withdrawn.
(If not signed by patient, check applicable box):

❏ Surrogate   ❏ Proxy (both as defined in Chapter 765, F.S.)
❏ Court appointed guardian   ❏ Durable power of attorney (pursuant to Chapter 709, F.S.)

_____   _____
(Applicable Signature)   (Print or Type Name)

PHYSICIAN'S STATEMENT

I, the undersigned, a physician licensed pursuant to Chapter 458 or 459, F.S., am the physician of the patient named above. I hereby direct the withholding or withdrawing of cardiopulmonary resuscitation (artificial ventilation, cardiac compression, endotracheal intubation and defibrillation) from the patient in the event of the patient's cardiac or respiratory arrest.

_____   _____   _____
(Signature of Physician)   (Date)   Telephone Number (Emergency)

_____   _____
(Print or Type Name)   (Physician's Medical License Number)

Fig. 3-3: DNRs are usually written for people with a terminal illness. *Courtesy of Lake-Sumter EMS.*

What Is a Do Not Resuscitate Order?

DNR orders are intended to direct the care of a patient in the specific setting of either respiratory or cardiac arrest. DNR orders are very specific orders that express a patient's denial of consent for specific interventions limited to CPR for either respiratory or cardiac arrest. As such, they only apply to the following specific interventions in the setting of respiratory or cardiac arrest:

- Airway—positioning, adjuncts and intubations
- Breathing—assisted ventilations
- Circulation—cardiac compressions, defibrillation and cardiac arrest medications

Up to the point of either respiratory or cardiac arrest, the DNR order would not apply and rescuers should provide the normal care for any conditions that they identify.

In most states, a DNR order is a physician's order not to resuscitate if a patient goes into cardiac or pulmonary (respiratory) arrest. It is part of the prescribed medical treatment plan and must have a physician's signature. Issues surrounding DNR orders are complex, and the laws and regulations regarding them vary from state to state. For these reasons, the American Red Cross advises all professional and certified lay rescuers to receive specific training from their employer, agency or medical director. In addition, rescuers are encouraged to check local laws and regulations. However, there are some general principles that all rescuers should be aware of, and can use to guide their practice.

End-of-life care legislation is in place across the country, and serves as a mechanism to address two equally valid, competing interests. Specifically, it allows patients to be involved in their own health care decision making and it protects health care personnel from liability for honoring patients' wishes. Ethical principles require that rescuers respect a person's right to make decisions regarding his or her own health care. This usually involves obtaining the patient's consent. However, sometimes a patient is either unconscious or otherwise incapacitated. In these cases, advance directives, such as health care proxies, living wills and DNR orders, provide mechanisms by which individuals can make their wishes known when they are unable to speak for themselves. In addition, advance directives allow those responsible for the care of others—such as a minor or an adult lacking the capacity for decisions—to make end-of-life decisions prior to the time when the decision is necessary. Of course, in the absence of an applicable advance directive, consent for emergency treatment is implied.

How Do You Know If There Is a DNR Order?

In most cases, the family, a caretaker or health care provider will inform you that a DNR order is in place.

A DNR order is written on a form developed, in most states, by the individual state's Department of Health or state EMS office to identify patients who do not wish to be resuscitated in the event of respiratory or cardiac arrest. In the case of in-patient admissions at hospitals and long-term care facilities, the DNR order may be on a form that complies with state laws and regulations but has been designed by the facility. In some states there are both hospital and in-patient forms. The properly completed form is signed by the competent patient or by the patient's representative, and then signed by a licensed physician on a specific form developed and approved by the respective state.

Unless provided with written documentation or unless your state laws and regulations allow acceptance of oral verification (which most states' laws do not), you must perform all procedures as you would in the absence of a DNR order.

In some states, there is a patient ID device in the form of a bracelet or a smaller version of the form that can be worn on a chain around the neck or clipped to a key chain or to clothing/bed so it can travel with the patient. It is equally as valid as a traditional DNR form and can be presented to EMS personnel when they arrive on scene; it is designed to allow the patient to move between settings with one document.

Can a DNR Order Be Revoked?

Review of individual state laws for specific criteria is necessary. Generally, the DNR order can be revoked at any time orally or in writing, by physical destruction, by failure to present it or by the oral expression of a contrary intent by the patient or the patient's health care proxy. In the out-of-hospital setting, it may be

(continued)

What Is a Do Not Resuscitate Order? *(continued)*

difficult to determine who the actual surrogate is and, likely, the question has arisen because the patient is in cardiac or respiratory arrest and cannot express his or her own wishes. If there is any doubt regarding revocation of the DNR order or someone verbally requests revocation, begin normal care procedures.

In What Health Care Settings Is the DNR Order Honored?

The DNR order is honored in most health care settings, including hospices, adult family care homes, assisted living facilities, emergency departments, nursing homes, home health agencies and in hospitals. State laws further provide that health care providers employed in these health care settings may withhold or withdraw CPR if presented with a DNR order and be immune from criminal prosecution or civil liability. In addition, most state laws and regulations allow DNR orders to be honored by prehospital providers. In those instances where the DNR order is presented to a prehospital emergency medical provider in a setting other than a health care facility, the form may be honored.

Review of individual state and local laws as well as local protocols is essential for compliance. Direct questions regarding DNR orders to the state regulating agency or state EMS office.

In the out-of-hospital setting, if there is any doubt as to whether a DNR order is valid or may have been revoked, care should proceed as it would in the absence of a DNR order; this includes activation of the EMS system and transport to a hospital. Usually, the hospital is better equipped and has additional resources to determine the validity and applicability of a DNR order then the resources that are available in the out-of-hospital setting.

Professional and workplace providers should receive specific training from their employer, agency or medical director regarding DNR orders.

Do EMRs Fail to Provide the Standard of Care If They Follow a DNR Order?

A professional rescuer who follows a DNR order is actually complying with the standard of care by respecting the patient's wishes, respecting the patient's denial of consent for CPR in the setting of either respiratory or cardiac arrest and complying with the physician's order for DNR. Follow local protocols and medical direction when presented with a DNR order.

Source: American Red Cross Advisory Council on First Aid, Safety, Aquatics and Preparedness—DNR answers, approved May 4, 2007

---

may be given this role for an elderly parent, an incapacitated spouse or an ill child, for example. You must be able to see the legal document, and the writing should be understandable, leaving no room for interpretation.

A **health care proxy** is the person named in a durable power of attorney for health care to make medical decisions on the patient's behalf. This person may also be known as an attorney-in-fact, an agent or a patient advocate. The health care proxy may be a friend, family member or other person designated at an earlier time by the patient or by the courts to be responsible for making health and medical decisions for the patient.

Next of kin refers to the closest relatives, as defined by state law, of a patient or deceased person. Most states recognize the spouse and the nearest blood relatives as next of kin, and these individuals may have certain legal authority regarding medical decisions for an incapacitated patient or the affairs of a deceased person.

OTHER LEGAL ISSUES
Assault

Assault is a threat or an attempt to inflict harm on someone. Assault can be physical, sexual or both. It may result in injury, and often results in emotional distress to the patient. If the patient feels threatened with bodily harm and the other person has the capability of inflicting harm, the act is considered assault.

Battery

Battery is the legal term used to describe the unlawful touching of a person without that person's consent. The EMR must obtain consent before providing care to a patient. Every patient has a legal right to determine what happens to and who touches that patient's body. If you try to provide care or check a pulse on a patient who has refused your care, you could be charged with battery. You must obtain consent, through the steps outlined earlier in this chapter, before even touching the patient.

Abandonment

Just as you must obtain the patient's consent before beginning care, you must also continue to provide care once you have begun. Once you have started emergency care, you are legally obligated to continue that care until a person with equal or higher training relieves you, you are physically unable to continue or the patient refuses care (**Fig 3-4**). Usually, your obligation for care ends when more advanced medical professionals take over. If you stop your care before that point without a valid reason, such as leaving momentarily to get the proper equipment, you could be legally responsible for the **abandonment** of a patient in need.

Negligence

Negligence refers to a failure to follow a reasonable standard of care, thereby causing or contributing to injury or damage to another. A person could be considered negligent by either acting wrongly or failing to act at all. For a lawsuit charging negligence to be successful, all four of the following must be proven:

1. The EMR had a duty to act. When an EMR is on duty, the duty to act is the obligation to respond to emergency calls and provide emergency care according to the expected level of knowledge and skills. Once care has begun, the duty is to continue providing care until the patient can be handed over to someone of equal or higher training.
2. The EMR breached that duty. Breach of duty refers to deviation from the standards of care expected for the rescuer's level of knowledge and skill. This can result in either simple negligence, which is what occurs when an error is made because of a deviation from standards, or gross negligence, which occurs if care is provided in such a manner that it can be considered dangerous or harmful to the patient.
3. The patient was injured because the EMR breached his or her duty. In legal terms, this is known as proximate cause. If injuries occurred to a patient due to breach of duty or negligence by the EMR, the patient must prove that these injuries were the direct result of the EMR's action or nonaction.
4. Harm or injury occurred. Harm to a patient is the end result of the actions of the EMR, either in pain or disability, physical or psychological.

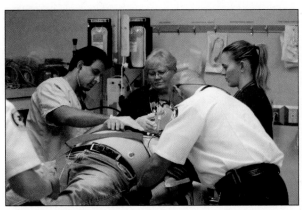

Fig. 3-4: Once you have started emergency care, you are legally obligated to continue that care until a person with equal or higher training relieves you, you are physically unable to continue or the patient refuses care.

CONFIDENTIALITY AND PRIVACY

While providing care to a patient, you may learn details about the patient that are private and confidential. Information such as medical issues, physical and mental conditions and any medications the patient is taking are personal to the patient and considered confidential. Respect the patient's privacy and obey the law by maintaining **confidentiality**. Exceptions to this rule include providing this information to the medical personnel who will take over care of the patient from you and any mandatory reporting requirements, public health issues or legal requirements.

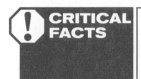

CRITICAL FACTS Personal information, such as the patient's medical issues, physical and mental conditions and medications they take, is considered confidential. Confidentiality can be broken only in cases where you must provide this information to medical personnel who will take over care, for mandatory reporting or in certain legal circumstances.

Health Insurance Portability and Accountability Act

Description

The *Health Insurance Portability and Accountability Act* (HIPAA) Privacy Rule is the first comprehensive federal protection for the privacy of *protected health information* (PHI). It makes provisions for aspects such as patient control over health information, the use and release of health records, appropriate disclosure of health information, and civil and criminal penalties for violation of patients' privacy rights.

Protected Health Information

Because of these privacy stipulations, you cannot relay any identifying information about the patient to anyone without the patient's specific consent. This includes media, employers, colleagues, friends and even other family members. Once your role with the patient has finished, you cannot speak of the patient with anyone else, including your co-workers, in a way that could somehow reveal the patient's identity. However, you may release information if you have written consent from the patient or the patient's parent or guardian. In the case of guardianship, you must have proof that the person is the child's or mentally incapacitated person's guardian before accepting consent.

The confidentiality of information refers not only to identity, but also to any medical issue or treatments that involved the patient, including primary assessments, physical or mental conditions as determined by your assessment, any treatment you provide and any medical history the patient discloses to you. The information should be written but may be given verbally by the patient or patient's guardian, though it is always better to get this information in writing.

Permitted Disclosures of PHI Without Written Patient Consent

By law, there are some circumstances when disclosure of PHI is permitted without patient consent. For example, when a patient is provided with emergency care and transported to a hospital or medical center, there are situations where information must be disclosed for payment for services. This information must be relayed to billing departments for the emergency services and the receiving institution. Insurance companies also require a certain amount of information. The information provided should be limited to what is required by law only.

Other situations where disclosure without consent is permissible include cases of mandatory reporting, situations involving public health issues and some law enforcement situations. For example, you must provide requested information if you have been legally summoned via a court-ordered subpoena.

There are other special situations where disclosure without permission is possible, including the following:

- PHI can be disclosed for purposes of research without authorization, under certain conditions.
- PHI may be disclosed to report abuse, neglect or domestic violence under specified circumstances.
- A covered entity may disclose PHI in the course of a judicial or an administrative proceeding under specified circumstances.
- Organ-procurement agencies may use PHI for the purposes of facilitating a transplant.
- Covered entities usually may disclose PHI to a health oversight agency for oversight activities authorized by law.
- The Privacy Rule permits disclosure of work-related health information as authorized by, and to the extent necessary to comply with, workers' compensation programs.

A valid authorization is required for any use or disclosure of PHI that is not required or otherwise permitted without authorization by the Privacy Rule.

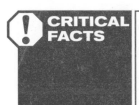
SPECIAL SITUATIONS

Medical Identification

Medical *identification* (ID) tags are designed to provide health care providers and EMS personnel with pertinent health information about a patient who may be unable to communicate in an emergency (**Fig. 3-5**). The tag may be included on a bracelet or necklace. Others may carry this information on a wallet card. These identifiers indicate special medical situations pertinent to a medical emergency. It is imperative that you look for them whenever you examine a patient. Examples of conditions you may be alerted to include allergies, diabetes and epilepsy. Some medical IDs may list a phone number to call to obtain further information.

Obvious Death

Although it is ultimately a physician's job to declare a patient dead, you will often be faced with situations in which death is obvious. In

these situations, resuscitative efforts may not be required. These situations include—

- Decapitation.
- Rigor mortis.
- Decomposition of the body.
- *Dependent lividity* (discoloration in the skin caused by the pooling of blood).

Organ Donors

Organs may only be donated when there is a signed, legal document that gives permission for the patient's organs to be harvested in the case of death (**Fig. 3-6**). Often this documentation is an organ donor card or a sticker on the patient's driver's license. Treat these patients as you would any other patient and provide the same lifesaving emergency care.

Evidence Preservation

Emergency medical care of the patient is the EMR's top priority. However, when faced with a crime scene, there are some precautions you must take to ensure the integrity of the scene is not disturbed. Do not disturb any item at the scene unless emergency medical care requires it. Observe and document

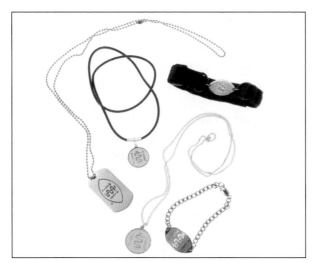

Fig. 3-5: Medical ID tags can be found on bracelets, necklaces and wallets. You must look for them whenever you examine a patient. *Courtesy of the Canadian Red Cross.*

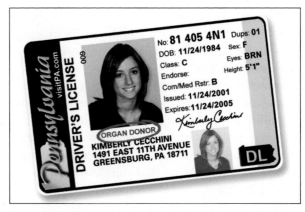

Fig. 3-6: Documentation about organ donation is often found on a patient's driver's license. *Courtesy of Donate Life Pennsylvania.*

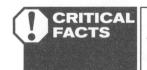

Mandated reporting must be done in cases of abuse and violence, but can also apply to certain infectious diseases, such as hepatitis B or HIV/AIDS. Know your state's requirements to ensure that you do not incur legal liability for failure to report or unauthorized disclosure.

anything unusual at the scene. Do not cut through bullet or knife holes in clothing, as they are part of the evidence collected during the investigation. Work closely with appropriate law enforcement authorities and obtain permission to do anything that may interfere with the investigation, including using the phone at the emergency scene.

Special Reporting Requirements

Mandated reporting usually refers to the practice of reporting situations in which a patient's injuries may have been caused through battery, abuse or other forms of violence. The requirements for reporting vary from state to state, and it is the EMR's responsibility to learn and follow specific state requirements for reporting incidents in which abuse is suspected.

Abuse or neglect of any kind must be reported in accordance with state requirements; this applies to children, the elderly and patients in domestic violence situations. Injuries that may be the result of a crime, such as gunshot and stab wounds, as well as poisoning or drug-related injuries, must also be reported. In some states, you also must report suspected sexual assaults.

Mandatory reporting can also apply to some infectious diseases such as tuberculosis, hepatitis B, HIV and AIDS.

Knowing the details of mandatory reporting is necessary to ensure that you do not incur legal liability for failure to report or unauthorized disclosure. You are responsible for fully documenting an objective report of your findings when you deem it necessary. However, most states will offer immunity for any potential liability that may result from reporting, such as slander or defamation of character. The most important things to remember are that you should act in good faith, report only what you know to be factual and avoid any speculation as to what you believe may have occurred or reporting how you feel.

PUTTING IT ALL TOGETHER

In your role as an EMR, you are guided by certain legal parameters, such as the duty to act and professional standards of care. Injured or ill persons have a right to expect competent initial care by an EMR. They also have a right to expect that you have a thorough understanding of the ethical and legal issues involved.

As a trained EMR, you have minimum standards for your performance, but it is important that you do not let your training stay at that minimum level. Practice your skills and increase your knowledge, taking the opportunity to learn as much as you can within your scope of practice. Most areas require that EMRs participate in a minimum number of continuing education or refresher courses to remain certified.

As an EMR, you are best protected legally by continually examining your role and skill level. By maintaining the legal requirements of explaining all actions, receiving consent before performing any procedure and carrying out those procedures to the best of your ability within your scope of practice, you will minimize the chances of a successful lawsuit against you.

You must be aware of the types of exceptional circumstances you may encounter, such as refusal of care and providing care for patients who may not be competent. By following the procedures set out by your state or region and by taking thorough notes of the events, with witnesses if possible, you should minimize the chances of a successful lawsuit.

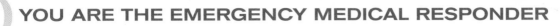

YOU ARE THE EMERGENCY MEDICAL RESPONDER

You advised the cyclist to go home and rest. At home, the cyclist loses consciousness and his roommate calls for an ambulance. Later, at the hospital, he is diagnosed as having a severe head injury that could have been minimized if medical care had been provided earlier. Do you believe there are any grounds for legal action against you? Why or why not?

4

The Human Body

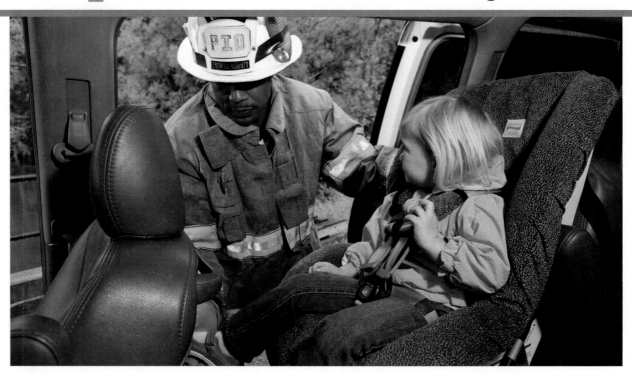

)))) YOU ARE THE EMERGENCY MEDICAL RESPONDER

Your fire rescue unit responds to the scene of a motor-vehicle collision involving a car with two people and a minivan driven by a woman who has two small children in car seats. As you size-up the scene, three people appear to be injured. The first person, a woman who was driving one of the vehicles, is going in and out of consciousness. You suspect her injuries may include possible fractured ribs. The second person, a passenger in the same vehicle, has injuries on the right side of his body. The third person, the driver of the minivan, appears to have chest and abdominal injuries, but she is conscious and you can speak with her. She is distraught because her children are in the back of the minivan and she is concerned about them. What would you do? How would you respond? How would you describe the injuries and the body systems involved to more advanced medical personnel?

Key Terms

Anatomy: The study of structures, including gross anatomy (structures that can be seen with the naked eye) and microscopic anatomy (structures seen under the microscope).

Body system: A group of organs and other structures that works together to carry out specific functions.

Cells: The basic units that combine to form all living tissue.

Circulatory system: A group of organs and other structures that carries oxygen-rich blood and other nutrients throughout the body and removes waste.

Digestive system: A group of organs and other structures that digests food and eliminates wastes.

Endocrine system: A group of organs and other structures that regulates and coordinates the activities of other systems by producing chemicals (*hormones*) that influence tissue activity.

Genitourinary system: A group of organs and other structures that eliminates waste and enables reproduction.

Integumentary system: A group of organs and other structures that protects the body, retains fluids and helps to prevent infection.

Musculoskeletal system: A group of tissues and other structures that supports the body, protects internal organs, allows movement, stores minerals, manufactures blood cells and creates heat.

Nervous system: A group of organs and other structures that regulates all body functions.

Organ: A structure of similar tissues acting together to perform specific body functions.

Physiology: How living organisms function (e.g., movement and reproduction).

Respiratory system: A group of organs and other structures that brings air into the body and removes wastes through a process called breathing, or respiration.

Tissue: A collection of similar cells acting together to perform specific body functions.

Vital organs: Those organs whose functions are essential to life, including the brain, heart and lungs.

Learning Objectives

After reading this chapter, and completing the class activities, you will have the information needed to—

- Identify various anatomical terms commonly used to refer to the body.
- Describe various body positions.
- Describe the major body cavities.
- Understand the basics of medical terminology and their application to emergency medical care.
- Identify and describe the fundamental anatomy and physiology of the major body systems.
- Give examples of how body systems interrelate.
- Describe the anatomical and physiological differences of children and infants and the resulting considerations for emergency care.

INTRODUCTION

As an *emergency medical responder* (EMR), you require a basic understanding of normal human structure and function. Knowing what the body's structures are and how they work will help you more easily recognize and understand injuries and illnesses. **Body systems** do not function independently. Each system depends on other systems to function properly. When your body is healthy, your body systems work well together. But an injury or illness in one body part or system will often cause problems in others. Knowing the location and function of the major **organs** and structures within each body system will help you to more accurately assess a patient's condition and provide the best care.

To remember the location of body structures, it is important to visualize the structures that lie beneath the skin. The structures you can see or feel are reference points for locating the internal structures you cannot see or feel. For example, to locate the pulse on either side of the neck, you can use the middle of the throat as a reference point. Using reference points will help you describe the location of injuries and other conditions you may find. This chapter provides you with an overview of important reference points, terminology and the functions of eight of the body systems. It also focuses on body structure (**anatomy**) and body function (**physiology**).

MEDICAL TERMINOLOGY

In order to have a common language with which health care providers can accurately communicate about patients, it is important to have a basic understanding of medical terminology. One of the key elements to understanding medical terminology is to break down the terms into their parts.

Medical terms often are constructed using a combining form (root word plus a combining vowel) that contains the meaning, plus a suffix (word ending) that has its own meaning and/or a prefix (word beginning).

Table 4-1:
Common Combining Forms

COMBINING FORM	WHAT DOES IT MEAN?
Cardi/o-	Heart, cardiac
Neur/o-	Nerve, neural
Oro-	Mouth
Arteri/o-	Artery, arterial
Hem/o-	Blood
Therm/o-	Heat
Vas/o-	Duct, vessel, vascular

For example, the medical term "endotracheal" is made up of the combining form "trache," which means trachea; the prefix "endo," which means within; and the suffix "al," which means pertaining to. By understanding the parts of the word, we understand the term endotracheal to mean "pertaining to something within the trachea." This term might be used with the word "tube," to describe a type of tube used within the trachea.

The easiest way to learn medical combining forms (**Table 4-1**), their prefixes and their suffixes is to memorize them. A few of the more common prefixes are: hypo- (below normal), hyper- (above normal), a- (without, no), tachy- (fast) and brady- (slow) (**Table 4-2**). A few of the more common suffixes are: -emic (pertaining to the blood), -emia (condition of the blood) and -a or -ia (condition).

ANATOMICAL TERMS
Directions and Locations

By knowing a few key locations of structures and how to describe them, you can more accurately recognize a serious injury or illness and communicate with other *emergency medical services*

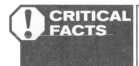 **CRITICAL FACTS**

Medical terms are often constructed from a root word and combining vowel, plus a suffix and/or a prefix. The easiest way to learn these medical combining forms, suffixes and prefixes is to memorize them.

Table 4-2:

Common Prefixes

COMBINING FORM	WHAT DOES IT MEAN?
Hyper-	Excessive, above, over, beyond
Hypo-	Less than normal, under
Tachy-	Fast, swift, rapid, accelerated
Brady-	Slow, dull

(EMS) personnel about a patient's condition **(Fig. 4-1, A–B)**.

- Anterior/posterior: Any part toward the front of the body is *anterior;* any part toward the back is *posterior.*

- Superior/inferior: *Superior* describes any part toward the patient's head; *inferior* describes any part toward the patient's feet.
- Frontal or coronal plane: That which divides the body vertically into two planes, anterior (the patient's front) and posterior (the patient's back).
- Sagittal or lateral plane: That which divides the body vertically into right and left planes.
- Transverse or axial plane: That which divides the body horizontally, into the superior (above the waist) and inferior (below the waist) planes.
- Medial/lateral: The terms *medial* and *lateral* refer to the midline, an imaginary line running down the middle of the body from the head to the ground and creating right and left halves. Any part toward the midline is medial; any part away from the midline is lateral.
- Proximal/distal: *Proximal* refers to any part close to the trunk (chest, abdomen and pelvis); *distal* refers to any part away from

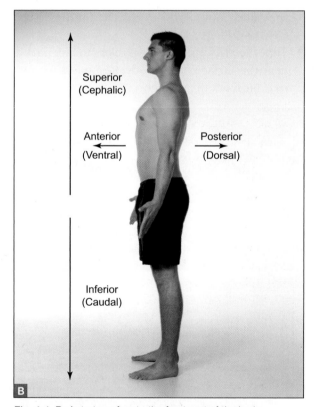

Fig. 4-1, A: Any part of the body toward the midline is medial; any part away from the midline is lateral. Any part close to the trunk is proximal; any part away from the trunk is distal. *Courtesy of the Canadian Red Cross.*

Fig. 4-1, B: Anterior refers to the front part of the body; posterior refers to the back of the body. Superior refers to anything toward the head; inferior refers to anything toward the feet. *Courtesy of the Canadian Red Cross.*

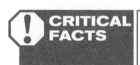

CRITICAL FACTS Knowing locations of anatomical structures and how to describe them will help you recognize a serious injury or illness and help you better communicate with other EMS personnel.

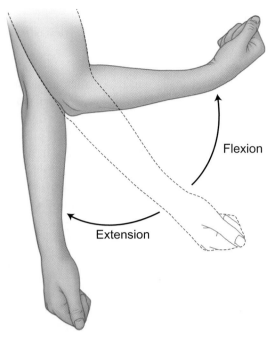

Fig. 4-2: Flexion and extension

the trunk and nearer to the extremities (arms and legs).

- Superficial/deep: *Superficial* refers to any part near the surface of the body; *deep* refers to any part far from the surface.

- Internal/external: *Internal* refers to the inside and *external* to the outside of the body.
- Right/left: *Right* and *left* always refer to the patient's right and left, not yours.

Movements

Flexion is the term used to describe flexing or a bending movement, such as bending at the knee or making a fist. *Extension* is the opposite of flexion—that is, a straightening movement (**Fig. 4-2**). The prefix "hyper" used with either term describes movement beyond the normal position.

Positions

As a rescuer, you will often have to describe a patient's position to other EMS personnel and health care providers. Using correct terms will help you communicate the extent of a patient's injury quickly and accurately.

Terms used to describe body positions include—

- Anatomical position. This position, where the patient stands with body erect and arms down at the sides, palms facing forward, is the basis for all medical terms that refer to the body.
- Supine position. The patient is lying face-up on his or her back (**Fig. 4-3, A**).

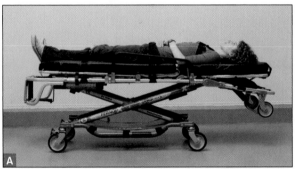
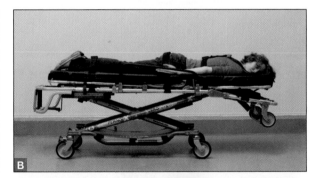
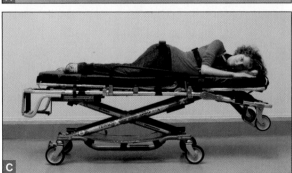
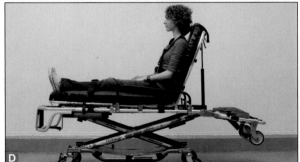

Fig. 4-3, A–D: Body positions include **(A)** supine position, **(B)** prone position, **(C)** right and left lateral recumbent position, and **(D)** Fowler's position.

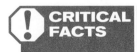

CRITICAL FACTS

Flexion is the term used to describe a bending movement. Extension describes a straightening movement.

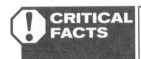 The organs of the body are located within hollow spaces in the body referred to as *body cavities* The five major cavities include the cranial, spinal, thoracic (chest), abdominal and pelvic cavity.

- Prone position. The patient is lying face-down on his or her stomach (**Fig. 4-3, B**).
- Right and left lateral recumbent position. The patient is lying on the left or right side (**Fig. 4-3, C**).
- Fowler's position. The patient is lying on his or her back, with the upper body elevated at a 45° to 60° angle (**Fig. 4-3, D**).

Body Cavities

The organs of the body are located within hollow spaces in the body referred to as *body cavities* (**Fig. 4-4**). The five major cavities include the—

- Cranial cavity. Located in the head and is protected by the skull. It contains the brain.
- Spinal cavity. Extends from the bottom of the skull to the lower back, is protected by the vertebral (spinal) column, and contains the spinal cord.
- Thoracic cavity (chest cavity). Located in the trunk between the diaphragm and the neck, and contains the lungs and heart. The rib cage, sternum and the upper portion of the spine protect it. The diaphragm separates this cavity from the abdominal cavity (**Fig. 4-5**).
- Abdominal cavity. Located in the trunk below the ribs, between the diaphragm and the pelvis. It is described using four quadrants created by imagining a line

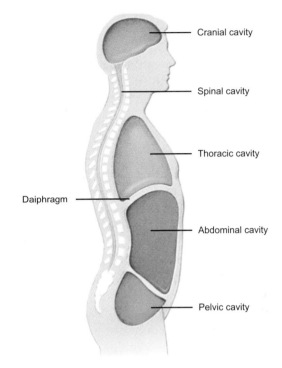

Fig. 4-4: The five major body cavities

from the breastbone down to the lowest point in the pelvis and another one horizontally through the navel. This creates the right and left, upper and lower quadrants. The abdominal cavity contains the organs of digestion and excretion, including the liver, gallbladder, spleen,

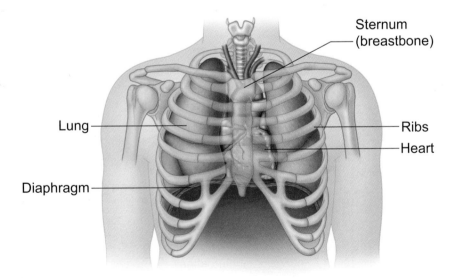

Fig. 4-5: The thoracic cavity is located in the trunk between the diaphragm and the neck.

pancreas, kidneys, stomach and intestines (**Fig. 4-6**).

- Pelvic cavity. Located in the pelvis, and is the lowest part of the trunk. Contains the bladder, rectum and internal female reproductive organs. The pelvic bones and the lower portion of the spine protect it.

Further description of the major organs and their functions are in the next section of this chapter and in later chapters.

BODY SYSTEMS

The human body is a miraculous machine. It performs many complex functions, each of which helps us live. The human body is made up of billions of different types of **cells** that contribute in special ways to keep the body functioning normally. Similar cells form together into **tissues**, and these in turn form together into organs. **Vital organs** such as the brain, heart and lungs are organs whose functions are essential for life. Each body system contains a group of organs and other structures that are especially adapted to perform specific body functions needed for life (**Table 4-3**).

For example, the **circulatory system** consists of the heart, blood and blood vessels. This system keeps all parts of the body supplied with oxygen-rich blood. For the body to work

properly, all of the following systems must work well together:

- Musculoskeletal
- Respiratory
- Circulatory
- Nervous
- Integumentary
- Endocrine
- Digestive
- Genitourinary

The Musculoskeletal System

The **musculoskeletal system** is a combination of two body systems, the muscular and skeletal systems, and consists of the bones, muscles, ligaments and tendons. This system performs the following functions:

- Supports the body
- Protects internal organs
- Allows movement
- Stores minerals
- Produces blood cells
- Produces heat

The adult body has 206 bones. Bone is hard, dense tissue that forms the skeleton. The skeleton forms the framework that supports the body. Where two or more bones join, they form a joint. Fibrous bands called *ligaments* usually hold bones together at joints. Bones vary in size and shape, allowing them to perform specific functions. Tendons connect muscles to bone.

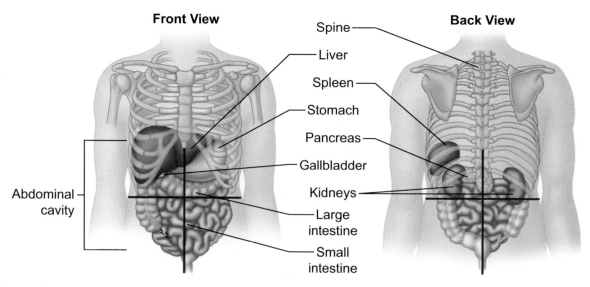

Fig. 4-6: The abdominal cavity contains the organs of digestion and excretion.

Table 4-3:
Body Systems

SYSTEMS	MAJOR STRUCTURES	PRIMARY FUNCTIONS	HOW THE SYSTEM WORKS WITH OTHER BODY SYSTEMS
Musculoskeletal system	Bones, ligaments, muscles and tendons	Provides body's framework; protects internal organs and other underlying structures; allows movement; produces heat; manufactures blood components.	Provides protection to organs and structures of other body systems; muscle action is controlled by the nervous system.
Respiratory system	Airway and lungs	Supplies the body with oxygen and removes carbon dioxide and other impurities through the breathing process.	Works with the circulatory system to provide oxygen to cells; is under the control of the nervous system.
Circulatory system	Heart, blood and blood vessels	Transports nutrients and oxygen to body cells and removes waste products.	Works with the respiratory system to provide oxygen to cells; works in conjunction with the urinary and digestive systems to remove waste products; helps give skin color; is under the control of the nervous system.
Nervous system	Brain, spinal cord and nerves	One of two primary regulatory systems in the body; transmits messages to and from the brain.	Regulates all body systems through a network of nerve cells and nerves.
Integumentary system	Skin, hair and nails	An important part of the body's communication network; helps prevent infection and dehydration; assists with temperature regulation; aids in production of certain vitamins.	Helps protect the body from disease-producing organisms; together with the circulatory system, helps regulate body temperature under control of the nervous system; communicates sensation to the brain by way of the nerves.
Endocrine system	Glands	Secretes hormones and other substances into the blood and onto the skin.	Together with the nervous system, coordinates the activities of other systems.
Digestive system	Mouth, esophagus, stomach and intestines	Breaks down food into a usable form to supply the rest of the body with energy.	Works with the circulatory system to transport nutrients to the body and remove waste products.
Genitourinary system	Uterus, genitalia, kidneys and bladder	Performs the processes of reproduction; removes wastes from the circulatory system and regulates water balance.	Assists in regulating blood pressure and fluid balance.

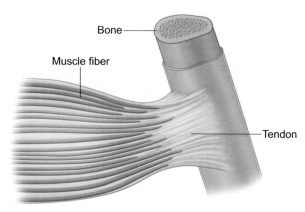

Fig. 4-7: Most of the body's muscles are attached to bones by tendons. Muscle cells, called fibers, are long and threadlike.

The Muscular System

The muscular system allows the body to move. Muscles are soft tissues. The body has more than 600 muscles, most of which are attached to bones by strong tissues called *tendons* (**Fig. 4-7**). Muscle tissue has the ability to contract (become shorter and thicker) when stimulated by a tiny jolt of an electrical or nerve impulse. Muscle cells, called *fibers*, are usually long and threadlike and are packed closely together in bundles, which are bound together by connective tissue.

There are three basic types of muscles, including—

- Skeletal. Skeletal, or voluntary, muscles are under the control of the brain and **nervous system**. These muscles help give the body its shape and make it possible to move when we walk, smile, talk or move our eyes.
- Smooth. Smooth muscles, also called *involuntary muscles*, are made of longer fibers and are found in the walls of tube-like organs, ducts and blood vessels. They also form much of the intestinal wall.
- Cardiac. Cardiac muscles are only found in the walls of the heart and share some of the properties of the other two muscle types: they are smooth (like the involuntary muscles) and striated (string-like, like the voluntary muscles). They are a special type of involuntary muscle that controls the heart. Cardiac muscles have the unique property of being able to generate their own impulse independent of the nervous system.

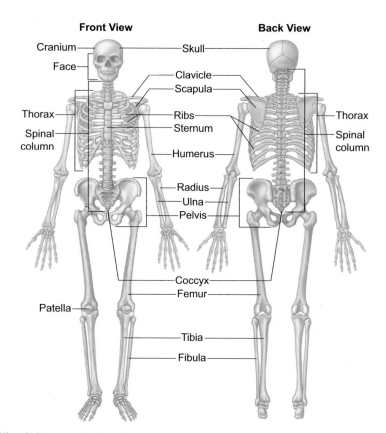

Fig. 4-8: The six parts of the skeleton are the skull, the spinal column, the thorax, the pelvis, and the upper and lower extremities.

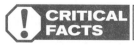 **CRITICAL FACTS** The three types of muscle are skeletal (voluntary), smooth (involuntary) and cardiac.

The Skeletal System

The skeleton is made up of six sections: the skull, spinal column, thorax, pelvis, and upper and lower extremities (**Fig. 4-8**).

- The skull: The skull is made up of two main parts: the cranium and the face. The cranium is made up of broad, flat bones that form the top, back and sides, as well as the front, which house the brain. Thirteen smaller bones make up the face, as well as the hinged lower jaw, or mandible, which moves freely.

- The spinal column: The spinal column, or spine, houses and protects the spinal cord. It is the principal support system of the body. The spinal column is made up of 33 small bones called *vertebrae*, 24 of which are movable. They are divided into five sections of the spine: 7 cervical (neck), 12 thoracic (upper back), 5 lumbar (lower back) and 9 sacral (lower spine with fused vertebrae) and coccyx (tailbone) (**Fig. 4-9**).

- The thorax: The *thorax*, also known as the *chest*, is made up of 12 pairs of ribs, the sternum (breastbone) and the thoracic spine. The 12 pairs of ribs are attached to the sternum with cartilage. Together, these structures protect the heart and lungs.

- The pelvis: The *pelvis*, also known as the *hip bones*, is made up of several bones, including the ilium, pubis and ischium. The pelvis supports the intestines and contains the bladder and internal reproductive organs.

- Upper extremities: The upper extremities, or upper limbs, include the shoulders, upper arms, forearms, wrists and hands. The upper arm bone is the humerus, and the two bones in the forearm are the radius and the ulna. The upper extremities are attached to the trunk at the shoulder girdle, made up of the clavicle (collarbone) and scapula (shoulder blade).

- Lower extremities: The lower extremities, or lower limbs, consist of the hips, upper and lower legs, ankles and feet. They are attached to the trunk at the hip joints. The upper bone is the femur or thigh bone, and the bones in the lower leg are the tibia and fibula. The kneecap is a small triangular-shaped bone, also called the *patella*.

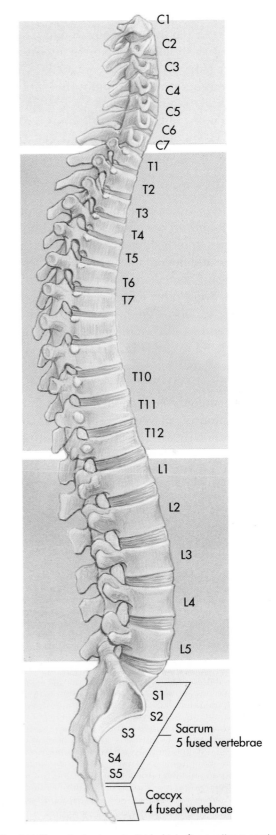

Fig. 4-9: The spinal column is divided into five sections: cervical, thoracic, lumbar, sacral and coccyx.

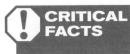

CRITICAL FACTS

The skeleton is made up of six sections: the skull, spinal column, thorax, pelvis, and upper and lower extremities.

- Joints: Joints are the places where bones connect to each other. Strong, tough bands called *ligaments* hold the bones at a joint together (**Fig. 4-10**). Most joints allow movement but some are immovable, as in the skull, and others allow only slight movement, as in the spine. All joints have a normal range of motion—an area in which they can move freely without too much stress or strain.

The most common types of moveable joints are the ball-and-socket joint, such as the hip and shoulder, and the hinged joint, such as the elbow, knee and finger joints. Different types of joints allow different degrees of flexibility and movement. Some other joint types include pivot joints (some vertebrae), gliding joints (some bones in the feet and hands), saddle joints (ankle) and condyloid joints (wrist) (**Fig. 4-11**).

The Respiratory System

The body can only store enough oxygen to last for a few minutes. The simple acts of inhalation and exhalation in a healthy person are sufficient

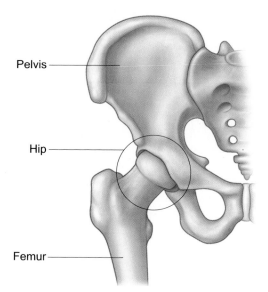

Pelvis

Hip

Femur

Fig. 4-10: Joints are the places where bones connect to each other.

to supply normal oxygen needs. If for some reason the oxygen supply is cut off, brain cells will begin to die in about 4 to 6 minutes. The **respiratory system** delivers oxygen to the body, and removes carbon dioxide from it, in a process called *respiration*.

Anatomy of the Respiratory System

Upper Airway

The upper airway includes the nose, mouth and teeth, tongue and jaw, pharynx (throat), larynx (voicebox) and epiglottis (**Fig. 4-12**). During inspiration (breathing in), air enters the body through the nose and mouth, where it is warmed and moistened. Air entering through the nose passes through the nasopharynx (part of the throat posterior to the nose) and air entering by the mouth travels through the oropharynx. The air then continues down through the larynx, which houses the vocal cords. The epiglottis, a leaf-shaped structure, folds down over the top of the trachea during swallowing, to prevent foreign objects from entering the trachea.

Lower Airway

The lower airway consists of the trachea (windpipe), bronchi, lungs, bronchioles and alveoli (**Fig. 4-12**). Once the air passes through the larynx, it travels down the trachea, the passageway to the lungs. The trachea is made up of rings of cartilage and is the part that can be felt at the front of the neck. Once air travels down the trachea it reaches the two bronchi, which branch off, one to each lung. These two bronchi continue to branch off into smaller and smaller passages called *bronchioles*, like the branches of a tree.

At the ends of each bronchiole are tiny air sacs called *alveoli*, each surrounded by capillaries (tiny blood vessels). These are the site of carbon dioxide and oxygen exchange in the blood. The lungs are the principal organs of respiration and house millions of tiny alveolar sacs.

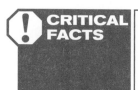

CRITICAL FACTS

Bones connect to each other at joints and are held together by ligaments. All joints have a normal range of motion, but some are immovable or allow only slight movement.

In a healthy person, respiration delivers oxygen the body needs. If that oxygen supply is cut off, brain cells will begin to die in about 4 to 6 minutes.

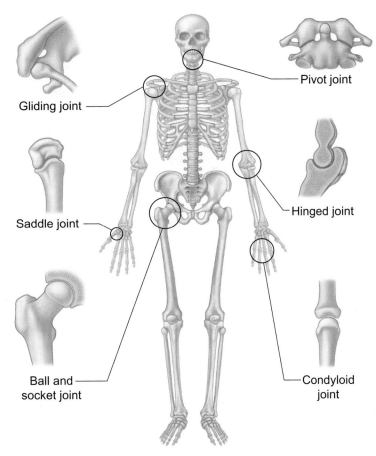

Gliding joint

Pivot joint

Saddle joint

Hinged joint

Ball and
socket joint

Condyloid
joint

Fig. 4-11: Common types of moveable joints

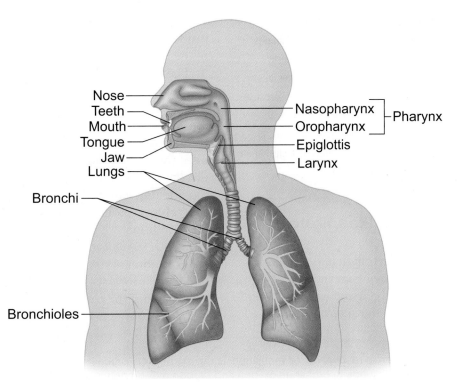

Nose

Teeth

Mouth

Tongue

Jaw

Lungs

Bronchi

Bronchioles

Nasopharynx

Oropharynx

Pharynx

Epiglottis

Larynx

Fig. 4-12: The upper and lower airways

Table 4-4:
Pediatric Considerations in the Respiratory System

ANATOMICAL DIFFERENCES IN CHILDREN AND INFANTS AS COMPARED WITH ADULTS	PHYSIOLOGICAL DIFFERENCES AND IMPACT ON CARE
Structures are smaller.	Mouth and nose are more easily obstructed by small objects, blood or swelling.
Primarily breathe through nose (especially infants).	Airway is more easily blocked.
Tongue takes up proportionately more space in the pharynx.	Tongue can block airway more easily.
Presence of "baby teeth"	Teeth can be dislodged and enter airway.
Face shape and nose are flatter.	Can make it difficult to obtain a good seal of airway with resuscitation mask.
Trachea is narrower, softer and more flexible.	Trachea can close off if the head is tipped back too far or is allowed to fall forward.
Have more secretions.	Secretions can block airway.
Use abdominal muscles to breathe.	This makes it more difficult to assess breathing.
Chest wall is softer.	Tend to rely more heavily on diaphragm for breathing.
More flexible ribs	Lungs are more susceptible to damage. Injuries may not be as obvious.
Breathe faster	Can fatigue more quickly, leading to respiratory distress.

Pediatric Considerations

The structures involved in respiration in children and infants differ from those of adults **(Table 4-4)**. They are usually smaller or less developed in children and infants. Some of these differences are important when providing care. Because the structures, including the mouth and nose, are smaller, they are obstructed more easily by small objects, blood, fluids or swelling. It is important to pay special attention to a child or an infant to make sure the airway stays open.

Physiology of the Respiratory System

External respiration, or ventilation, is the mechanical process of moving air in and out of the lungs to exchange oxygen and carbon dioxide between body tissues and the environment. It is primarily influenced by changes in pressure inside the chest that cause air to flow into or out of the lungs.

The body's chemical controls of breathing are dependent on the level of carbon dioxide in the blood. If carbon dioxide levels increase, the respiration rate increases automatically so that twice the amount of air is taken in until the carbon dioxide is eliminated. It is not the lack of oxygen but the excess carbon dioxide that causes this increase in respiratory rate. Hyperventilation may result from this condition.

Internal respiration, or *cellular respiration,* refers to respiration at the cellular level. These metabolic processes at the cellular level, either within the cell or across the cell membrane, are carried out to obtain

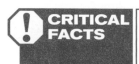

CRITICAL FACTS

External respiration, or ventilation, is the mechanical process of moving air in and out of the lungs to exchange oxygen and carbon dioxide between body tissues and the environment. It is primarily influenced by changes in pressure inside the chest that cause air to flow into or out of the lungs.

energy. This occurs by reacting oxygen with glucose to produce water, carbon dioxide and ATP (energy).

Structures That Support Ventilation

During inspiration, the thoracic muscles contract, and this moves the ribs outward and upward. At the same time, the diaphragm contracts and pushes down, allowing the chest cavity to expand and the lungs to fill with air. The intercostal muscles, the muscles between the ribs, then contract. During expiration (breathing out), the opposite occurs: the chest wall muscles relax, the ribs move inward and the diaphragm relaxes and moves up. This compresses the lungs, causing the air to flow out.

Accessory muscles are secondary muscles of ventilation only used when breathing requires increased effort. Limited use can occur during normal strenuous activity, such as exercising, but pronounced use of accessory muscles signals respiratory disease or distress. These muscles include the spinal and neck muscles. The abdominal muscles may also be used for more forceful exhalations. Use of abdominal muscles represents abnormal or labored breathing and is a sign of respiratory distress.

Vascular Structures That Support Respiration

Oxygen and carbon dioxide are exchanged in the lungs through the walls of the alveoli and capillaries. In this exchange, oxygen-rich air enters the alveoli during each inspiration and passes through the capillary walls into the bloodstream. On each exhalation, carbon dioxide and other waste gases pass through the capillary walls into the alveoli to be exhaled.

The Circulatory System

The circulatory system consists of the heart, blood vessels and blood. It is responsible for delivering oxygen, nutrients and other essential chemical elements to the body's tissue cells and removing carbon dioxide and other waste products via the bloodstream (**Fig. 4-13**).

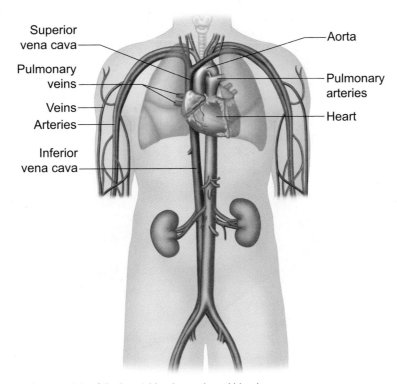

Fig. 4-13: The circulatory system consists of the heart, blood vessels and blood.

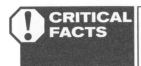

CRITICAL FACTS The circulatory system consists of the heart, blood vessels and blood. It is responsible for delivering oxygen, nutrients and other essential chemical elements to the body's tissue cells and removing carbon dioxide and other waste products via the bloodstream.

Anatomy of the Circulatory System

The heart is a highly efficient, muscular organ that pumps blood through the body. It is about the size of a closed fist and is found in the thoracic cavity, between the two lungs, behind the sternum and slightly to the left of the midline.

The heart is divided into four chambers: right and left upper chambers called *atria*, and right and left lower chambers called *ventricles* (**Fig. 4-14**). The right atrium receives oxygen-depleted blood from the veins of the body and, through valves, delivers it to the right ventricle, which in turn pumps the blood to the lungs for oxygenation. The left atrium receives this oxygen-rich blood from the lungs and delivers it to the left ventricle, to be pumped to the body through the arteries. There are arteries throughout the body, including the blood vessels that supply the heart itself, which are the coronary arteries.

There are four main components of blood: red blood cells, white blood cells, platelets and plasma. The red blood cells carry oxygen to the cells of the body and take carbon dioxide away. This is carried out by hemoglobin, on the surface of the cells. Red blood cells give blood its red color. White blood cells are part of the body's immune system and help to defend the body against infection. There are several types of white blood cells. Platelets are a solid component of blood used by the body to form blood clots when there is bleeding. Plasma is the straw-colored or clear liquid component of blood that carries the blood cells and nutrients to the tissues, as well as waste products away to the organs involved in excretion.

There are different types of blood vessels that serve different purposes: arteries, veins and capillaries. Arteries carry blood away from the

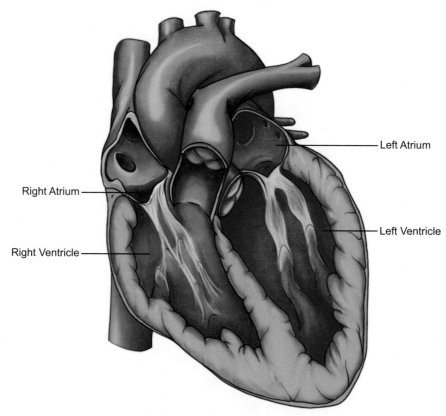

Right Atrium

Right Ventricle

Left Atrium

Left Ventricle

Fig. 4-14: The heart's four chambers

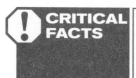

CRITICAL FACTS

There are three different types of blood vessels: arteries, veins and capillaries. Arteries carry mostly oxygenated blood away from the heart. Veins carry deoxygenated blood back to the heart. Capillaries are the tiny blood vessels that connect the systems of arteries and veins.

heart, mostly oxygenated blood. The exception is the arteries that carry blood to the lungs for oxygenation, the pulmonary arteries. The aorta is the major artery that leaves the heart. It supplies all other arteries with blood. As arteries travel further from the heart, they branch into increasingly smaller vessels called *arterioles*. These narrow vessels carry blood from the arteries into capillaries (**Fig. 4-15**).

The venous system includes veins and venules. Veins carry deoxygenated blood back to the heart. The one exception is the pulmonary veins, which carry oxygenated blood away from the lungs. The superior and inferior vena cavae are the large veins that carry the oxygen-depleted blood back into the heart. Like arteries, veins also branch into smaller vessels the further away they are from the heart. Venules are the smallest branches and are connected to capillaries. Unlike arterial blood, which is moved through the arteries by pressure from the pumping of the heart, veins have valves that prevent blood from flowing backward and help move it through the blood vessels.

Capillaries are the tiny blood vessels that connect the systems of arteries and veins. Capillary walls allow for the exchange of gases, nutrients and waste products between the two systems. In the lungs, there is exchange of carbon

dioxide and oxygen in the pulmonary capillaries. Throughout the body, there is exchange of gases and nutrients and waste at the cellular level.

Physiology of the Circulatory System

As the heart pumps blood from the left ventricle to the body, this causes a wave of pressure we refer to as the *pulse*. We can feel this pulse at several points throughout the body. These "pulse points" occur where the arteries are close to the surface of the skin, and over a bone (e.g., carotid pulse point in the neck, brachial pulse point on the inside of the upper arm).

As the blood flows through the arteries, it exerts a certain force that we call *blood pressure* (BP). BP is described using two measures, the systolic pressure (when the left ventricle contracts) and the diastolic pressure (when the left ventricle is at rest). Oxygen and nutrients are delivered to cells throughout the body, and carbon dioxide and other wastes are taken away, all through the delivery of blood. This continuous process is called *perfusion*.

The primary gases exchanged in perfusion are oxygen and carbon dioxide. All cells require oxygen to function. Most of the oxygen

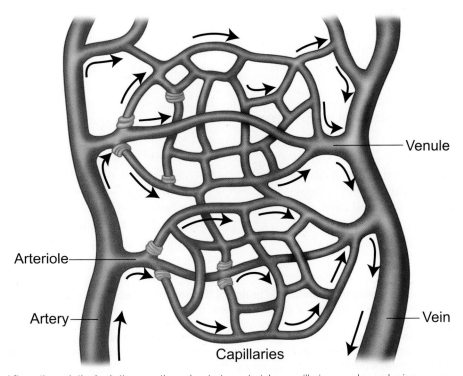

Fig. 4-15: As blood flows through the body it moves through arteries, arterioles, capillaries, venules and veins.

Blood Clotting

One of blood's characteristics is its ability to clot. Normally, blood flows freely though the blood vessels but if there is any trauma, blood must be capable of clotting so that bleeding will stop.

The clotting mechanism is made up of platelets and the thrombin system. Platelets are small cell fragments made in the bone marrow that become sticky when bleeding occurs. They adhere to the blood vessel wall at the site of bleeding. The thrombin system is made up of several proteins that use chemical reactions to create fibrin. The fibrin clumps and, together with the platelets, forms the clot.

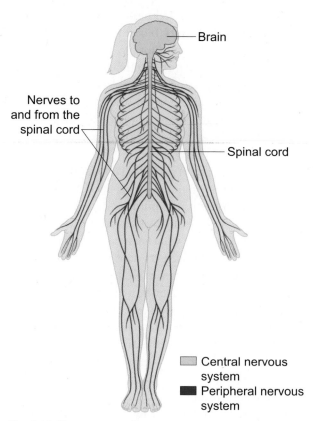

Fig. 4-16: The nervous system

is transported to the cells attached to the hemoglobin, but a tiny amount is also dissolved in the liquid component of the blood, the plasma. The major waste product in the blood, carbon dioxide, is transported mostly in the blood as bicarbonate and transported by the hemoglobin molecule. A tiny amount of carbon dioxide is dissolved in the plasma.

The Nervous System

The nervous system is the most complex and delicate of all the body systems. The center of the nervous system, the brain, is the master organ of the body and regulates all body functions. The primary functions of the brain are the sensory functions, motor functions and the integrated functions of consciousness, memory, emotions and use of language.

Anatomy of the Nervous System

The nervous system can be divided into two main anatomical systems: the central nervous system and the peripheral nervous system (**Fig. 4-16**). The central nervous system consists of the brain and spinal cord. Both are encased in bone (the brain within the cranium and the spinal cord within the spinal

column), are covered in several protective layers called *meninges* and are surrounded by cerebrospinal fluid.

The brain itself can be further subdivided into the cerebrum, the largest and outermost structure; the cerebellum, also called "*the small brain*," which is responsible for coordinating movement; and the brainstem, which joins the rest of the brain with the spinal cord. The brainstem is the control center for several vital functions including respiration, cardiac function and vasomotor control (dilation and constriction of the blood vessels), and is the place of origin for most of the cranial nerves (**Fig. 4-17**).

The peripheral nervous system is the portion of the nervous system located outside the brain and spinal cord, which includes the nerves to and from the spinal cord. These nerves carry sensory

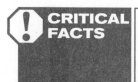

CRITICAL FACTS

The primary functions of the brain are the sensory functions, motor functions and the integrated functions of consciousness, memory, emotions and use of language.

The nervous system is divided into two functional systems. The voluntary system controls movement of the muscles and sensation from the sensory organs. The autonomic system controls the involuntary muscles of the organs and glands.

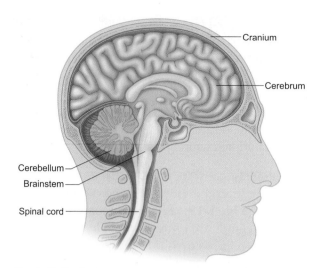

Fig. 4-17: The brain

information from the body to the spinal cord and brain, and motor information from the spinal cord and brain to the body.

Physiology of the Nervous System

The nervous system can also be divided into two functional systems, the voluntary and autonomic systems. The voluntary system controls movement of the muscles and sensation from the sensory organs.

The autonomic system is involuntary, and controls the involuntary muscles of the organs and glands. It can be divided into two systems: the sympathetic and parasympathetic systems. The sympathetic system controls the body's response to stressors such as pain, fear or a sudden loss of blood. These actions are sometimes referred to as the *"fight-or-flight" response*. The parasympathetic system works in balance with the sympathetic system, by controlling the body's return to a normal state.

The Integumentary System

The **integumentary system** consists of the skin, hair, nails, sweat glands and oil glands. The skin separates our tissues, organs and other systems from the outside world.

The skin is the body's largest organ (**Fig. 4-18**). It has three major layers, each consisting of other layers. The epidermis, or outer layer, contains the skin's pigmentation, or melanin. The dermis, or second layer, contains the blood vessels that supply the skin, hair, glands and nerves, and is what contributes to the skin's elasticity and

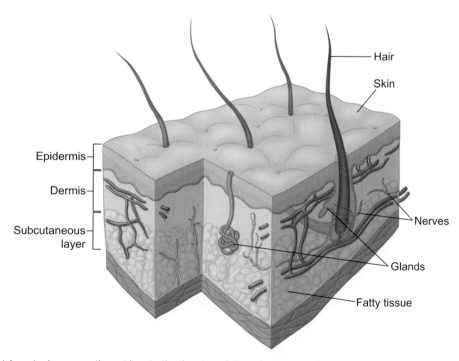

Fig. 4-18: The skin's major layers are the epidermis, the dermis and the subcutaneous layer.

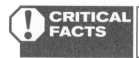 **CRITICAL FACTS** The skin is the largest organ in the human body. It protects against injury and pathogens, regulates fluid balance and body temperature, produces vitamin D and stores minerals.

strength. The deepest layer, the subcutaneous layer, is made up of fatty tissue and may be of varying thicknesses depending on its positioning on the body.

The skin serves to protect the body from injury and from invasion by bacteria and other disease-producing pathogens. It helps regulate fluid balance and body temperature. The skin also produces vitamin D and stores minerals. Blood supplies the skin with nutrients and helps provide its color. When blood vessels dilate (become wider), the blood circulates close to the skin's surface, making some people's skin appear flushed or red and making the skin feel warm. Reddening or flushing may not appear in darker skin. When blood vessels *constrict* (become narrower), not as much blood is close to the skin's surface, causing the skin to appear pale or ashen, and feel cool. This pallor can be found on the palms of the hands of darker-skinned people.

The Endocrine System

The **endocrine system** is one of the body's regulatory systems, and is made up of ductless glands. These glands secrete hormones, which are chemical substances that enter the bloodstream and influence activity in different parts of the body (e.g., strength, stature, hair growth and behavior).

Anatomy of the Endocrine System

There are several important glands within the body (**Fig. 4-19**). The hypothalamus and pituitary glands are in the brain. The *pituitary gland*, also referred to as the *"master gland,"* regulates growth as well as many other glands. The hypothalamus secretes hormones that act on the pituitary gland. The thyroid gland is in the anterior neck, and regulates metabolism, growth and development. It also regulates nervous system activity. The adrenal glands are located on the top of the kidneys, and secrete several

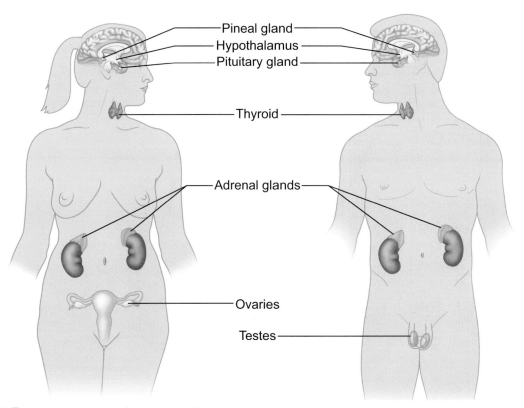

Pineal gland
Hypothalamus
Pituitary gland
Thyroid
Adrenal glands
Ovaries
Testes

Fig. 4-19: The endocrine system in females and males

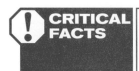

CRITICAL FACTS One of the critical functions controlled by the body's endocrine system is the control of blood glucose levels. The sympathetic nervous system is also regulated through the endocrine system.

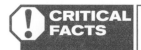

CRITICAL FACTS

The digestive system, or gastrointestinal system, consists of the organs that work together to break down food, absorb nutrients and eliminate waste.

hormones, including epinephrine (adrenalin) and norepinephrine (noradrenaline). The gonads (ovaries and testes) produce hormones that control reproduction and sex characteristics. The pineal gland is a tiny gland in the brain that helps regulate wake/sleep patterns.

Physiology of the Endocrine System

One of the critical functions controlled by the body's endocrine system is the control of blood glucose levels. The Islets of Langerhans, located in the pancreas, make and secrete insulin, which controls the level of glucose in the blood and permits cells to use glucose and glucagon (a pancreatic hormone), which raises the level of glucose in the blood.

The sympathetic nervous system is also regulated through the endocrine system. Adrenaline and noradrenaline, produced by the adrenal glands, cause multiple effects on the sympathetic nervous system. Effects include vasoconstriction (constricting of vessels), increased heart rate and dilation of smooth muscles, including those that control respiration.

The adrenal glands and pituitary gland are also involved in kidney function, and regulate water and salt balance. The body works to keep water and levels of electrolytes in the body in balance.

The Digestive System

The **digestive system**, or gastrointestinal system, consists of the organs that work together to break down food, absorb nutrients and eliminate waste. It is composed of the alimentary tract (food passageway) and the accessory organs that help prepare food for the digestive process (**Fig. 4-20**).

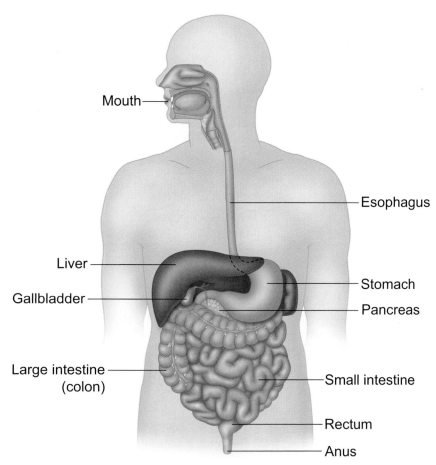

Fig. 4-20: The digestive system

Food enters the digestive system through the mouth and then the esophagus, the passageway to the stomach. The stomach and other major organs involved in this system are contained in the abdominal cavity. The stomach is the major organ of the digestive system, and the location where the majority of digestion, or breaking down, takes place. Food travels from the stomach into the small intestine, where further digestion takes place and nutrients are absorbed. The hepatic portal system collects blood from the small intestine and transfers its nutrients and toxins to the liver for absorption and processing before continuing on to the heart. Waste products pass into the large intestine, or colon, where water is absorbed and the remaining waste is passed through the rectum and anus.

The liver is the largest solid organ in the abdomen and aids in the digestion of fat through the production of bile, among other processes. The gallbladder serves to store the bile. The pancreas secretes pancreatic juices that aid in the digestion of fats, starches and proteins. It is also the location of the Islets of Langerhans, where insulin and glucagon are produced.

Digestion occurs both mechanically and chemically. *Mechanical digestion* refers to the breaking down of food that begins with chewing, swallowing and moving the food through the alimentary tract, and ends in defecation. *Chemical digestion* refers to the chemical process involved when enzymes break foods down into components the body can absorb, such as fatty acids and amino acids.

The Urinary System

Part of the **genitourinary system**, the urinary system consists of organs involved in the elimination of waste products that are filtered and excreted from the blood. It consists of the kidneys, ureters, urethra and urinary bladder (**Fig. 4-21**).

The kidneys are located in the lumbar region behind the abdominal cavity just beneath the chest, one on each side. They filter wastes from the circulating blood to form urine. The ureters

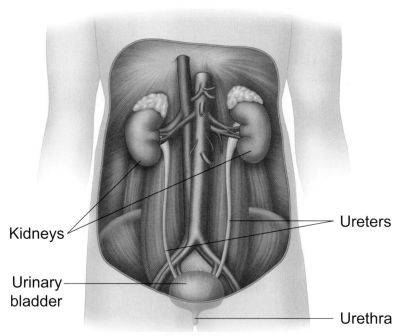

Kidneys

Ureters

Urinary bladder

Urethra

Fig. 4-21: The urinary system

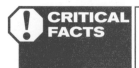

The urinary system consists of organs involved in the elimination of waste products that are filtered and excreted from the blood. It consists of the kidneys, ureters, urethra and urinary bladder.

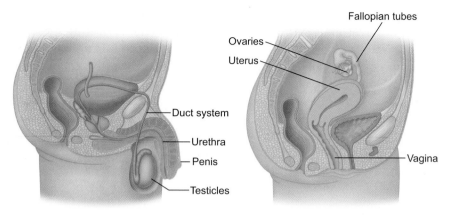

Fig. 4-22, A–B: **(A)** The male reproductive system; **(B)** The female reproductive system

carry the urine from the kidneys to the bladder. The bladder is a small, muscular sac that stores the urine until it is ready to be excreted. The urethra carries the urine from the bladder and out of the body.

The urinary system removes wastes from the circulating blood, thereby filtering it. The system helps the body maintain fluid and electrolyte balance. This is achieved through buffers, which control the pH (amount of acid or alkaline) in the urine.

The Reproductive System

Part of the genitourinary system, the reproductive system of both men and women includes the organs for sexual reproduction.

Male Reproductive System

The male reproductive organs are located outside of the pelvis and are more vulnerable to injury than those of the female. They include the testicles, a duct system and the penis (**Fig. 4-22, A**).

Puberty usually begins between the ages of 10 and 14 and is controlled by hormones secreted by the pituitary gland in the brain. The testes produce sperm and testosterone, the primary male sex hormone. The urethra is part of the urinary system and transports urine from the bladder; it is also part of the reproductive system through which semen is ejaculated. The sperm contributes half the genetic material to an offspring.

Female Reproductive System

The female reproductive system consists of the ovaries, fallopian tubes, uterus and vagina, and is protected by the pelvic bones (**Fig. 4-22, B**).

Glands in the body, including the hypothalamus and pituitary glands in the brain, and the adrenal glands on the kidneys, interact with the reproductive system by releasing hormones that control and coordinate the development and functioning of the reproductive system.

The menstrual cycle is approximately 28 days in length. Approximately midway through the cycle, usually a single egg is released which, if united with a sperm, will attach to the lining of the uterus, beginning pregnancy. The female's ovum contributes half the genetic material to the characteristics of a fetus.

PUTTING IT ALL TOGETHER

By having a fundamental understanding of body systems and how they function and interact, coupled with knowledge of basic medical terminology, you will be more likely to accurately identify and describe injuries and illnesses.

Each body system plays a vital role in survival. All body systems work together, to help the body maintain a constant healthy state. When the environment changes, body systems adapt to these new conditions. For example, the musculoskeletal system works harder during exercise; the respiratory and circulatory systems must also work harder to meet the body's increased oxygen demands. Body systems also react to the stresses caused by emotion, injury or illness.

Body systems do not work independently. The impact of an injury or a disease is rarely restricted to one body system. For example, a broken bone may result in nerve damage that will impair movement and feeling. Injuries to the ribs can make breathing difficult. If the heart stops beating for any reason, breathing will also stop.

In any significant injury or illness, body systems may be seriously affected. This may result in a progressive failure of body systems called *shock*. Shock results from the inability of the circulatory system to provide oxygenated blood to all parts of the body, especially the vital organs.

Generally, the more body systems involved in an emergency, the more serious the emergency.

Body systems depend on each other for survival. In serious injury or illness, the body may not be able to keep functioning. In these cases, regardless of your best efforts, the patient may die.

Fortunately, basic care is usually all you need to provide support to injured body systems until more advanced care is available. By learning the basic principles of care described in later chapters, you may be able to make the difference between life and death.

))) YOU ARE THE EMERGENCY MEDICAL RESPONDER

As you get closer to the woman in the car, you see that she is clutching one side of her abdomen, just below the ribcage. Her passenger is holding his right hip and looks dazed. The woman in the minivan now exhibits shallow breathing and her pulse is weak. What do you suspect is happening to the woman in the car?

5

Lifting and Moving Patients

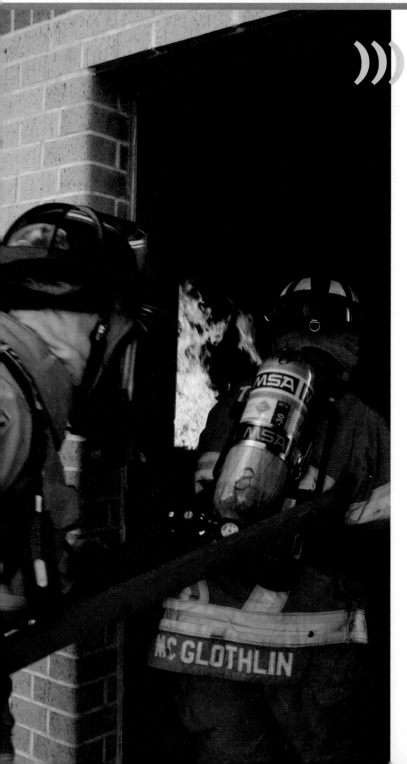

))) **YOU ARE THE EMERGENCY MEDICAL RESPONDER**

Your fire rescue unit is summoned to a recently remodeled building in response to a 9-1-1 call for a reported fire. You arrive to find smoke filling the area. Two people carry a man through a doorway. Three others stagger through and collapse to the ground. Smoke is blowing over them. Flames flicker inside the structure. You quickly size-up the scene and determine that the structure should be secure for the next few minutes. There is a large grassy area that extends at least 200 feet in front of the building. Should you move victims away from the vicinity of the burning building? Why or why not?

Key Terms

Ankle drag: A method of moving a patient by grasping the patient's ankles; also known as the foot drag.

Backboard: A piece of equipment used to immobilize a patient's head, neck and spine during transport.

Blanket drag: A method of moving a patient, using a blanket, in an emergency situation where equipment is limited and the patient is suspected of having a head, neck or spinal injury.

Body mechanics: The field of physiology that studies muscular actions and the function of the muscles in maintaining posture.

Clothes drag: A type of emergency move that uses the patient's clothing; used for a patient suspected of having a head, neck or spinal injury.

Direct carry: A method of moving a patient from a bed to a stretcher or vice-versa; performed by two responders.

Direct ground lift: A non-emergency method of lifting a patient directly from the ground; performed by several responders.

Draw sheet: A method of moving a patient from a bed to a stretcher or vice-versa by using the stretcher's bottom sheet.

Extremity lift: A two-responder, non-emergency lift in which one responder supports the patient's arms and the other the patient's legs.

Firefighter's carry: A type of carry during which the patient is supported over the responder's shoulders.

Firefighter's drag: A method of moving a patient in which the patient is bound to the responder's neck and held underneath the responder; the responder moves the patient by crawling.

Log roll: A method of moving a patient while keeping the patient's body aligned because of a suspected head, neck or spinal injury.

Pack-strap carry: A type of carry in which the patient is supported upright, across the responder's back.

Position of comfort: The position a patient naturally assumes when feeling ill or in pain; the position depends on the mechanism of the injury or nature of the illness.

Power grip: A hand position for lifting that requires the full surface of the palms and fingers to come in contact with the object being lifted.

Power lift: A lift technique that provides a stable move for the patient and protects the person lifting from serious injury.

Reasonable force: The minimal force necessary to keep a patient from harming him- or herself or others.

Recovery position: A posture used to help maintain a clear airway in an unresponsive, breathing patient.

Restraint: A method of limiting a patient's movements, usually by physical means such as a padded cloth strap; may also be achieved by chemical means, such as medication.

Shoulder drag: A type of emergency move that is a variation of the clothes drag.

Squat lift: A lift technique that is useful when one of the lifter's legs or ankles is weaker than the other.

Stair chair: Equipment used for patient transport in a sitting position.

Stretcher: Equipment used for patient transport in a supine position.

Supine: The body position of lying flat on the back; used when the patient has suspected head, neck or spinal injuries.

Two-person seat carry: A non-emergency method of carrying a patient by creating a "seat" with the arms of two responders.

Walking assist: A method of assisting a patient to walk by supporting one of the patient's arms over the responder's shoulder (or each of the patient's arms over the shoulder of one responder on each side).

Learning Objectives

After reading this chapter, and completing the class activities, you will have the information needed to—

- Define body mechanics.
- Explain the safety precautions to follow when lifting and moving a patient.
- Describe the conditions that require an emergency move.
- Describe the indications for assisting in non-emergency moves.
- Describe the various devices associated with moving a victim in the out-of-hospital setting.
- Explain the guidelines for patient positioning and packaging for transport.
- Explain the indications for when to use restraints.
- Describe the types of restraints.
- Make appropriate decisions regarding the use of equipment for moving a victim in the out-of-hospital setting.

Skill Objectives

After reading this chapter, and completing the class activities, you should be able to—

- Demonstrate an emergency move.
- Demonstrate a non-emergency move.

INTRODUCTION

At some point in many emergency situations, you will need to lift and move a patient. Sometimes this will be to provide easier access to administer first aid. At other times, you will need to move the patient to a safer location. You may also need to move a patient to transport him or her to the hospital. This chapter will teach you how to quickly and safely lift and move patients.

ROLE OF THE EMERGENCY MEDICAL RESPONDER

When providing care, you will usually not face hazards that require you to immediately move patients. In most cases, you can provide care where you find the patient. Moving a patient needlessly can lead to further injury. For example, moving a patient who has a painful, swollen, deformed leg without taking the time to immobilize it could result in an open fracture if the end of the bone were to tear the skin. Soft tissue damage, damage to the nerves, blood loss and infection could all result unnecessarily. Needless movement of a patient with a head, neck or spinal injury could cause paralysis or even death. Therefore, only move a patient if the scene is too dangerous to remain, if you need to reach another patient to provide care or if you need to move the patient in order to provide proper care.

Safety Precautions

Before you act, always size-up the scene and consider the factors affecting the situation:
- Any dangerous conditions at the scene
- The distance a patient must be moved
- The size of the patient
- Your physical ability
- Whether others can help you
- The *mechanism of injury* (MOI) and patient's possible condition
- Any aids or equipment to facilitate patient transport at the scene

Failing to consider these factors could cause injury. If you were to become injured, you might be unable to move the patient and could risk complicating the situation and making things worse.

Know Your Own Physical Limitations

Lifting and moving a patient requires physical strength and a high level of fitness. If you improperly lift a patient, you can permanently injure yourself. Adequate weight training, stretching and cardiovascular exercises will help ensure that you are ready for the physical demands of an emergency situation. You should only move a patient by yourself if you can do so safely and comfortably. Know your own physical limitations and, when in doubt, ask for assistance from other responders.

Body Mechanics

Body mechanics refers to the field of physiology that studies muscular actions and the function of the muscles in maintaining the posture of the body. In other words, it is the study of using your body in the safest and most efficient way to achieve a desired outcome.

Make sure to employ the following principles of body mechanics when lifting and moving a patient:
- Keep your back straight. Lift with the legs, not the back. Use the muscles in the legs, hips and buttocks and contract the muscles of your abdomen.
- Maintain a firm grip on the **stretcher** or the patient, being sure to never let go of the stretcher. Keep the patient's weight as close to your body as possible and maintain a low center of gravity. Follow the manufacturer's operating instructions for the stretcher you are using.
- Avoid twisting your body as you lift.
- Maintain a firm footing and walk in small measured steps.
- When possible, move forward rather than backward.
- Use good posture. Poor posture can fatigue your back and abdominal muscles, making you more prone to injuries. When standing, your ears, shoulders and hips should be aligned vertically, your knees should be bent slightly and your pelvis tucked slightly forward. When sitting, your weight should be distributed evenly and your ears, shoulders and hips should be aligned.

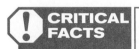
CRITICAL FACTS Before you act, always size-up the scene and consider the factors affecting the situation, including any dangerous conditions, your physical ability and the patient's possible condition.

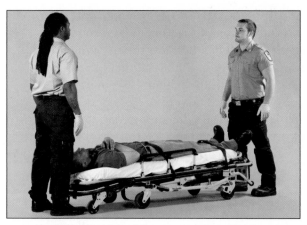

Fig. 5-1: When lifting patients, keep your back in a locked-in position, with your head up, back straight and shoulders square to the patient.

PRINCIPLES OF MOVING PATIENTS

There are a number of different ways to move a patient to safety and no one way is best. Any of the following moves is acceptable, providing that you can move a patient without injuring yourself or causing further injury to the patient. All team members should be trained in the proper techniques and have practiced them until the moves become automatic. Communicate your next moves clearly and frequently with your partner, the patient and other *emergency medical services* (EMS) personnel. If the patient is conscious, explain what you are doing or what you are about to do. Tell the patient what is expected of him or her, such as not reaching out to grab anything.

Back in Locked-In Position

Always begin your lift facing the patient or object and with your back in a locked-in position. Keep your legs shoulder-width apart, head up, back straight and shoulders square

(Fig. 5-1). Keep the weight of the patient or object as close to your body as possible. Tighten the muscles in your back and abdomen and keep your back straight while you lift. Keep your arms locked and avoid twisting while carrying.

Power Grip

The **power grip** allows for maximum stability and strength from your hands. To perform the power grip, grab the object so that both palms and fingers come in complete contact with the object **(Fig. 5-2)**. All of your fingers should be bent at the same angle.

Power Lift

The **power lift** technique provides a stable move for the patient while protecting you from serious injury. To perform the power lift correctly, remember to keep your back locked and avoid bending at the waist.

- Position your feet, making sure they are on a flat surface and are a comfortable distance apart (usually shoulder width), and turned slightly outward to provide maximum comfort and stability.
- Bend your knees. You should not feel like you are falling forward.
- Tighten your back and abdominal muscles. Keep your back as straight as possible and do not twist or turn. Make sure your feet are flat and your weight is evenly distributed.
- Position your hands. Use the power grip once your hands are in position. Grip the object in the way that is most comfortable and stable. For most people, that is approximately 10 inches apart.
- Lift, keeping your back locked, and make sure your upper body lifts before your hips do **(Fig. 5-3)**.
- Reverse the process to lower.

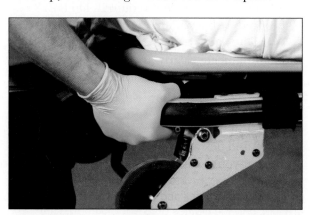

Fig. 5-2: In a power grip, both palms and fingers should be in complete contact with the object being lifted.

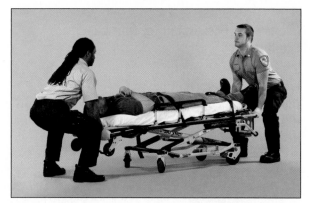

Fig. 5-3: Perform the power lift with your back locked to provide stability for the patient and to prevent injuring yourself.

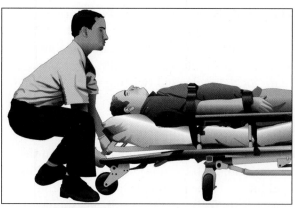

Fig. 5-4: The squat lift is a useful alternative to the power lift if one of your ankles or legs is weaker than the other.

Squat Lift

The **squat lift** is an alternative to the power lift, and is useful if one of your legs or ankles is weaker than the other. Remember to avoid bending at the waist when performing this lift.

- Stand with your weaker leg slightly forward. The foot on the weaker side should remain flat on the ground throughout the lift sequence.
- Squat down until you can grasp the object. Use the power grip.
- Push yourself up with your stronger leg (**Fig. 5-4**). Keep your back locked and lead with your head, lifting your upper body before your hips.
- Reverse the procedure to lower.

Reaching
General Guidelines

Emergency medical responders (EMRs) will often have to reach for equipment or patients. To minimize the risk of injury, try to reposition the object to avoid reaching and lifting. If that is not possible, reach no more than 20 inches in front of your body. When reaching, keep your back in the locked position and do not twist. Support your upper body with your free arm. When reaching overhead, do not lean back from the waist (hyperextending).

Correct Reaching for Log Rolling

The **log roll** is usually performed when the patient is suspected of having a spinal injury. Ideally, *four* people working in tandem perform it. One responder is located at the patient's head, while two or three others perform the actual move (**Fig. 5-5, A–E**). The patient's arms should be at his or her sides with the legs straight and together. The responder at the patient's head directs the movement and maintains in-line stabilization of the head and neck until the patient is secured on the **backboard**. The other responders roll the patient onto the side, and onto the backboard.

When performing a log roll, keep your back straight and lean from the hips, not the waist. Use the shoulder muscles whenever possible.

Pushing and Pulling

There may be instances when you will need to push or pull an object. Push rather than pull whenever possible. If pulling an object is necessary, keep your back locked and bend your knees slightly. Keep the load between your shoulders and hips and close to your body. This will keep the pull line centered with your body (**Fig. 5-6**).

If you need to push an object, try to push from the area between your waist and shoulders whenever possible. If the weight is below waist level, push from a kneeling position, keeping your elbows bent and your arms close to your body. This will increase the force you can apply. Avoid pushing or pulling objects overhead, as there is an inherent risk and likelihood of injury.

Carrying

To minimize injury both to yourself and to the patient, follow these guidelines when carrying a patient:

- Before lifting or carrying, estimate the total weight to be lifted or carried. Do not forget to include the weight of any equipment used in addition to the weight of the patient.
- Know your own physical abilities and limitations. Do not overestimate your abilities or those of your team members. Call for additional assistance if required. Do not proceed with a patient move until you can do so safely, regardless of your first instinct.
- Communicate clearly and frequently with your partner, the patient and other EMRs.
- When you carry, keep the weight as close to your body as possible, with your back in the locked-in position.
- Bend and flex at your hips and knees rather than at your waist.

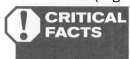

CRITICAL FACTS In any emergency move, take care to protect the head, neck and spine. If you suspect the patient of having a head, neck or spinal injury, only the clothes drag or blanket drag are safe ways to move the patient.

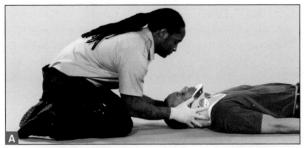

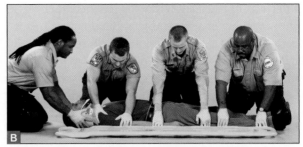

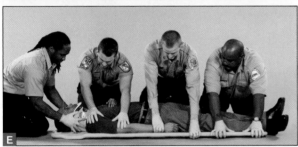

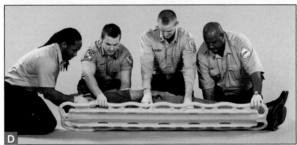

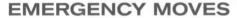

Fig. 5-5, A–E: To perform a log roll: **(A)** Have one responder maintain in-line stabilization of the head while **(B)** three responders perform the actual move. **(C)** Roll the patient in tandem, **(D)** placing the backboard against the patient and **(E)** returning the patient in tandem, always maintaining in-line stabilization.

EMERGENCY MOVES

In any emergency move, take care to protect the head, neck and spine. If you suspect the patient of having a head, neck or spinal injury, only the **clothes drag** or **blanket drag** are safe ways to move the patient.

Indications for Emergency Moves

In general, treat patients at the scene rather than moving them to provide care. However, some situations require emergency moves. These include the following:

- Immediate danger: Danger to you or the patient from fire, close proximity of explosives or other imminent hazards, lack of oxygen, risk of drowning, possible explosion, collapsing structure or other reasons such as uncontrolled traffic hazards, civil unrest or extreme weather conditions.
- Gaining access to other patients: A person with minor injuries may need to be moved quickly to allow you to reach other patients who may have life-threatening conditions.
- Providing proper care: A patient with a medical emergency, such as cardiac arrest or heat stroke, may need to be moved to provide proper care.

For example, someone in cardiac arrest needs CPR, which should be performed on a firm, flat surface with the patient positioned on the back. If the person collapses on a bed or in a small bathroom, the surface or space may not be adequate to provide appropriate care.

Moves used by EMRs include assists, carries and drags. One or two people can do most of these moves and most of them do not require equipment (the exception is the **direct ground lift**, which calls for *three* people). This is important because, with most emergency moves, equipment is not often immediately available and time is critical.

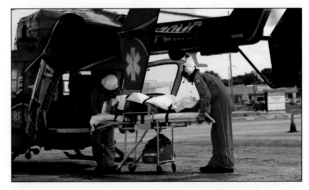

Fig. 5-6: When pulling, keep the pull line centered with your body. When pushing, push from the area between your waist and shoulders, if possible.

The greatest danger in moving a patient quickly is the possibility of aggravating a spinal injury. In an emergency, make every effort to pull the patient in the direction of the long axis of the body to provide as much protection to the head, neck and spine as possible. It is impossible to remove a patient from a vehicle quickly and at the same time provide much protection to the head, neck and spine.

Clothes Drag

The clothes drag is an appropriate emergency move for a person suspected of having a head, neck or spinal injury. This move helps keep the head and neck stabilized. To carry out a clothes drag, gather the patient's clothing behind the neck. Using the clothing, pull the patient to safety. During the move, cradle the patient's head by both the clothing and your hands. Move carefully, since you will be moving backward. Keep your back as straight as possible and bend your legs (**Fig. 5-7**). This type of emergency move is exhausting and may result in back strain for the responder, even when done properly.

Blanket Drag

The blanket drag is a good way to move a patient in an emergency situation when stabilization equipment is unavailable or the situation dictates that there is not enough time or space to use stabilization equipment. The blanket drag is appropriate for a patient suspected of having a head, neck or spinal injury. Position a blanket (or tarp, drape, bedspread or sheet) next to the patient. Keep the patient between you and the blanket. Gather half the blanket and place it against the patient's side. Being careful to keep about 2 feet of blanket above the patient's head, roll the patient toward your knees, reach across and position the blanket directly next to the patient. Gently roll the patient as a unit onto the blanket, being careful not to twist the patient's spinal column. After smoothing out the blanket, wrap it around the patient, gather up the excess at the patient's head, and drag, being sure

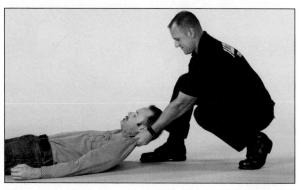

Fig. 5-7: Clothes drag

to keep the patient's head as low as possible. Move carefully because you are moving backward, and keep your back as straight as possible (**Fig. 5-8**).

Shoulder Drag

The **shoulder drag** is a variation of the clothes drag, in which you reach under the patient's armpits (from the back), grasp the patient's forearms and drag the patient (**Fig. 5-9**). Keep

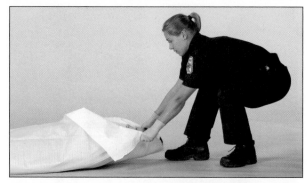

Fig. 5-8: Blanket drag

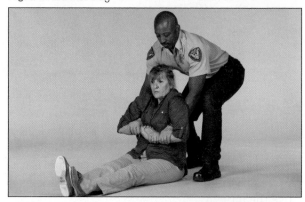

Fig. 5-9: Shoulder drag

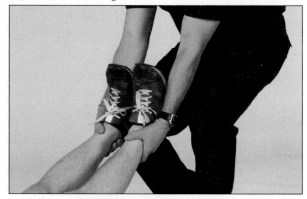

Fig. 5-10: Ankle drag

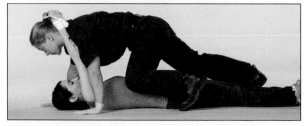

Fig. 5-11: Firefighter's drag

your back as straight as possible and do not twist. This move is exhausting and should be done carefully, since you are moving backward. The move may result in back strain. This move is *not* safe for a patient suspected of having a head, neck or spinal injury.

Ankle Drag

For the **ankle drag** (also known as the *foot drag*), firmly grasp the patient's ankles and move backward. Be careful to pull on the long axis of the body and not bump the patient's head. Keep your back as straight as possible and do not twist. Move carefully because you are moving backward, which may result in back strain (**Fig. 5-10**). This move is *not* safe for a patient suspected of having a head, neck or spinal injury.

Firefighter's Drag

For the **firefighter's drag**, position the patient on the back. Bind the patient's hands together gently at the wrists. Alternatively, you can strap a belt or other device behind the patient's shoulder blades, loop it through the straps on your air pack and fasten. Straddle the patient on your hands and knees and slip your head through the patient's arms. Place the patient's bound wrists behind your head. Keeping your back as straight as possible, and keeping the patient centered under you, slowly crawl forward, carrying the patient with you (**Fig. 5-11**). Be careful not to bump the patient's head. This move is *not* safe for a patient suspected of having a head, neck or spinal injury.

Firefighter's Carry

The **firefighter's carry** is *not* appropriate for patients with suspected head, neck, spinal or abdominal injuries, since the patient's body is twisted, the head is not supported and the patient's abdomen bears the weight during the movement. To perform the carry for a patient who is lying face-up, grasp the patient's wrists. While standing on the patient's toes, pull the patient over a shoulder. Finally, pass an arm between the legs and grasp the arm nearest you. Alternatively, you can kneel in front of a seated patient, place one shoulder against the patient's abdomen and hoist the patient across your shoulders. Pull the patient over a shoulder. The patient's feet should be on one side and the head on the other. Pass your arm between the patient's legs and grasp the patient's arm that is closest to you. Keep your back as straight as possible, lift with your legs and stand up (**Fig. 5-12**).

Pack-Strap Carry

The **pack-strap carry** can be used on both conscious and unconscious patients. Using it on an unconscious patient requires a second responder to help position the patient on your back. To perform the pack-strap carry, have the patient stand, or have a second responder support the patient. Position yourself with your back to the patient, back straight and knees bent so that your shoulders fit into the patient's armpits. Cross the patient's arms in front of you and grasp the patient's wrists (**Fig. 5-13**). Lean

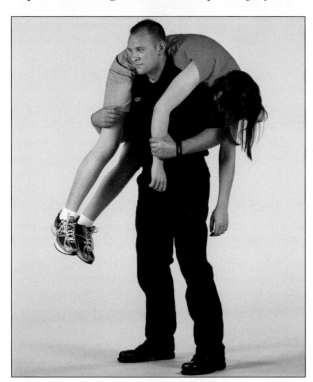

Fig. 5-12: Firefighter's carry

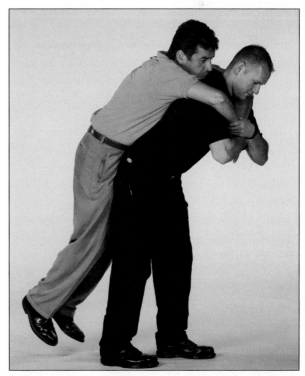

Fig. 5-13: Pack-strap carry

forward slightly and pull the patient up onto your back. Stand and walk to safety). Depending on the size of the patient, you may be able to hold both the patient's wrists with one hand. This leaves your other hand free to help maintain balance, open doors and remove obstructions. This move is *not* safe for a patient suspected of having a head, neck or spinal injury.

NON-EMERGENCY MOVES
Uses

A non-emergency move requires no special equipment, and is generally performed with other responders. Do not use non-emergency moves if there is a possibility of a spinal injury. A non-emergency move is used to move a patient from one location to another, such as from the accident scene to an ambulance or other transport vehicle or to a stretcher, from a bed to a stretcher or from the floor to a chair. It may also be used to move a patient to a different position as part of the medical treatment. The best way to move a patient in a non-emergency situation is the easiest way that will not cause injury or pain.

Non-emergency moves are used most frequently with patients with altered mental status, patients with inadequate breathing, patients who are in shock or patients in other situations that are potentially dangerous. Examples include a patient who is on a beach with the tide coming in or one who is lying on the ground in a busy traffic area.

Techniques
Walking Assist

The most basic move is the **walking assist**. It is frequently used to help patients who simply need assistance to walk to safety. Either one or two responders can use this method with a conscious patient.

To carry out a walking assist, place the patient's arm across your shoulders and hold it in place with one hand. Support the patient with your other hand around the patient's waist (**Fig. 5-14, A**). In this way, your body acts as a crutch, supporting the patient's weight while you both walk. A second responder, if present, can support the patient in the same way from the other side (**Fig. 5-14, B**).

Two-Person Seat Carry

The **two-person seat carry** is a method of moving a patient that requires a second responder.

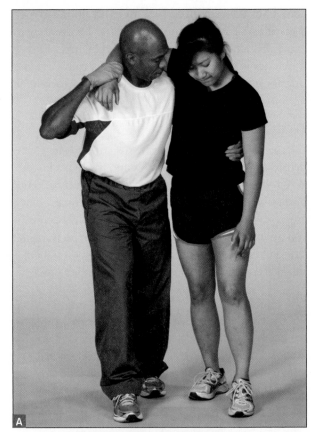

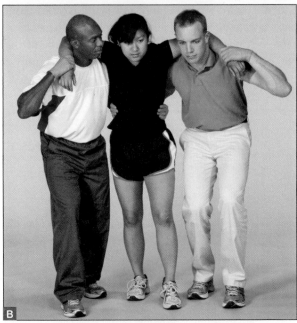

Fig. 5-14, A–B: Walking assist with (A) one responder and (B) two responders

To perform the two-person seat carry, put one arm under the patient's thighs and the other across the patient's back. Interlock your arms with those of a second responder, under the patient's legs and across the patient's back. The patient places his or her

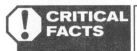
A non-emergency move is used to move a patient from one location to another. Do not use non-emergency moves if there is a possibility of a spinal injury.

arms over the responders' shoulders. The patient is then lifted in the "seat" formed by the responders' arms (**Fig. 5-15**). Keep your back straight and lift with your legs. Do *not* use this move for a patient suspected of having a head, neck or spinal injury.

Direct Ground Lift

The direct ground lift requires at least *three* responders. The three responders line up on one side of the patient and kneel close to the patient. The patient should cross arms over the chest. The responder kneeling at the patient's head places one arm under the patient's shoulders, cradling the head, and places the other arm under the patient's upper back. The next responder places one arm under the patient's waist and the other under the buttocks. The third responder cradles the patient's hips and legs. On a signal from the responder at the patient's head, all three responders lift the patient to their knees and support the patient by rolling the patient against their chests (**Fig. 5-16**). On the next signal, all will rise to their feet and move the patient to the stretcher. Reverse the steps to lower the patient. Responders should keep their backs straight and lift with their legs.

Extremity Lift

In the **extremity lift**, one responder kneels behind the patient, keeping the back straight,

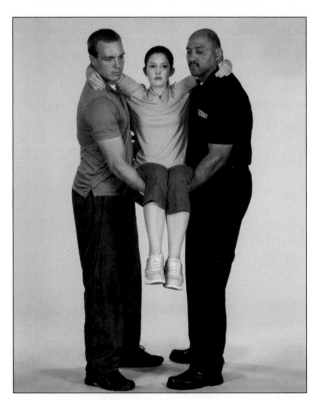

Fig. 5-15: Two-person seat carry

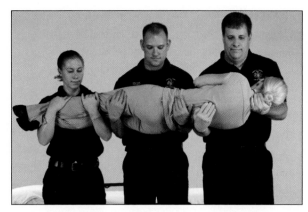

Fig. 5-16: Direct ground lift

reaches under the patient's arms and grasps the patient's opposite wrist. The second responder kneels between the patient's legs and firmly grasps around the patient's knees and thighs. On a signal from the responder at the patient's head, both responders move from a crouching position to a standing position. The responders then move the patient to a stretcher (**Fig. 5-17**).

Moving Patients From a Bed to a Stretcher

There are two techniques designed for moving a patient from a bed to a stretcher or vice versa: the **direct carry** and the **draw sheet**.

Direct Carry

Position the stretcher at a right angle to the bed, with the head of the stretcher at the foot of the bed. Two responders position themselves beside the bed on the same side as the stretcher. One responder slides his or her arms around the patient's shoulders and back, and the second responder cradles the patient's waist and hips. On a signal from the responder at the patient's head, the responders lift the patient simultaneously and curl the patient's body in

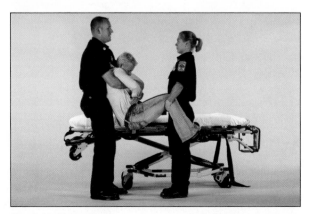

Fig. 5-17: Extremity lift

toward their chest. With a minimum of steps, the responders can then turn and place the patient on the stretcher (**Fig. 5-18, A–C**). Responders should keep their backs straight, lift with their legs and not twist their bodies.

Draw Sheet

To transfer a patient from the stretcher to the bed, the responders loosen the bottom sheet on the stretcher and position the stretcher along the side of the bed. Responders stand beside the

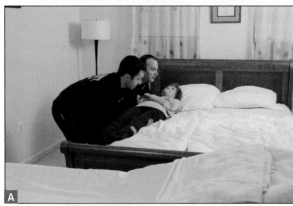

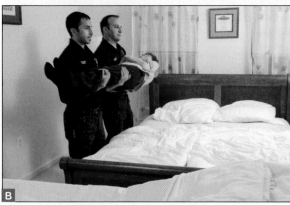

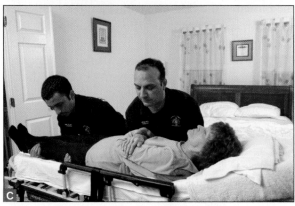

Fig. 5-18, A–C: To perform a direct carry: On a signal from the responder at the patient's head, **(A)** the responders lift the patient simultaneously, **(B)** the responders curl the patient's body in toward their chest and **(C)** place the patient on the stretcher.

stretcher and on the other side of the bed. The responders on the bed side of the patient lean over the bed and grasp the sheet firmly at the patient's head and hips. The responders on the stretcher side grasp the sheets in the same place. They then slide the patient into the bed. If there are more responders available, they should be positioned to help support the patient's legs by grasping the sheet in the same manner as the initial responders (**Fig. 5-19**).

EQUIPMENT

To best decide on the most suitable equipment for patients under different conditions, it is important to familiarize yourself with the different types available and match the appropriate equipment for the size and condition of each patient.

Stretchers

There are several types of stretchers designed to deal with patient transport.

- Standard wheeled stretchers are most commonly used when moving patients from a situation in which transport by ambulance for more advanced medical care is required (**Fig. 5-20, A**). They are equipped with a collapsible undercarriage for ease of loading.
- Portable stretchers are lightweight and often are used as auxiliary stretchers in ambulances (**Fig. 5-20, B**). They are designed for use with additional patients, as well as for maneuvering in areas where space is limited.
- The bariatric stretcher was designed to accommodate a weight of up to 1600 pounds (**Fig. 5-20, C**).

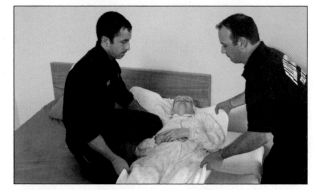

Fig. 5-19: Draw sheet technique

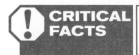
CRITICAL FACTS   There are two techniques designed for moving a patient from a bed to a stretcher or vice versa: the direct carry and the draw sheet.

- Basket stretchers, also known as *Stokes baskets,* get their name because of their basket-like shape (**Fig. 5-20, D**). They are capable of safely transporting and securing patients requiring a backboard. There are two types: a welded metal frame with a chicken wire web and a tubular aluminum frame that has been riveted to a molded polyethylene shell.
- Flexible stretchers are made of canvas or synthetic materials and are designed to allow easy transport of patients from confined spaces, narrow hallways and in

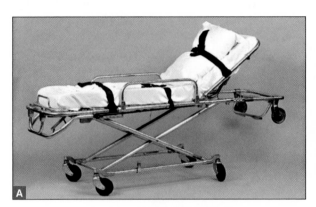

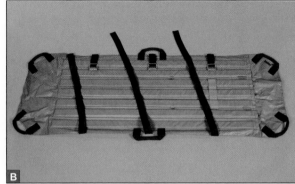

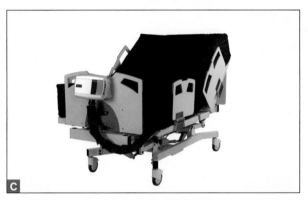

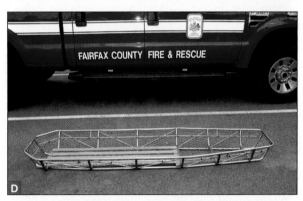

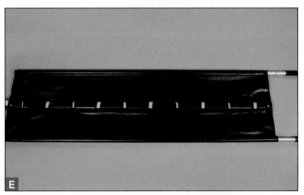

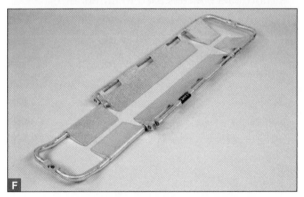

Fig. 5-20, A–G: Types of stretchers include **(A)** standard wheeled stretcher, **(B)** portable stretcher, **(C)** bariatric stretcher *(Courtesy of Stryker)*, **(D)** basket stretcher, **(E)** flexible stretcher, **(F)** scoop or orthopedic stretcher and **(G)** pneumatic or electronic stretcher.

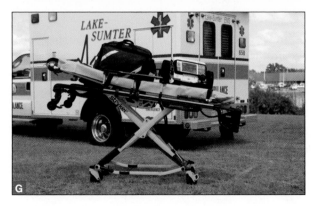

situations with multiple steps or rough terrain (**Fig. 5-20, E**).

- Scoop or orthopedic stretchers are designed for patients weighing up to 300 pounds, and are made to be assembled and disassembled around the patient (**Fig. 5-20, F**). A scoop stretcher is *not* recommended for a patient with a suspected head, neck or spinal injury because it does not support those areas.
- A pneumatic or electronic stretcher reduces the amount of manual lifting involved in patient transport (**Fig. 5-20, G**). It uses a hydraulic lift system to raise and lower the frame.

Stair Chair

A **stair chair** is used when a wheeled stretcher is deemed too long for the rescue or extrication (**Fig. 5-21**). It is especially useful when there is a small elevator or staircase in which a long stretcher will not fit. It is recommended that *three* responders be present when using the stair chair to ensure patient safety, two to act as carriers and one to serve as a spotter to watch for potential difficulties.

Backboards

Backboards are used to immobilize a patient's head, neck and spine during transport and are considered a standard piece of EMS equipment (**Fig. 5-22, A–B**).

A short backboard is used to immobilize non-critical patients who are already in a sitting position. The vest type and/or corset design is most commonly used to secure patients in this

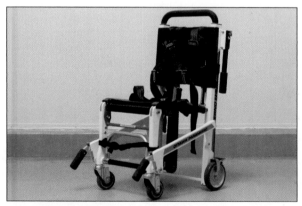

Fig. 5-21: Stair chair. *Courtesy of the Canadian Red Cross.*

situation, and allows the patient's head, chest and lower back to be strapped in. They are used with a long backboard, which provides complete stabilization and immobilization of the patient's head, neck, torso, pelvis and extremities. Both long and short boards are lightweight and come in several styles. The *Kendrick Extrication Device* (KED) is a vest-type device that is commonly used to stabilize patients in vehicle collisions who are in an upright position. It is used together with a cervical collar (**Fig. 5-23**).

The full-body vacuum mattress can be used as either a backboard or moving device once the patient is secured. This design allows the mattress to conform to whatever shape is required to accommodate the patient's condition. It avoids the need for additional padding and becomes rigid once fully deflated.

PATIENT POSITIONING AND PACKAGING FOR TRANSPORT

Make patients as comfortable as possible while awaiting transport. Unless a life-threatening emergency dictates the necessity, do not move an injured patient. A patient is usually moved by EMRs once the patient has been examined, evaluated and stabilized. There are times when a patient's condition will dictate the position you place the patient in.

Position of Comfort
Indications for Use

Patients with various injuries or illnesses may be placed in a **position of comfort**, which is the position that is most comfortable, unless the injury or illness prevents it. This might include a patient who is in pain, is experiencing breathing problems, is nauseated or is vomiting.

Techniques

Someone with abdominal pain will be more comfortable on the side with knees drawn up. If a patient is experiencing breathing difficulties, the patient may be more comfortable sitting

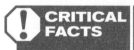
CRITICAL FACTS Patients with various injuries or illnesses may be placed in a position of comfort, which is the position that is most comfortable, unless the injury or illness prevents it.

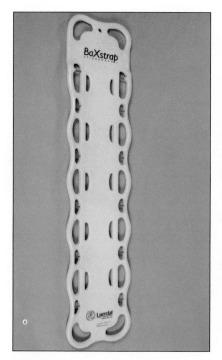
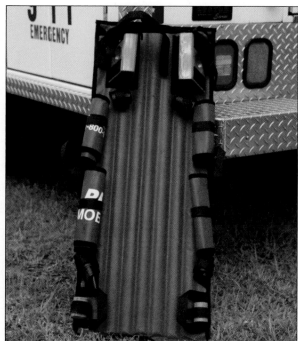

Fig. 5-22, A–B: **(A)** Adult backboard; **(B)** Pediatric backboard

up rather than lying down, and is normally transported in a sitting up position of comfort.

A patient who is nauseated or vomiting should be allowed to remain in whatever position is most comfortable. However, you should monitor the patient closely and position yourself to monitor and manage the patient's airway. An alert but nauseated person should be transported in a sitting-up position. If the patient is unconscious and you are alone and have to leave the person (e.g., to call for help), or you cannot maintain an open and clear airway because of fluids or vomit, transport the patient on the side, in the modified *high arm in endangered spine* (H.A.IN.E.S.) recovery position.

Recovery Positions
Indications for Use

The patient's condition should guide the EMR's decision regarding patient position while awaiting transport. In some cases, the person may be unconscious but breathing. Generally that person should not be moved from a face-up position and an open airway should be maintained, especially if there is a suspected spinal injury. However, there are a few situations when you should move a person into a modified H.A.IN.E.S recovery position whether or not a spinal injury is suspected. Examples of these situations include if you are alone and have to leave the person (e.g., to call for help), or you cannot maintain an open and clear airway because of fluids or vomit. Placing a person in a modified H.A.IN.E.S. recovery position will help keep the airway open and clear.

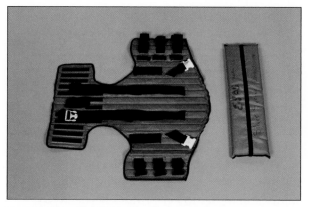

Fig. 5-23: Kendrick Extrication Device

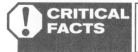

CRITICAL FACTS A person who is unconscious but breathing should not be moved from a face-up position, especially if there is a suspected spinal injury.

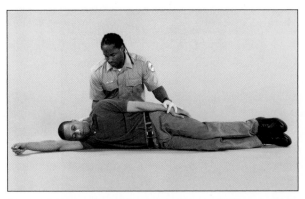

Fig. 5-24: For a patient with a suspected spinal injury, use the modified H.A.IN.E.S. recovery position.

Techniques

To place an adult or a child in a modified H.A.IN.E.S. recovery position (**Fig. 5-24**):

- Kneel at the person's side.
- Reach across the body and lift the arm farthest from you up next to the head with the person's palm facing up.
- Take the person's arm closest to you and place it next to his or her side.
- Grasp the leg farthest from you and bend it up.
- Using your hand that is closest to the person's head, cup the base of the skull in the palm of your hand and carefully slide your forearm under the person's shoulder closest to you. Do not lift or push the head or neck.
- Place your other hand under the arm and hip closest to you.
- Using a smooth motion, roll the person away from you by lifting with your hand and forearm. Make sure the person's head remains in contact with the extended arm and be sure to support the head and neck with your hand.
- Stop all movement when the person is on his or her side.
- Bend the knee closest to you and place it on top of the other knee so that both knees are in a bent position.
- Make sure the arm on top is in line with the upper body.
  - If you must leave the person to get help, place the hand of the upper arm palm side down with the fingers under the armpit of the extended lower arm.

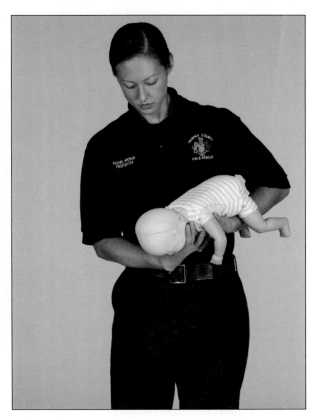

Fig. 5-25: An infant recovery position

To place an infant in a **recovery position**—

- Place the infant in a recovery position as would be done for an older child.
- You also can hold an infant in a recovery position by—
  - Carefully positioning the infant face-down along your forearm.
  - Supporting the infant's head and neck with your other hand while keeping the infant's mouth and nose clear (**Fig 5-25**).

Supine Position
Indications for Use

In a **supine** position, the patient is lying face-up. The supine position should be used when assessing an unconscious patient, when a patient needs CPR or assisted ventilation or when a patient has suspected head, neck or spinal injuries. In order to perform CPR effectively, for example, a patient must be lying in a supine position. Transport a patient in shock in a supine position. Immobilize a patient with a suspected head, neck or spinal injury in the supine position on a backboard. The patient then can be placed on the side by tilting the backboard to ensure the airway stays open and fluids drain from the mouth and are not aspirated (inhaled or sucked into the lungs).

Techniques

A log-roll reach is performed to transfer a patient to a supine position. At least *four* responders should perform it. The most experienced member of the team should be at the patient's head. The responder at the head will be the lead for the move and will stabilize the head and neck during the move. To stabilize the head, place your hands on either side of the patient's head at the jaw line, with your fingers behind the head at the base of the skull. The second responder stands at the patient's shoulders and upper back area. The third responder stands at the patient's hips. The fourth responder stands on the opposite side to position the backboard. The responder at the patient's head leads the move. On that responder's count, the other responders roll the patient as a team onto the patient's side, while the lead responder keeps the patient's head stable. The responder on the opposite side of the patient positions the backboard under the patient (**Fig. 5-26, A–C**).

MEDICAL RESTRAINT

If a patient is aggressive or violent and in need of emergency care, he or she may need to be restrained. However, an EMR should avoid restraining a patient unless the patient presents a danger to him- or herself or to others. Also, be aware that some state laws require EMRs to have police authorization before they can use **restraints**. If you are not authorized to use restraints, wait for someone with proper authority to arrive at the scene.

Even if you are authorized to use restraints, it is still best to have police present, if possible. Seek approval from medical direction. Be aware of and follow local protocols involving the use of patient restraints. Remember, as discussed in **Chapter 3**,

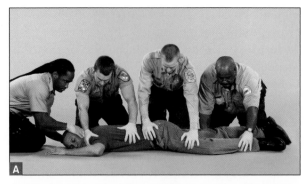
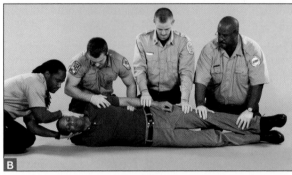
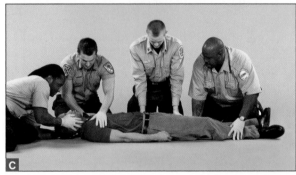

Fig. 5-26, A–C: To perform a log-roll reach: **(A)** One responder stabilizes the head while three others perform the move, **(B)** one responder maintains in-line stabilization of the head while **(C)** the others reach across and roll the patient onto his or her back.

restraining a patient without justification can give rise to a claim of assault and battery.

Altered Mental Status

Patients sometimes become aggressive or violent as a result of illness or trauma. Any condition that reduces the amount of oxygen to the brain, such as some head injuries, can cause a significant change in behavior. Too little oxygen could make a normally calm patient suddenly become anxious or even

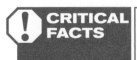 **CRITICAL FACTS** Restraint should be reserved only for situations where the patient presents a danger to him- or herself or to others. If state laws prohibit you from using restraints, wait for proper authorities to arrive on the scene.

violent. Physical illness as a result of substance abuse, diabetic emergencies, heat or cold exposure, or problems with the nervous system associated with aging can lead to alterations in behavior. Patients who are in an altered mental state may need to be restrained.

Reasonable Force

When restraining a patient, an EMR should always use **reasonable force**—the minimum force necessary to keep a patient from injuring him- or herself or others. A force is considered reasonable if it is as great as or minimally greater than the force the patient is exerting to resist. The amount of force you should use depends on—
- The height and weight of the patient.
- The mental state of the patient.
- The type of behavior the patient is manifesting.
- The type of restraint to be used (e.g., humane restraints that are padded and made of cloth, leather or wide roller gauze versus metal handcuffs, which are not considered humane).

Using Restraints

If restraints must be used, be sure that you have adequate assistance. You will need at least *four* responders trained in the use of restraints, plus an additional EMR who can advise the patient what is taking place. Plan out your actions before you take them. You must know ahead of time what each responder will be doing so you can act quickly and safely. Try to use responders of the same gender as the patient if possible. Remember that both medical and law enforcement personnel need to be consulted prior to the use of restraints. Always follow local protocols.

Use only the force necessary to successfully apply the restraint. Estimate the range of motion of the patient's arms and legs and stay beyond range until ready. Once the decision has been made to restrain the patient, act quickly. Have one EMR talk to the patient throughout restraining. Approach the patient with four responders simultaneously, one preassigned to each limb. Use only restraints that have been preapproved by medical direction. Restraints should be humane—made of leather or cloth. In addition, use only commercial wrist- and ankle-restraining straps.

Never secure a patient in a prone position. You must have access to the patient's airways at all times. A patient in a prone position will not be able to adequately breathe because the weight of the body will force the organs toward the diaphragm, which could lead to hypoxia (lack of oxygen) and other conditions. The lack of oxygen may cause the patient to become more aggressive. Consider the use of emergency oxygen to ensure the patient has adequate airflow. Be sure to monitor the patient's condition frequently.

Carefully and completely document, in detail, the events surrounding your use of force and the techniques that you used.

Types of Restraints

In circumstances where you need to restrain a patient, you will be using physical restraints, such as soft leather or cloth straps. There are also medications that act as a chemical form of restraint, but these must only be administered under medical authorization and by personnel trained to do so. Patients who are chemically restrained must be transported in an *advanced life support* (ALS) unit and should be given emergency oxygen and monitored closely. *Never* leave any restrained patient unattended.

PUTTING IT ALL TOGETHER

Take the time to size-up the scene upon arrival and determine if moving the patient is necessary before attempting to do so. Remember that your safety and the safety of your team always come first. This is especially true in incidents involving hazardous materials.

Avoid the common mistake of moving an injured or ill person unnecessarily. If you recognize a potentially life-threatening situation that requires the patient be moved immediately, use one of the techniques described in this chapter. Use the safest and

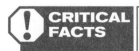

CRITICAL FACTS When restraining a patient, use reasonable force. Force is considered reasonable if it is as great as or minimally greater than the force the patient is exerting to resist.

easiest method to rapidly move the patient without causing injury to either yourself or the patient. Practice the lifts, moves and carries ahead of time so that they will be automatic to you when you need to use them.

It is important for you to familiarize yourself with some of the typical equipment used in local EMS systems. Practice using the different types of stretchers and backboards, as you could be called on to use them at any time.

If it becomes necessary to restrain a patient, follow the prescribed protocol carefully and ensure you have law enforcement and medical authorization before restraining a patient. Document the situation carefully to avoid future legal problems.

YOU ARE THE EMERGENCY MEDICAL RESPONDER

You and two other firefighters get to the collapsed victims. Two of the victims are unconscious. One man indicates his lower left leg may have been fractured. You recognize the immediate danger to the two unconscious victims and to the others who have escaped from the building. Time is critical. You need to get everyone to a safer place. Additional fire rescue units and EMS personnel have been called but have not arrived yet and the fire continues to build. How would you move the unconscious patients? How would you move the man with the lower leg injury?

SKILLsheet

Clothes Drag

NOTE: The clothes drag is an appropriate emergency move for a person suspected of having a head, neck or spinal injury.

STEP 1
Position the patient on his or her back.

STEP 2
Kneel behind the patient's head.

STEP 3
Gather the patient's clothing behind the neck.

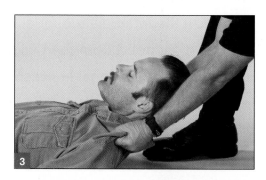

STEP 4
Using the clothing, pull the patient to safety.
◆ During the move, cradle the patient's head by both the clothing and your hands.
◆ Move carefully, since you will be moving backward.
◆ Keep your back as straight as possible and bend your legs.

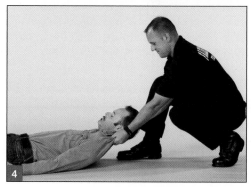

SKILLsheet

Blanket Drag

NOTE: The blanket drag is appropriate for a patient suspected of having a head, neck or spinal injury.

STEP 1

Position a blanket (or tarp, drape, bedspread or sheet) next to the patient.

STEP 2

Keep the patient between you and the blanket.

STEP 3

Gather half the blanket and place it against the patient's side.

◆ Keep about 2 feet of blanket above the patient's head.

STEP 4

Roll the patient toward your knees, reach across and position the blanket directly next to the patient.

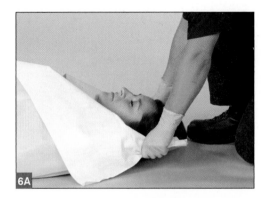

STEP 5

Gently roll the patient as a unit onto the blanket, being careful not to twist the patient's spinal column.

STEP 6

After smoothing out the blanket, wrap it around the patient.

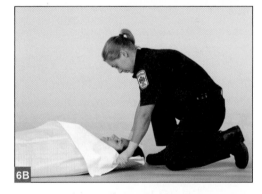

STEP 7

Gather up the excess at the patient's head, and drag the blanket.

◆ Be sure to keep the patient's head as low as possible.

◆ Move carefully backward, keeping your back as straight as possible.

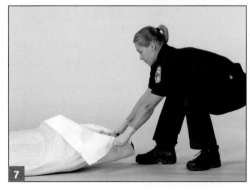

SKILLsheet

Shoulder Drag

NOTE: This move is **not** safe for a patient suspected of having a head, neck or spinal injury.

STEP 1

Reach under the patient's armpits (from the back), grasp the patient's forearms and drag the patient.
- ◆ Keep your back as straight as possible and do not twist.

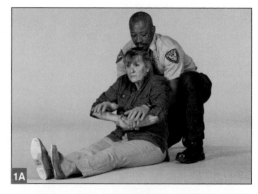

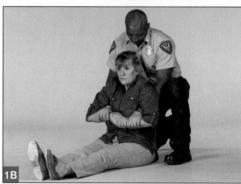

STEP 2

Carefully move backward.

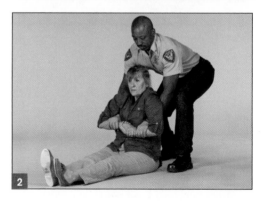

SKILLsheet

Ankle Drag (also known as the Foot Drag)

NOTE: This move is **not** safe for a patient suspected of having a head, neck or spinal injury.

STEP 1

Firmly grasp the patient's ankles and move backward.
◆ Be careful to pull on the long axis of the body and not bump the patient's head.

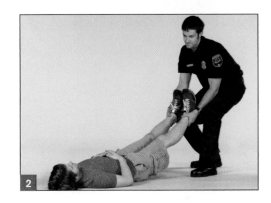

STEP 2

Carefully move backward.
◆ Keep your back as straight as possible and do not twist.

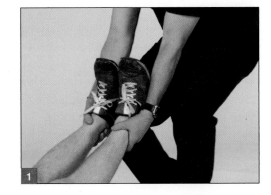

SKILLsheet

Firefighter's Drag

NOTE: This move is **not** safe for a patient suspected of having a head, neck or spinal injury.

STEP 1

Position the patient on the back. Bind the patient's hands together gently at the wrists.

STEP 2

Straddle the patient on your hands and knees, and slip your head through the patient's arms.

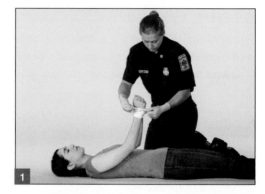

STEP 3

Place the patient's bound wrists behind your head.

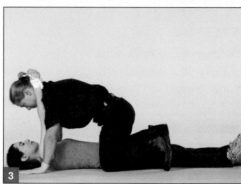

STEP 4

Slowly crawl forward, carrying the patient with you.
- Keep your back as straight as possible.
- Keep the patient centered under you.
- Do not bump the patient's head.

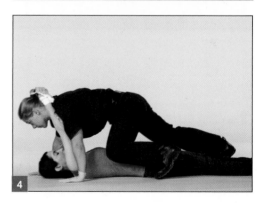

SKILLsheet

Firefighter's Carry

NOTE: The firefighter's carry is **not** appropriate for patients with suspected head, neck, spinal or abdominal injuries.

To perform the firefighter's carry on a patient who is lying face-up—

STEP 1

Grasp the patient's wrists.

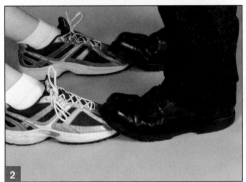

STEP 2

While standing on the patient's toes, pull the patient over a shoulder.

STEP 3

Pass an arm between the legs and grasp the arm nearest you.
◆ Alternatively, kneel in front of a seated patient, place one shoulder against the patient's abdomen and hoist the patient across your shoulders.

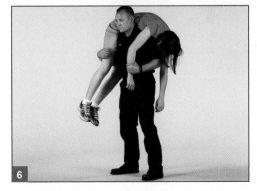

STEP 4

Pull the patient over a shoulder.

STEP 5

The patient's feet should be on one side and the head on the other.

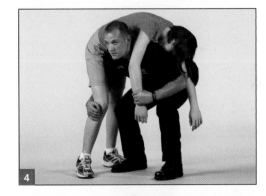

STEP 6

Lift with your legs and stand up.
◆ Keep your back as straight as possible.

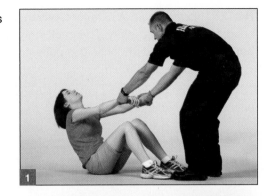

SKILLsheet

Pack-Strap Carry

NOTE: This move is **not** safe for a patient suspected of having a head, neck or spinal injury. The pack-strap carry can be used on both conscious and unconscious patients.

To perform the pack-strap carry on either a conscious or unconscious patient—

STEP 1

Have the patient stand, or have a second responder support the patient.

STEP 2

Position yourself with your back to the patient.
◆ Keep your back straight and knees bent so that your shoulders fit into the patient's armpits.

STEP 3

Cross the patient's arms in front of you and grasp the patient's wrists.

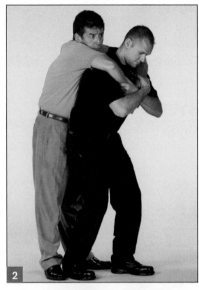

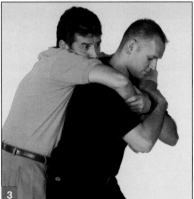

STEP 4

Lean forward slightly and pull the patient up onto your back.

STEP 5

Stand and walk to safety.

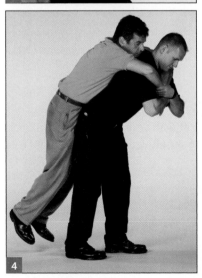

SKILLsheet

Walking Assist

NOTE: Either one or two responders can use this method with a conscious patient.

STEP 1

Place the patient's arm across your shoulders and hold it in place with one hand.

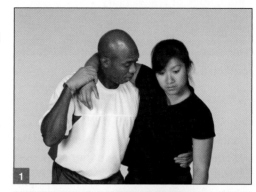

STEP 2

Support the patient with your other hand around the patient's waist.

NOTE: A second responder, if present, can support the patient in the same way from the other side.

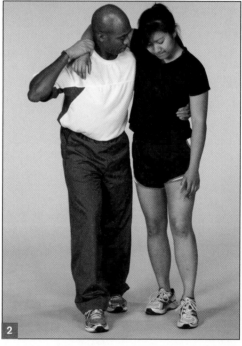

SKILLsheet

Two-Person Seat Carry

NOTE: Do **not** use this move for a patient suspected of having a head, neck or spinal injury.

STEP 1

Put one arm under the patient's thighs and the other across the patient's back.

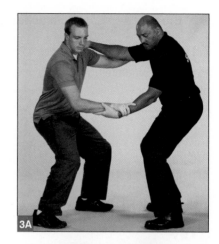

STEP 2

Interlock your arms with those of a second responder, under the patient's legs and across the patient's back.

◆ The patient places his or her arms over the responders' shoulders.

STEP 3

Lift the patient in the "seat" formed by the responders' arms.

◆ Keep your back straight and lift with your legs.

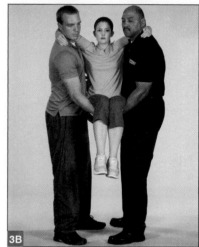

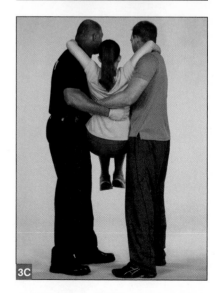

SKILLsheet

Direct Ground Lift

NOTE: The direct ground lift requires at least three responders.

STEP 1

All responders line up on one side of and kneel close to the patient.
◆ The patient should cross arms over the chest.

STEP 2

The responder kneeling at the patient's head places one arm under the patient's shoulders, cradling the head, and places the other arm under the patient's upper back.

STEP 3

The next responder places one arm under the patient's waist and the other under the buttocks.

STEP 4

The third responder cradles the patient's hips and legs.

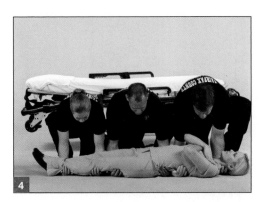

Continued on next page

Direct Ground Lift *continued*

STEP 5

On a signal from the responder at the patient's head, all three responders lift the patient to their knees.

◆ Provide support by rolling the patient against the responders' chests.

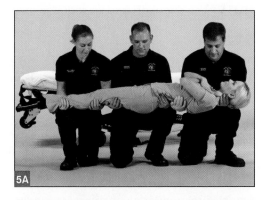

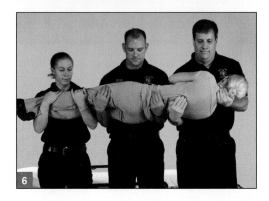

STEP 6

On the next signal, all carefully rise to a standing position and then move the patient to the stretcher.

◆ Reverse the steps to lower the patient.
◆ Keep backs straight and lift with the legs.

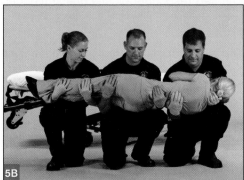

SKILLsheet

Extremity Lift

NOTE: The extremity lift requires two responders.

STEP 1

One responder kneels behind the patient, keeping the back straight, reaches under the patient's arms and grasps the patient's opposite wrist.

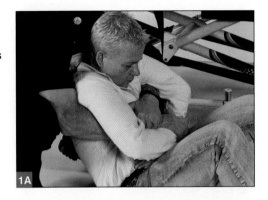

STEP 2

The second responder kneels between the patient's legs, firmly grasps around the patient's knees and thighs.

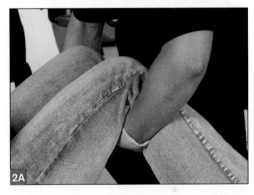

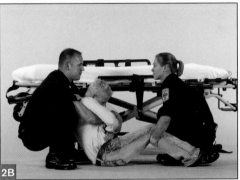

Continued on next page

Extremity Lift *continued*

STEP 3

On a signal from the responder at the patient's head, both responders move from a crouching position to a standing position.

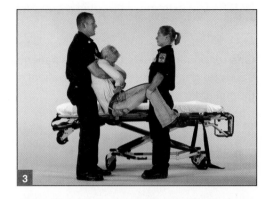

STEP 4

The responders then move the patient to the stretcher.

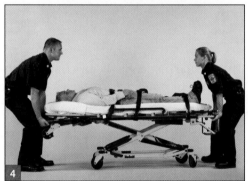

UNIT

2

ASSESSMENT

6

Scene Size-Up

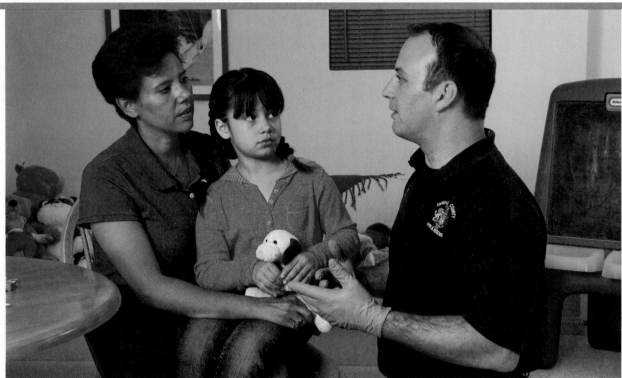

))) YOU ARE THE EMERGENCY MEDICAL RESPONDER

You are summoned to a neighbor's home after the 43-year-old mother and her two children from next door were apparently overcome by carbon monoxide from using a gas oven. The power went out earlier and has not been restored. The family members were found by a concerned neighbor. When you arrive, you see the mother and one of the children who are conscious and complaining of nausea and severe headaches. You also see a 6-year-old boy who appears to be unresponsive and not breathing. What should you be concerned with prior to conducting an assessment and providing care? Are there other services, such as fire or police, you should summon to the scene?

Key Terms

Blast injury: An injury caused by an explosion; may occur because of the energy released, the debris or the impact of the person falling against an object or the ground.

Blunt trauma: An injury in which a person is struck by or falls against a blunt object such as a steering wheel or dashboard, resulting in an injury that does not penetrate the body, may not be evident and may be more widespread and serious than suspected.

Chocking: The use of items such as wooden blocks placed against the wheels of a vehicle to help stabilize it.

Dispatch: Personnel trained in taking critical information from emergency callers and relaying it to the appropriate rescue personnel.

Hazardous material (HAZMAT): Any chemical substance or material that can pose a threat or risk to health, safety and property if not properly handled or contained.

Hematoma: A mass of usually clotted or partially clotted blood that forms in soft tissue space or an organ as a result of ruptured blood vessels.

Kinematics of trauma: The science of the forces involved in traumatic events and how they damage the body.

Mechanism of injury (MOI): The force or energy that causes a traumatic injury (e.g., a fall, explosion, crash or attack).

Nature of illness: The medical condition or complaint for which the person needs care (e.g., shock, difficulty breathing), based on what the patient or others report as well as clues in the environment.

Penetrating injury: An injury in which a person is struck by or falls onto an object that penetrates or cuts through the skin, resulting in an open wound or wounds, the severity of which is determined by the path of the object (e.g., a bullet wound).

Tripod position: A position of comfort that a person may assume automatically when breathing becomes difficult; in a sitting position, the person leans slightly forward with outstretched arms, and hands resting on knees or an adjacent surface for support to aid breathing.

Learning Objectives

After reading this chapter, and completing the class activities, you will have the information needed to—

- Explain the rationale for sizing up a scene.
- Identify the elements of a scene size-up.
- Determine when a scene is safe to enter.
- Describe common hazards found at the scene of a trauma or medical emergency.
- Have a basic understanding of scene and traffic control and related safety issues.
- Describe the principles of personal safety at an emergency scene.
- Identify standard and specialized *personal protective equipment* (PPE).

- Describe common *mechanisms of injury* (MOIs) and natures of illness.
- Recognize an unstable vehicle.
- Explain the safety fundamentals of vehicle stabilization.
- Know when to request and what types of additional resources may be necessary at the scene.
- Describe other dangerous situations and *hazardous materials* (HAZMAT).

INTRODUCTION

It is natural when you arrive at the scene of an emergency to want to rush in and start helping people who may be in obvious pain or distress. But, no matter what the situation, it is essential to take the time to carefully and systematically prepare for and size-up the scene. By doing this, you may save time later, prevent further harm to yourself and the patient and reduce the risk of overlooked injuries.

In this chapter, you will learn about the priority of preparation, ensuring your personal safety, determining the number of patients, identifying the *mechanism of injury* (**MOI**) or **nature of illness** and assessing the possible need for additional resources.

DISPATCH INFORMATION

As an *emergency medical responder* (EMR), it is important that you come prepared with the best available information before arriving at any emergency scene. Therefore, paying close attention to the information **dispatch** has provided to you is essential. This information gives you the first clues as to what you may encounter, including hazards you may need to take into consideration. It will also effect the *personal protective equipment* (PPE) and other equipment you may need.

Keep in mind that the information provided by dispatch is likely to be incomplete and may not be entirely accurate. The caller may have only given a location and some indication that medical assistance was needed. Hazards may be present that were not relayed by the person who reported the emergency, or the person may deliberately lie or exaggerate the severity of the condition in order to get medical attention. However, never undervalue the information dispatch can provide you as a foundation for your preparations.

SAFETY
Scene Safety

Almost every emergency response carries a certain risk to the safety of the EMR. Upon arrival at an emergency scene, safety should be your first priority. Safety includes both personal safety and the safety of others, including patients and bystanders. Begin with assessment of the scene and the surroundings, both of which provide valuable information about the emergency situation and will help ensure your own well-being.

Use each of your senses to size-up the scene. In addition to seeing and feeling for hazards, listen for unusual sounds, for example loud explosions or crackling sounds. Use your sense of smell to detect any unusual or unexpected odors, such as gasoline or other chemicals.

Always observe the scene thoroughly for dangers such as traffic, unstable structures, downed electrical lines, leaking fuels or fluids, smoke or fire, broken glass, swift-moving water, violence, explosions or toxic gas exposure. Some emergency scenes are immediately dangerous; others may become dangerous while you are providing care. Sometimes the dangers are obvious, such as at a fire or with the presence of hostile patients or bystanders. Other dangers may be less obvious, such as the presence of *hazardous materials* (**HAZMAT**) or unstable structures.

Take safety measures that are appropriate to the situation. In some cases, this might mean leaving or moving away from the scene if it is too dangerous, and may require a call for specialized personnel or other additional resources.

Controlling the Scene
Traffic Control

Once you have eliminated or removed the current dangers, you need to prevent new hazards from affecting the scene as you provide care for the patient(s). This is frequently a concern when dealing with emergencies on or near a road, and traffic control may be needed. Always pay attention to the road. Keep your eyes and ears open to avoid becoming a victim yourself.

Usually, the police will take responsibility for directing traffic at a scene. However, if the police have not yet arrived, you may need to manage this task. Always follow local protocols or guidelines

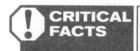 **CRITICAL FACTS** Safety includes both personal safety and the safety of others, including patients and bystanders.

but, in general, one person should be designated to be in charge of traffic control. If possible, traffic should be directed onto an entirely different road. If another route is not possible, the blocked-off area should be arranged so that any moving traffic is at least 50 feet from the scene.

The redirection of the vehicles needs to start well back from the scene. Traffic may be moving quickly and you need to provide plenty of time for vehicles to slow down and move over. Flares, reflective cones, signs and other warning devices should be put in position, about 10 to 15 feet apart in a slanting line (**Fig. 6-1, A–C**). Avoid placing a flare near puddles of fluid that may have spilled or leaked out of the involved vehicles, as the fluid may be flammable. On a curve, start the line of flares at the beginning of the curve; on a hill, start at the top of the hill. If the crash happened on a two-way road, put up flares or warning devices in both directions. Any rescuers setting out the flares or waving traffic away should be wearing reflective clothing and always be walking toward traffic. Do not turn your eyes away from oncoming traffic.

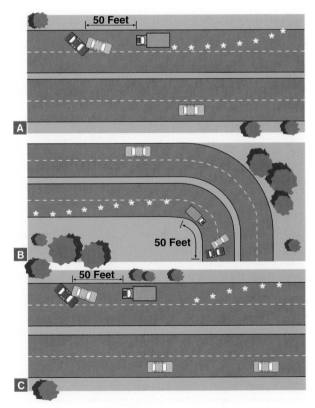

Fig. 6-1, A–C: **(A)** Proper position of flares on a straight road; **(B)** Proper position of flares on a curved road; **(C)** Proper position of flares on a hill

Ambulances or other transport and emergency vehicles should be positioned to help control the scene. If there are other emergency vehicles present, ambulances should be parked in front of the scene with the tires angled away from where care is being provided and with the loading doors facing away from traffic. Ambulances should be blocking the road as much as possible. If other emergency vehicles are present, they should park down from the scene with their tires angled away from where care is being provided. If there is a fire, park at least 100 feet away; in a HAZMAT situation, aim for a distance of 2000 feet. Also look for a location that is uphill and upwind if there are HAZMATs or fire. Leave emergency lights on to provide another warning to drivers approaching the scene, and turn headlights to a lower setting.

Crowd Control

You can help keep the situation calm at the scene by staying calm yourself. For example, walk quickly to patients rather than run. Walking is not only safer but also sends a message to the crowd that you are in control and confident. In very chaotic situations, it may help to set up a barrier around the scene and designate one person to ensure people stay behind the barrier.

Re-Evaluating the Scene

Continually reassess the situation for new dangers that may arise. For example, a building or structure that seemed stable when you arrived may begin to crumble or become unstable. True scene safety and control is a continuous, not an initial, process.

Personal Safety

Of your primary responsibilities, safety should always be foremost. You should always ensure your own safety. When you arrive on the scene, your first priority is to determine your own personal safety needs. The only safe scene is one that does not represent a threat to you or to the response team. A cornerstone of personal safety is the use of appropriate PPE.

Approach all emergency scenes cautiously until you can size-up the situation. If you arrive at the scene by vehicle, park a safe distance away.

If the scene appears safe, continue to evaluate the situation as you approach (**Fig. 6-2**).

Pay particular attention to the—

- Location of the emergency.
- Extent of the emergency.
- Apparent scene dangers.
- Apparent number of injured or ill people.
- Behavior of the patient(s) and any bystanders.

If at any time the scene appears unsafe, move to a safe distance. Notify additional personnel and wait for their arrival. Never enter a dangerous scene unless you have the training and equipment to do so safely. Well-meaning rescuers have been injured or killed because they forgot to watch for hazards. If your training has not prepared you for a specific emergency, such as a fire or an incident involving HAZMATs, notify appropriate personnel.

When arriving at an emergency scene, always follow these four guidelines to ensure your personal safety and that of bystanders:

1. Take time to evaluate the scene. Doing so will enable you to recognize existing and potential dangers.
2. Wear appropriate PPE for the situation. Be a constant advocate for the use of appropriate protective equipment.
3. **Do not** attempt to do anything you are not trained to do. Know what resources are available to help.
4. Get the help you need by notifying additional personnel. Be prepared to describe the scene and the type of additional help you require.

Another important aspect of personal safety is protecting yourself from exposure to infectious diseases. This is especially important if you are providing care for a patient when blood or other body fluids may be present. Since it is impossible to know if a patient may be infected or not, you should always take protective measures. These protective measures are discussed in detail in **Chapter 2**.

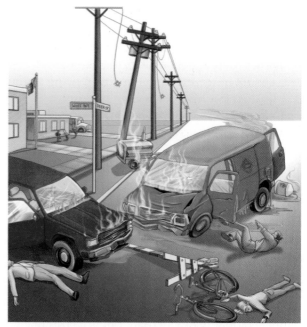

Fig. 6-2: Continue to evaluate the scene as you approach for the extent of the emergency, apparent danger, and number and behavior of patients and bystanders.

Personal Protective Equipment
Standard Precautions Overview

PPE is an important component of standard precautions, which are based on the principle that all blood, body fluids, secretions, excretions (except sweat), nonintact skin and mucous membranes may contain transmissible infectious agents. Standard precautions include a group of infection prevention practices that apply to all patients, regardless of suspected or confirmed infection status, in any health care delivery setting. They are based on universal precautions, which were developed for protection of health care personnel. Standard precautions focus on protection of responders and patients.

Implementation of Standard Precautions

The extent of standard precautions used is determined by the anticipated blood, body fluid or pathogen exposure, and includes the use of—

- Hand washing. Keeping hands clean is one of the best ways to keep from getting sick and spreading illnesses.

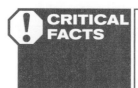

CRITICAL FACTS

Once you determine the scene is safe, approach and continue to evaluate the scene. Evaluation should include location and extent of the emergency, scene dangers, number of patients, and behavior of patients and bystanders.

To ensure the safety of all involved, always evaluate the scene, wear PPE, call for additional personnel if needed and only treat within the scope of your training.

- Gloves. Gloves should be worn whenever you touch or are in contact with a patient. Gloves are essential for any rescue situation.
- Gowns. A gown may provide further protection from body fluids that could otherwise be splashed onto your clothing or skin.
- Masks. Masks block potentially infectious body fluids from reaching your face; most germs and viruses can enter the body easily through the mouth or nose.
- Protective eyewear. In hazardous situations, these protect your eyes from debris and heat as well as body fluids.
- CPR breathing barriers (e.g., resuscitation masks and *bag-valve-mask resuscitators* [BVMs]). Use when providing ventilations to the patient is necessary.

Personal Protective Equipment

PPE includes clothing or specialized equipment that provide some protection to the wearer from substances that may pose a health or safety risk. The specific PPE is appropriate for the potential hazard, such as steel-toe boots, helmets, heat-resistant outerwear, self-contained breathing apparatus and leather gloves (**Fig. 6-3**).

Specialized protective equipment and gear are designed to protect appropriately trained responders, and include items such as—
- Chemical and biological suits.
- Specialized rescue equipment for difficult or complicated extrications.
- Ascent or descent gear for specialized rescue situations.

In addition to using appropriate PPE, do not forget the role that frequent hand washing or use of hand sanitizers play to keep you—and those around you—safe, by reducing the spread of germs.

Safety of Others

You have a responsibility for the safety of others at the scene, as well as for your own personal safety. Discourage bystanders, family members or unprepared responders from entering an area that appears unsafe. You can ask well-intentioned individuals to help you keep unauthorized people away from unsafe areas and summon more appropriate help. Some dangers may require you to take special measures, such as placing physical barriers to

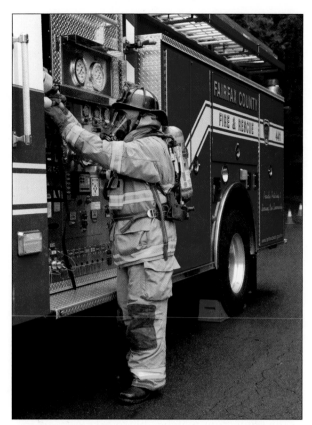

Fig. 6-3: Protect yourself from substances that may be harmful or contaminated by using appropriate PPE specific for the potential hazard.

prevent onlookers from getting too close. Other situations may require you to act quickly to free someone who is trapped or to move a patient in immediate danger.

Patient Safety

Once you are confident of your own safety and the safety of the general scene, turn to the safety of the patient. As you approach the patient, continue to scan the area for possible dangers. Do not move a patient unless there is an immediate danger.

Ideally, you should move patients only after you have assessed and properly cared for them. If the patient does not seem to be seriously injured, and the area is dangerous, you can ask the patient to move to safety where you can provide care. If, however, immediate dangers threaten a patient's life, you must decide whether to move the person. If the area is dangerous and the patient is not able to move, move the patient as quickly and safely as possible without making the injuries or illness worse. If the situation is so dangerous that you cannot reach or move the patient, move to safety yourself and call for additional assistance. If there is no immediate danger, tell the patient not to move.

Situations that may require an emergency move include—

- The presence of explosives or other HAZMATs that present an immediate danger (such as a natural gas or gasoline/fuel leak or fire).
- The inability to make the scene safe (such as a structure about to collapse).
- The need to get to other patients who have a more serious problem to provide the appropriate care.
- When it is necessary to provide appropriate care (such as moving a patient to the top or bottom of a flight of stairs to perform CPR).

Chapter 5 provides more detailed information on how to safely move injured or ill patients.

Bystander Safety

Look for bystanders who are in potential danger at the scene. You may be able to take steps to reduce the danger, but if not, tell them to move to safety.

If the scene is safe and you need help, look for bystanders who may be able to assist you. They may be able to tell you what happened, how many people were involved or may help in other ways. A bystander who knows a patient may know whether there are any medical conditions or allergies you should be aware of. Bystanders can meet and direct an ambulance to your location, help keep the area free of unnecessary traffic and even help you provide care if it is appropriate.

Number of Patients

Another important aspect when you are sizing up the scene is the number of patients at the scene. Often this is quick and easy to determine. But in some cases—for example, a multiple-vehicle crash or a significant explosion—it can be quite challenging. Patients may be trapped inside motor vehicles or may have been forcefully ejected from their vehicles and away from the immediate scene. An open door provides a clue that a patient has left the vehicle or was thrown from it. If one patient is bleeding or screaming loudly, you may overlook another patient who is unconscious. It is also easy in any emergency situation to overlook a small child or an infant if he or she is not crying. Accounting for the number of patients who require care is also important for determining the number of ambulances needed.

If it appears that there are more patients than you and the others with you can care for, call for additional help immediately. If you start helping the patients right away, you are likely to forget to make the call. Once you have called for additional help, you can quickly assess the patients to determine which ones you will begin caring for first.

MECHANISM OF INJURY AND NATURE OF ILLNESS

Once you are able to work safely with the patient, observe the scene and the patient to gather information about what has happened and the MOI or nature of the illness. As you gain experience, you will be able to arrive at a scene and quickly scan the area to make a rough determination of the injuries or illnesses you can expect to be dealing with.

Mechanism of Injury

MOI refers to the physical events that caused the injury. It is important to determine MOI because it can alert rescuers to possible hidden or more serious injuries that may not be immediately visible. Some of the most common MOIs an EMR will encounter are vehicle crashes, **blunt trauma**, falls and **penetrating trauma**.

Vehicle Crashes

The science of the energy of motion (kinetics), and the resulting damage to the human body (trauma), is called the **kinematics of trauma**.

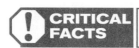 **CRITICAL FACTS** | Common MOIs include motor-vehicle crashes, falls and blunt or penetrating trauma.

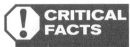

CRITICAL FACTS Motor-vehicle collisions clearly demonstrate the impact that the energy of motion has to cause damage to the human body. This is referred to as the *kinematics of trauma.*

Nowhere is the kinematics of trauma more apparent than in motor-vehicle crashes, which demonstrate all too vividly the effects of speed and rapid changes in speed (acceleration and deceleration) on the human body. When a car crashes into another vehicle or an object such as a tree, the people inside will continue moving at the same speed the car was traveling until something stops them. That "something" may be a seat belt, a car seat harness, the steering wheel, dashboard or airbag. Even when the person's body collides with the steering wheel, the person's internal organs continue to move until they are stopped by the body's framework—such as the ribs or skull. In a sense, there are *three* separate events, or *collisions*: first, the car hits another vehicle or an object and its forward motion is stopped; second, the person hits the interior of the car and stops; and finally the person's internal organs hit the skeleton or muscular framework of the body and stop **(Fig. 6-4, A–C)**.

Just as the first collision can cause both obvious damage to the car—the crumpled fender—and hidden damage—the leaking radiator—so the last two collisions can cause both visible and invisible damage to the people in the vehicle. The extent of the damage will depend in part on the speed and weight of the vehicles and the kinetic energy of motion that is absorbed.

The wreckage of cars, aircraft or machinery may contain hazards such as sharp pieces of metal or glass, fuel and moving parts. Therefore, do not try to rescue someone from wreckage unless you have the proper training and equipment, such as turnout (or "bunker") gear, safety glasses, gloves and a helmet. Specialized rescue teams can be called in for extensive or heavy rescue. Care for the patient is provided only after the wreckage has been stabilized. Gather as much information as you can, and make sure more advanced medical personnel have been called.

There are five types of motor-vehicle crashes and each yields a different possible pattern of injuries: head-on, rear-end, side impact, rotational impact and rollover.

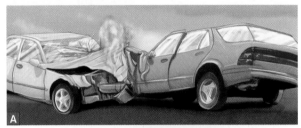

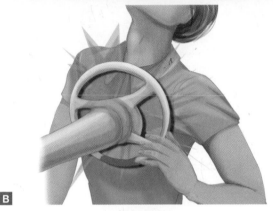

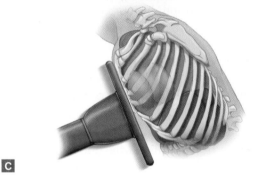

Fig. 6-4, A–C: The kinematics of trauma are apparent in motor-vehicle crashes. **(A)** The car hits another vehicle or an object and its forward motion is stopped. **(B)** The person hits the interior of the car and is stopped. **(C)** The person's internal organs hit the skeleton or muscular framework of the body and stop.

Head-On Crash

In a head-on crash, the driver will keep moving when the vehicle stops, and either will be thrown upward against the steering wheel and windshield, or downward under the steering wheel. In some cases, the driver may actually be thrown partially or completely through the windshield. If you see damage to the dashboard and windshield, you should anticipate that the driver may have abdominal injuries to the liver and spleen. The person may also have serious chest injuries, including broken ribs, ruptured lungs and torn arteries. Facial

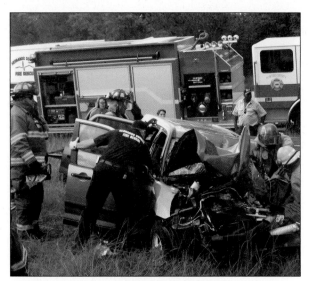

Fig. 6-5: A head-on car crash. *Courtesy of Captain Phil Kleinberg, EMT-P, Lake-Sumter EMS.*

injuries are common and will be obvious, but keep in mind that the person's neck and brain may also be injured, and this sometimes happens without any bleeding or bruising on the face (**Fig. 6-5**).

Rear-End Crash

In a rear-end collision, the rear vehicle pushes the vehicle in the front forward. The driver and any passengers will feel their heads and necks whipped back at first, and then they will be jolted forward as the car stops. The backward motion of the head and neck often leads to a strained neck, or what is often called a *whiplash injury*. After this sudden acceleration, the car will usually come to an abrupt stop because of the damage to the vehicle. This sudden stopping may cause injuries similar to those in a head-on crash.

Side Impact

If a vehicle hits the side of another car, the door and frame of the car can be pushed into the bodies of the driver and passengers. There may be injuries to any parts of the person's body, especially if the crash was forceful enough to crush the side of the car. If the person was not wearing a seat belt, the person may have been thrown against other passengers or against the far side of the car, so injuries can be found on both sides of the body.

Rotational Impact

Rotational impact occurs when the vehicle is thrown off center. It is the result of the vehicle striking an object and rotating around it. This can cause a variety of injury patterns, usually due to the person being struck by stationary objects inside the vehicle, such as the steering wheel, doorposts, windows or dashboard.

Rollover

When a car rolls over, the driver and/or passenger(s) inside experiences a series of impacts (**Fig. 6-6**). Each time the car starts to turn, the person is thrown in a new direction, possibly colliding with the door, the steering wheel, the roof of the car and any passengers. Injuries to many parts of the body are possible. If the person was not wearing a seat belt, the person may be ejected from the car through an open or broken window or door. This puts the person at greater risk, because the car may roll onto him or her. If the crash takes place on a road, the person may be ejected in front of oncoming traffic. Responders should check around the scene in case there are other people who have been ejected. Sometimes these individuals can land at some distance from the car. They may also be under the car.

Unstable Vehicles

Any movement of the vehicle during patient care or extrication can prove dangerous or even deadly to patients with severe spinal injuries, or could result in injury to rescue personnel. Local fire department and rescue squad personnel specially trained in vehicle stabilization and extrication will respond to the scene when notified.

To make the rescue setting as safe as possible, it is important to ensure the vehicle is stable. You can assume a vehicle is *unstable* if it is—

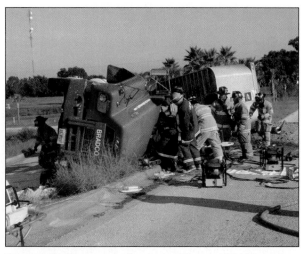

Fig. 6-6: A rollover crash. *Courtesy of Captain Phil Kleinberg, EMT-P, Lake-Sumter EMS.*

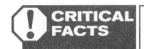

- Positioned on a tilted surface.
- Stacked on top of another vehicle, even partly.
- Positioned on a slippery surface.
- Overturned or on its side.

Vehicles must be stabilized in order to attempt to remove a patient. Placing blocks or wedges against the wheels of the vehicle will greatly reduce the chance of the vehicle moving. This process is called **chocking.** You can use items such as rocks, logs, wooden blocks and spare tires. If a strong rope or chain is available, it can be attached to the frame of the vehicle and then secured to strong anchor points, such as large trees, guardrails or another vehicle. Letting the air out of the vehicle's tires also reduces the possibility of movement. For further details on how to stabilize a vehicle, see **Chapter 30**.

Seat Belts and Airbags

In all types of motor-vehicle crashes, the benefits of seat belts and airbags far outweigh the risks, but there are also possible injuries associated with them.

If the lap belt is fastened too low on the person's body, across the base of the pelvis, it can dislocate the hips. If it is fastened too high, it can cause injury to the abdomen. Worn without a shoulder strap, a lap belt will keep the person from being ejected from the car but still allows a person's head to strike the dashboard; a back seat passenger can also strike the back of the front seat as a result of lap belt-only usage. A shoulder strap prevents these injuries but can cause injuries to the shoulder, chest and abdomen.

Airbags may be in the front of the car only, or may be in the door panels, roof rails and the side of seat backs. They are designed to inflate very rapidly just before impact and then deflate again just as quickly. Because they deflate so fast, they may not stop all forward motion of the driver's head and chest, so it is important to check to see if the driver also hit the steering wheel. If the steering wheel is damaged or deformed, the driver may have serious abdominal or chest injuries, even if the airbag was activated. Airbags can also cause injuries to the head, face, eyes, spine and arms, especially if the person is less than 5'2" tall. These injuries can prove fatal.

In some collisions, the airbag is not deployed and may present a hazard during extrication. If the patient is pinned directly behind an undeployed airbag, both of the vehicle's battery cables should be disconnected following established safety protocols. Ideally, the system should be deactivated before any attempts are made to extricate the patient. Do not mechanically cut through or displace the steering column until the system has been deactivated. The airbag module should not be cut or drilled into. Also, heat should not be applied to the area of the steering wheel hub; an undeployed airbag inflates in a normal manner if the chemicals sealed inside reach a temperature above 350° F. For further details on an undeployed airbag, see **Chapter 30**.

Additional Hazards

Other hazards at a motor-vehicle crash include fire, leaking fluids, downed power lines and special considerations for hybrid vehicles. For further details on hybrid and alternative fuel vehicles, see **Chapter 30**.

Motorcycle Crashes

Motorcycle riders do not have the protection of a vehicle body around them, so in a crash situation they are at particular risk for severe injuries. Motorcycle crashes may result in head-on impact, angular impact, ejection from the motorcycle or injury from "laying the bike down" (sliding down on one side of the bike).

If a crash is head-on, the sudden deceleration causes the rider to be thrown into or over the handlebars. Hitting the handlebars may cause injuries to the chest, abdomen or legs, depending on the rider's position. If the person is completely ejected from the bike, there may be internal injuries and head, neck, back and extremity injuries. Without a helmet, the rider is more likely to have serious or fatal head injuries.

Often when motorcycles crash, it is because the bike and rider come in contact with a protruding object, such as a tree branch, road sign or fence post, or another vehicle and often at high speeds. The rider may be injured by the object and then suffer further injuries as the bike falls or slides.

When a motorcycle rider realizes that a crash is likely, the rider may try to slow down the bike and reduce the risk by deliberately laying the bike down on its side, placing a leg between the bike and the road. This leads to abrasions of the soft tissues of the leg, which can go quite deep, depending partly on what protective clothing the rider is wearing. If the lower leg is trapped against the exhaust pipe, the patient can also have serious burns.

Recreational Vehicle Crashes

Since *all-terrain vehicles* (ATVs) are frequently ridden off-road or on uneven ground and are not very stable, they are prone to tipping over. In an ATV crash, expect to see injuries similar to those seen in motorcycle crashes. The rider is often ejected from the vehicle and the ATV may roll over onto the rider.

Snowmobile riders involved in a crash often experience serious head and neck injuries, and the snowmobile may roll over onto the rider. Winter weather may make it difficult for the rider to see protruding objects or wires and this can lead to collisions and injuries.

Blunt Injuries

When someone is struck by or falls against a blunt object—one with no sharp edges or points—the resulting injuries are often closed wounds. This type of wound is known as a **blunt injury** or blunt trauma. This means that although the soft tissues of skin, muscle, nerves and blood vessels may be damaged, the skin is not broken and there is no visible bleeding. The patient may look unharmed, but there may be serious, even fatal, injuries to the internal organs as well as significant internal bleeding. The extent of the injuries may not be visible immediately after, but may only appear after a few hours. The injuries may be more extensive than they appear.

The rescuer should look for—
- Contusions or bruises—Swelling, discoloration and pain where the person was hit.
- **Hematoma**—A large, bluish lump formed by blood collecting under the skin **(Fig. 6-7)**.

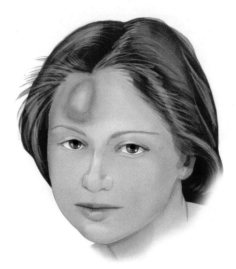

Fig. 6-7: A hematoma may indicate more serious hidden injuries.

Small- or medium-sized contusions only need to have cold compresses applied. Larger contusions and bruising or hematomas may indicate that there are more serious hidden injuries. It is also important to check for possible bone fractures, especially if there is a lot of swelling or pain or if the body part is deformed.

Falls

Falls are another common cause of injury. The severity of the injuries caused by a fall is determined by—
- The distance the patient fell (the speed of the fall increases when the person falls from a greater height).
- The surface the patient landed on (a soft, yielding surface will reduce the injuries).
- Any objects in the way that might have slowed the fall or, on the other hand, injured the patient during the fall.
- The position of the patient's body on landing.

If the patient falls from a height of more than 15 feet onto a hard surface, injuries may be severe, even if the patient looks unharmed at first glance. You may discover fractured bones in the feet, ankles, legs, pelvis and spine. In falls from a greater height, the patient may also have damage to internal organs.

It is a natural reflex to throw out your hands when you are falling. When a fall involves the hands hitting the ground, the person's wrists may be fractured and, if the person falls from a great enough height, there also might be a fracture or injury to the elbow and shoulder.

A person falling head first usually throws out the arms, so injuries or fractures in the arms and shoulders are typical. The head may be pushed forward or backward on landing, or may be pressed down by the person's body, and any of these can cause serious injury to the head and spine. The rest of the body will then hit the ground, and injuries to the chest and pelvis can happen during this phase of the fall.

Penetrating Injuries

A **penetrating injury** occurs when the patient is hit by or falls onto something that can penetrate or cut through the skin. This will cause an open wound (or wounds, as there may be both an entrance and exit wound) and bleeding.

The path of the projectile through the body usually determines the severity of the injury. For example, if a knife or bullet does not damage any internal organs or major blood vessels, the resulting injuries may be fairly minor, but a stabbing or shotgun blast that hits the heart or lungs or severs an artery can quickly lead to a fatality.

In addition to the path of the object, the speed with which the projectile travels through the body is also a determining factor: the faster the object is moving, the more widespread the damage done. If the patient falls onto something sharp, or is stabbed with a knife or another object, this is termed a *low-velocity penetrating trauma*. If the weapon or object used is available at the scene, it can provide some hints as to the extent of the injuries. A knife, for example, only harms the tissues it actually contacts, so knowing how long the knife is will indicate how deep the injuries may be.

Because it hits the body at greater speed, a bullet or pellet fired from a handgun, rifle or shotgun will cause damage to the body well beyond its actual pathway through the body. This is because it carries with it a wave of pressure that compresses tissues around it as it speeds through the body (**Fig. 6-8, A–B**). Always check for an exit wound, which may be larger than the entrance wound, because this helps to determine

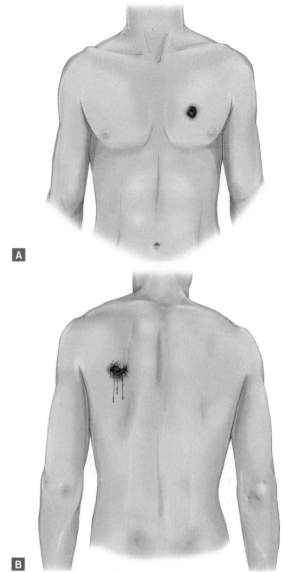

Fig. 6-8, A–B: For a penetrating injury, always check for an **(A)** entrance wound and **(B)** exit wound.

the bullet's pathway through the body. The most serious, and most often fatal, gunshots are to the head, chest and abdomen. While bullets that hit the arms and legs are less likely to be quickly fatal, they can cause serious bleeding and permanent damage to the limbs. Keep in mind that a small entrance hole, which may not bleed very much, may hide dramatic and serious internal injuries.

Blast Injuries

Another type of injury is a **blast injury**, which is caused by an explosion. There are three phases to an explosion, and

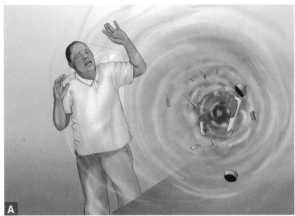

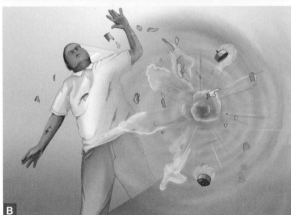

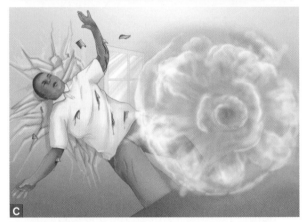

Fig. 6-9, A–C: There are three phases of a blast injury. **(A)** Primary phase: Energy sends a wave of pressure expanding outward from the center of the blast. **(B)** Secondary phase: Debris around the center of the blast blows outward, causing blunt or penetrating injuries and sometimes burns. **(C)** Tertiary phase: Force of the explosion knocks a person to the ground, against a wall or into other objects.

therefore, three possible MOIs from it (**Fig. 6-9, A–C**):

- In the primary phase, the energy released during the explosion sends a wave of pressure expanding outward from the center of the blast. Individuals hit by this pressure can experience injury to any body part that is air-filled, especially the lungs, stomach, intestines and inner ears. In some cases, this can be fatal, even though the person may show no external injuries.
- In the secondary phase, the debris around the center of the blast is blown outward and can cause injury when it strikes the person—often with considerable speed and force. These blunt or penetrating injuries will generally be visible and easily recognized. If some of the debris is on fire, the person may be burned.
- In the tertiary phase, the person is knocked to the ground or against a wall or other objects by the force of the explosion. Depending on how far away the person is, and how large the explosion, the injuries may be similar to those sustained by someone ejected during a car crash.

Nature of the Illness

In some situations, you may be called to a scene because a person is ill. Or, if you are called to an emergency and there is no evidence of trauma, but the patient has signs and symptoms of a problem, you may suspect an illness or a medical condition. Recognizing the nature of the illness helps you to plan the steps to provide immediate care.

A conscious patient may be able to describe the symptoms, or there may be obvious signs (e.g., labored breathing, vomiting). If the patient is unable to speak, ask any bystanders or family what they have observed about the patient, and about any pre-existing conditions.

Determining the nature of the illness can be made more difficult if the patient or others do not tell the truth. If a person overdosed on drugs, for example, the family may deny knowing what caused the problem, and may lie about drug use if you ask about it directly. It is important to scan the scene for items that may provide clues about the problem. Look for prescription and non-prescription medications, evidence of alcohol or recreational drug use and medical equipment in regular use.

Consider the patient's location and environment as well. For example, has the patient been in the woods or long grass? Then you might need to examine the patient for snake or spider bites. Is the weather extremely hot and humid? Heat stroke or other heat-related illnesses are a possibility.

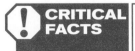

CRITICAL FACTS You may be called to a scene because a person is ill and there is no evidence of trauma. Recognizing the nature of illness helps you to plan the steps to provide immediate care.

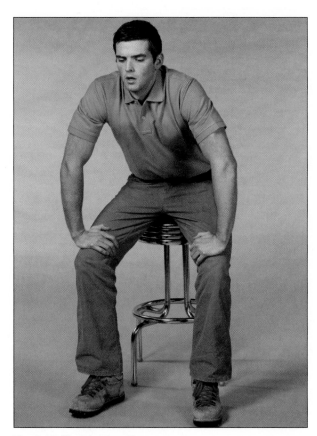

Fig. 6-10: The tripod position

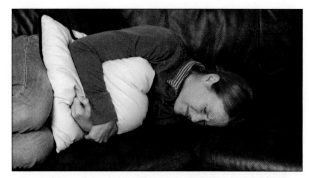

Fig. 6-11: Patients with abdominal pain might pull the knees in toward the chest or clutch at the abdomen.

Simply observing the patient can also tell you a great deal. Patients with chest pain or breathing problems often lean forward while sitting in what is called the **tripod position (Fig. 6-10)**. Patients with abdominal pain often pull their knees up toward their chest, either lying down or sitting with their back against a hard surface (**Fig. 6-11**). Loss of bladder or bowel control can indicate that the patient has had a stroke or a seizure.

Any observations should be recorded, as they not only help you evaluate the situation, but may help the health care provider who will see the patient in an entirely different environment.

ADDITIONAL RESOURCES

Once you have sized-up the scene and determined the mechanism or injury or nature of illness, you will be able to decide what additional resources are needed to keep you and the patient safe or to provide care. The number of resources will depend on any hazards at the scene, the number of injured or ill persons as well as the nature of the injuries or illnesses.

Chemical and biological suits can provide protection against HAZMATs and biological threats of varying degrees. Specialized rescue equipment may be necessary for difficult or complicated extrications.

Calling for Additional Resources

You may need to call for—
- *Advanced life support* (ALS), to provide a higher level of care for patients with a severe illness or trauma.
- Air medical transport (e.g., helicopter), to provide the fastest transport to the appropriate hospital or trauma center.
- Utilities (e.g., power/gas company), to assess, turn off or isolate dangerous downed power lines or leaking pipes.
- Fire department, to contain or extinguish fires from any source.
- Law enforcement, to direct or reroute traffic, or to maintain control with any potentially violent bystanders, patients or perpetrators.

Hazardous Materials

HAZMATs are any chemical substances or materials that can pose a threat to the health, safety and property of an individual. Any

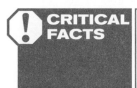

CRITICAL FACTS

Once you have sized-up the scene and determined the mechanism or injury or nature of illness, you will be able to decide what additional resources are needed to keep you and the patient safe or to provide care. The number of resources will depend on any hazards at the scene, the number of injured or ill persons as well as the nature of the injuries or illnesses.

HAZMAT poses a special risk for responding personnel. When you approach an emergency scene, look for clues that indicate the presence of HAZMATs. These include—

- Signs (placards) on vehicles, storage facilities or railroad cars identifying the presence of hazardous materials.
- Clouds of vapor.
- Spilled liquids or solids.
- Unusual odors.
- Leaking containers, bottles or gas cylinders.
- Chemical transport tanks or containers.

Those who transport or store HAZMATs in specific quantities are required by the U.S. Department of Transportation to post placards identifying the specific hazardous material, by name or number, and its specific dangers.

In order to identify the material, it is helpful to have binoculars on hand. Binoculars allow you to view the scene from a safe distance. If you do not see a placard but suspect a HAZMAT is present, try to get information before you approach the scene. Do not approach a HAZMAT scene unless you are trained to do so and have appropriate PPE such as a *self-contained breathing apparatus* (SCBA) and chemical protective suit.

If you find clues that there may be HAZMATs on the scene—

- Notify dispatch so that the appropriate personnel may be brought to the scene.
- Do not approach the scene.
- Remain uphill and upwind a safe distance from the scene.
- Await specialized resources.

For more information on HAZMATs emergencies, including training and guides that are available, refer to **Chapter 29**.

Violence

Violence can take place in a wide variety of settings, but certain factors make it much more likely to occur. These include scenes of domestic violence, fights in bars, gang fights, street fights, potential suicide or any situation where angry bystanders or family members are present. At scenes where there has been arguing, fighting or threats, the potential for violence is increased. Look for anything that indicates violence has taken place, such as broken glass, overturned furniture, weapons, or alcohol or drug use. The risk of violence may be increased in situations where there is yelling, swearing, threatening, pacing or when a person is using clenched fists or throwing objects. There may be other signs of tension, for example an awkward silence in a situation where you expect a lot of activity and noise. You may also discover a history of aggressive behavior, which increases the risk of violence.

There are times when restraining a patient may be necessary, to ensure the safety of the patient, yourself and bystanders. Restraint should be used as a last resort, however, and must be carried out only after consultation with law enforcement and medical direction. Use only as much force as is necessary to restrain the patient, and always follow local protocols. Always keep your personal safety in mind when restraining patients. For further information on the use of restraint, refer to **Chapter 5**.

If you arrive at the scene of violence or a crime, do not try to reach any patient until you are sure the scene is safe. Someone who has been shot, stabbed or sustained other injuries from violence may have severe injuries but, until the scene is safe, there is nothing you can do to provide care. For the scene to be safe, law enforcement personnel must make it secure. Wait for law enforcement to arrive and secure the scene before attempting to provide care.

Police usually gather evidence at a crime scene, so do not touch anything except what you must to provide care. Once law enforcement secures the crime scene and allows you to enter to provide care, make sure that they are aware of your presence and actions. Always have and use appropriate PPE (**Table 6-1**).

Domestic Violence

Domestic violence situations are among the most potentially dangerous scenes you may encounter as an *emergency medical responder* (EMR). Domestic violence crosses all boundaries, affecting people of all ages, races, education, socioeconomic classes and sexual orientations. However, there are certain circumstances that may indicate that domestic violence may be a factor. Any of the following conditions should lead you to suspect domestic violence and respond accordingly:

- The injured person will not admit to being abused.
- The injuries sustained do not fit the history, and the patient seems to be ashamed or embarrassed about the injuries.
- You observe injuries that involve contusions and lacerations of the face, head, neck, breasts and abdomen.
- The suspected perpetrator of the violence is unwilling to allow the injured person to give a history or be alone with *emergency medical services* (EMS) personnel.
- There are excessive delays between the injury and seeking treatment.
- The patient repeatedly uses EMS services.
- The injuries occur during pregnancy.
- Substance abuse is involved.
- There are frequent suicide gestures.

Law enforcement agencies generally send two officers to answer domestic disturbances, to reduce the potential of danger. EMRs should take a similar approach to domestic disturbances, with heightened awareness to all possible clues. For example, the calling party denies calling EMS personnel when you arrive at the door. This may be a clue that should lead you to suspect potential danger and heighten your awareness when responding to the scene.

If law enforcement has not been called, call them right away and do not approach until the police arrive and secure the scene. Your personal safety always outweighs the need to respond.

Once inside, your awareness must continue. While the police may have already secured the scene, it is appropriate for you to do so also; visually check everyone for weapons. Determine who is in the residence and where they are. Once identified, any bystanders should be asked to leave. Do not allow residents to get between you and an exit route and do not let yourself be backed into a corner. Know where your partner is at all times and ensure that your partner is equally aware of what else is going on. Look at body cues such as clenched fists, flared nostrils and flushed cheeks. If there are weapons present, ask law enforcement to intervene.

Remember that, while you were originally called to help, your presence, along with that of law enforcement, changes the dynamics of the scene.

Stay calm. Take your time and take nothing for granted. Assume control of the situation slowly. Introduce yourself, speaking directly to the patient. Explain what you are doing. Ask open-ended questions, allowing the patient to talk. Restore control to the patient. Do not be judgmental. If you can, separate yourself and the patient from the suspected perpetrator.

Table 6-1:
Responding to Specific Emergency Situations

SITUATION	APPROPRIATE BEHAVIOR
Hazardous materials	If you suspect hazardous materials, stay a safe distance away, upwind and uphill. Do not create sparks. Notify dispatch immediately.
Motor-vehicle crashes	Do not attempt a rescue until wreckage has been stabilized.

PUTTING IT ALL TOGETHER

Use the information you received from dispatch to begin your planning, but remember that it may be inaccurate or outdated. Make sure you have whatever protective equipment you will need available. Your first priority is your own safety, so look first for any hazards that might put you at risk.

After your own safety, your next priority is to keep patients and bystanders safe. This may mean redirecting traffic or preventing people from intruding on the scene. In some cases, it may mean moving the patient. A safe scene may change to a dangerous one quickly. As you care for the patient, be aware of your surroundings and be prepared to take any necessary steps to ensure your safety.

Analyze the scene to determine the number and locations of patients and also the MOI or nature of the illness. Then create a plan to provide appropriate care. If your assessment tells you that you will need help, call the appropriate personnel before beginning to provide care for the patient.

YOU ARE THE EMERGENCY MEDICAL RESPONDER

You have taken the proper precautions to make it safe for you to enter the scene and begin assessing and providing care for carbon monoxide poisoning. What if the mother and children lived in a place other than a single-family home? What additional considerations or actions might there be?

Enrichment
Dealing with Hazards at the Scene

In addition to the specific emergency situations already discussed, other hazardous scenes require special consideration **(Table 6-2)**. Remember to always expect the unexpected and make sure the scene is safe before entering. If it is not, notify the necessary agencies to do what is necessary to provide you with a safe working environment.

Table 6-2:
Additional Emergency Situations

SITUATION	APPROPRIATE BEHAVIOR
Traffic	Leave a path for arriving emergency vehicles. Put up reflectors, traffic cones, flares or lights to direct dangerous traffic away from the scene.
Fire	Never approach a burning vehicle or enter a burning building without proper equipment and training. If in a burning building, do not open hot doors or use elevators, and stay close to the floor.
Electricity	Assume all downed wires are dangerous. Do not attempt to move them. Do not touch any metal fence, metal structure or body of water in contact with a wire. Notify the fire department and power company immediately.
Water and Ice	Follow the rule of reach, throw, row then go. Never enter water or go on ice unless you are trained to do so and have proper rescue equipment.
Unsafe Structures	Do not enter structures that you suspect are unsafe. Call for trained and equipped personnel. Gather as much information as possible about the victim(s).
Natural Disasters	Report to the person in charge. Follow the rescue plan and standard operating procedures. Avoid obvious hazards and be cautious when using equipment.
Multiple Victims	Report to the person in charge. Care for victims with the most life-threatening conditions first.
Hostile Situations	If the victim or bystanders threaten you, retreat to safety. Never try to restrain, argue with or force care on a victim. Summon law enforcement personnel.
Suicide	Do not enter until summoned by law enforcement personnel. Do not touch anything except what you must to provide care.
Hostage Situations	Do not enter until summoned and cleared by law enforcement personnel. Gather as much information as possible about the victims.

Traffic

Traffic is often the most common danger you and other emergency personnel will encounter. If you drive to a collision scene, always try to park where your vehicle will not block other traffic, such as an ambulance that needs to reach the scene. The only time you should park in a roadway or block traffic is—

Continued on next page

Enrichment
Dealing with Hazards at the Scene (continued)

- To protect an injured person.
- To protect any rescuers, including yourself.
- To warn oncoming traffic, if the situation is not clearly visible.

Others can help you put reflectors, traffic cones, flares or lights along the road. These items should be placed well back of the scene to enable oncoming motorists to stop or slow down in time **(Fig. 6-12)**.

Emergency personnel are sometimes injured or killed by traffic at emergency scenes. In fact, hazards on the roadway are the number-one cause of death among EMS workers. If you are not a law enforcement officer, and dangerous traffic makes the scene unsafe, wait for more help to arrive before providing care.

There are several important reasons to control traffic at the scene: to protect the crash scene from further potential collisions, prevent injury to the rescue team, ensure minimal

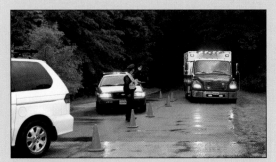

Fig. 6-12: You may have to control traffic to maintain a safe scene if the emergency occurs on or near a roadway.

disruption and allow emergency vehicles to reach the scene. On arrival, request the assistance of additional law enforcement and fire services to help control the scene.

Fire

Any fire can be dangerous. Make sure the local fire department has been summoned. Only firefighters, who are highly trained and properly equipped against fire and smoke, should approach a fire. Do not let others approach. Gather information to help the responding fire and EMS units. Find out the possible number of people trapped, their location, the fire's cause and whether any explosives or chemicals are present. Give this information to emergency personnel when they arrive. If you are not trained to fight fires or lack the necessary equipment, follow these basic guidelines:

- Do not approach a burning vehicle.
- Never enter a burning or smoke-filled building.
- If you are in a building that is on fire, always check doors before opening them with the back of your hand. If a door is hot to the touch, do not open it.
- Avoid smoke and fumes by staying close to the floor.
- Never use an elevator in a building that may be burning.

Downed Electrical Lines

Downed electrical lines also present a major hazard to responders. Always look for downed wires at a scene, and always treat them as dangerous. If you find downed wires, follow these guidelines:

- Move the crowd back from the danger zone. The safe area should be established at a point twice the length of the span of the wire (i.e., the distance between the poles).
- Never attempt to move downed wires.
- Notify the fire department and the power company immediately. Always assume that downed wires are energized, or live. Even if they are not energized at first, they may become energized later.
- If downed wires are in contact with a vehicle, do not touch the vehicle and do not let others touch it. Tell anyone in the vehicle to stay still and stay inside the vehicle. Never attempt to remove people from a vehicle with downed wires across it, no matter how seriously injured they may seem.
- Do not touch any metal fence, metal structure or body of water in contact with a downed wire. Wait for the power company to shut off the power source.

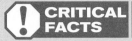 **CRITICAL FACTS** | Hazards on the roadway are the number-one cause of death among EMS workers.

Water and Ice

Water and ice also can be serious hazards. To help a conscious person in the water, always follow the basic rule of *"reach, throw, row then go."* You may reach out to someone in trouble with a branch, a pole or even your hand, being careful not to be pulled into the water. When the person grasps the object, lean back and pull the person to safety.

If you cannot reach the person, try to throw the person something nearby that floats. If you have a rope available, attach an object that floats to one end, such as a life jacket, plastic jug, ice chest or empty gas can. Never enter a body of water to rescue someone unless you have been trained in water rescue, and then only as a last resort. If possible, you can use a boat to get closer (row), but not close enough that the patient can grab the side of the boat and tip it. The "go" part of this technique is only for those who can perform deep-water rescue.

Fast-moving water is extremely dangerous and often occurs with floods, hurricanes and low head dams. Ice is also treacherous. It can break under your weight, and the cold water beneath can quickly overcome even the best swimmers. Never enter fast-moving water or venture out on ice unless you are trained in this type of rescue. Such rescues require careful planning and proper equipment. Wait until trained personnel arrive.

Unsafe Structures

Buildings and other structures, such as mines, wells and unreinforced trenches, can become unsafe because of fire, explosions, natural disasters, deterioration or other causes. An unsafe building or structure is one in which—
- The air may contain debris or hazardous gases.
- There is a possibility of being trapped or injured by collapsed walls, weakened floors and other debris.

Try to establish the exact or probable location of anyone in the structure. Gather as much information as you can, call for appropriate help and wait for the arrival of personnel who are properly trained and equipped.

Natural Disasters

Natural disasters include tornadoes, hurricanes, earthquakes, forest fires and floods **(Fig. 6-13)**. Rescue efforts after a natural disaster are usually coordinated by local resources until they become overwhelmed. Then the rescue efforts are coordinated by a government agency such as the Federal Emergency Management Agency (FEMA). Typically, you first would report to the person or people in charge at the scene; then, work with the disaster response team and follow the rescue plan.

Natural disasters pose more risks than you might realize. Often, more injuries and deaths result from electricity, HAZMATs, rising water and other dangers than from the disaster itself. When responding to a natural disaster, be sure to carefully size-up the scene, avoid obvious hazards and use caution when operating rescue equipment. Never use gasoline-powered equipment, such as chain saws, generators and pumps in confined spaces.

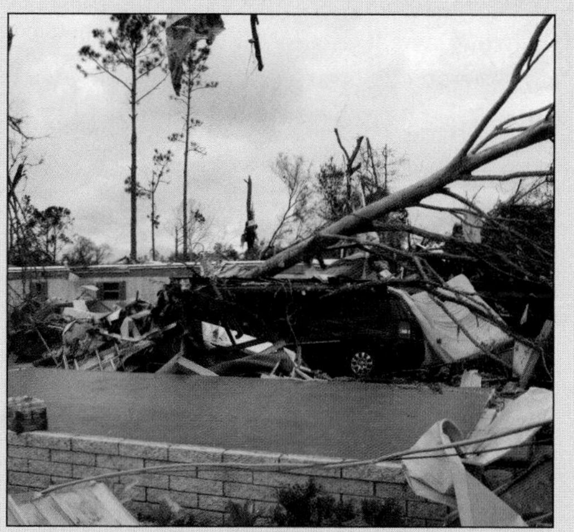

Fig. 6-13: When responding to a natural disaster, be sure to carefully size-up the scene and avoid obvious hazards. *Courtesy of Captain Phil Kleinberg, EMT-P, Lake-Sumter EMS.*

Multiple Patients

Scenes that involve more than one patient are referred to as *multiple-casualty incidents* (MCIs). Such scenes make your task more complex, since you must determine who needs immediate care and who can wait for more help to arrive. MCIs are covered in more detail in **Chapter 30**.

Hostile Situations

Environmental factors, such as HAZMAT, electricity and unsafe structures, are not the only dangers you may encounter. You may sometimes encounter a hostile patient or family member. Any unusual or hostile behavior, including rage, may be a result of the emergency, injury, illness or fear. Many patients are afraid of losing control

Continued on next page

Enrichment
Dealing with Hazards at the Scene (continued)

and may show this as anger. Hostile behavior also may result from the use of alcohol or other drugs, lack of oxygen or an underlying medical condition **(Fig. 6-14)**.

If a patient needing care is hostile toward you, try to calmly explain who you are and that you are there to help. Remember that you cannot provide care without the patient's consent. If the person accepts your offer to help, keep talking as you assess the patient's condition. When the patient realizes you are not a threat, the hostility usually goes away.

If the patient refuses your care or threatens you, withdraw from the scene. Never try to restrain, argue with or force care on a patient. If the patient does not let you provide care, wait for more advanced medical care. Sometimes a close friend or a family member will be able to reassure a hostile patient and convince the patient to accept your care.

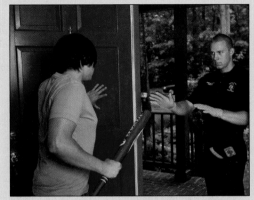

Fig. 6-14: If a patient or person with the patient becomes hostile, remain calm and remember that you cannot provide care without consent.

However, family members or friends who are angry or hysterical can make your job more difficult. Sometimes they may not allow you to provide care. At other times, they may try to move the patient before he or she has been stabilized. A terrified parent may cling to a child and refuse to let you help. When family members act this way, they often feel confused, guilty and frightened. Be understanding and explain the care you are providing. By remaining calm and professional, you will help calm them.

Hostile crowds are a threat that can develop when you least expect it. As a rule, you cannot reason with a hostile crowd. If you decide the crowd at a scene is hostile, wait at a safe distance until law enforcement and EMS personnel arrive. Approach the scene only when police officers declare it safe and ask you to help. Never approach a hostile crowd unless you are trained in crowd management and supported by other trained personnel.

Suicide

Never enter a suicide scene unless police have made it secure. If the person is obviously dead, be careful not to touch anything at the scene such as a weapon, medicine bottle, suicide note or other evidence. If the scene is safe and the person is still alive, provide emergency care as needed. Concentrate on your care for the patient and leave the rest to law enforcement personnel.

Never approach an armed suicidal person unless you are a law enforcement officer trained in crisis intervention. Approach only if you have been summoned to provide care once the scene has been secured.

If you happen to be on the scene when an unarmed individual threatens suicide, try to reassure and calm the person. Make sure that appropriate personnel have been notified. You cannot physically restrain a suicidal person without medical or legal authorization. Listen to the person and try to keep the person talking until help arrives. Try to be understanding. Do not dare the person to act, or trivialize the person's feelings. Unless your personal safety is threatened, never leave a suicidal person alone.

Hostage Situation

If you encounter a hostage situation, your first priority is to not become a hostage yourself. Do not approach the scene unless you are specially trained to handle these situations. Assess the scene from a safe distance and call for law enforcement personnel. A police officer trained in hostage negotiations should take charge.

Try to get any information from bystanders that may help law enforcement personnel. Ask about the number of hostages, any weapons seen and other possible hazards. Report any information to the first law enforcement official on the scene. Remain at a safe distance until law enforcement personnel summon you.

7 Primary Assessment

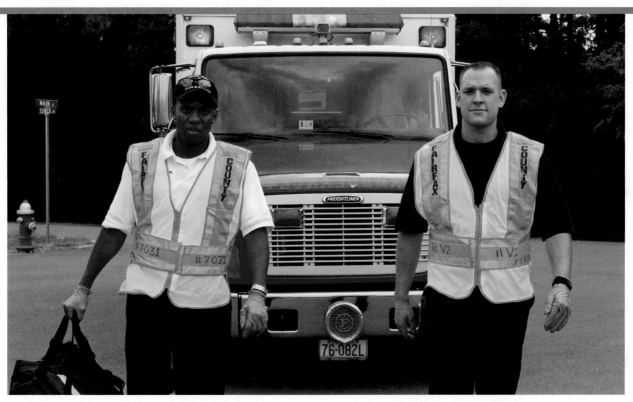

))) YOU ARE THE EMERGENCY MEDICAL RESPONDER

Your rescue unit arrives at a scene to find a distraught mother who says, "I can't wake my baby up." The infant appears to be unconscious and is turning blue. How would you respond? What are your immediate priorities? What should you do first?

Key Terms

Agonal gasp: Isolated or infrequent gasping in the absence of other breathing in an unconscious person; can occur after the heart has stopped beating. Agonal gasps are not breathing.

Airway: The pathway for air from the mouth and nose through the pharynx, larynx and trachea and into the lungs.

AVPU: Mnemonic describing the four levels of patient response: Alert, Verbal, Painful and Unresponsive.

Brachial artery: The main artery of the upper arm; runs from the shoulder down to the bend of the elbow.

Breathing rate: Term used to describe the number of breaths per minute.

Capillary refill: A technique for estimating how the body is reacting to injury or illness by checking the ability of the capillaries to refill with blood.

Carotid artery: The major artery located on either side of the neck that supplies blood to the brain.

CPR breathing barrier: Devices that allow for artificial ventilations without direct mouth-to-mouth contact; includes resuscitation masks and *bag-valve-mask resuscitators* (BVMs).

Cyanotic: Showing bluish discoloration of the skin, nailbeds and mucous membranes due to insufficient levels of oxygen in the blood.

Glasgow Coma Scale (GCS): A measure of *level of consciousness* (LOC) based on eye opening, verbal response and motor response.

Hypoxic: Having below-normal concentrations of oxygen in the organs and tissues of the body.

Level of consciousness (LOC): A person's state of awareness, ranging from being fully alert to unconscious; also referred to as mental status.

Minute volume: The amount of air breathed in a minute; calculated by multiplying the volume of air inhaled at each breath (in mL) by the number of breaths per minute.

Perfusion: The circulation of blood through the body or through a particular body part for the purpose of exchanging oxygen and nutrients with carbon dioxide and other wastes.

Primary (initial) assessment: A check for conditions that are an immediate threat to a patient's life.

Pulse: The beat felt from each rhythmic contraction of the heart.

Respiratory arrest: A condition in which there is an absence of breathing.

Respiratory distress: A condition in which a person is having difficulty breathing or requires extra effort to breathe.

Signs: Term used to describe any observable evidence of injury or illness, such as bleeding or unusual skin color.

Signs of life: A term sometimes used to describe breathing and a pulse in an unresponsive patient.

Stoma: A surgical opening in the body; a stoma may be created in the neck following surgery on the trachea to allow the patient to breathe.

Symptoms: What the patient reports experiencing, such as pain, nausea, headache or shortness of breath.

Vital signs: Important information about the patient's condition obtained by checking respiratory rate, pulse and blood pressure.

Learning Objectives

After reading this chapter, and completing the class activities, you will have the information needed to—

- Summarize the reasons for forming a general impression of the patient.
- Explain the purpose of the primary (initial) assessment.
- Describe methods for assessing a patient's *level of consciousness* (LOC).
- Explain the differences in assessing the LOC of an adult, a child and an infant.
- Describe methods of assessing whether a patient is breathing.
- Distinguish a patient with adequate breathing from a patient with inadequate breathing.
- Describe the methods used to assess circulatory status.
- Explain the differences in obtaining a pulse in an adult, a child and an infant.
- Explain the need to assess a patient for external bleeding.
- Describe how to assess a patient for severe bleeding.
- Describe how to assess breathing rate and quality, pulse rate and quality, and skin appearance.
- Describe how to establish priorities for care including recognition and management of shock.

Skill Objectives

After reading this chapter, and completing the class activities, you should be able to—

- Perform a primary assessment.
- Demonstrate how to assess LOC.
- Demonstrate how to open the airway using the jaw-thrust (without head extension) maneuver.
- Demonstrate how to use a resuscitation mask.

INTRODUCTION

In previous chapters, you learned how to prepare for an emergency, the precautions to take when approaching the scene and how to recognize a dangerous situation. You also learned about your roles and responsibilities. As an *emergency medical responder* (EMR), you can make a difference in an emergency—you may even save a life. But to do this, you must learn how to provide care for an injured or ill person, and set priorities for that care.

When an emergency occurs, one of the most essential aspects of your job is the **primary (initial) assessment**. The primary assessment is the process used to quickly identify those conditions that represent an immediate threat to the patient's life, so that you may properly treat them as they are found. An effective primary assessment includes creating a general impression of the patient, checking for responsiveness and checking **airway**, breathing and circulatory status.

THE IMPORTANCE OF SCENE SIZE-UP

Once you recognize that an emergency has occurred and decide to act, always remember the importance of sizing up the scene first. A primary assessment should never occur until after the scene size-up. The four main components to consider during a scene size-up include—

1. Scene safety.
2. The *mechanism of injury* (MOI) or nature of illness.
3. The number of patients involved.
4. The resources needed.

Ensuring Scene Safety

Always begin by making sure the scene is safe for you, other rescuers, the patient(s) and any bystanders, as discussed in **Chapter 6**. Take the necessary precautions when working in a dangerous environment. If you do not have the necessary training and equipment, do not approach the patient—summon the appropriate personnel. Keep assessing the situation, and, if conditions change, you then may be able to approach the patient. Remember, nothing is gained by risking your safety. An emergency that begins with one injured or ill person could end up with two if you are hurt.

Determining Mechanism of Injury or Nature of the Illness

When attempting to determine the MOI or nature of the illness, you must look around the scene for clues to what caused the emergency and the extent of the damage (**Fig. 7-1**). Consider the force that may have been involved in creating an injury. These considerations will help you to think about the possible types and extent of the patient's injuries. Take in the whole picture. How a motor vehicle is damaged or the presence of nearby objects, such as shattered glass, a fallen ladder or a spilled medicine container, may suggest what happened. If the patient is unconscious, determining the MOI or nature of the illness may be the only way you can identify what occurred.

Recognizing Patients

When you size-up the scene, look carefully for more than one patient. You may not see everyone at first. For example, in a motor-vehicle collision,

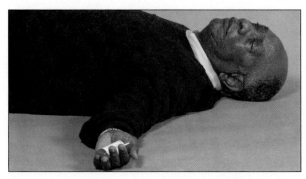

Fig. 7-1: Search the scene for clues to determine what caused the emergency or injury and the extent of the damage.

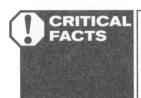

CRITICAL FACTS

Primary assessment is essential to the job of an EMR to ensure proper care. However, a scene size-up to evaluate safety, MOI or nature of illness, number of patients and resources needed should always be done first.

To determine the MOI or nature of illness, check the scene for clues and consider the force that may have been involved.

an open door may be a clue that someone has left the vehicle or was thrown from it. If one patient is bleeding or screaming loudly, you may overlook another patient who is unconscious. It is also easy in an emergency situation to overlook small children or infants if they are not crying.

Summoning More Advanced Personnel

At times, you may be unsure if more advanced medical personnel are needed. For example, the patient may ask you not to call an ambulance or transport vehicle to avoid embarrassment about creating a scene. Your training as an EMR will help you make the decision. As a general rule, summon more advanced medical personnel for any of the following conditions:

- Unconsciousness or altered *level of consciousness* (**LOC**)
- Breathing problems (difficulty breathing or no breathing)
- Chest pain, discomfort or pressure lasting more than a few minutes, that goes away and comes back or that radiates to the shoulder, arm, neck, jaw, stomach or back
- Persistent abdominal pain or pressure
- No **pulse**
- Severe external bleeding (bleeding that spurts or gushes steadily from a wound)
- Vomiting blood or passing blood
- Severe (critical) burns
- Suspected poisoning
- Seizures
- Stroke (sudden weakness on one side of the face/facial droop, sudden weakness on one side of the body, sudden slurred speech or trouble getting words out or a sudden severe headache)
- Suspected or obvious injuries to the head, neck or spine
- Painful, swollen, deformed areas (suspected broken bone) or an open fracture

It is impossible to provide a complete or definitive list—there are always exceptions. Trust your instincts and follow local protocols. It is better to have more advanced medical personnel respond to a non-emergency than arrive at an emergency too late to help.

The Role of Bystanders

Do not underestimate the role of bystanders in an emergency situation. Scene safety is always first and foremost, so look for bystanders who are in potential danger and instruct them to move to safety. Ask anyone present how many people may be involved in the emergency; bystanders may provide essential information to help you identify patients. Bystanders may also be able to tell you what happened or help in other ways. A bystander who knows the patients may know whether they have any medical conditions or allergies. Bystanders can also meet and direct ambulance to your location.

GENERAL IMPRESSION OF THE PATIENT

Once you have conducted a scene size-up and assessed that the scene is safe for you and your colleagues, your first step in the primary assessment is to determine what has occurred and what is happening with the patient—a general impression. This initial general impression will determine your immediate course of action.

Questions to ask yourself include—
- Does the patient look sick or injured?
- Is there a noticeable MOI?
- Is the patient conscious or alert?
- Does the patient appear to be breathing?
- Is the patient bleeding?
- What is the patient's approximate age?

Your general impression may alert you to a serious problem that requires additional resources or to a minor problem you can care for easily. You will discover these problems by looking for any **signs** and **symptoms** the patient may have. Signs are evidence of injury or illness that you can observe, such as bleeding or unusual skin appearance. Symptoms are what the patient reports experiencing, such as pain, nausea, headache or shortness of breath.

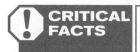 **CRITICAL FACTS**
Many conditions warrant summoning advanced medical personnel. These include breathing problems, prolonged chest pain, seizures and suspected head, neck or spinal injuries—to name a few.

As you perform the primary assessment, check for immediate life-threatening conditions. This means assessing whether the patient—

- Is conscious.
- Has an open and clear airway.
- Is breathing.
- Has a pulse.
- Is not bleeding severely.

As you assess the patient, determine if spinal precautions are necessary based on your general impression and the suspected MOI. If the scene suggests an MOI in which the patient may have a head, neck or spinal injury, you must ensure that the patient's head and neck do not move by using manual stabilization and the jaw-thrust (without head extension) maneuver.

First, speak to the patient. This may be to warn the patient to remain still if there is a situation that could cause damage to the head, neck or spine. For example, in a motor-vehicle collision or a fall off a ladder the patient would need to remain still. Identify yourself as a rescuer and state that you are there to help. Obtain consent from the patient before beginning the primary assessment and providing care.

When approaching a patient, you should try to approach from the front so that the patient can see you without needing to turn his or her head **(Fig. 7-2)**. This is especially important in the case of a suspected head, neck or spinal injury.

Ask questions such as—

- What happened?
- What is your name?
- Where are you?
- What day of the week is it?

Age Delineation

As part of gaining a general impression, attempt to determine the patient's age. For the purpose of this text, an adult is considered anyone approximately 12 years old or older. A child is considered 1 to about 12 years of age, and an infant is under 1 year of age. The approximate age of the patient will have an effect on the care you provide.

For use of *automated external defibrillators* (AEDs)–based on *Food and Drug Administration* (FDA) approval of these devices–a child is considered to be between the ages of 1 and 8 or weighing less than 55 pounds. If precise age or weight is not known, the responder should use his or her best judgment and not delay care in determining age.

RESPONSIVENESS
Establishing Responsiveness

When approaching a patient, check for responsiveness and assess his or her LOC. A person's LOC can range from being fully alert to being unconscious.

Fig. 7-2: When approaching a patient, approach from the front so the patient can see you without needing to turn his or her head.

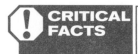

CRITICAL FACTS Always check for life-threatening conditions: lack of consciousness, abnormal breathing, blocked airway, no pulse or severe bleeding.

The answers to these questions will give you an idea of the patient's LOC and orientation. Keep in mind that certain pre-existing conditions and diseases may be responsible for a patient's orientation. If possible, speak with family members to establish if this is usual behavior for the patient or if it represents a change.

Pediatric Considerations

Be aware that children and infants may be fully aware of you but unable to answer your questions. This response can be for a variety of reasons. Children may not be able to speak or understand your questions, they may not speak or understand English, they may be too frightened of the situation or of you as a stranger or they may be crying too hard and be unable to stop. If possible, try to assess a young child or an infant in a parent's or guardian's arms or lap. Approach slowly and gently, and give the child or infant some time to get used to you, if possible. Use the child's name, if you know it.

Geriatric Considerations

In elderly patients, certain conditions and diseases may be responsible for changes in LOC. For example, a patient with dementia may be confused by your questions. The patient also may not speak or understand English. When you think this might be the case, speak with family members if possible to establish if this is usual behavior for the patient or if it represents a change. Also, do not assume that difficulty responding to questions about time and current events necessarily means the patient is disoriented. It is not unusual for people who live alone to lose track of time, and some may not follow current events. In this case, alter your questions so that they address information related to the patient's immediate environment and the circumstances surrounding why you were called in order to truly gauge the patient's orientation.

Patient Response—AVPU

In describing a patient's LOC, a four-level, mnemonic scale is traditionally used, referred to as **AVPU**. The letters A, V, P and U each refer to a stage of awareness (**Table 7-1**).

Table 7-1:
Levels of Consciousness

LEVEL	CHARACTERISTIC BEHAVIOR
Alert	Able to respond appropriately to questions
Verbal	Responds appropriately to verbal stimuli
Painful	Only responds to painful stimuli
Unresponsive	Does not respond

- **A**lert: Patients who are alert are aware of their surroundings, able to acknowledge your presence and able to respond to your questions.
- **V**erbal: Sometimes the patient is only able to react to sounds, such as your voice. The patient's eyes may be closed but they open when hearing your voice or when the patient is told to open them. The patient may appear to be lapsing into unconsciousness. A patient who has to be stimulated by sound to respond is described as responding to verbal stimuli.
- **P**ainful: A patient who does not respond to verbal stimuli or commands, but does respond when someone inflicts pain, is described as responding to painful stimuli. Pinching the earlobe or the skin above the collarbone are examples of painful stimuli used to try to get a response (**Fig. 7-3**). Be cautious however

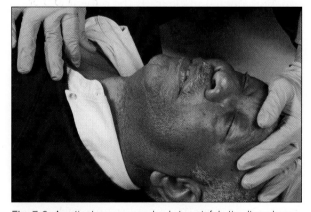

Fig. 7-3: A patient may respond only to painful stimuli, such as a pinch or pull of the skin above the collarbone.

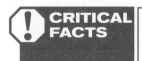 **CRITICAL FACTS** To assess LOC, ask simple questions such as "What is your name?" LOC can range from being fully alert to unconsciousness. Always approach a patient from the front to avoid head turning.

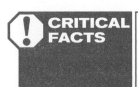
about pinching the earlobe in patients who may have neck trauma, as they may try to move their head away from an irritating stimulus. Instead, forcefully pinch or squeeze the fleshy section of skin between the patient's thumb and forefinger.

- **U**nresponsive: Patients who do not respond to any stimuli are described as being unconscious or unresponsive to stimuli.

Once you have assessed the victim's LOC, the next thing you must do is to check the victim's airway, breathing and circulation (pulse, severe bleeding and skin characteristics).

AIRWAY STATUS

The pathway for air passage between the mouth and nose to the lungs is called the *airway*. Without an open airway, the patient cannot breathe. A patient who can speak or cry is conscious, has an open airway, is breathing and has a pulse. However, the patient may still be at risk of a compromised airway.

Assess the airway with the unconscious patient face-up. First, verify if the airway is patent (open and clear). If the patient is breathing (chest is rising and falling) or the patient is speaking to you and aware of the surroundings, then you need to ensure that the airway remains open and clear. Continue to assess the patient's respiratory status throughout the period that you provide care. The airway can become blocked by fluids, solid objects, the tongue or swollen tissue caused by trauma or severe allergic reaction.

Determine whether there is a need for any interventions to establish or maintain patency. For example, does the patient require suctioning to remove fluids or a finger sweep to remove solid objects or debris? Will an oral (or nasal) airway be necessary to prevent the tongue from falling back in the throat and blocking the airway? Refer to **Chapter 11** for information on suctioning and the use of airways.

If the victim is wearing dentures, leave them in place unless they become loose and block the airway. Dentures help support the victim's mouth and cheeks, making it easier to seal the resuscitation mask if you need to provide ventilations.

Opening the Mouth

If you need to open the mouth to clear the airway of fluids or debris and the patient is unresponsive, use the cross-finger technique to open the patient's mouth with a gloved hand:

- Kneel beside the patient near his or her head.
- Cross the thumb and forefinger of one hand.
- Put your thumb on the patient's lower teeth and your forefinger on the patient's upper teeth (**Fig. 7-4**).
- Use a scissors motion to open the mouth.

Assessing Airway and Breathing in the Responsive Patient

If the patient speaks, you know that the airway is functional, but the patient may still be at risk. If a patient's breathing is noisy, the sounds can indicate the type of problem. For example, stridor (high-pitched whistling sound) can indicate that the airway is narrowing through swelling, a foreign body or trauma. Continually reassess and monitor the patient's breathing because breathing status, rate and quality can change suddenly.

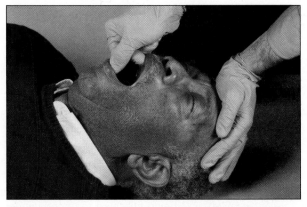

Fig. 7-4: The cross-finger technique uses a scissoring motion of the thumb and forefinger to open an unresponsive patient's mouth.

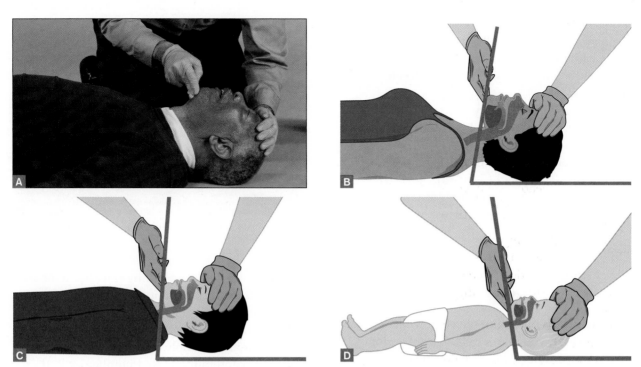

Fig. 7-5, A–D: **(A)** Head-tilt/chin-lift technique; **(B)** Correct angling of head-tilt/chin-lift technique in an adult; **(C)** Correct angling of head-tilt/chin-lift technique in a child; **(D)** Correct angling of head-tilt/chin-lift technique in an infant

Assessing Airway and Breathing in the Unresponsive Patient

It is more difficult to tell if an unconscious patient has an open airway. To open the airway for a patient who has not suffered an injury to the head, neck or spine, open and maintain the airway using the head-tilt/chin-lift technique. For patients of all ages, tilt the head back and lift the chin to open the airway. Do not tilt a child's or an infant's head back as far as an adult's. Tilt a child's head slightly past the neutral position and tilt an infant's head to the neutral position.

Opening the Airway—Head-Tilt/Chin-Lift Technique

To open the airway with the head-tilt/chin-lift technique—
1. Kneel beside the patient's head and neck.
2. Place one hand on the patient's forehead.
3. Place the fingertips of two or three fingers of your other hand under the bony part of the patient's lower jaw near the chin. If the patient is a child or an infant, use only one or two fingers.
4. Use firm backward pressure from the palm of your hand to tilt the head back while lifting the jaw up with the fingertips to extend the

chin forward (**Fig. 7-5, A–B**). If the patient is a child, only tilt the head slightly past neutral (**Fig. 7-5, C**). For an infant, only tilt the head to a neutral position (**Fig. 7-5, D**).
5. Keep pressure on the patient's forehead to help maintain the airway in an open position.

Opening the Airway—Jaw-Thrust (Without Head Extension) Maneuver

To open the airway for someone who has a suspected head, neck or spinal injury, use the jaw-thrust (without head extension) maneuver (**Fig. 7-6**).

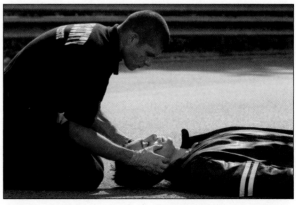

Fig. 7-6: Jaw-thrust (without head extension) maneuver without a mask

This technique moves the tongue away from the back of the throat, allowing air to enter the lungs without moving the head and neck. After opening the airway, look, listen and feel for breathing.

If you suspect an injury to the head, neck or spine, open the airway by using the jaw-thrust (without head extension) maneuver, to keep the head and neck in a neutral position. Do not move the head to the side, forward or back. Note that if you cannot establish an open airway using the jaw-thrust (without head extension) maneuver; use the head-tilt/chin-lift technique instead.

BREATHING STATUS

If the patient is breathing the chest will rise and fall. However, you must also *listen* and *feel* for signs of breathing. Position your ear over the patient's mouth and nose so you can hear and feel air as it escapes. At the same time, watch the chest rise and fall. Look, listen and feel for breathing for *no more than 10 seconds*.

Check the patient's neck to see if he or she breathes through a **stoma**. A stoma is an opening in the neck to allow a person to breathe after surgery to remove part or all of the larynx (voice box) or other structures of the airway (**Fig. 7-7**). The person may breathe *partially* through this opening, or may breathe *entirely* through the stoma instead of through the nose and mouth. Use a round, pediatric mask if you need to provide ventilations.

Isolated or infrequent gasping in the absence of other breathing in an unconscious person may be **agonal gasps** which can occur after the heart has stopped beating. Agonal gasps are not breathing. Do not confuse this with breathing. Care for the patient as if there is no breathing at all.

If the patient is breathing, assess the *rate* and *depth* of the breathing. A healthy adult breathes regularly, quietly and effortlessly. The normal **breathing rate** for an adult is between 12 and 20 breaths per minute. However, some people breathe slightly slower or faster. You can usually observe the chest rising and falling.

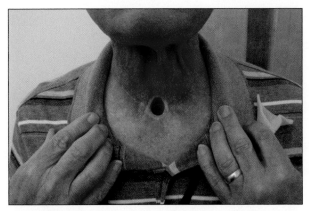

Fig. 7-7: A stoma is an opening in the neck that allows a person to breathe. *Courtesy of the International Association of Laryngectomees.*

To determine the breathing rate, listen for the sounds as the patient inhales and exhales. Count the number of times the patient breathes (inhaling and exhaling is one breath) for either 15 seconds and multiply that number by 4 or 30 seconds and multiply that number by 2. If the patient is awake and alert, do not to let the patient know or disclose when you are observing breathing, as the patient may become self-conscious. This can cause a change in breathing pattern and not provide an accurate assessment. If the patient is breathing, continue to maintain an open airway.

Pediatric Considerations

Children and infants breathe more quickly than adults. Children can breathe up to 30 breaths per minute, while infants can have a respiratory rate up to 50 breaths per minute. While counting the breaths, assess whether breathing is shallow, deep or normal, and whether the child or infant appears to be having difficulty breathing. Normal (effective) breathing appears effortless. Keep in mind that infants have periodic breathing, so changes in the pattern of breathing are normal. Also, agonal gasps do not occur frequently in children.

As with adults, if a child or an infant is breathing spontaneously, you must still reassess regularly to ensure that the breathing status does not change.

Breathing rate may be abnormal for the patient's age, meaning either too slow or too

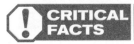 **CRITICAL FACTS** | Look, listen and feel for breathing for no more than 10 seconds.

Table 7-2:
Normal Breathing Rates

AGE	NUMBER OF BREATHS PER MINUTE	ADDITIONAL NOTES
Adults (12 years old or older)	12 to 20	• Normal chest rise and fall • Quiet breathing (no abnormal breathing sounds) • No great effort of breathing • Rates may alter due to emotional and physical conditions
Children (1 to about 12 years old)	15 to 30	• Sometimes breathe irregularly, so may need to assess for 1 minute and repeat frequently • Rates may alter due to emotional and physical conditions
Infants (under 1 year of age)	25 to 50	• Have periodic breathing (periods of rapid, shallow breathing that occurs during sleep; normal for infants)

fast. Respirations may be too slow: less than 8 per minute for adults, less than 10 per minute for children and less than 20 per minute for infants. Or they may be too fast: greater than 20 per minute for adults, greater than 30 per minute for children and greater than 60 per minute for infants.

Depth of breathing may also be abnormal, with shallow movement of the chest as it rises and falls. Abnormal breathing may be noisy. There may be a gurgling noise without secretions in the mouth or wheezing. Other abnormal breath sounds include whistling sounds, crowing sounds or snoring.

The amount of effort a conscious patient puts into breathing can be observed by watching to see if the patient is using the accessory muscles, the muscles in the neck, between the ribs and/or the abdomen, to breathe. Nasal flaring is another indication of difficulty breathing, as is the tripod position, where the patient sits and leans forward, bracing both arms on knees or an adjacent surface for support to aid breathing.

Administer emergency oxygen or provide ventilations as appropriate if the patient is having trouble breathing. This would be necessary if the patient is—

- Unresponsive. Monitor the patient's airway to ensure that respirations are continuing and are effective.
- **Hypoxic.** Pale, cool, clammy, moist skin is an early sign of inadequate oxygenation.
- **Cyanotic.** The patient is not receiving adequate oxygen. This is a clear but late sign of inadequate oxygenation. The mouth, lips and nailbeds would appear blue in color.
- Breathing very shallow respirations. The patient is likely not receiving an adequate supply of oxygen.
- Breathing increasingly slow. Oxygen intake will be dropping and the patient is likely not receiving an adequate supply of oxygen.
- Tolerant of assisted ventilation. For those who are not tolerant of assisted ventilation, you can use a blow-by technique. Refer to **Chapter 12** for more information.

It is important to remember that the respiratory status of a patient can change suddenly.

If the victim is not breathing and the cause is the result of a drowning or another respiratory cause such as hypoxia or a drug overdose, give 2 ventilations. Also give 2 ventilations for children and infants unless it is a witnessed sudden collapse. For a witnessed

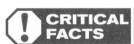 **CRITICAL FACTS** | It is important to remember that the respiratory status of a patient can change suddenly.

sudden collapse, skip the 2 initial ventilations. Provide ventilations using a resuscitation mask or BVM. These **CPR breathing barriers** can help protect against disease transmission when performing CPR or giving ventilations to a patient.

Resuscitation Mask

To use a resuscitation mask, select the proper size for the patient (adult, child or infant), then—

- Position yourself beside the patient's head and neck and assemble the mask by attaching the one-way valve to the mask if necessary.
- Position the resuscitation mask over the patient's mouth and nose.
- Seal the mask.
- Open the airway by tilting the head back and lifting the chin.
- Blow into the mask (**Fig. 7-8**).
  - Each ventilation should last about 1 second and make the chest clearly rise.

See **Chapter 10** for more information about use of breathing devices and artificial ventilations.

If breathing is too slow for the age of the patient, speak to the patient; response to verbal stimuli may increase breathing. If the patient is unresponsive, painful stimuli may increase breathing. If these work in regulating the respirations, monitor the patient to ensure the respiratory rate does not drop again. If the patient is not breathing, the patient will likely need assistance. Assist breathing by either giving ventilations or administering emergency oxygen, if available.

Someone with asthma or emphysema who is in **respiratory distress** may try to do

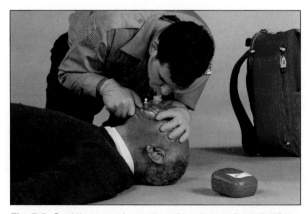

Fig. 7-8: Seal the properly positioned mask over the patient's mouth and nose, use the head-tilt/chin-lift technique to open the airway and blow into the mask.

Bag-Valve-Mask Resuscitators

Bag-valve-mask resuscitators (BVMs) are difficult to use by a single rescuer. Two *emergency medical responders* (EMRs) should provide ventilations with a BVM: one to establish and maintain the airway and seal of the mask, and the other to deliver ventilations by squeezing the bag. EMRs should not use the BVM during one-rescuer CPR. Instead, they should use a technique, such as mouth-to-mask, that minimizes the need for changes in position and minimizes interruptions of chest compressions during CPR.

Only responders who are well trained in—and have frequent opportunities to perform—one-rescuer BVM should consider using this technique. These responders need to continuously monitor their efforts to ensure adequate ventilations and change to an alternate method if necessary.

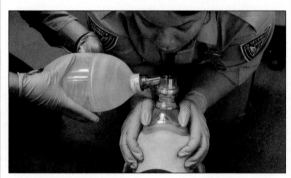

When providing BVM ventilations, one responder maintains the airway and seals the mask while the other delivers ventilations.

pursed-lip breathing. Have the person assume a position of comfort. After he or she inhales, have the person slowly exhale out through the lips, pursed as though blowing out candles. This creates back pressure, which can help open airways slightly until more advanced medical personnel arrive.

If the patient is not breathing at all (**respiratory arrest**), but has a pulse, provide ventilations with a resuscitation mask and administer emergency oxygen, if available. If additional EMRs and equipment are available, use a BVM. Once you have begun giving ventilations, continue until the patient begins to breathe spontaneously and adequately or until more advanced medical personnel take over.

Table 7-3:
Artificial Ventilation Rates

AGE	NUMBER OF VENTILATIONS PER MINUTE*
Adult (12 years old and older)	About 12 (1 ventilation about every 5 seconds)
Child (1 year to about 12 years old)	About 20 (1 ventilation about every 5 seconds)
Infant (under 1 year of age)	About 20 (1 ventilation about every 5 seconds)
Newborn	30 to 60 (1 ventilation about every 1–2 seconds)

*Each ventilation should be approximately 1 second in duration.

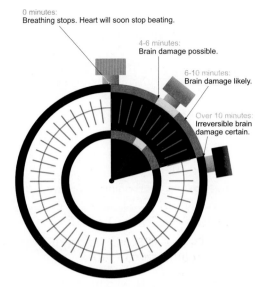

0 minutes:
Breathing stops. Heart will soon stop beating.

4-6 minutes:
Brain damage possible.

6-10 minutes:
Brain damage likely.

Over 10 minutes:
Irreversible brain damage certain.

Fig. 7-9: Time is critical in life-threatening emergencies.

Table 7-4:
Respiratory Status and Providing Care

SIGNS	RESPIRATORY STATUS	PROVIDING CARE
• Normal rate and depth of breathing • Absence of abnormal breath sounds • Air moves freely in and out of the chest. • Normal skin color	• Breathing is adequate.	• Monitor breathing for any changes. • Administer emergency oxygen, if available.
• Rate and/or depth of breathing is slower or faster than normal range. • Breathing is shallow. • There are no breath sounds or breath sounds are diminished. • Breathing is noisy: crowing, stridor, snoring, gurgling or gasping. • Cyanosis (blue or gray skin color) • Decreased **minute volume**	• Breathing is inadequate. • Breathing is either slow or shallow. • Patient is moving some air in and out of the chest. • Breathing is not enough to sustain life.	• Assist ventilations. • Administer emergency oxygen, if available.
• The chest does not rise. • No evidence of air moving in through mouth or nose. • There are no breath sounds.	• Patient is not breathing.	• Provide ventilation. • Administer emergency oxygen, if available.

CIRCULATORY STATUS

While assessing the patient's airway and breathing, you should assess blood circulation. If the heart has stopped, blood will not circulate throughout the body. If blood does not circulate, the patient will suffer severe brain damage or die because of a lack of oxygen (**Fig. 7-9**).

After checking for breathing and a pulse, quickly scan for severe bleeding. This is the quickest way to evaluate whether or not the patient has any circulation.

Pulse

The most commonly used method of checking for adequate circulation is to check for a pulse. With every heartbeat, a wave of blood moves through the blood vessels. This creates a beat called the *pulse*. You can feel it with your fingertips in the arteries near the skin.

Table 7-5:
Normal Pulse Rates

AGE	NUMBER OF BEATS PER MINUTE	ADDITIONAL NOTES
Adults (12 years old or older)	60 to 100	• A well-conditioned athlete may have a pulse of 50 beats per minute or lower. • An adolescent (11–14 years old) may have a pulse rate of 60 to 105.
Children (1 to about 12 years old)	Toddler (1–3 years): 80 to 130 Preschool-age (3–5 years): 80 to 120 School-age (6–10 years): 70 to 110	• Normal pulse rates vary based on the child's age. • An adolescent (11–14 years old) may have a pulse rate of 60 to 105.
Infants (under 1 year old)	Newborn: 120 to 160 Infant (1–5 months): 90 to 140 Infant (6 months to 1 year): 80 to 140	• Normal pulse rates vary based on the infant's age.

When the heart is healthy, it beats with a steady rhythm. This beat creates a regular pulse. A normal pulse for an adult ranges from 60 to 100 beats per minute. A well-conditioned athlete may have a pulse of 50 beats per minute or lower. A pulse of greater than 100 beats per minute is too fast for an adult at rest. Certain medications, such as beta-blockers, can cause the heart to beat at slower rates, which would be considered normal for that person.

Pediatric Considerations

A normal pulse in a child varies according to age, from 80 to 130 for children ages 1–3, to 60 to 105 in adolescents ages 11–14. An infant can have a normal pulse ranging from 80 to 140 beats per minute. A slow or fast pulse for a child and an infant varies according to age.

If the heartbeat changes, so does the pulse. An abnormal pulse may be a sign of a potential problem. Signs of an abnormal pulse include—
- Irregular pulse.
- Weak and hard-to-find pulse.
- Excessively fast or slow pulse.

When someone is severely injured or ill, the heart may beat unevenly, producing an irregular pulse. The rate at which the heart beats can also change. The pulse speeds up when a person is excited, anxious, in pain, losing blood or under stress. It slows down when a person is relaxed. Some heart conditions or medications can also speed up or slow down the pulse rate. Sometimes changes may be very subtle and difficult for you to detect. The most important change to note is a pulse that changes from being present to no pulse at all. It is important to remember that the definition of what is a "normal" pulse may be different for some. Be sure to ask if there are known congenital disorders or other natural explanations for a seemingly slow or irregular heartbeat as part of the patient history.

Checking a pulse involves placing two fingers on top of a major artery located close to the skin's surface and over a bony structure. Pulse sites that are easy to locate are the **carotid arteries** in the neck, the radial arteries in the wrists and the **brachial arteries** in the upper arms (**Fig. 7-10, A–C**). There are also other pulse sites you may use. To check the pulse rate, count the number of beats in either 15 seconds and multiply that number by 4 or in 30 seconds and multiply

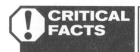

CRITICAL FACTS A "normal" pulse is relative. Ask about any known congenital disorders or other natural explanations for an irregular pulse as part of your patient history.

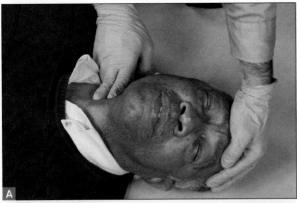

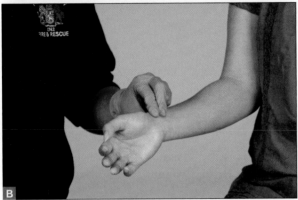

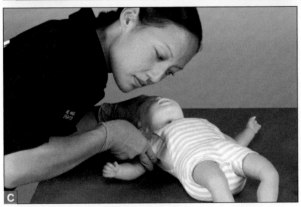

Fig. 7-10, A–C: A pulse can be checked in arteries located close to the skin's surface and over a bony structure. These include the **(A)** carotid, **(B)** radial and **(C)** brachial arteries.

that number by 2. The number you get is the number of heartbeats per minute.

An injured or ill patient's pulse may be hard to find. If you have trouble finding a pulse, keep checking for one periodically. If a patient is breathing, the heart is also beating. There may be a loss in circulation to the injured area, however, causing a loss of pulse. If you cannot find the pulse in one place, try another location, such as in the other wrist.

If the patient is conscious and breathing, check the pulse to determine the rate and quality of the pulse. For conscious adults and children, you usually check the radial pulse on the thumb side of the patient's wrist. For infants, you should check the brachial artery located on the inside of the upper arm, midway between the shoulder and elbow.

If the patient is unconscious, remember, find out whether the patient has an open and clear airway, whether the patient is breathing and whether there is a pulse. If the patient is not breathing, you should only be concerned whether the pulse is present or absent and not with the rate and quality. Check the pulse for an adult or a child at either of the carotid arteries located in the neck. Check the brachial pulse of an infant in the middle of the upper arm.

To find the carotid pulse, place two fingers on the front of the neck, then slide your fingers toward you and down into the groove at the side of the neck. Feel for *no more than 10 seconds*. Sometimes the pulse may be difficult to find, since it may be slow or weak. However, if you do not find a definite pulse after 10 seconds, do not waste any more time attempting to find one. Assume there is no pulse and begin resuscitation immediately.

In some cases, the person may be unconscious but breathing. Generally that person should not be moved from a face-up position and an open airway should be maintained, especially if there is a suspected spinal injury. However, there are a few situations when you should move a person into a modified *high arm in endangered spine* (H.A.IN.E.S.) recovery position whether or not a spinal injury is suspected. Examples of these situations include if you are alone and have to leave the person (e.g., to call for help), or you cannot maintain an open and clear airway because of fluids or vomit. Placing a person in a modified H.A.IN.E.S. recovery position will help keep the airway open and clear. Treat for shock (hypoperfusion). Administer emergency oxygen, if available.

If the patient does not have a pulse, you need to keep blood containing oxygen circulating. This involves providing ventilations to get oxygen into the patient's lungs and performing chest compressions to circulate the oxygen to the brain. This procedure is called *CPR* and is described in **Chapter 13**.

Severe Bleeding

Checking circulation also means looking for severe bleeding. Bleeding is severe when blood spurts from the wound or cannot be controlled. Severe bleeding is life threatening and steps should be taken to control it immediately. Check for it by looking from head to toe for signs of external bleeding, including underneath the patient (**Fig. 7-11**). Techniques for controlling severe bleeding are described in **Chapter 19**.

Perfusion

The next step is to establish whether the patient is maintaining adequate blood flow. **Perfusion** describes the circulation of blood through the body or through a particular body part. The appearance of the skin and its temperature can be helpful in providing information about the patient's circulation. Checking the skin characteristics requires you to look at and feel the skin. There are four aspects of skin conditions to note, including—

- Color. Is it pale and ashen, or flushed and pink?
- Temperature. Is it hot or cold?
- Moisture. Is it moist or dry?
- **Capillary refill**. Is it normal or slow?

Skin Color

In some people, the skin looks red when the body is forced to work harder. The heart pumps faster to get more blood to the tissues and this increased blood flow causes reddened skin or a flushed appearance. In contrast, the skin may look pale or bluish if blood flow is inadequate. Pale skin may indicate low body temperature, blood loss, shock or poor blood flow to a body part. For a dark-skinned patient, check the palms. When a person with darker skin becomes pale, the skin turns ashen, a grayish color. Blue or gray (cyanotic) skin may indicate a problem with airway, ventilation or respiration, or it may be a sign of poor blood flow.

Skin Temperature

Skin temperature is also a sign of blood circulation. Increased blood flow makes the skin feel warm. Cool skin may indicate low body temperature or shock (**Fig. 7-12**).

Skin Moisture

You can also gain information from the degree of moisture on the skin. Normal skin is dry or slightly moist. Wet or sweaty skin may indicate physical exertion, stress, severe pain or shock.

Capillary Refill

One technique for estimating how the body is reacting to injury or illness is to check the ability of the capillaries to refill with blood. This technique, known as *capillary refill*, is more reliable in children and infants up to the age of 6 than it is in adults.

Capillary refill is an estimate of the amount of blood flowing through the capillary beds, such as those in the fingertips. The capillary beds in the fingertips are normally rich with blood, which causes the pink color under the fingernails. When a serious injury or illness occurs, the body attempts to conserve blood in the vital organs. As a result, capillaries in the fingertips are among the first blood vessels to constrict, thereby limiting their blood supply.

Environmental temperature can play a role in the effectiveness of capillary refill. If the patient is exposed to cold temperatures, the capillary refill will normally be slow. Refill slows because blood is directed away from the peripheral areas of the body, like the limbs, in an effort to maintain core body temperature.

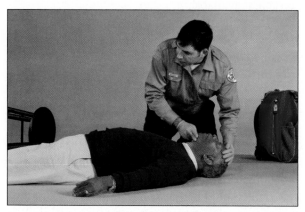

Fig. 7-11: Assessing circulation includes quickly scanning the patient for severe bleeding.

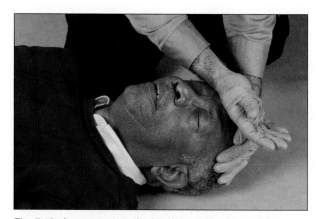

Fig. 7-12: Assess a person's skin temperature by partially removing your glove and feeling the skin.

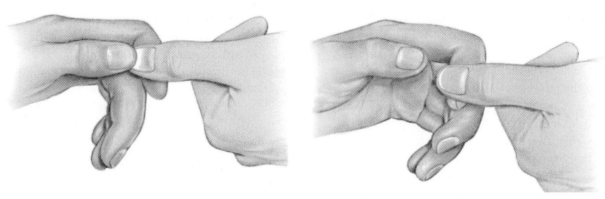

Fig. 7-13: To check capillary refill, squeeze the tip of a finger or thumb for about 2 seconds and then release.

Pediatric Considerations

In children, check capillary refill in fingernails or toenails. In infants, check capillary refill in the forearm or over the kneecap.

To check capillary refill, squeeze the body part (tip of a finger or thumb) for about 2 seconds and then release. In a healthy child, the normal response is for the area to turn pale as you press it and immediately turn pink again as you release (**Fig. 7-13**). If the area does not return to pink within 2 seconds (the time it takes to say "capillary refill"), this indicates insufficient circulation and a potentially serious injury or illness. Remember that environmental temperature can play a role in the effectiveness of this technique. If the child is exposed to cold temperatures, the capillary refill normally will be slow as the body is attempting to maintain core body temperature.

IDENTIFYING LIFE THREATS

Consciousness, breathing and circulation, including pulse and skin characteristics, are called **vital signs**. They are sometimes referred to as "**signs of life**." Check the vital signs often as you monitor a patient while you wait for more advanced medical personnel to take over. Assess the patient to determine if it is a life-threatening condition. If the patient is unstable, care for the life-threatening condition

as soon as it is discovered. For stable patients (vital signs within normal range), assess the patient's condition and provide care as necessary. Patients who are unstable should be reassessed every 5 minutes or more often if indicated by the patient's condition. Reassess stable patients every 15 minutes, or as deemed appropriate by the patient's condition.

Pediatric Considerations

The APGAR scoring system is the universally accepted method of assessing a newborn at 1 minute after birth, at 5 minutes after birth and again at 10 minutes after birth. APGAR stands for Appearance, Pulse, Grimace, Activity and Respiration. The term APGAR also stands for the person who developed it, Virginia Apgar, MD. For more information on assessing a newborn, refer to **Chapter 24**.

SHOCK

If the patient shows signs of shock, you will need to provide care for shock during the primary assessment. In order to determine whether shock should be treated immediately, watch for—
- Decreased responsiveness.
- Unresponsiveness to verbal commands.
- A heart rate that is too fast or too slow.
- Skin signs of shock.
- A weak or no radial pulse (brachial pulse for infants).

Other signs that indicate a person may be going into shock include restlessness or irritability;

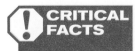 **CRITICAL FACTS** | Check vital signs, such as pulse and respiratory rate, often while you wait for more advanced medical personnel to take over.

altered LOC; nausea or vomiting; pale, ashen, cool, moist skin; rapid breathing and pulse; and excessive thirst. In particular, restlessness and irritability is often the first sign of shock.

If the patient is in shock, control any external bleeding as soon as possible to minimize blood loss and administer emergency oxygen, if it is available. Lay the patient flat (supine). Keep the patient from geting chilled or overheated.

PUTTING IT ALL TOGETHER

The primary assessment helps to identify any life-threatening conditions so they can be cared for rapidly. Problems that are not an immediate threat can become serious if you do not recognize them and provide care. By following the proper steps when conducting the primary assessment, you will give the patient with a serious injury or illness the best chance for survival. Before you proceed with a primary assessment, be certain to size-up the scene to make sure there are no dangers to you, the patient and bystanders and to consider the MOI, nature of illness, the number of patients involved and additional resources you may need.

The essential aspects to the primary assessment are making a general impression of the patient and checking responsiveness, airway, breathing and circulation. Determine if there are any immediate threats to life, such as the absence of breathing or pulse or the presence of severe external bleeding.

Although this plan of action can help you decide what care to provide in any emergency, providing care is not an exact science. Because each emergency and each patient is unique, an emergency may not occur exactly as it did in a classroom setting. Even within a single emergency, the care needed may change from one moment to the next.

YOU ARE THE EMERGENCY MEDICAL RESPONDER

As you begin a primary assessment, you verify that the infant is unconscious. What are your next steps in the primary assessment? Should you call for more advanced medical personnel? Why or why not?

Jaw-Thrust (Without Head Extension) Maneuver

NOTE: Always follow standard precautions when providing care.

After sizing up the scene and establishing that the patient is unresponsive, lying face-up and a head, neck or spinal injury is suspected—

STEP 1

Kneel above the patient's head.

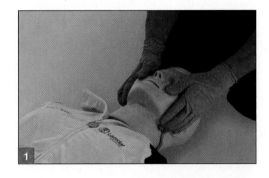

STEP 2

Put one hand on each side of the patient's head, with your thumbs near the corners of the mouth pointed toward the chin.

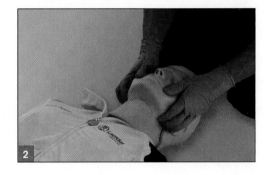

STEP 3

Use your elbows for support.

STEP 4

Slide your fingers into position under the angles of the patient's jawbone.
◆ For a child or an infant, only use two or three fingers of each hand.

STEP 5

Without moving the patient's head, apply downward pressure with your thumbs and lift the jaw.

NOTE: If the patient's lips close, pull back the lower lip with your thumbs.

SKILLsheet

Using a Resuscitation Mask—Adult, Child and Infant

NOTE: Always follow standard precautions when providing care. Size-up the scene for safety. Always select a properly sized mask for the patient.

STEP 1

Assemble the resuscitation mask.

◆ Attach the one-way valve to the resuscitation mask, if necessary.

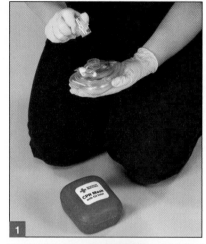

STEP 2

Position the mask.

◆ Kneel to the side of or above the patient's head and place the rim of the mask between the lower lip and chin.

◆ Lower the resuscitation mask until it covers the patient's mouth and nose.

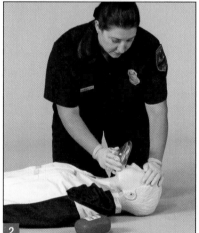

STEP 3

Seal the mask.

◆ From the *side* of the patient's head—
  • With your top hand, place your thumb and fingers around the top of the resuscitation mask to create a "C."
  • With your other hand, slide your first two fingers into position on the bony part of the patient's chin.
  • Apply even, downward pressure with your top hand and the thumb of your lower hand to seal the top and bottom of the mask.

◆ From *above* the patient's head—
  • Place your thumbs and index fingers along each side of the resuscitation mask to create a "C."
  • Slide your fingers into position behind the angles of the patient's jawbone to create an "E" on both sides of the patient's jawbone.
  • Apply even, downward pressure with your thumbs.

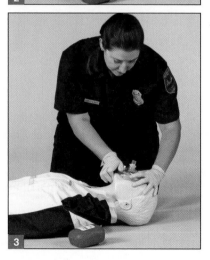

STEP 4

Open the airway.

◆ From the *side* of the patient's head—
   • Tilt the head back and lift the chin to open the airway.
◆ From *above* the patient's head—
   • Tilt the head back and lift the jaw to open the airway.

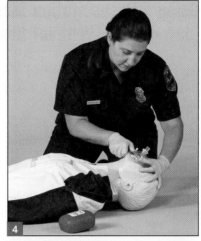

STEP 5

Blow into the mask.

◆ Give **2** ventilations to the patient.
◆ Each ventilation should last about **1** second and make the chest clearly rise.

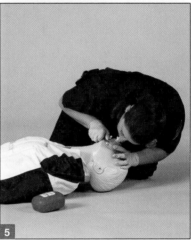

SKILLsheet

Using a Resuscitation Mask–Head, Neck or Spinal Injury Suspected (Jaw-Thrust [Without Head Extension] Maneuver)–Adult or Child

NOTE: Always follow standard precautions when providing care. Size-up the scene for safety. Always select a properly sized mask for the patient.

If a head, neck or spinal injury *is suspected*–

STEP 1
Assemble the resuscitation mask.
◆ Attach the one-way valve to the resuscitation mask, if necessary.

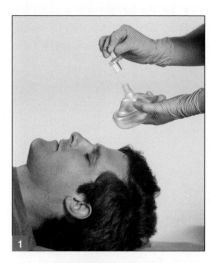

STEP 2
Position the mask.
◆ Kneel above the patient's head.
◆ Place the rim of the mask between the lower lip and chin.
◆ Lower the resuscitation mask until it covers the patient's mouth and nose.

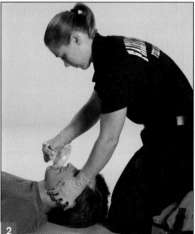

STEP 3
Seal the mask.
◆ Place your thumbs along each side of the resuscitation mask.
◆ Use your elbows for support.
◆ Slide your fingers into position under the angles of the patient's jawbone.
◆ Without moving the patient's head, apply even, downward pressure with your thumbs to seal the mask.

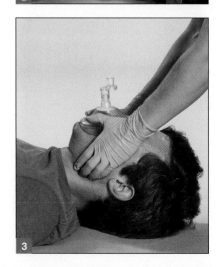

STEP 4

Open the airway.

◆ Without tilting the head back, open the airway by pushing or *thrusting* the lower jaw up with your fingers along the jawbone.

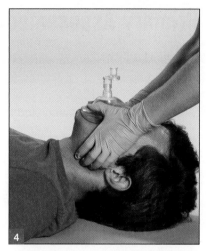

STEP 5

Blow into the mask.

◆ Give **2** ventilations to the patient.
◆ Each ventilation should last about **1** second and make the chest clearly rise.

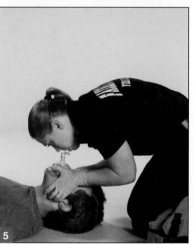

SKILLsheet

Primary Assessment

NOTE: Always follow standard precautions when providing care.

Size-up the scene for safety and then–

STEP 1

Check for responsiveness–
- Tap the shoulder and ask "Are you okay?"
- For an infant, tap the shoulder or flick the underside of the foot.

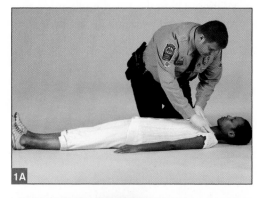

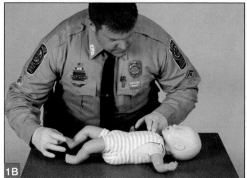

STEP 2

If no response–
- Summon more advanced medical personnel.
- If the patient is face-down, roll the patient onto his or her back while supporting the head, neck and back.

STEP 3

Open the victim's airway and check for breathing and a definite pulse for no more than **10** seconds.
- To open the airway from the side, use the head-tilt/chin-lift technique. To open the airway from above the victim's head, use the jaw-thrust (with head extension) maneuver. If a head, neck or spinal injury is suspected, use the jaw-thrust (without head extension) maneuver.
- Look, listen and feel for breathing.
- For an adult or a child, feel for a carotid pulse by placing two fingers in the middle of the victim's throat and then sliding them into the groove at the side of the neck closest to you. Press in lightly; pressing too hard can compress the artery.

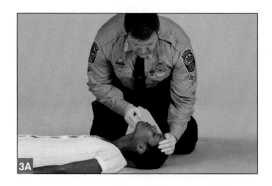

◆ For an infant, feel for the brachial pulse on the inside of the upper arm between the infant's elbow and shoulder. Press in lightly; pressing too hard can compress the artery.

NOTE: For a breathing emergency (e.g., drowning, hypoxia) or for a child or an infant whom you did not see suddenly collapse, give **2** ventilations prior to Step 4.

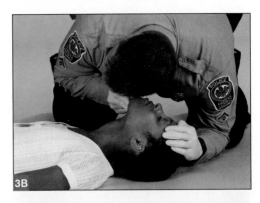

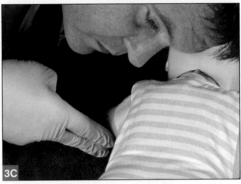

STEP 4
Quickly check for severe bleeding.

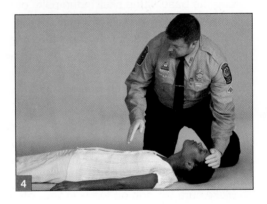

Continued on next page

Primary Assessment *continued*

STEP 5

Provide care based on the conditions found.

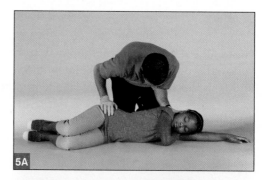

NOTE: If a person is unconscious but breathing, in general, leave that person in a face-up position, especially if there is a suspected spinal injury. However, if you are alone and have to leave the person (e.g., to call for help), or you cannot maintain an open and clear airway because of fluids or vomit, place the person in a modified H.A.IN.E.S. recovery position. Do this whether or not a spinal injury is suspected. To place an adult or a child in a modified H.A.IN.E.S. recovery position—

♦ Kneel at the person's side.
♦ Reach across the body and lift the arm farthest from you up next to the head with the person's palm facing up.
♦ Take the person's arm closest to you and place it next to his or her side.
♦ Grasp the leg farthest from you and bend it up.
♦ Using your hand that is closest to the person's head, cup the base of the skull in the palm of your hand and carefully slide your forearm under the person's shoulder closest to you. Do not lift or push the head or neck.

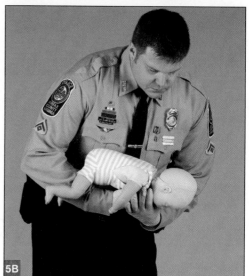

♦ Place your other hand under the arm and hip closest to you.
♦ Using a smooth motion, roll the person away from you by lifting with your hand and forearm. Make sure the person's head remains in contact with the extended arm and be sure to support the head and neck with your hand.
♦ Stop all movement when the person is on his or her side.
♦ Bend the knee closest to you and place it on top of the other knee so that both knees are in a bent position.
♦ Make sure the arm on top is in line with the upper body.
  • If you must leave the person to get help, place the hand of the upper arm palm side down with the fingers under the armpit of the extended lower arm.

To place an infant in a recovery position—
♦ Place the infant in a recovery position as would be done for an older child.
♦ You also can hold an infant in a recovery position by—
  • Carefully positioning the infant face-down along your forearm.
  • Supporting the infant's head and neck with your other hand while keeping the infant's mouth and nose clear.

Enrichment
Glasgow Coma Scale

The **Glasgow Coma Scale (GCS)** is a tool used to assess a patient's LOC. Originally intended to assess LOC following a head injury, it is now considered valuable for primary and ongoing assessments of any medical or trauma patient.

A GCS score is based on three parameters: eye opening (**E**), verbal response (**V**) and motor response (**M**). The total score will range from 3 to 15 (E+V+M = 3–15), with 3 representing coma or death and 15 representing a fully awake patient. A GCS score of 8 or less indicates severe brain injury, 9–12 indicates moderate brain injury and 13–15 indicates mild brain injury.

For patients more than 5 years of age, use the standard scale. For children under the age of 5, the verbal responses must be adjusted using the *Pediatric Glasgow Coma Scale* (PGCS).

Table 7-6:
Glasgow Coma Scale

RESPONSE	STATUS	SCORE
Eye Opening (E)	Spontaneous	4 points
	Opens to verbal command	3 points
	Opens to pain	2 points
	No response	1 point
Verbal Response (V)	Oriented and speaks	5 points
	Confused conversation, but able to answer questions	4 points
	Inappropriate responses, words discernible	3 points
	Incomprehensible speech or sounds	2 points
	No response	1 point
Motor Response (M)	Obeys verbal commands	6 points
	Purposeful movement to painful stimulus	5 points
	Withdraws from pain (flexion)	4 points
	Abnormal flexion from pain	3 points
	Extension in response to pain	2 points
	No response	1 point

Continued on next page

Enrichment
Glasgow Coma Scale (continued)

Table 7-7:
Pediatric Glasgow Coma Scale[1]

AREA ASSESSED	CHILDREN	INFANTS	SCORE
Eye Opening (E)	Open spontaneously	Open spontaneously	4 points
	Open in response to verbal stimuli	Open in response to verbal stimuli	3 points
	Open in response to pain only	Open in response to pain only	2 points
	No response	No response	1 point
Verbal Response (V)	Oriented, appropriate	Coos and babbles	5 points
	Confused	Irritable cries	4 points
	Inappropriate words	Cries in response to pain	3 points
	Incomprehensible words or nonspecific sounds	Moans in response to pain	2 points
	No response	No response	1 point
Motor Response (M)	Obeys commands	Moves spontaneously and purposefully	6 points
	Localizes painful stimulus	Withdraws to touch	5 points
	Withdraws in response to pain	Withdraws in response to pain	4 points
	Responds to pain with decorticate posturing (abnormal flexion)	Responds to pain with decorticate posturing (abnormal flexion)	3 points
	Responds to pain with decerebrate posturing (abnormal extension)	Responds to pain with decerebrate posturing (abnormal extension)	2 points
	No response	No response	1 point

[1]Adapted from Davis RJ et al: Head and spinal cord injury. In *Textbook of Pediatric Intensive Care,* edited by MC Rogers. Baltimore, Williams & Wilkins, 1987; James H, Anas N, Perkin RM: *Brain Insults in Infants and Children.* New York, Grune & Stratton, 1985; and Morray JP et al: Coma scale for use in brain-injured children. *Critical Care Medicine* 12:1018, 1984.

8

History Taking and Secondary Assessment

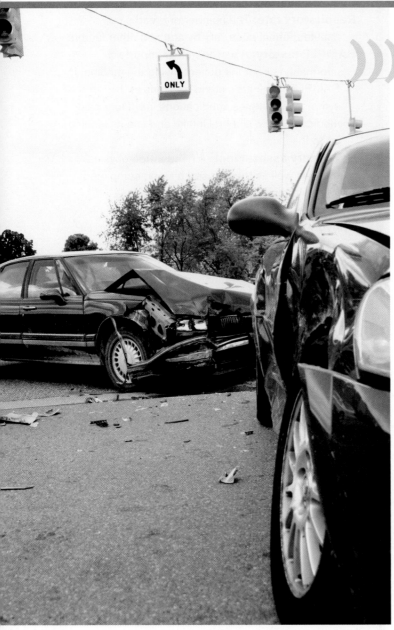

YOU ARE THE EMERGENCY MEDICAL RESPONDER

You arrive at the scene of a motor-vehicle collision, a fender bender, in which a woman who was driving her husband to the hospital because he was complaining of chest pain, rammed into the car in front of her. A police unit is on the scene assisting the husband, who collapsed and apparently is unconscious. Your partner proceeds to help the police officer with the unconscious patient. You notice that the woman is clutching one of her arms. As a responding firefighter, how would you respond to and assess the injured woman?

Key Terms

Auscultation: Listening to sounds within the body, typically through a stethoscope.

Blood pressure (BP): The force exerted by blood against the blood vessel walls as it travels throughout the body.

Chief complaint: A brief description, usually in the patient's own words, of why *emergency medical services* (EMS) personnel were called to the scene.

DCAP-BTLS: A mnemonic to help remember the components of a rapid trauma assessment; the initials stand for deformities, contusions, abrasions, punctures/penetrations, burns, tenderness, lacerations and swelling.

Detailed physical exam: An in-depth head-to-toe physical exam; takes more time than the rapid assessment and is only done when time and the patient's condition allow.

Diastolic blood pressure: The force exerted against the arteries when the heart is between contractions, or at rest.

DOTS: A mnemonic to help remember what to look for during the physical exam; the initials stand for deformities, open injuries, tenderness and swelling.

Focused medical assessment: A physical exam on a *medical* patient, focused only on the area of the chief complaint, e.g., the chest in a patient complaining of chest pain.

Focused trauma assessment: A physical exam on a *trauma* patient, focused only on an isolated area with a known injury such as a hand with an obvious laceration.

Ongoing assessment: The process of repeating the primary assessment and physical exam while continually monitoring the patient; performed while awaiting the arrival of more highly trained personnel or while transporting the patient.

OPQRST: Mnemonic to help remember the questions used to gain information about pain; the initials stand for onset, provoke, quality, region/radiate, severity and time.

Palpation: Examination performed by feeling part of the body, especially feeling for a pulse.

Physical exam: Exam performed after the primary assessment; used to gather additional information and identify signs and symptoms of injury and illness.

Pulse oximetry: A test to measure the percentage of oxygen saturation in the blood using a pulse oximeter.

Rapid medical assessment: A term describing a quick, head-to-toe exam of a medical patient.

Rapid trauma assessment: A term describing a quick, head-to-toe exam of a trauma patient.

Respiratory rate: The number of breaths per minute; normal rates vary by age and other factors.

SAMPLE history: A way to gather important information about the patient, using the mnemonic SAMPLE; the initials stand for signs and symptoms, allergies, medications, pertinent past medical history, last oral intake and events leading up to the incident.

Secondary assessment: A head-to-toe physical exam as well as the focused history; completed following the primary assessment and management of any life-threatening conditions.

Sphygmomanometer: A device for measuring BP; also called a BP cuff.

Stethoscope: A device for listening, especially to the lungs, heart and abdomen; may be used together with a BP cuff to measure BP.

Systolic blood pressure: The force exerted against the arteries when the heart is contracting.

Vial of Life: A community service program that provides *emergency medical services* (EMS) personnel and other responders with vital health and medical information (including any advance directives) when a person, who suffers a medical emergency at home, is unable to speak; consists of a label affixed to the outside of the refrigerator to alert responders and a labeled vial or container that has pertinent medical information, a list of medications, health conditions and other pertinent medical information regarding the occupant(s).

Learning Objectives

After reading this chapter, and completing the class activities, you will have the information needed to—

- Explain the purpose of the patient history.
- Explain the components of the SAMPLE history.
- Explain the purpose of the secondary assessment.
- Explain the importance of properly assessing a patient's vital signs.
- Explain the components of a physical exam.
- State the areas of the body that are evaluated during the physical exam.
- Identify further questions that may be asked during the physical exam.
- Identify the components of the ongoing assessment.
- Explain the importance of properly assessing a patient's *blood pressure* (BP).
- Describe the techniques used to measure BP.

Skill Objectives

After reading this chapter, and completing the class activities, you should be able to—

- Demonstrate how to obtain a SAMPLE history.
- Demonstrate how to obtain baseline vital signs.
- Demonstrate how to obtain BP by auscultation and palpation.
- Demonstrate how to perform a secondary assessment.

INTRODUCTION

In **Chapter 7**, you learned how to conduct a primary assessment, which helps you to determine if the patient has any life-threatening conditions through checking *level of consciousness* (LOC), airway, breathing and circulatory status. However, as you will learn in this chapter, you can obtain more information about the patient through history taking and the **secondary assessment**, which includes interviewing the patient and bystanders, monitoring vital signs and conducting a **physical exam**. As with the primary assessment in the case of serious injury or illness, performing and documenting a thorough history and secondary assessment can increase the patient's chance of survival.

OBTAINING THE FOCUSED/ MEDICAL HISTORY

A crucial aspect of your job is to find out as much as possible about the emergency situation, so that you can communicate this information to more advanced medical personnel. In addition to your close observation of the scene and patient, interviews with those involved are generally your best sources of information. Remember never to enter a scene unless you are sure you can do so safely.

Asking the patient about the incident and any existing medical conditions is called obtaining a history. Obtaining a history should not take much time and may be done before or during the physical exam. Keep in mind that, for a trauma patient or an unresponsive medical patient, the history will likely be performed after the physical exam. For a medical patient who is responsive, the history will likely be performed first.

Under ideal circumstances, patients will be able to tell you themselves all you need to know about what happened and any related medical issues. Help relieve the patient's anxiety by explaining who you are and that you are there to help. Also ask the patient's name and use

it. Always obtain consent before touching or providing care to a patient.

Pediatric Considerations

If a child or an infant does not respond to your questions, it does not always mean the child or infant is unable to respond. Children and infants may be frightened of you or the situation, may not understand the question or may not be able to speak. Position yourself at or below eye-level with the child to avoid being intimidating. Do not separate the child from a parent or guardian, unless absolutely necessary.

Geriatric Considerations

Keep in mind that older people usually prefer to be addressed more formally, as in "Mr. or Mrs. Smith." Position yourself at eye-level with the patient and speak slowly. Older patients may sometimes appear confused. This can be caused by conditions such as dementia or Alzheimer's disease. It can also be the result of an acute medical condition and may not be typical behavior for that person. Make sure the patient can see and hear you, as an older patient may have vision or hearing problems. Allow time for the elderly patient to respond. Always treat the patient with dignity and respect **(Fig. 8-1)**.

Necessary information cannot always be obtained from the patient. The patient may be unconscious, disoriented, agitated or otherwise uncooperative or the patient may not understand and/or speak English. In these cases, interviews

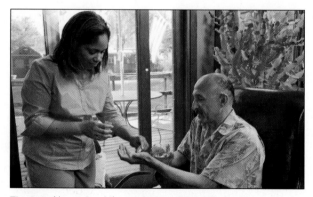

Fig. 8-1: Always treat the geriatric patient with dignity and respect.

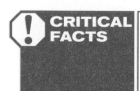

CRITICAL FACTS

A crucial aspect of your job is to find out as much as possible about the emergency situation, so that you can communicate this information to more advanced medical personnel.

Asking the patient about the incident and any existing medical conditions is called obtaining a history. Obtaining a history should not take much time and may be done before or during the physical exam.

with family, friends, caregivers, bystanders or public safety personnel may be helpful.

Sources of information may also be all around you. Be sure to check the patient for a medical *identification* (ID) tag or bracelet or other medical information sources, such as wallet cards or kits for treating anaphylaxis or diabetes. Other hints include the presence of pill containers or a service animal. If you are in the patient's home, you should also look for a **Vial of Life** label on the outside of the refrigerator door—it signifies that a vial or container, such as a sealable plastic bag, contains vital medical information and has been placed on the top shelf of the refrigerator door. Some people keep their medications in the refrigerator, so it also is a good idea to look for these items.

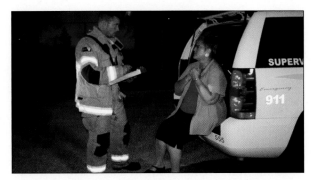

Fig. 8-2: Understanding the chief complaint will help you determine if you are dealing with someone who is injured or someone who is ill. *Courtesy of Terry Georgia.*

COMPONENTS OF A PATIENT HISTORY

Obtaining a full patient history involves several components. Key among them is the **chief complaint**, which will allow you to make the important distinction of whether you are dealing with a trauma or medical emergency. Other components to consider are the *mechanism of injury* (MOI) or nature of illness, the presence and assessment of pain, as well as an evaluation of any relevant medical information.

Chief Complaint

The most important component of a patient history is the chief complaint. This is the reason why *emergency medical services* (EMS) personnel were called to the scene. The best way to determine the chief complaint is to ask the patient, "Why did you call for EMS personnel?" Record the chief complaint in the patient's own words (**Fig. 8-2**).

Keep in mind that the most obvious problem is not always the chief complaint. For instance, if a patient's arm is mangled in a car accident, it may

appear to be the chief complaint, until you find out the patient is having chest pain and crashed the car after blacking out. When interviewing the patient about the chief complaint, remember to ask the "who, what, when, where and how" of the incident.

Understanding the chief complaint generally makes it clear whether you are dealing with a trauma patient—someone who is injured—or a medical patient—someone who is ill—or a combination. This primary division will guide how you manage the patient.

Mechanism of Injury or Nature of Illness

The next piece of information to determine is the MOI for a trauma patient or the nature of the illness for a medical patient.

Mechanism of Injury

In the case of an injury, it is important to find out how the injury occurred and determine what the forces were that caused the injury. This may help predict the specific type of injuries the patient may have.

It will also help you determine whether there is any risk of a spinal injury. If the MOI suggests there is, tell the patient not to move and provide manual stabilization by restricting

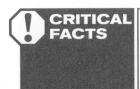

CRITICAL FACTS

Necessary information cannot always be obtained from the patient. The patient may be unconscious, disoriented, agitated or otherwise uncooperative or the patient may not understand and/or speak English. In these cases, interviews with family, friends, caregivers, bystanders or public safety personnel may be helpful.

The most important component of a patient history is the chief complaint. This is the reason why EMS personnel were called to the scene.

motion and supporting the head and neck in the position in which you found it. Once you have dealt with the risk of spinal injury, follow the steps for trauma patients. These steps depend on whether there is a significant MOI or not.

Examples of a significant MOI include—
- Being ejected from a vehicle or thrown from a motorcycle.
- A fall from greater than 15 feet or three times the patient's height.
- A vehicle rollover.
- A vehicle collision.
- A pedestrian struck by a vehicle.
- A blunt or penetrating trauma that causes a change in mental status.
- A penetrating injury to the head, neck, chest or abdomen.
- A blast injury.

Nature of Illness

In the case of a medical patient, ask the patient, family, friends or any bystanders why EMS personnel were called. If no one is available to interview, observe the scene. Look for clues such as a very hot or very cold environment or the presence of drugs or poisons (**Fig. 8-3**).

The steps involved in conducting a secondary assessment on a medical patient depend on whether the patient is responsive or unresponsive.

If the medical patient is responsive, obtain the history first and then perform your exam. In this situation, the history is your first priority because it may be the most valuable information you obtain and also because it is prudent to speak immediately with a responsive patient, since this status might change.

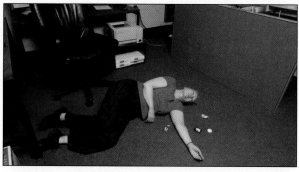
Fig. 8-3: If no one is available to interview, look for clues on the scene to determine what might have happened. *Courtesy of the Canadian Red Cross.*

SAMPLE HISTORY

Using the mnemonic SAMPLE, determine the following six items for the history:
- **S**igns and symptoms
- **A**llergies
- **M**edications
- **P**ertinent past medical history
- **L**ast oral intake
- **E**vents leading up to the incident

In addition to the **SAMPLE history**, ask the patient to explain what happened. Ask questions such as—
- What happened?
- Are you having any pain?
- How would you describe the pain? You can expect to hear descriptions such as burning, throbbing, aching or sharp pain.
- Is the pain spreading or radiating?
- On a scale of 1 to 10, with 1 being lowest and 10 being highest, how bad is the pain?
- When did the pain start? (See **OPQRST.**)

Sometimes the patient will be unable to give you the information. This is often the case with a child or with an adult who momentarily lost

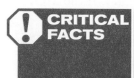
CRITICAL FACTS

Assessing the MOI may help predict the specific type of injuries the patient may have. Significant MOIs include events such as being ejected or thrown from a vehicle, a fall from greater than 15 feet or three times a patient's height or receiving a penetrating injury to the head, neck, chest or abdomen.

In the case of a medical patient, ask the patient, family, friends or any bystanders why EMS personnel were called.

The mnemonic SAMPLE refers to what essential information to obtain when taking a history. It refers to signs and symptoms, allergies, medications, pertinent past medical history, last oral intake and event leading up to the incident.

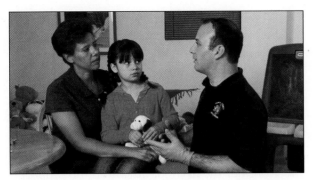

Fig. 8-4: Family members or friends may be able to provide information about children.

consciousness and may not be able to recall what happened or is disoriented. Ask family members, friends or bystanders what happened (**Fig. 8-4**). They may be able to give you helpful information, such as telling you if a patient has a medical condition you should be aware of. They may also be able to help calm the patient, if necessary.

Obtain consent before approaching or touching the patient. Patients may be frightened; offer reassurance. Be calm and patient and, if possible, ensure you are in a comfortable and private location where you will not be interrupted. Use open-ended questions, and encourage the patient to talk using verbal and nonverbal cues. Show you are listening by repeating and paraphrasing the patient's replies. Maintain eye contact and speak slowly, deliberately and in simple terms.

Signs and Symptoms

Signs include any medical or trauma assessment findings you can see, feel, hear or smell. For example, this would include measuring **blood pressure** (**BP**), seeing an open wound or feeling skin temperature. Symptoms refer to what the patient reports, for example, "I'm having trouble breathing," "I have a headache" or "My chest hurts." For further symptoms, ask the patient to describe the current problem. Ask questions such as—

- Where do you have pain?
- Are you feeling nauseated?
- Do you have a headache?
- Are you having any difficulty breathing?

Allergies

Ask the patient whether he or she is allergic to any medications, food or environmental elements, such as dust, pollen or bees.

Medications

Ask the patient questions to determine whether he or she is currently using any medications, whether prescription or *over-the-counter* (OTC). Ask additional questions such as—

- Do you take any vitamins or herbal remedies?
- Have you taken someone else's medications?
- Did you take any recreational drugs?
- Are you using any medication patches?

Pertinent Past Medical History

Determine whether the patient is under a health care provider's care for any condition, if the patient has had a similar problem in the past or if the patient has been recently hospitalized or had recent surgeries. If the patient is female, ask if she is or could be pregnant.

Last Oral Intake

Determine when the patient last had something to eat or drink and what it was. Also, ask if the patient has recently taken any medication, and if so, what.

Events Leading Up to the Incident

Determine what the patient was doing before and at the time of the incident. The events leading up to the incident could help identify the MOI or nature of the illness.

THE SECONDARY ASSESSMENT

The purpose of the secondary assessment is to locate and further assess the signs and symptoms of an injury or illness. The secondary assessment consists of a head-to-toe physical exam. It may only consist of a rapid assessment (**rapid trauma assessment** or **rapid medical assessment**) or it may also include a **detailed physical exam** at a later stage.

If you find life-threatening injuries or medical conditions during the primary assessment, such as unconsciousness, no breathing, no pulse or severe bleeding, do not waste time with the physical exam. Instead, focus your attention on providing care for the life-threatening conditions. Complete a secondary assessment following the primary assessment, once all life-threatening conditions are addressed and have been stabilized, if time and resources permit.

For patients with a significant MOI or other critical finding such as altered mental status, take the following steps during the secondary assessment:

1. Continue to maintain spinal stabilization and an open airway.
2. Consider the need for advanced life support backup and the need for transport (e.g., for life-threatening conditions, such as airway trauma).
3. Reassess the patient's mental status, as this may change at any time.
4. Perform a rapid trauma assessment, which is a rapid head-to-toe physical exam. (See sidebar on **DCAP-BTLS**, page 172.)
5. Assess baseline vital signs.
6. Obtain a SAMPLE history. If the patient is responsive, ask some history questions simultaneously with the physical exam.
7. Prepare the patient for transport (simultaneously as assessment is being conducted).
8. Provide emergency care.
9. Obtain trauma score (e.g., Glasgow Coma Scale [GCS]), if trained.

Your major concern during the rapid trauma assessment is any potentially life-threatening injuries that you must manage immediately.

For the trauma patient who does not have a significant MOI such as those outlined above, follow these steps:

1. Perform a **focused trauma assessment** (e.g., for a laceration to the leg).
2. Obtain a SAMPLE history and baseline vital signs.
3. Perform components of a detailed physical exam, as needed.
4. Provide emergency care.

For a responsive medical patient, follow these steps for the secondary assessment:

1. Assess the patient's complaints (**OPQRST**—**o**nset, **p**rovoke, **q**uality, **r**egion/**r**adiate, **s**everity and **t**ime).

2. Obtain the SAMPLE history.
3. Perform a **focused medical assessment** unless signs and symptoms make the focus unclear, in which case you would perform a rapid medical assessment (head to toe).
4. Assess baseline vital signs.
5. Perform components of the detailed physical exam, as needed.
6. Provide emergency care.
7. Consider the need for advanced life support backup and the need for transport (e.g., for life-threatening conditions, such as anaphylaxis).

If the medical patient is unresponsive, consider the patient as critical, requiring that you begin with a rapid medical assessment, to gain as much information as possible on the nature of the illness.

For an unresponsive medical patient, take the following steps for the secondary assessment:

1. Consider the need for advanced life support backup and the need for transport (e.g., for life-threatening conditions, such as heart attack).
2. Perform a rapid medical assessment (head to toe).
3. Assess baseline vital signs.
4. Position a patient who is unresponsive, but breathing, face-up and ensure protection of the airway.
5. Obtain a SAMPLE history from the family or any bystanders, if available.
6. Provide emergency care.

Physical Exam

Many patients view a physical exam with apprehension and anxiety—they feel vulnerable and exposed. Maintain professionalism throughout the physical exam and display compassion toward the patient. Explain what areas you are going to assess. If you have questions about an area and the patient is responsive, ask questions prior to examining the area. Maintain the patient's privacy during the physical exam, such as by conducting the exam in an area that cannot be seen by bystanders. When you need to remove the patient's clothing,

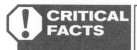 **CRITICAL FACTS** There are several steps that are essential to follow when conducting the secondary assessment.

cut it away rather than manipulating the patient to remove it. Cover each area after you have examined it. Try to keep the patient calm, and keep the patient from moving the head, neck and spine and any body part that hurts to move.

Pediatric Considerations

You may find it helpful to use distracting measures, such as a teddy bear or doll, to gain the trust of a child. Keeping the child with the parent or guardian can also help ease the child's fear. If the child becomes extremely agitated or upset, conduct a toe-to-head assessment of the child.

Geriatric Considerations

When assessing geriatric patients, consider that they may have glasses and/or hearing aids and will be better able to participate in the assessment process if they are wearing them. Expect the assessment to take longer with geriatric patients than with a younger adult. Keep in mind that it might take geriatric patients a little longer to respond. For other geriatric considerations, refer to **Chapter 26**.

Your exam may focus on a specific area, based on the patient's chief complaint, or be specific to a particular injury or illness. As you discover certain signs and symptoms, there may be specific relevant questions you should ask.

For the rapid assessment, be sure to examine the patient systematically, placing special emphasis on areas suggested by the chief complaint, but remembering to examine the whole body. The patient may focus on a bothersome complaint or a painful one, and fail to identify a more serious problem.

The physical exam for trauma and medical patients is similar, in that the purpose is to gather additional information. However, the type of information you are assessing for may be different in the two different types of patients. With the trauma patient, you are looking for evidence of injury; with the medical patient, you are trying to determine the severity of the condition. For example, if you are examining a limb in the trauma patient, you may be most interested in tenderness, pain, swelling and deformities, as well as pulse and motor/sensory function, as an indication of injury. For the medical patient, you may be looking for signs of inadequate circulation, discoloration or swelling, as well as motor/sensory function, as a sign of the status of the brain or heart.

When you perform the physical exam, gather additional information on the patient's condition. As you examine the patient, compare each body part on one side of the body to the other. You can gain information by inspecting visually as well as palpating (feeling) areas of the body.

DOTS

The mnemonic **DOTS** may be helpful during the physical exam for patients who have been injured. It stands for—

- **D**eformities. Deformities may include depressions or indentations, parts that have shifted away from their usual position, parts that are more rigid or less rigid than normal (e.g., abdomen) or obvious signs of broken bones.
- **O**pen injuries. Open injuries may include anywhere there is bleeding, including the scalp. These may be serious, such as open injuries to the chest, or less serious, as in cuts and scrapes. Open injuries also include penetrating wounds, such as knife or gunshot wounds.
- **T**enderness. Tenderness may be experienced even when there are no obvious signs of injury. When there is tenderness of the abdomen, it is important to determine in which quadrant the patient feels pain. Begin in the quadrant where the patient feels the least pain so this does not influence the remaining assessment of the abdomen.
- **S**welling. Swelling may indicate an accumulation of blood, air or other fluid in the tissues below the skin. In an extremity, it may indicate that the bone is broken.

OPQRST

As part of the physical exam, if the patient is responsive, ask questions to gain information about pain. One method of questioning can be remembered using the mnemonic OPQRST, which stands for Onset, Provoke, Quality, Region/Radiate, Severity and Time. It can be

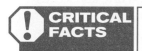
CRITICAL FACTS | As part of the physical exam of a responsive patient, ask questions using the OPQRST mnemonic.

DCAP-BTLS

During the rapid trauma assessment, the mnemonic **DCAP-BTLS** may help you remember the components of assessment to include. The letters stand for—

- **D**eformities.
- **C**ontusions.
- **A**brasions.
- **P**unctures/penetrations.
- **B**urns.
- **T**enderness.
- **L**acerations.
- **S**welling.

Keep these types of injuries in mind as you check each major area. Remember to use each of your senses. Many of these types of injuries can be seen on exam. By palpating (feeling) for injuries, you can determine if there are any deformities or swelling and if the patient is experiencing any pain or tenderness. Even if the patient cannot tell you, you can observe any grimacing on the patient's face. In addition to seeing and feeling for signs of injury, listen for abnormal breathing sounds, for example gurgling or stridor in the upper airway. Auscultate (listen) to the lungs with a stethoscope for breath sounds. You can also listen for the sound of broken bones rubbing against each other. Use your sense of smell. This is one way you can detect any unusual or unexpected odors such as the presence of alcohol or a fruity-smelling breath, as well as the possible presence of urine or feces.

As with any physical exam, try to keep the patient calm and comfortable. Rather than focusing on your findings, explain what you are doing to minimize any distress about the injuries. Do not move the patient unnecessarily in case there is a neck or spinal injury.

If there is a serious MOI, it is crucial to completely expose the patient to look for additional injuries. Protect the patient's privacy by covering all patients, male or female of any age, with a sheet and only expose the area you are examining.

When you need to remove clothing, cut it away rather than manipulating the patient to remove it. Cover each area after you have examined it.

Your major concern during the rapid trauma assessment is any potentially life-threatening injuries that you must manage immediately.

---

used for both patients who have been injured and those who have a medical condition.

- **O**nset: What were you doing when the pain started? Was the onset abrupt or gradual?
- **P**rovocation or palliation: What makes it worse? What makes it better?
- **Q**uality: Is the pain blunt, sharp, burning, crushing or tearing?
- **R**egion/**R**adiate: Where is the pain and does it radiate (spread)? Do you have pain or discomfort somewhere else?
- **S**everity: On a scale of 1 to 10, how intense is the pain?
- **T**ime: When did it start? How long has it been present? How has it changed since it started?

For trauma patients, the mnemonic DCAP-BTLS will remind you of the most common signs and symptoms you may find.

DETAILED PHYSICAL EXAM

Once the focused history and physical exam have been completed and any life-threatening conditions have been managed, a detailed physical exam may be conducted. This exam is not carried out on every patient. It requires much more time than a rapid assessment to conduct, as it is more detailed, and so can only be performed when time and the patient's condition allow. Often, it is conducted in the ambulance or other transport vehicle, en route to the hospital.

The detailed physical exam is a systematic head-to-toe exam that helps you gather additional information about injuries or conditions that may need care. These injuries or conditions are not immediately life threatening but could become so if not cared for. For example, you might find minor bleeding or possible broken bones as you conduct your exam of the patient. As you conduct the physical exam, tell the patient what you are going to do.

The physical exam process involves looking (inspection), listening (**auscultation**) and feeling (**palpation**). You may even smell something you can gather as information, such as the smell of bleach on the breath, which may indicate poisoning. After telling the patient exactly what you are going to do and asking the patient to hold still, inspect and palpate each part of the body, starting with the head, before you move on to the next area.

Ask the patient to tell you if any areas hurt. Avoid touching any painful areas or having the patient move any area that causes discomfort. Watch facial expressions and listen for a tone of voice that may reveal pain. Look for a medical ID tag or bracelet (**Fig. 8-5**). This tag may help you determine what is wrong, who to call for help and what care to provide.

As you do the head-to-toe exam, think about how the body normally looks and feels. Be alert for any sign of injuries—anything that looks or feels unusual. If you are uncertain whether your finding is unusual, check the other side of the body for symmetry. Once the detailed physical exam is complete, reassess the vital signs and continue emergency care.

Head

To check the head, look for blood or clear fluid in or around the ears, nose and mouth. Blood or clear fluid can indicate a serious head injury. Is there presence of vomit around the mouth? Look at the teeth (**Fig. 8-6**).

Check the LOC again and note any change. Look at facial symmetry. Check the pupils. If they are unequal, this is an abnormal finding. Do they react to light by constricting and to darkness by dilating? This reaction is normal. If they remain constricted or dilated, this is an abnormal finding. Does the shape of the eyes look unusual? Look for bruising on the face, especially around the eyes.

Neck

To check the neck, look and feel for any abnormalities (**Fig. 8-7, A–C**). Does the patient breathe through a stoma? A stoma is an opening

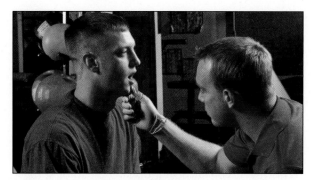

Fig. 8-6: Blood or clear fluid in the ears, mouth or nose can indicate a serious head injury.

in the neck to allow a person to breathe after surgery to remove part, or all, of the larynx (voice box) or other structures of the airway. The person may breathe *partially* through this opening, or may breathe *entirely* through the stoma instead of through the nose and mouth.

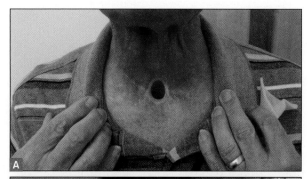

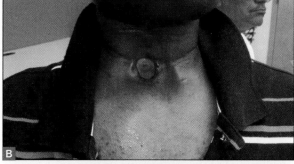

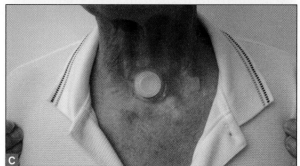

Fig. 8-7, A–C: **(A)** A stoma without a prosthesis. **(B)** A stoma with tracheoesophageal prosthesis. Prosthesis should not be removed by an EMR. **(C)** A stoma with a heat and moisture exchange filter. The filter should be removed in an emergency. *Courtesy of the International Association of Laryngectomees.*

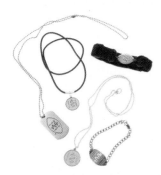

Fig. 8-5: A medical ID tag or bracelet may help determine what is wrong, what care to provide and whom to call. *Courtesy of the Canadian Red Cross.*

Are there any open wounds? Is the patient using the accessory muscles for breathing (a sign of difficulty)? Is the jugular vein distended (enlarged and protruding) **(Fig. 8-8)**?

If the patient has not suffered an injury involving the head or trunk and does not have any pain or discomfort in the head, neck or back, then there is little likelihood of spinal injury. You should proceed to check other body parts. If, however, you suspect a possible head or spine injury because of the MOI, such as a motor-vehicle collision or a fall from a height, minimize movement to the patient's head and spine. If you suspect head or spine injuries, take care of these first. Do not be concerned about finishing the physical exam. You will learn techniques for stabilizing and immobilizing the head and spine in **Chapter 23**.

Chest

Check the collarbones and shoulders by feeling for deformity **(Fig. 8-9)**. Ask the patient to shrug the shoulders. Check the chest by asking the patient to take a deep breath and then blow the air out. Ask the patient if there is any pain. Auscultate for lung sounds if you are trained to do so. Look and listen for more subtle signs of breathing difficulty, such as wheezing or diminished lung sounds. Feel the ribs for deformity. Examine the chest. Does it rise and fall without effort or is there evidence of an effort to breathe? Are there any open wounds? Is the chest symmetrical?

Abdomen

Next, ask if the patient has any pain in the abdomen. Expose the abdomen and look for discoloration, open wounds or distension (swelling). Are there any scars or protruding organs? Does the patient look pregnant? Look

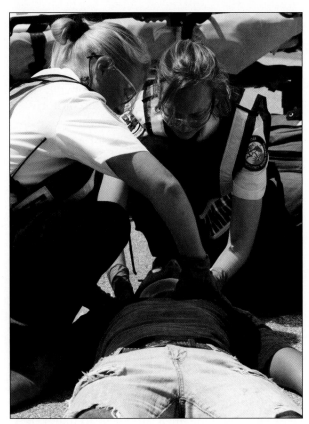

Fig. 8-9: Examine the chest, looking for deformities or signs that the patient is having difficulty breathing. *Courtesy of Terry Georgia.*

at the abdomen for any pulsating. If there is no pulsating, apply slight pressure to each of the abdominal quadrants **(Fig. 8-10)**, avoiding any areas where the patient had indicated pain.

Back

Examine the back for any injuries by palpating equally along the spine from neck downward, with your fingertips. Check for any reaction to pain. Look for discoloration, open wounds and any signs of bleeding. Your exam should be methodical and purposeful so that you do not overlook any details **(Fig. 8-11)**.

Pelvis

Check the hips, asking the patient if there is any pain. Place your hands on both sides of the pelvis and push in on the sides and down on the hips. Check for any reaction to pain.

Extremities

Check only one extremity at a time. Look at and feel each leg for any deformity. If there is no apparent sign of injury, ask the patient to move the

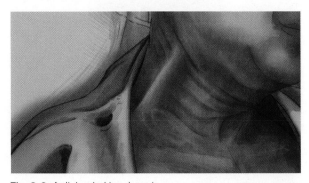

Fig. 8-8: A distended jugular vein

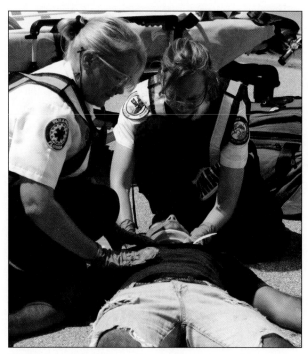

Fig. 8-10: Look for discoloration, open wounds, swelling or pulsating in the abdomen. *Courtesy of Terry Georgia.*

toes, foot and leg. Repeat this procedure on the other leg. Finally, determine if the patient has any pain in the arms or hands. Feel the arms for any deformity. Check limbs for symmetry and check the pulse. Look at color. If there is no apparent sign of injury, ask the patient to move the fingers,

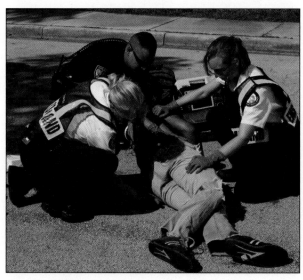

Fig. 8-11: Examine the back methodically, looking for discoloration, open wounds, bleeding or reactions to pain. *Courtesy of Terry Georgia.*

hand and arm. Repeat this procedure on the other arm. Check for distal circulation and sensation in both arms and legs. Check capillary refill.

Pediatric Considerations

Capillary refill is a method for assessing adequate blood flow. It is more reliable in children and infants 6 years of age and younger.

If the patient can move all body parts without pain or discomfort and there are no other apparent signs or symptoms of injury, have the patient attempt to rest for a few minutes in a sitting position. If more advanced help is not needed, continue to check the signs and symptoms and monitor the patient's condition.

Take note of the information you find during the physical exam. Sometimes you may need to have a partner fill out the form with the information you gather. This will help you when it is time to give a verbal report to the next level of care as you transfer the patient. Immediately treat any life-threatening problems found in the detailed physical exam.

OBTAINING BASELINE VITAL SIGNS

Vital signs provide a starting point for judging the effectiveness of prehospital care. They can tell you how the body is responding to injury or illness. Look for changes in vital signs and note anything unusual.

Vital signs are taken after managing life-threatening problems found during the primary assessment. They are normally taken after the rapid assessment is complete; however, if several responders are on scene, they may be taken simultaneously. Note that absolute values are not as important as trends.

There are three major vital sign measures to be taken:

- **Respiratory rate**
- Pulse
- BP

You may also measure LOC, skin characteristics and pupils at this stage.

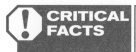

CRITICAL FACTS When obtaining baseline vital signs, respiratory rate, pulse and BP are essential. LOC, skin characteristics and pupils can be assessed as well.

Respiratory Rate

A healthy person breathes regularly, quietly and effortlessly. The normal breathing rate for an adult is between 12 and 20 breaths per minute. However, some people breathe slightly slower or faster.

Excitement, fear and exercise cause breathing to increase and become deeper. Certain injuries or illnesses can also cause both the rate and quality of breathing to change.

As you assess the patient, watch and listen for any changes in breathing. Abnormal breathing may indicate a potential problem. The signs and symptoms of abnormal breathing include—

- Gasping for air.
- Noisy breathing, including whistling sounds, crowing, gurgling or snoring.
- Excessively fast or slow breathing.
- Painful breathing.

In the primary assessment, the goal is to determine whether a patient is breathing at all, whereas in the secondary assessment, you are concerned with the rate, rhythm and quality of breathing. Look, listen and feel again for breathing (**Fig. 8-12**). Look for the rise and fall of the patient's chest or abdomen. Listen for sounds as the patient inhales and exhales. Count the number of times a patient breathes (inhales and exhales) in 30 seconds and multiply that number by 2 or in 15 seconds and multiply that number by 4. This is the number of breaths per minute. As you check for the rate and quality of breathing, try to do it without the patient's knowledge. If the patient realizes you are checking breathing, this may cause a change in breathing pattern without the patient being

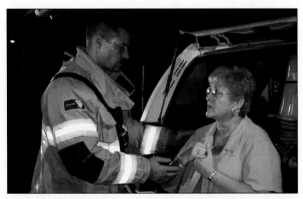

Fig. 8-12: Take note of rate, rhythm and quality when evaluating breathing in the secondary assessment. *Courtesy of Terry Georgia.*

aware of it. Maintain the same position you would when you are checking the pulse.

Pediatric Considerations

Respiratory rates in children and infants vary by age. The following are the normal respiratory rates by age category:

- Newborns: 30 to 50 breaths per minute
- Infants (0 to 5 months): 25 to 40 breaths per minute
- Infants (6 to 12 months): 20 to 30 breaths per minute
- Toddlers (1 to 3 years): 20 to 30 breaths per minute
- Preschoolers (3 to 5 years): 20 to 30 breaths per minute
- School age (6 to 10 years): 15 to 30 breaths per minute
- Adolescents (11 to 14 years): 12 to 20 breaths per minute

Refer to **Chapter 7** for more information on breathing rate and quality.

Lung sounds, or breath sounds, are the noises produced by the lungs during breathing. Some are normal and others are abnormal. The most common abnormal breath sounds are crackles, rhonchi, stridor and wheezing. *Crackles*, also called *rales*, are small popping, rattling or bubbly sounds that are produced when closed spaces pop open. They can be described as fine or coarse. *Rhonchi* are low-pitched snoring sounds caused by the narrowing of the airway and the presence of secretions in the airway. *Stridor* is a harsh, high pitched sound due to obstruction in the air passages. *Wheezing* is a high-pitched, whistling sound created by air flowing through narrow airways and can be heard on exhalation.

Absent or decreased normal sounds can also be an indication of problems with breathing, for example because of air or fluid around the lungs, or reduced air flow to part of the lungs.

Pulse

With every heartbeat, a wave of blood moves through the blood vessels. This creates a beat called the pulse. You can feel it with your fingertips in arteries near the surface of the skin. In the primary assessment, the goal is to determine whether a pulse is present. To determine this, you check the carotid arteries. In the secondary assessment, you are trying to determine pulse rate, rhythm and quality. This is most often done by checking the radial pulse located on the thumb side of the patient's wrist.

When the heart is healthy, it beats with a steady rhythm. This beat creates a regular pulse.

A normal pulse for an adult is between 60 and 100 beats per minute. A well-conditioned athlete may have a pulse of 50 beats per minute or lower. Refer to **Chapter 7**, **Table 7-5** for average pulse rates by age. If the heartbeat changes, so does the pulse. An abnormal pulse may be a sign of a potential problem. These signs include—

- An irregular pulse.
- A weak and hard-to-find pulse.
- An excessively fast or slow pulse.

When severely injured or unhealthy, the heart may beat unevenly, producing an irregular pulse. The rate at which the heart beats can also change. The pulse speeds up when a patient is excited, anxious, in pain, losing blood or under stress. It slows down when a patient is relaxed. Some heart conditions can also speed up or slow down the pulse rate. Sometimes changes may be subtle and difficult to detect. The most important change to note is a pulse that changes from being present to no pulse at all.

Checking a pulse is a simple procedure. Place two fingers on top of a major artery where it is located close to the skin's surface and over a bony structure. Pulse points that are easy to locate include the carotid arteries in the neck, the radial artery in the wrist and, for infants, the brachial artery in the inside of the upper arm (**Fig. 8-13**). To check the pulse rate, count the number of beats in 30 seconds and multiply that number by 2, or the number of beats in 15 seconds and multiply that number by 4. The result is the number of heartbeats per minute. If you find the pulse is irregular, you may need to check it for more than 30 seconds.

An injured or ill patient's pulse may be hard to find. Remember, if a patient is breathing, the heart is also beating. However, there may be a loss in circulation to the injured area, causing a loss of pulse. If you cannot find the pulse in one place, check it in another location, such as in the other wrist.

Pediatric Considerations

When measuring the pulse in an infant, use the brachial artery rather than the radial artery, as in adults. Pulse measurement in children and infants varies by age:

- Newborns: 120 to 160 *beats per minute* (bpm)
- Infants (0 to 5 months): 90 to 140 bpm
- Infants (6 to 12 months): 80 to 140 bpm

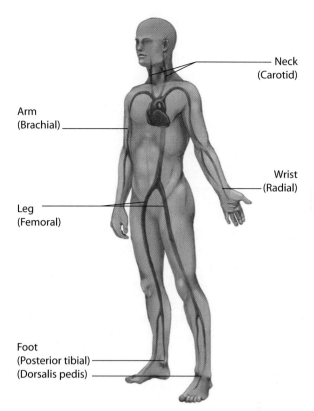

Fig. 8-13: Easily located pulse sites

- Toddlers (1 to 3 years): 80 to 130 bpm
- Preschoolers (3 to 5 years): 80 to 120 bpm
- School age (6 to 10 years): 70 to 110 bpm
- Adolescents (11 to 14 years): 60 to 105 bpm

Blood Pressure

Another vital sign used to assess a patient's condition is BP. BP measures the force of blood against the walls of the artery as it travels through the body. It is a good indicator of how the circulatory system is functioning.

Because a patient's BP can vary greatly, it is only one of several factors that give you an overall picture of a patient's condition. Stress, excitement, injury and illness can affect BP.

When a person is injured or ill, a single BP measurement is often of little value. A more accurate picture of a patient's condition immediately after an injury or the onset of an illness is whether BP changes over time while you provide care. For example, a patient's initial BP reading could be uncommonly high as a result of the stress of the emergency. It can also be temporarily elevated just because the patient is in the presence of a medical professional, a phenomenon called *"white coat hypertension."* Providing care, however, usually relieves some of the fear, and BP may return to within a normal range. At other times, BP will remain unusually high or low. For example, an injury resulting in a severe loss of blood may cause BP to remain unusually low. You should be concerned about unusually high or low BP or a large change in BP whenever signs and symptoms of injury or illness are present.

Equipment for Measuring Blood Pressure

To measure BP, you need two pieces of equipment: a **sphygmomanometer** (BP cuff) and a **stethoscope (Fig. 8-14)**. A sphygmomanometer is made up of two main parts: an inflatable cuff that is wrapped around the patient's arm and a manometer. The cuff is made of fabric and comes in several sizes. It has a rubber bladder inside, which is connected at the end to a hose with a rubber ball, called a bulb. A valve in the bulb opens and closes to control the flow of air into the bladder. The valve is controlled by a screw. If you turn the screw to the left, it opens the valve and lets the air escape from the bladder. If you turn the screw to the right, it closes the valve so that when you pump air into the bladder with the bulb, the valve keeps the air inside the bladder, making the cuff tight.

When you pump air into the cuff, the bladder pressure increases until it is strong enough to stop the blood flow through the brachial artery. At this point, you do not hear anything through the stethoscope. As you turn the valve to release pressure on the brachial artery, the cuff pressure eventually matches and then drops below the **systolic blood pressure**. When the cuff pressure reaches this point, you begin to hear the pulse sounds. As the cuff pressure drops to equal the **diastolic blood pressure** in the artery, the sounds change or fade away.

The second part to the sphygmomanometer is the manometer, a gauge that measures systolic and diastolic pressure. The numbers on the gauge show the pressure in millimeters; the higher the number,

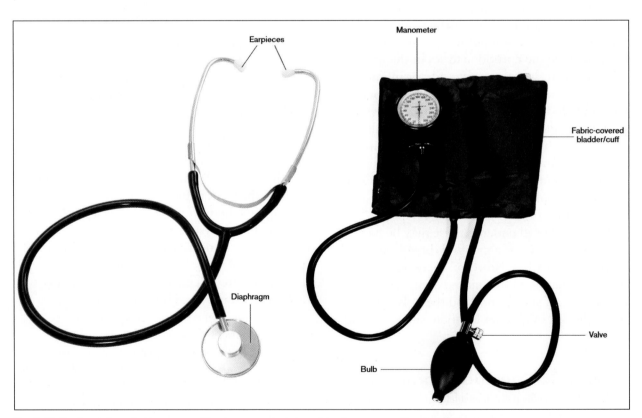

Fig. 8-14: Equipment needed to measure blood pressure includes a blood pressure cuff and a stethoscope.

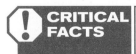 **CRITICAL FACTS** To measure BP, you need two pieces of equipment: a sphygmomanometer (BP cuff) and a stethoscope.

the greater the pressure. There are three types of manometers: mercury, aneroid and electronic.

The aneroid manometer shows the pressure readings on a round dial with an arrow that points to the numbers (**Fig. 8-15, A**). Although there is no mercury column, the numbers on the dial are equal to *millimeters of mercury* (mmHg). The arrow moves from zero to the higher numbers as you inflate the cuff.

The electronic manometer (**Fig. 8-15, B**) eliminates the need for using a stethoscope and listening for the pulse sounds, because it takes the BP readings for you and displays them on a digital screen like the one on an electronic thermometer.

The stethoscope is used together with the sphygmomanometer to allow you to hear the BP sounds. It consists of two pieces of tubing that are connected at one end to a flat disk called a diaphragm. The earpieces, which are connected to the other end of the tubing, fit into your ears and allow you to hear sounds. Some stethoscopes have a bell-shaped end in addition to the diaphragm. Before taking a person's BP, check the tubing and diaphragm for cracks and holes that could make it difficult to hear and could cause you to make an error in the BP reading. To prevent the spread of infection, use alcohol to clean the diaphragm after each contact with a person. If you use a stethoscope that is used by other caregivers and is used on a regular basis, clean the earpieces with alcohol before putting them in your ears.

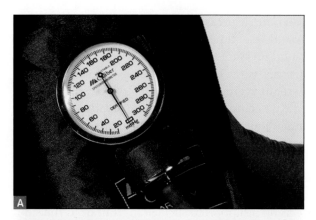

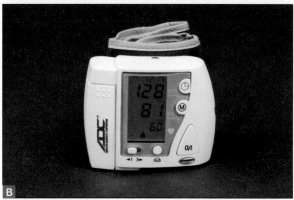

Fig. 8-15, A–B: (**A**) An aneroid manometer; (**B**) An electronic manometer.

Measuring Blood Pressure

BP is measured in millimeters of mercury, or mmHg. It is reported as two numbers, systolic BP over diastolic blood pressure. Systolic blood pressure is the force exerted against the arteries

Table 8-1:
Categories for Blood Pressure Levels in Adults in Millimeters of Mercury (mmHg)[1]

CATEGORY	SYSTOLIC (TOP NUMBER)	DIASTOLIC (BOTTOM NUMBER)
Normal	Less than 120	Less than 80
Prehypertensive	120–139	80–89
High blood pressure		
Stage 1	140–159	90–99
Stage 2	160 or higher	100 or higher

[1]For adults 18 and older who are not on medication for high blood pressure, are not having a short-term serious illness and do not have other conditions, such as diabetes or kidney disease. When systolic and diastolic blood pressures fall into different categories, the higher category should be used to classify blood pressure level. For example, 160/80 mmHg would be stage 2 high blood pressure. http://www.nhlbi.nih.gov/health/dci/Diseases/Hbp/HBP_WhatIs.html

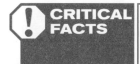

CRITICAL FACTS

BP is measured in millimeters of mercury, or mmHg. It is reported as two numbers, systolic blood pressure over diastolic blood pressure. Systolic blood pressure is the force exerted against the arteries when the heart is contracting. Diastolic blood pressure is the force exerted against the arteries when the heart is between contractions.

when the heart is contracting. An average adult systolic blood pressure is 120 mmHg. Diastolic blood pressure is the force exerted against the arteries when the heart is between contractions, with an average adult reading of 80 mmHg.

An accurate reading can be acquired through auscultation (listening) or by palpation (feeling).

To measure BP by auscultation, use the BP cuff together with the stethoscope, as follows:

- Have the patient sit or lie down in a comfortable position. Make sure the forearm is on a supported surface in front or to the side of the patient and not hanging down or raised above the level of the heart.
- Select an appropriately sized cuff for the patient. The cuff should cover approximately two-thirds of the patient's upper arm. Place the cuff so that the bladder is centered over the brachial artery and the bottom edge of the cuff is about 1 inch above the crease of the elbow.
- Place the stethoscope earpieces in your ears, with the earpieces facing forward. Center the *diaphragm* of the stethoscope firmly over the brachial artery, about 1 inch above the crease of the elbow (**Fig. 8-16**).
- Close the thumb valve by rotating the knob *clockwise* and then squeeze the rubber bulb to inflate the cuff. This compresses the brachial artery, momentarily stopping the blood flow. Stop inflating when you can no longer hear the pulse.
- Next, slowly release the air in the cuff at approximately 2 to 4 mmHg per second by turning the valve *counterclockwise* and listen with the stethoscope. Watch the pressure gauge and note the number, recorded in even numbers, when you first hear the pulse again. This is the *systolic* pressure, or the pressure of the blood when the heart beats.

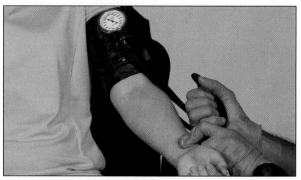

Fig. 8-17: Estimating a systolic blood pressure requires you to feel for the radial pulse.

- Continue to release the air from the bulb and watch the manometer. Once you hear the last sound, record the reading on the gauge. This is the *diastolic* pressure, or the pressure between heartbeats.

Palpation can prove particularly helpful and recommended in noisy environments where auscultation may prove difficult or potentially inaccurate. Measuring BP by palpation requires you to feel the radial artery as you inflate the BP cuff (**Fig. 8-17**).

- Have the patient sit or lie down in a comfortable position. Make sure the forearm is on a supported surface in front or to the side of the patient and not hanging down or raised above the level of the heart.
- Select an appropriately sized cuff for the patient (**Fig. 8-18**). The cuff should cover approximately two-thirds of the patient's upper arm. Place the cuff so that the bladder is centered over the brachial artery and the bottom edge of the cuff is about an inch above the crease of the elbow.
- Locate the patient's radial pulse, then close the thumb valve by rotating the knob *clockwise* and then squeeze the rubber bulb to inflate

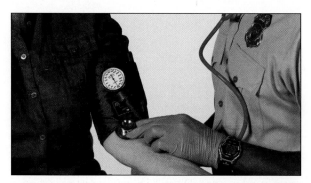

Fig. 8-16: When measuring blood pressure by auscultation, center the diaphragm of the stethoscope firmly over the brachial artery.

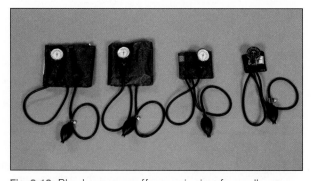

Fig. 8-18: Blood pressure cuffs come in sizes for small, average and large arms.

Table 8-2:

Precautions for Taking a Person's Blood Pressure

PRECAUTION	REASON
Place the cuff on the person's bare arm or lightly clothed arm.	Heavy clothing may give an incorrect reading. When the diaphragm is placed on heavy clothing, it creates noises that make it difficult to hear pulse sounds.
Select the correct cuff size: adult-size for most adults, extra-large for some adults and child-size for small people.	Using the correct size results in an accurate reading.
Wrap the cuff smoothly and snugly.	A smooth wrap gives an accurate reading.
Position the cuff correctly, with the center of the bladder over the brachial artery.	Correct positioning gives an accurate reading.
Do not place the cuff on a cast.	The cuff cannot compress the cast, which results in no reading.
Do not place the cuff on an arm with an IV in place.	The pressure from the cuff could stop the flow of fluid and possibly cause the needle to clog or dislodge from the vein.
Do not place the cuff on the weak arm of a person who has had a stroke or on a person's paralyzed arm. For a woman who has had a mastectomy, do not place the cuff on the arm that is on the same side as the mastectomy.	Circulation in these conditions is impaired, resulting in an inaccurate reading. Also, an inflated cuff decreases circulation in the arm and may cause some damage.
Do not place the cuff on an arm that has an AV fistula which is used for hemodialysis.	Placing and inflating the blood pressure cuff over this site can cause low blood flow, blood clot formation within the fistula as well as collapse of the fistula making the site unusable. This could lead to surgical intervention for the patient.

the cuff. This compresses the brachial artery which in turn compresses the radial artery, momentarily stopping the blood flow. Stop inflating when you can no longer feel the radial pulse. Record the reading on the manometer.

- Continue to inflate the cuff for another 20 mmHg beyond this point. Release the pressure slowly by turning the regulating valve *counterclockwise*, and allow it to deflate at about 2 to 4 mmHg per second. Continue to feel for the radial pulse as the cuff deflates. The point at which the pulse returns is the approximate *systolic* blood pressure. This BP reading should be shown with an even number followed by the letter P to indicate palpation, for example, 130/P. It is important to note whether the patient was lying or sitting when the reading was taken.

When the proper equipment is not available, you can approximate the systolic blood pressure in certain pulse locations. For example, the radial artery, located at the wrist, indicates a systolic pressure of about 80 mmHg. The femoral artery indicates a systolic pressure of at least 70 mmHg. The carotid artery in the neck indicates a systolic pressure of about 60 mmHg. Two options for approximating the systolic blood pressure include asking the patient what his or her normal BP is or inflating the cuff to 160 mmHg.

Pediatric Considerations

It is difficult to obtain an accurate BP reading on a child. First, the cuff must fit correctly, and it is difficult to have the correct size for a wide range of children. However, determining BP in children is not as important as it is with adults. In general, children under 3 years of age do not have their BP taken. What

Table 8-3:
Normal Blood Pressure Ranges in Children and Infants

AGE	SYSTOLIC	DIASTOLIC
Children (1 to 12 years old)	90 + (2 × age in years) mmHg	2/3 of systolic pressure
Infants (1 to 12 months)	70 + (2 × age in years) mmHg	2/3 of systolic pressure
Newborns (ages 1 to 28 days)	>60 mmHg (varies depending on birth weight and gestation)	>14 mmHg (varies depending on birth weight and gestation)

is more important in assessing children is adequate airway management. Children's BP may not drop until there has been a significant loss of blood. Therefore, provide care for shock if the MOI calls for it, regardless of BP.

BP may be *estimated* in children. The formula for the *average* BP for a child is 90 + (2 × the age of the child in years). This formula can be used for children up to the age of 12.

BP numbers in children and infants vary by age.
• Infants (1 to 12 months): systolic 70 mmHg (lower limit of normal); diastolic 2/3 of systolic pressure. Ranges for newborns vary depending on birth weight and whether the newborn is full term or premature.
• Children (1 to 12 years):
  • Lower limit of normal: systolic 70 mmHg + (2 × age in years); diastolic 2/3 of systolic pressure
  • Upper limit of normal: systolic 90 mmHg + (2 × age in years); diastolic 2/3 of systolic pressure
• Adolescents: systolic 90 mmHg (lower limit of normal); diastolic 2/3 of systolic pressure

For other pediatric considerations, see **Chapter 25**.

ONGOING ASSESSMENT

Once you have completed the secondary assessment and provided care for any injuries and illnesses, provide **ongoing assessment** and care while you wait for more advanced medical care to arrive. The purpose of the ongoing assessment is to identify and treat any changes in

the patient's condition in a timely manner and to monitor the effectiveness of interventions or care provided. Record additional findings and turn this information over to the next level of care.

Table 8-4:
Vital Signs by Age

ADULTS (ABOUT 12 YEARS AND OLDER)	
Pulse	60 to 100 beats per minute
Blood pressure	90–140 mmHg (systolic) 60–90 mmHg (diastolic)
Respirations	12 to 20 breaths per minute
CHILDREN (AGE 1 TO ABOUT 12 YEARS)	
Pulse	80 to 100 beats per minute
Blood pressure	80–110 mmHg systolic
Respirations	15 to 30 breaths per minute
INFANTS (AGE 1 TO 12 MONTHS)	
Pulse	100 to 140 beats per minute
Blood pressure	70–95 mmHg systolic
Respirations	25 to 50 breaths per minute
NEONATAL/NEWBORN (FULL-TERM TO 28 DAYS)	
Pulse	120 to 160 beats per minute
Blood pressure	>60 mmHg systolic
Respirations	40 to 60 breaths per minute

Source: www.emsresource.net

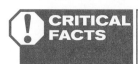 **CRITICAL FACTS** — Ongoing assessment should be done after the secondary assessment. Its purpose is to identify and care for any changes in the patient's condition and to monitor the effectiveness of care provided.

The patient's condition can gradually worsen, or a life-threatening condition, such as respiratory or cardiac arrest, can occur suddenly. Do not assume that the patient is out of danger just because there were no serious problems at first. Reassess the patient at regular intervals. Patients who are unstable should be reassessed at least every 5 minutes or more often if indicated by the patient's condition. Reassess stable patients every 15 minutes, or as deemed appropriate by the patient's condition.

The physical exam and history do not need to be repeated unless there is a specific reason to do so. If any life-threatening conditions develop, stop whatever you are doing and provide appropriate care immediately.

Reassessment includes the—
- Primary assessment.
- Vital signs.
- Chief complaint.
- Interventions, or care provided.

Reassess Primary Assessment

Reassess each aspect of the primary assessment and compare to the patient's baseline status. For LOC, is the patient maintaining the same level of responsiveness or becoming more or less alert? Recheck the airway to ensure it is open and clear. Reassess the adequacy of breathing by monitoring breathing rate, depth and effort. Reassess the adequacy of circulation by checking both carotid and radial pulses. Recheck skin characteristics (color, temperature and moisture).

Reassess Vital Signs

Repeat vital signs as necessary each time you reassess the patient. Repeat BP, pulse and respiration.

Reassess Chief Complaint

Constantly reassess the patient's chief complaint or major injury. Determine if the pain or discomfort is remaining the same, getting worse or getting better. Ask the patient whether there are any new or previously undisclosed complaints.

Reassess Interventions

Reassess the effectiveness of each intervention performed. Consider the need for new interventions or modifications to care already being provided.

THE NEED FOR MORE ADVANCED MEDICAL PERSONNEL

While waiting for more advanced medical care (**Table 8-5**), help the injured or ill patient stay calm and as comfortable as possible. These conditions are by no means a complete list. It is impossible to describe every possible condition since there are always exceptions. Trust your instincts. If you think there is an emergency, there probably is. It is better to call for more advanced medical care than to wait.

PUTTING IT ALL TOGETHER

Once you have sized-up the scene and performed a primary assessment, you are ready to move on to the secondary assessment. This requires you to perform a physical exam to find and care for any other problems that are not an immediate threat to life but might become serious if you do not recognize them and provide care. This head-to-toe physical exam involves looking at and feeling the body for abnormalities. Use the mnemonic DOTS as you perform the physical exam. For many patients, this will be a rapid medical or trauma assessment.

Obtain pertinent history from the patient. This is especially important if the patient is suffering from an illness that has already been diagnosed and is being cared for by a health care provider. Whether you obtain the history before, after or during the physical exam depends on the MOI or nature of the illness and whether the patient is responsive or unresponsive. Use the mnemonic SAMPLE to gather all of the necessary information. For some patients, if there is time and the patient's condition warrants it, you will go back and complete a detailed physical exam.

Once the assessment is complete, perform ongoing assessments until more advanced personnel take over. Reassess every 5 minutes for unstable patients and every 15 minutes for stable ones, or as dictated by the patient's condition.

Although this plan of action can help you decide what care to provide in any emergency, providing care is not an exact science. Because each emergency and each patient are unique, an emergency may not occur exactly as it did in a classroom setting. The care needed may change

Table 8-5:

When to Call for More Advanced Medical Personnel

CONDITION	SIGNS AND SYMPTOMS
Unconscious or decreased level of consciousness	• Patient does not respond to tapping, loud voices or other attempts to awaken.
Trouble breathing	• Breathing is noisy (sounds such as wheezing or gasping). • Patient feels short of breath. • Skin has a flushed, pale or bluish appearance.
No breathing	• You cannot see the patient's chest rise and fall. • You cannot hear and feel air escaping from the nose and/or mouth.
No pulse	• You cannot feel the carotid pulse in the neck or the pulses in other pulse points.
Severe bleeding	• Patient has bleeding that spurts or gushes steadily from the wound.
Persistent pain or pressure in the chest	• There is chest pain, discomfort or pressure lasting more than a few minutes; that goes away and comes back; or that radiates to the shoulder, arm, neck, jaw, stomach or back.
Persistent pain or pressure in the abdomen	• Patient has persistent pain or pressure in the abdomen that is not relieved by resting or changing positions.
Vomiting blood or passing blood	• You can see blood in vomit, urine or feces.
Severe (critical) burns	• Burns that cover a large surface area; cover more than one body part; involve the head, neck, mouth or nose or affect the airway. Burns other than localized superficial burns to a small child or elderly patient; those affecting the hands, feet or genitals; or those resulting from chemicals, explosions or electricity.

from one moment to the next. For example, the primary assessment may indicate the patient is conscious, breathing, has a pulse and no severe bleeding is evident. However, during your physical exam, you may notice that the patient begins to experience difficulty breathing. At this point, there is a need to summon more advanced medical personnel, if this has not already been done, and provide appropriate care. Provide necessary information about the patient's condition once more advanced medical personnel arrive.

Many variables exist when dealing with emergencies. You do not need to "diagnose" what is wrong with the patient to provide appropriate care. Treat the conditions you find, always caring for life-threatening conditions first. Perform the primary and secondary assessments as a guideline to help you assess the patient's condition.

As you read the remaining chapters, remember the steps of the assessments. They form the basis for providing care in any emergency.

Table 8-5:
(continued)

CONDITION	SIGNS AND SYMPTOMS
Suspected poisoning	• Patient shows evidence of swallowed, inhaled, absorbed or injected poison, such as presence of drugs, medications, cleaning agents or hypodermic needles and syringes. • Mouth or lips may be burned.
Sudden illness requiring assistance	• Patient has seizures, severe headaches, slurred speech or changes in the level of consciousness; unusually high or low blood pressure; or a known diabetic condition.
Stroke	• Sudden weakness on one side of the face/facial droop, sudden weakness on one side of the body, sudden slurred speech or trouble getting words out or a sudden severe headache.
Head, neck or back (spinal) injuries	• Consider how the injury happened: for example, a fall, severe blow or collision suggests a head injury. • Patient complains of severe headaches or neck or back pain. • Patient is unconscious. • Blood or clear fluid is detected in the ears, mouth or nose. • There is bleeding or deformity of the scalp, face or neck.
Possible broken bones	• Consider how the injury happened: for example, a fall, severe blow or collision suggests a fracture. • There is evidence of damage to blood vessels or nerves: for example, slow capillary refill, no pulse below the injury or loss of sensation in the affected part. • Patient is unable to move the body part without pain or discomfort. • There is a swollen or deformed limb. • Fractures are associated with open wounds.

YOU ARE THE EMERGENCY MEDICAL RESPONDER

The injured woman accompanies you to a separate area so you can assess her for injuries. She is still clutching her arm. What steps would you take to identify any injuries or conditions that may need medical care? After assessing this patient, you find no life-threatening conditions. How often would you reassess her and why?

SKILLsheet

How to Obtain a SAMPLE History

STEP 1

Using the mnemonic SAMPLE, determine the following six items for the history:

1. Signs and symptoms: Signs include seeing bleeding, hearing breathing distress, and feeling cool, moist skin. Symptoms include pain, nausea, headache, and difficulty breathing.
2. Allergies: Determine if the victim is allergic to any medications, food, or environmental elements, such as pollen or bees.
3. Medications: Determine if the victim is presently using any medications, prescription or non-prescription.
4. Pertinent past medical history: Determine if the victim is under a health care provider's care for any condition or if the victim has had a similar problem in the past or been recently hospitalized.
5. Last oral intake: This intake includes solids or liquids and can include food, fluid and medication.
6. Events leading up to the incident: Determine what the victim was doing before and at the time of the incident.

SKILLsheet

How to Perform a Secondary Assessment for a Responsive Medical Patient

NOTE: Always follow standard precautions when providing care.

STEP 1
Assess the patient's complaints (use the mnemonic OPQRST—onset, provoke, quality, region/radiate, severity and time).

STEP 2
Obtain a SAMPLE history (see Skill Sheet on page 186).

STEP 3
Perform a focused medical assessment unless signs and symptoms make the focus unclear, in which case you would perform a rapid medical assessment (head to toe).

STEP 4
Assess baseline vital signs.

STEP 5
Perform components of the detailed physical exam, as needed.

STEP 6
Provide emergency care.

NOTE: Consider the need for advanced life support backup and the need for transport (e.g., for life-threatening conditions, such as anaphylaxis).

If the medical patient is unresponsive, consider the patient as critical, requiring that you begin with a rapid medical assessment, to gain as much information as possible on the nature of the illness.

SKILLsheet

How to Perform a Secondary Assessment for an Unresponsive Medical Patient

NOTE: Always follow standard precautions when providing care.

STEP 1

Consider the need for advanced life support backup and the need for transport (e.g., for life-threatening conditions, such as heart attack).

STEP 2

Perform a rapid medical assessment (head to toe).

STEP 3

Assess baseline vital signs.

STEP 4

Position a patient who is unresponsive, but breathing, face-up and ensure protection of the airway.

STEP 5

Obtain a SAMPLE history (see Skill Sheet on page 186) from the family or any bystanders, if available.

STEP 6

Provide emergency care.

SKILLsheet

Physical Exam and Patient History

STEP 1
Perform physical exam beginning with the head and neck.

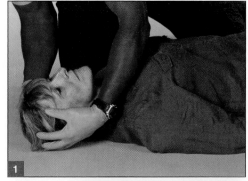

STEP 2
Check the shoulders.

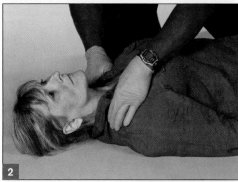

STEP 3
Check the chest.

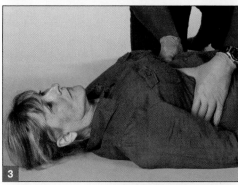

STEP 4
Check the abdomen.

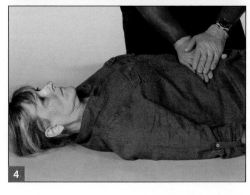

Continued on next page

Physical Exam and Patient History *continued*

STEP 5
Check the pelvis.

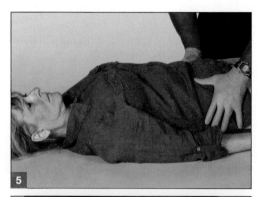

STEP 6
Check the arms and hands.

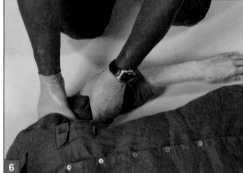

STEP 7
Check the legs and feet.

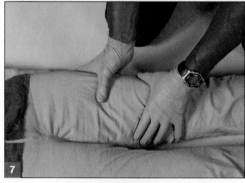

STEP 8
Check the patient's back.

STEP 9
Interview the patient to obtain a SAMPLE history (see Skill Sheet on page 186).

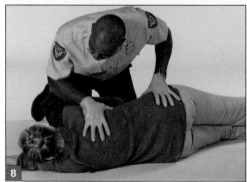

SKILLsheet

How to Obtain Baseline Vital Signs

NOTE: Always follow standard precautions when providing care. When assessing breathing, look for a stoma or other signs of a neck breather.

STEP 1

Check respirations for rate, rhythm and quality of breathing.

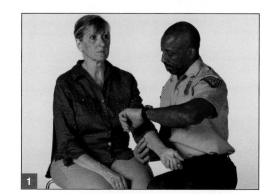

- ◆ Look, listen and feel for breathing.
  - Look for the rise and fall of the patient's chest or abdomen.
  - Listen for sounds as the patient inhales and exhales.
- ◆ Count the number of times a patient breathes in **30** seconds.
  - Multiply that number by **2** (or in **15** seconds by **4**). This is the number of breaths per minute.
- ◆ Record your findings.

NOTE: As you check for the rate and quality of breathing, try to do it without the patient's knowledge. If the patient realizes you are checking breathing, this may cause a change in breathing pattern without the patient being aware of it. Maintain the same position you would when you are checking the pulse.

STEP 2

Check for a pulse.

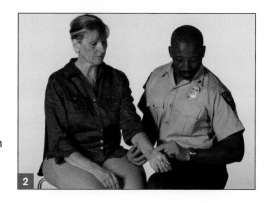

- ◆ Place two fingers on top of a major artery near the skin's surface and over a bony structure.
  - Pulse points include the carotid arteries in the neck, the radial artery in the wrist and, for infants, the brachial artery in the inside of the upper arm.
  - To check the pulse rate, count the number of beats in **30** seconds and multiply that number by **2** (or in **15** seconds by **4**).
- ◆ Record your findings.

NOTE: An injured or ill patient's pulse may be hard to find. If a patient is breathing, the heart is also beating. There may be a loss in circulation to the injured area, causing a loss of pulse. If you cannot find the pulse in one place, check it in another, such as in the other wrist.

Continued on next page

How to Obtain Baseline Vital Signs *continued*

STEP 3

Check skin characteristics.

NOTE: Checking the skin characteristics requires you to look at and feel the skin. You may need to partially remove a disposable glove in order to determine skin moisture and temperature. Be careful not to come in contact with any blood or open wounds.

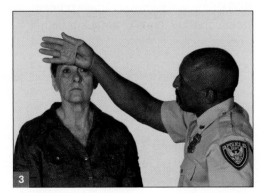

◆ To check skin characteristics look or feel for–
  • Color. Is it pale and ashen, or flushed and pink?
  • Temperature. Is it hot or cold?
  • Moisture. Is it moist or dry?
  • Capillary refill. Is it normal or slow?
  • Record your findings.

SKILLsheet

Taking and Recording a Patient's Blood Pressure (by Auscultation)

STEP 1
Approximate systolic blood pressure.
◆ Either ask the patient what his or her BP is or use **160** mmHg as an alternative.

NOTE: The radial artery, located at the wrist, indicates a systolic pressure of about **80** mmHg. The femoral artery in the leg indicates a systolic pressure of at least **70** mmHg. The carotid artery in the neck indicates a systolic pressure of about **60** mmHg.

STEP 2
Select an appropriately sized cuff for the patient.

STEP 3
Position the cuff.

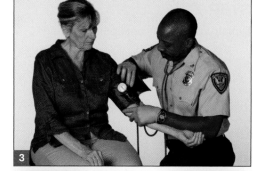

STEP 4
Locate brachial pulse.

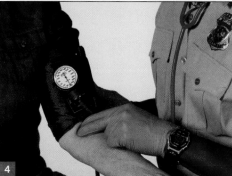

STEP 5
Position the diaphragm of the stethoscope over the pulse point.

NOTE: Hold the diaphragm in place with your fingers, not your thumb, because you may hear the pulse in your thumb instead of the patient's brachial pulse.

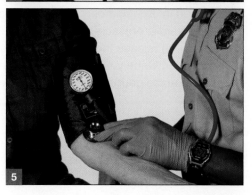

Continued on next page

Taking and Recording a Patient's Blood Pressure (by Auscultation) *continued*

STEP 6

Inflate cuff. Stop inflating when you can no longer hear the pulse.

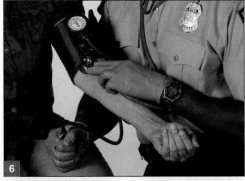

STEP 7

Deflate cuff slowly until pulse is heard.

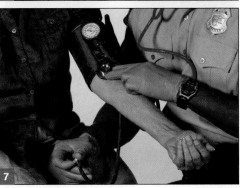

STEP 8

Continue deflating cuff until the pulse is no longer heard.

STEP 9

Quickly deflate cuff by opening the valve.

STEP 10

Record findings.
- ◆ Watch the pressure gauge and note the number, recorded in even numbers, when you first hear the pulse again (systolic pressure).
- ◆ Continue to release the air from the bulb and watch the manometer. Once you hear the last sound, record the reading on the gauge (diastolic pressure).

SKILLsheet

Taking and Recording a Patient's Blood Pressure (by Palpation)

STEP 1

Select an appropriately sized cuff for the patient's arm and position the cuff.

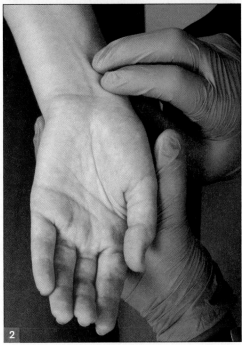

STEP 2

Locate the radial pulse.

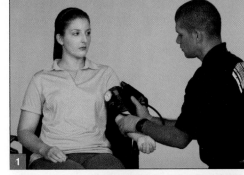

Continued on next page

Taking and Recording a Patient's Blood Pressure (by Palpation) *continued*

STEP 3

Inflate the cuff beyond where pulse disappears.

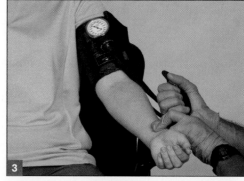

STEP 4

Deflate the cuff slowly until pulse returns; the point where the pulse returns is the approximate systolic blood pressure.

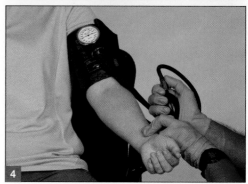

STEP 5

Quickly deflate the cuff by opening the valve.

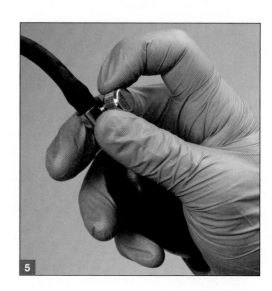

STEP 6

Record the approximate systolic blood pressure with a "P" for palpation method (e.g., **130**/P).

Enrichment
Pulse Oximetry

PURPOSE

Pulse oximetry is used to measure the percentage of oxygen saturation in the blood. The reading is taken by a pulse oximeter **(Fig. 8-19)** and appears as a percentage of hemoglobin saturated with oxygen. Normal saturation is approximately 95 to 99 percent. The reading is recorded as 95 to 99 percent SpO_2.

Pulse oximetry also is used to assess the adequacy of oxygen delivery during positive pressure ventilation and the impact of other medical care provided.

When monitoring a conscious victim's oxygen saturation levels using a pulse oximeter, you may reduce the flow of oxygen and change to a lower-flowing delivery device if the oxygen level of the victim reaches 100 percent.

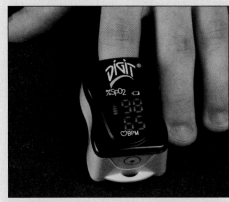

Fig. 8-19: A pulse oximeter measures the oxygen saturation level in a patient's blood.

The percent of oxygen saturation always should be documented whenever vital signs are recorded and in response to therapy to correct hypoxia. A reading below 94 percent may indicate hypoxia. Pulse oximetry should be used as an added tool for patient evaluation, as it is possible for patients to show a normal reading but have trouble breathing, or have a low reading but appear to be breathing. When treating the patient, all symptoms should be assessed, along with the data provided by the device. The pulse oximeter reading never should be used to withhold oxygen from a patient who appears to be in respiratory distress or when it is the standard of care to apply oxygen despite good pulse oximetry readings, such as in a patient with chest pain.

Indications

Pulse oximetry should be applied whenever a patient's oxygenation is a concern and for the following situations:
* All patients with neurologic, respiratory or cardiovascular complaints
* All patients with abnormal vital signs
* All patients who receive respiratory depressants (morphine, diazepam, midazolam)
* Critical trauma patients

Pulse oximetry should be taken and recorded with vital signs for stable patients at least every 15 minutes and reassessed and recorded every 5 minutes for unstable patients.

Table 8-6:
Pulse Oximetry

RANGE	VALUE	TREATMENT
Normal	95 to 100 percent	None
Mild hypoxia	91 to 94 percent	Administer emergency oxygen using a nasal cannula or resuscitation mask.
Moderate hypoxia	86 to 90 percent	Administer emergency oxygen using a non-rebreather mask or bag-valve-mask resuscitator.
Severe hypoxia	≤85 percent	Administer emergency oxygen using a non-rebreather mask or bag-valve-mask resuscitator with positive pressure.

Source: www.emsresource.net

Continued on next page

Enrichment
Pulse Oximetry (continued)

Procedure

When using a pulse oximeter, refer to the manufacturer's directions to ensure proper use. In general, the procedure for measuring pulse oximetry is the same.

Once the machine is turned on, allow for self-tests. If the patient is wearing nail polish, remove it using an acetone wipe, as it can interfere with the reading. Then apply the probe to the patient's finger. The manufacturer also may recommend alternative measuring sites, such as the finger and then the ear lobe on the next measurement.

Pediatric Considerations

The manufacturer may recommend alternative measuring sites for pulse oximetry in infants, such as the foot.

The machine will register the oxygen saturation level. Once it begins to register, record the time and the initial saturation percent, if possible, on the prehospital care report. Verify the patient's pulse rate on the oximeter with the actual pulse of the patient. Be sure to monitor critical patients continuously until more advanced medical personnel are available. If you are recording a one-time reading, be sure to monitor the patient for a few minutes, as oxygen saturation can vary. As mentioned above, document the percent of oxygen saturation whenever vital signs are recorded and in response to therapy to correct hypoxia.

Limitations

Some factors may reduce the reliability of the pulse oximetry reading, including—
* Hypoperfusion, poor perfusion (shock).
* Cardiac arrest (absent perfusion to fingers).
* Excessive motion of the patient during the reading.
* Fingernail polish.
* Carbon monoxide poisoning (carbon monoxide saturates hemoglobin).
* Hypothermia or other cold-related illness.
* Sickle cell disease or anemia.
* Cigarette smokers (due to carbon monoxide).
* Edema (swelling).
* Time lag in detection of respiratory insufficiency. (The pulse oximeter could warn too late of a decrease in respiratory function based on the amount of oxygen in circulation.)

9

Communication and Documentation

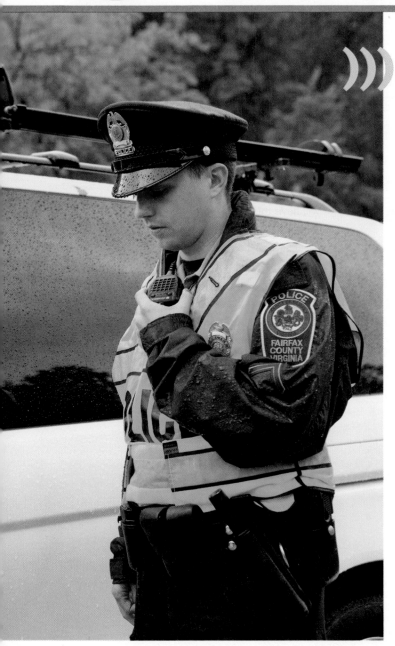

))) **YOU ARE THE EMERGENCY MEDICAL RESPONDER**

As the closest responders in the area, your police unit is called to the scene where an elderly woman has collapsed in front of her home. When you arrive, a neighbor tells you that the woman suddenly collapsed and tripped on the concrete step in the walkway in front of her home. She is now conscious but a little dazed, and you find that she is also very frightened and apprehensive. What can you do to try to ease the woman's fears and reduce her anxiety as you assess her for injuries?

Key Terms

Communications center (dispatch): The point of contact between the public and responders (also known as a *9-1-1 call center* or *Public Service Answering Point*, or [PSAP]); responsible for taking basic information from callers and dispatching the appropriate personnel; in some communities may also provide prearrival instructions to the 9-1-1 caller.

Echo method: A communication technique in which the listener repeats orders word for word to ensure the message was heard and understood accurately.

Medical control: Direction given to *emergency medical responders* (EMRs) by a physician when EMRs are providing care at the scene of an emergency or are en route to the receiving facility; may be provided either directly via radio or indirectly by pre-established local medical treatment protocols.

Minimum data set: A standardized set of details about patients; this information is included in the *prehospital care report* (PCR).

Patient narrative: A section on the prehospital care report where the assessment and care provided to the patient are described.

Prehospital care report (PCR): A document filled out for all emergency calls; used to keep medical personnel informed so they can provide appropriate continuity of care; also serves as a record for legal and billing purposes; may be written or electronic; if electronic, it is then an E-PCR.

Run data: A section on the PCR where information about the incident is documented.

Learning Objectives

After reading this chapter, and completing the class activities, you will have the information needed to—

- Recognize the importance of effective communication within the *emergency medical services* (EMS) system.
- Recognize the need for compassion and empathy when caring for a patient's physical and mental needs.
- Communicate willingly and with sensitivity in the care of all patients.
- Identify the components of the *prehospital care report* (PCR).
- Describe the fundamental components of documentation and related issues.
- Explain the importance of maintaining confidentiality about the condition, circumstances and care of the patient.
- Describe the elements of a verbal report given during the transfer of care.

INTRODUCTION

When you arrive on the scene to assist injured or ill persons, what you think you see and what has actually happened may not be the same thing. It is easy to make judgments that may turn out to be incorrect. Communication may be difficult in times of stress, particularly if there are other factors involved, such as language barriers or fear. For this reason, the *emergency medical responder* (EMR) must be able to assess the situation and work out the best methods of obtaining the needed information. Other factors such as background noise may also inhibit communication between the EMR and other members of the team or patient. Effective communication with the patient and bystanders is of utmost importance to understand what took place. By using various techniques to gain the trust and confidence of the public, an EMR can discover details of the injury or illness that may otherwise go undiscovered.

Communication among response team members is also a major part of responding to a medical or trauma emergency. Communication is important for EMRs, as they may need to call for additional resources to transfer patient care to other responders or to the receiving facility. Communication is also important as it facilitates interaction within the team structure. By using the appropriate communication techniques, understanding the equipment used and the type of information that needs to be relayed, the EMR improves the quality of care provided to the patient.

The final element of emergency care is documentation. Records of all that has occurred, from the beginning of the call for help to the point at which the patient has been transported to the receiving facility, are extremely important. Proper and thorough documentation will assist more advanced medical personnel in providing care and can help prevent inappropriate lawsuits.

COMMUNICATING WITHIN THE EMERGENCY COMMUNICATIONS SYSTEM

For an *emergency medical services* (EMS) system to run properly, constant communication must be a priority among its key components, which include—

- The **communications center (dispatch)**, which is responsible for taking basic information from callers and dispatching the appropriate personnel. In some communities, the communications center may also provide prearrival instructions to the 9-1-1 caller.
- The medical director and receiving facility, often a hospital.
- The EMS personnel in the field.

To work efficiently, the EMS system must have a communications system geared toward its particular needs. Often, this involves a radio communication system and/or a mobile phone system for communication among members of its network.

Radio Communication System Components

Radio communication for an EMS system is comprised of four key components, including the base station, mobile radios, portable radios and repeaters. All radios in the United States, including those used by EMS personnel, are regulated and licensed by the *Federal Communications Commission* (FCC).

The base station is the hub of communications and should be situated in the best possible location for sending and receiving signals. It must have access to power and an antenna for maximum quality reception.

Mobile radios are mounted in emergency vehicles. Their ability to send and receive messages varies and is affected by terrain and objects, such as tall buildings, which may be in the vicinity.

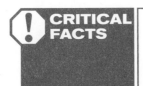
CRITICAL FACTS

For an EMS system to run properly, constant communication among the communication center, the medical director, the receiving facility and EMS personnel must be a priority.

Radio communication for an EMS system is comprised of four key components, including the base station, mobile radios, portable radios and repeaters.

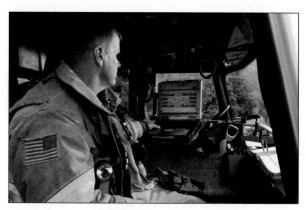

Fig. 9-1: A mobile data terminal is situated in the emergency vehicle and displays information in text that has been relayed from the base.

Portable radios are handheld radios that are particularly useful when you must be out of your vehicle. Their range is limited, but can be boosted by use of a repeater, a device that receives a low-powered radio signal and rebroadcasts it at a higher power. Repeaters increase the amount of territory you can access through radio communication.

Digital equipment uses an encoder and a decoder, which allow emergency personnel to communicate more easily, without overutilizing bandwidth. A mobile data terminal uses written data rather than voice instructions. The terminal is situated in the emergency vehicle and information is relayed from the base to the terminal (**Fig. 9-1**). The information is then displayed in text, to be read off the screen. To respond, emergency personnel can transmit in the same manner, or push a button to switch to voice mode.

Rules for Radio Communication

The FCC regulates the use of radio communication systems. Therefore, those who use these systems must follow FCC rules. Ground rules for use of an EMS radio communication system help ensure that information is communicated as completely and accurately as possible. (The FCC website can be found at *www.fcc.gov.*)

Here are some important FCC rules to follow when using an EMS radio communication system:

- Use EMS frequencies only for EMS communication.

- Before speaking, listen to make sure the channel you are using is clear.
- Close your vehicle windows to avoid distortions.
- To communicate, press the *push-to-talk* (PTT) button and wait 1 second before speaking.
- Speak slowly, with your lips about 2–3 inches from the microphone.
- Address the unit you are calling by its name and number, and then identify yourself by your unit name and number.
- Wait for the unit to let you know they are ready to receive your communication.
- Use concise, clear and plain language in your communications. Because of a lack of uniformity across jurisdictions and the need for rapid and clear communications from different responding agencies in a major crisis, the 10 code system (operational/brevity codes) is being phased out in favor of plain language as required by the *Department of Homeland Security* (DHS) and in support of the *National Incident Management System* (NIMS).
- Keep transmissions brief, organized and to the point. Omit courtesy terms like "please" and "thank you."
- When saying numbers that might be confused with other numbers, say the number, then the individual digits (e.g., to avoid confusing 15 with 50, say "fifteen," then "one-five").
- Give only objective, verifiable information and remember that others can listen in on radio communications. Do not use patients' names in your communications.
- Use "affirmative" and "negative" rather than "yes" and "no."

Communicating with Dispatch

The communications center (dispatch) is also known as a *9-1-1 call center* or *Public Service Answering Point* (PSAP). The role of dispatch is to receive emergency calls and send the appropriate team to respond. Dispatch is the point of contact between the public and responders (**Fig. 9-2**). In the 9-1-1 system, *emergency medical dispatchers* (EMDs) must decide which emergency service resources are required.

EMDs (and the call takers who assist them) must gather as much information as possible

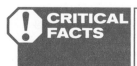

CRITICAL FACTS Ground rules for use of a radio communication system, as set forth by the FCC, help ensure that information is communicated completely and accurately throughout the EMS system.

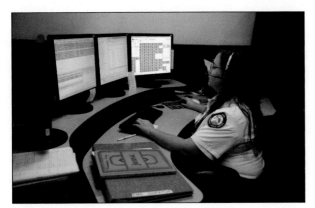

Fig. 9-2: Dispatch serves as a liaison between the public and emergency response personnel.

regarding the emergency. They also may advise callers about what the callers may be able to do while awaiting your arrival. Dispatchers note the time the call was received and the time they dispatched emergency services. Also, they usually record all conversations and radio dispatches, in order to have an indisputable record of the events. (For more information on EMDs, refer to **Chapter 27**.)

As an EMR and depending on the work setting, you are responsible for—

- Receiving instructions from dispatch and acknowledging receipt.
- Providing an *estimated time of arrival* (ETA) to dispatch, if requested, and reporting any delays along the route that may change the ETA.
- Announcing your arrival at the scene to dispatch and providing your assessment of whether more emergency services should be sent or if assigned resources can be released.
- Informing dispatch when you leave for transport to the hospital or when your role is finished, if you have been relieved by more advanced medical personnel. When relaying information about transport, you must inform dispatch of how many patients you have, the name of the receiving facility and your ETA.
- On arrival, notifying dispatch that you have arrived on scene.
- When the patient transfer is complete and you are able to leave the hospital, letting dispatch

know you are once again available for service. You may have to contact dispatch again once you return to your station or home base.

Communicating with Medical Control

Depending on your EMS system, **medical control** may or may not be located at the receiving facility. There may be times when you must speak to medical control while you are on scene. This would most likely be in a situation in which standing orders or protocols would not be sufficient and you have questions about the care provided to the patient. Communications with medical control must be thorough but brief.

When communicating with medical control, provide the following information:

- Who you are (unit, level of service and your role)
- Patient characteristics (age, gender, chief complaint)
- The patient's mental status
- SAMPLE (signs and symptoms, allergies, medications, pertinent past medical history, last oral intake, events leading up to the incident) history
- Relevant information about past illnesses
- Vital signs and results of your physical assessment
- Any care you provided and the patient's response to the care
- Your questions

Ask whether you should perform any further actions and estimate when you will arrive at the receiving facility. Whenever you receive medical direction, repeat the order *word-for-word*. This is called the **echo method**. Write down important or lengthy medical instructions.

Communicating with Medical Personnel

When other EMS personnel arrive on the scene, identify yourself and give a verbal report. Interact within the team structure, communicating any

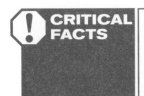
CRITICAL FACTS

When communicating with medical control, always identify yourself and give all relevant information on the patient and the care provided.

Successful interpersonal communication with patients and their families means being empathetic, having awareness of cultural differences, showing sensitivity to an individual's emotions and listening effectively.

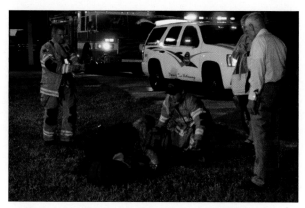

Fig. 9-3: Communicate any information regarding the patient and the scene to other EMS personnel who arrive, working within the team structure. *Courtesy of Terry Georgia.*

information concerning the patient and the scene to law enforcement and other responders (**Fig. 9-3**).

Communicating with the Receiving Facility

As soon as possible, the transport crew notifies the receiving facility about the patient and the ETA. The receiving facility (medical control) or operator is informed if there are any changes in the patient and the ETA, and communicates any changes in the patient's condition.

When communicating with the receiving facility, give the following information:

- Who you are (unit and role)
- How many patients will be arriving
- Patient characteristics (age, gender, chief complaint)
- Immediate history (events leading to the injury or illness)
- Any care you provided and the patient's response to the care
- Any vital information such as the need for isolation
- ETA

At the receiving facility, crew members will provide additional information about the scene and the patient(s). They will also complete whatever documentation is necessary to meet local or state standards and their organization's protocols.

Mobile Phone Communication

Mobile or cellular phones are becoming more popular in some EMS districts. They can be useful for covering longer distances than radio communication and their sound clarity

in communication is usually superior. Since mobile phones are fairly maintenance-free and provide the ability for direct communication between parties, they are also often used as back-up sources of communication should the radio system fail. However, there are drawbacks to mobile phones. For example, in cases of emergencies that involve multiple people, mobile phone service can be compromised due to system overload. Mobile phones are also impractical for multiunit coordination.

INTERPERSONAL COMMUNICATION

To be empathetic means to understand, be culturally sensitive and be sensitive to the thoughts, feelings and experiences of another person. In order to listen effectively to what is being said to you, it is important that you have empathy for the people involved.

Communicate with patients in a way that achieves a positive relationship. Before doing anything, unless it is a life-threatening situation, introduce yourself to the patient and family members, if present. Tell the patient what your role is and what you will do. Introducing the other members of your team is also important.

Medical and trauma emergencies can be frightening to those involved. When speaking to an injured or ill person and family members, be sure to speak slowly and clearly (**Fig. 9-4**). Avoid using medical terms and abbreviations, and speak in words that are easily understandable.

If possible, try to adapt the physical environment to facilitate communication by making sure there is adequate lighting and that you have minimized distractions such as noises, interference from others and noisy equipment nearby. Get down to the patient's eye level to avoid appearing threatening. Make eye contact and use body language that shows you are open and interested in what people have to say, for example, standing with arms at your sides instead of crossed, and with hands open rather than in closed fists.

One way to put people at ease is to address them by name, whenever possible. Note, however, that if the patients are older adults, as a matter of showing respect, you should not call them by their first names unless invited to do so. A general rule of thumb is to address individuals in

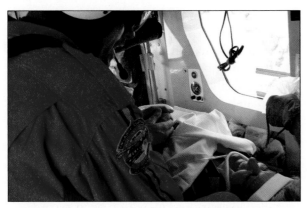
Fig. 9-4: Medical or trauma emergencies can be frightening. Speak clearly and slowly. *Courtesy of Ted Crites.*

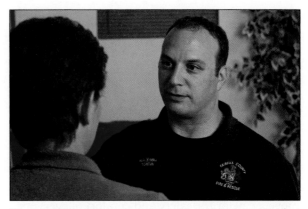
Fig. 9-5: Making eye contact with a patient helps him or her feel more comfortable.

the way that they introduce themselves to you. For example, if the patient and family member introduce themselves as Mr. and Mrs. Smith, you should address them as such.

If possible, have the patient tell you his or her name and what problems he or she is having. It may be instinctive for family members or friends to do so, but it is best if you can have the patient speak, so you can observe the patient's ability to communicate, *level of consciousness* (LOC) and mental status. You can also learn a lot about physical problems just by observing people while they are talking. If someone can only speak a few words before needing to take a breath, for example, that may mean there is a respiratory emergency. Someone clutching the stomach or chest may be doing so without being aware of it and this can give you information. Someone who winces with pain should be asked about the pain. If the patient cannot speak or is unable to give you information, then ask bystanders for the information.

Listen carefully to what the injured or ill person is telling or trying to tell you. Observe the patient as you listen (**Fig. 9-5**). Provide reassurance if there seems to be some reluctance to speak about a topic. Mention that any information you are told about the problem may be important and will remain confidential, even if it is upsetting to talk about. Attempt to gather patient information in a private setting that is away from bystanders. Individuals may feel uncomfortable giving information about the situation in front of others.

Because of the stressful nature of the situation, it is always best to ask one question at a time so the person answering can concentrate while giving the answers. Also, the answer to one

question may lead you to another related one. Asking more than one question at a time may provide confused responses. Avoid interruptions as much as possible. Allow the patient to finish a thought. If you need clarification, ask questions at the end of the patient's statement.

Depending on the type of information you are trying to find out, you may want to ask closed or direct questions, to which patients should be able to give you a "Yes" or "No" answer or a short answer. For example, you might ask "Did you have something to eat?" or "What time was it when you last ate?" For more detailed information, you may need to ask more open-ended questions, which allow for more detailed answers. This type of question may be a little more difficult for patients to answer, but can provide answers with greater depth. A typical open-ended question might be "How are you feeling right now?"

From the patient's perspective, there is nothing more annoying than not being listened to. Consider the last time you had to repeat information to someone several times; it is not a pleasant experience. Listening lets people know you believe they are important. If you ask a question, listen for the answer. Make notes, if necessary, so you do not forget what was said. If you forget too often, the patient may stop answering your questions.

As you interview the patient or bystanders, be careful to avoid the pitfalls of interviewing. For example, be sure to word questions so that you do not provide false assurance or reassurance. Avoid giving advice or asking leading or biased questions. Try to let the person you are interviewing do most of the talking and do not interrupt. Avoid asking "Why" questions, which can be perceived as judgmental; in most circumstances you do not need to know why something happened, only *what* happened.

Listen to what bystanders tell you; they may have seen or heard something that will help you determine how to care for the patient. But, after they have provided the information you require, you must consider the patient's privacy while you continue to assess the situation and provide care. Often, bystanders want to stay and watch. Be firm but reasonable with bystanders. Ask them to move away for the safety and comfort of everyone. If a crowd appears that could become hostile, explaining your role may set the crowd at ease. If, however, the crowd appears to be threatening, call for backup from the appropriate service.

Everyone deserves equal care, dignity and respect, regardless of age, language, culture or socioeconomic status. It is important not to make judgments about the patient on the basis of these differences or others, such as the patient's physical appearance. Your physical appearance is also important. By being neat and well groomed, you help give both patients and their family members a sense of confidence in you.

If you are providing care for someone who speaks a language you do not understand, call for someone who can translate. A family member or neighbor, for example, may be able to speak both your language and that of the patient. Some dispatch centers and hospitals also offer language line services which may be useful.

Watch the patient's body language, whether your language is spoken or not. Nonverbal clues can help determine what is wrong. Be sensitive to cultural differences; in some cultures, it may be inappropriate to make eye contact, or for someone of the opposite gender to help the patient. There are also cultural differences that relate to the appropriate distance to stand apart from another person. Respect these differences and do what you can to help.

THE IMPORTANCE OF DOCUMENTATION

Documentation procedures are established by state regulations or local policy, and may vary from state to state and one EMS system to another. Documenting your care is as important as the care provided. Your record will help more advanced medical personnel to assess the patient

and continue care. It is important to write the record as soon as possible after the emergency, while the information is fresh. Because a patient's condition may change before arriving at the receiving facility, a record of the condition immediately after the emergency will provide useful information for responders and emergency department staff. They can compare the current condition with what you recorded earlier.

Your record is a legal document and is important if legal action occurs. Should you be called to court for any reason, your record will support what you saw, heard and did at the emergency scene. Documentation of injuries and illnesses is also useful when analyzing current response practices and protocols and planning preventative action for the future. Records are also used for *quality assurance* (QA) practices within a department.

PREHOSPITAL CARE REPORT
Description and Uses of the Prehospital Care Report

A *prehospital care report* (**PCR**), also called a *run report* or *trip sheet*, is the essential documentation for each emergency call (**Fig. 9-6**). The primary function of this report is to ensure high-quality patient care. Hospital and other more advanced medical personnel need to know what transpired during a call in order to provide the patient with appropriate continuity of care. This information allows medical personnel to determine what treatment the patient needs and which complaints must be addressed first. The PCR can also be used to evaluate care provided and identify areas where quality of care requires improvement in future scenarios. Keeping good records allows EMRs to learn from both successes and failures.

The PCR has multiple functions. As mentioned before, the PCR also serves as a legal document, particularly if the responder was present at the scene of a crime or if the incident leads to a lawsuit. It is not uncommon to be called to testify in court years after the response. In addition, the PCR is a valuable educational and research tool. The information may be used in research projects on a variety of issues, including studies on the safety and efficacy of certain interventions, the cost-

PREHOSPITAL CARE REPORT

PCR# _____

Call Date	Provider Number	Unit Number	Incident Number	Interfacility Transfer Number	Call Disposition
___/___/___					

Response	Transport	Time of Call	Time Enroute	Time First ALS on Scene	Time Arrived on Scene	Time Left Scn / Call Canceled	Time Arrived at Destination	Contact Made with:	Time of Contact
☐ 1 Code ☐ 1 ☐ 2 ☐ 3	☐ 1 ☐ 2 ☐ 3	:	:	:	:	:	:	☐ Base Hospital ☐ Receiving Facility ☐ Control Facility ☐ None	:

Patient Name (Last, First, Mi) _____

Patient Address _____

Incident Location _____

Patient Age	Patient DOB	Patient Gender	Est. Patient Weight	County	Map Zone	No. Pts. At Scene
Mos Yrs	___/___/___	☐ Male ☐ Female	kg			

Chief Complaint _____ Pain Level: ___ **Allergies** _____

Medical History _____ **Medications** _____

Initial Physical Examination

Unremarkable

Head	☐	
Neck	☐	
Chest	☐	
Abdomen	☐	
Back	☐	
Pelvis	☐	
Limbs	☐	
Neuro	☐	
Skin Signs	☐	

GCS

Eye	Verbal	Motor
4 spont	5 oriented	6 obeys
3 voice	4 confused	5 localizes
2 pain	3 inapprop	4 withdrwl
1 none	2 incompr	3 flexion
	1 none	2 extensn
		1 none

Time	E	V	M	Total
:	___	+ ___	+ ___	= _____
:	___	+ ___	+ ___	= _____
:	___	+ ___	+ ___	= _____

Mechanism of Injury

Types of Illness/Injury

Field Clinical Impression: _____

Care Giver FD/PD/BS/PH	Time	Procedure / Medication (with dose, route) CODE / DESCRIPTION	Response / Comments / ECG (MD Signature: Base Order)	Resp Rate	Blood Pressure	Pulse Rate	Pain Level
	:				/		
	:				/		
	:				/		
	:				/		
	:				/		
	:				/		
	:				/		
	:				/		
	:				/		
	:				/		
	:				/		
	:				/		

☐ Medication Wasted: _____ Time: _____ Signature: _____ Witness Signature: _____

Special Scene Conditions:
- ☐ ALS w/o base contact
- ☐ Complicated extrication
- ☐ DNR
- ☐ Drug use suspected
- ☐ ETOH use suspected
- ☐ Hazardous materials
- ☐ MCI
- ☐ Multiple EMS providers
- ☐ Possible provider exposure
- ☐ Unsafe scene
- ☐ Other:

Safety Eq Used:
- ☐ Lap Restraint
- ☐ Lap/Shoulder restraint
- ☐ Child Safety seat
- ☐ Airbag
- ☐ Helmet
- ☐ Protective Clothing

MVA Conditions:
- ☐ Bent steering wheel
- ☐ Death in same vehicle
- ☐ Ejection
- ☐ Passenger comptmnt intrusn
- ☐ Rollover

Destination Decision Reason
- ☐ Nearest Rec. Facility
- ☐ MCI/DCF
- ☐ Physician request
- ☐ Pt/Family request
- ☐ Triage to trauma center
- ☐ Triage to other specialty center
- ☐ Other _____

Receiving Hosp

Base Hospital

Tier I Trauma Triage:
- ☐ GCS Motor Score < 5
- ☐ Systolic BP < 85
- ☐ Penetrating Trauma: Head, Neck, Chest, Torso
- ☐ Paramedic Judgement

Tier II Trauma Triage
- ☐ Flail Chest
- ☐ Combo Burn/Trauma
- ☐ 2 or more long bone fx.
- ☐ Pelvic fracture
- ☐ pedestrian thrown/run over
- ☐ Judgement of the paramedic or flight nurse
- ☐ Open/depress. skull fx
- ☐ Paralysis
- ☐ Amput. Prox. wrist/ankle
- ☐ Fall > 20 ft.
- ☐ Pregnancy

Pediatric Trauma Triage
- ☐ Glasgow Coma Score Motor Component < 5 AND
- ☐ BP < 80 if patient over age 6; < 70 if under 6
- ☐ Advanced airway or continuous support of airway
- ☐ Penetrating trauma: head, neck, chest, torso or proximal to elbow/knee with vascular compromise
- ☐ Flail Chest
- ☐ Amput. Prox. wrist/ankle
- ☐ Pelvis Fracture
- ☐ Traumatic paralysis

Base MD _____

MICN _____

Care Transferred To		Cert. Number	Name (print)	Signature
		A)		
Agency	Time :	B)		
Name		C)		

☐ Continuation form used

Fig. 9-6: The PCR is essential for proper documentation of an emergency.

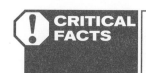
effective implementation of patient care or the typical presentation of certain injuries or illnesses. The PCR also has an administrative function—serving as an important part of the patient's medical record. It may be used for billing, insurance reimbursement or maintaining statistics on hospital emergency services.

Given the importance and multiple functions of the PCR, it is crucial that the PCR is filled out accurately, completely and correctly. Some PCRs are completed with pen and paper, while others are filled out electronically, called an *E-PCR* (**Fig. 9-7**).

Sections of the PCR

Typically, the four sections of a PCR include—

1. **Run data**. The run data section contains administrative information, including the time the incident was reported, when the unit was notified, when the unit arrived and left the scene, when the unit arrived at its destination and when the transfer of care was made. It also includes such information as the EMS unit number, names of the EMS crew members and their levels of certification and the address to which the unit was dispatched.
2. Patient data. The patient data section contains all the background information on the patient, including legal name, age, gender, birth date, home address, Social Security Number (where required) and billing and insurance information. It also contains the time the incident occurred, address where the patient was picked up and

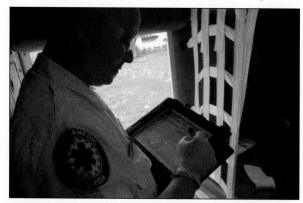

Fig. 9-7: PCRs should be filled out accurately, completely and correctly, regardless of whether they are written or electronic. *Courtesy of Captain Phil Kleinberg, EMT-P, Lake-Sumter EMS.*

any care the patient received before EMS personnel arrived.

3. Check boxes. The check boxes section, as the name implies, contains a series of boxes that are checked in accordance with the patient's condition. The check boxes refer to information about the patient, including vital signs (often more than one set must be taken), chief complaint, level of responsiveness, appearance and respiration rate.
4. **Patient narrative**. The patient narrative section is an open-ended portion of the PCR in which a description of the assessment and care is provided. The goal is to provide a complete and thorough picture of what went on and what the patient's condition is. This section must include the SAMPLE history, the patient's chief complaint (in the patient's own words, if possible), how the chief complaint began and how it progressed and the mechanism of the injury or nature of the illness. It should also include relevant details of the patient's medical history. It is important to remain objective in this section: that is, describe what happened but do not draw any conclusions about the situation.

Minimum Data Set

The **minimum data set** refers to all the information that must be included in the PCR. It consists of the following:

- Patient information gathered by the EMR
  - Time of events
  - Assessment findings, including the following:
    - Chief complaint
    - LOC
    - Systolic blood pressure for patients more than 3 years old
    - Skin perfusion (capillary refill)
    - Skin color and temperature
    - Pulse rate
    - Respiratory rate and effort
  - Emergency medical care provided
  - Patient demographics, such as age and gender
  - Changes in the patient after care and who the patient was turned over to

- Observations at the scene
- Disposition (e.g., whether the patient refused care or was transported to a hospital)
- Administrative information
  - Time the incident was reported
  - Time the unit was notified
  - Time unit en route to the call
  - Time the unit arrived at the scene
  - Time the unit left the scene
  - Time of arrival at the receiving facility
  - Time of transfer of care
  - Time unit available for next call

Note that it is important to use accurate and synchronous clocks to allow all involved to gather accurate medical information. For example, it is important to know details such as how long the patient was in cardiac arrest. The *National EMS Information System* (NEMSIS), which is a system to gather data on the local and state level of EMS systems and prehospital care, can be a helpful tool for tracking data in the local area.

Confidentiality

Control of the contents of a PCR falls within the *Health Insurance Portability and Accountability Act* (HIPAA). HIPAA has strict rules about how patient information is used and distributed. Violation of HIPAA rules can have severe penalties. The contents of the PCR must be kept confidential, as it contains personal and potentially sensitive information about the patient. While in your care, it is your responsibility to ensure that the PCR is in appropriate hands. (For more information on HIPAA and confidentiality, refer to **Chapter 3**.)

Refusal of Treatment

While any competent adult has the right to refuse treatment, questions may come up later as to whether the patient was truly competent at the time of refusing treatment. Therefore, it is important to perform as complete an assessment of the patient as is possible, given the situation. For a patient who refuses treatment, record on the PCR exactly what care you wished to provide to the patient, and make one last effort to convince the patient to accept this care before leaving the scene. Be sure to include in the PCR that the patient received a complete explanation of the possible consequences of refusing care, including the risk of death if this is appropriate. Offer the patient alternative methods of obtaining care, such as visiting the patient's family health care provider. Tell patients that you or another EMS team is willing to return to the scene should they change their decision. Make sure this is all documented in the PCR and is signed by the patient and a witness, if available. Always follow local protocols for refusal of care as they may differ from state to state. (For more information on refusal of treatment, see **Chapter 3**.)

Falsification

The PCR must be a thorough and accurate record of what occurred during a call. Any error of omission or commission in care must be highlighted in the PCR, along with any steps that were made to correct the situation. Only document the facts on the PCR. Do not leave anything out and do not add anything that was not done.

Be aware that falsification of a PCR is a serious offense. It can lead to revocation of your certification and even to criminal charges. More seriously, it can significantly compromise patient care.

Parts of the PCR that are most frequently falsified are vital signs and treatment. EMRs who forget to measure vital signs have been known to make them up, or those who forget certain crucial treatments, such as administering emergency oxygen to a patient with chest pain, may fail to mention this error. Be honest; it is far better for you and the patient if you own up to your mistakes up front.

TRANSFER OF CARE

When more advanced medical personnel arrive on the scene, you will need to give a verbal report on the number of patients involved, their conditions and the emergency situation. If a multipart PCR is available, the copy should be transferred with the patient. This relieves the transferring provider from having to collect redundant information, thus saving time.

Specifically, you will need to provide the following information about the patient(s):
- Current condition

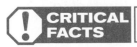 **CRITICAL FACTS** Control of the contents of a PCR falls within HIPAA.

- Age and gender
- Chief complaint
- Brief, pertinent history of what happened
- How you found the patient(s)
- Major past injuries or illnesses
- Vital signs
- Pertinent findings of the physical exam(s)
- Emergency care provided and the response to care

SPECIAL SITUATIONS

Documentation of the emergency situation and the care you provided is not only important for the patient, but also may prove essential for local authorities when legal matters are involved. It is particularly important to report any abuse, exposure to dangerous situations or injuries.

Once your report is complete, it should be submitted to the proper authorities in the proper time frame and should include the names of all agencies, people and facilities involved in the emergency response.

As always when writing these legal documents, be objective. Write only the facts and your observations; do not write your own subjective comments or opinions and do not draw any of your own conclusions. The only subjective comments or opinions should be those of the patient. Be sure to sign and date the document. Always keep a copy for your own records while making copies to distribute to the proper authorities based on local protocols. Your region or location will have its own standards and procedures, which will indicate which authorities are authorized to receive this documentation.

PUTTING IT ALL TOGETHER

Communication and documentation are a major part of providing emergency care. It is important for everyone on the team to understand what is going on and what happened before they arrived on the scene. This is only possible through good communication with patients, bystanders and colleagues.

Although emergency situations may make it difficult for some patients to effectively communicate, the EMS team, by showing confidence and encouragement, can successfully elicit the required information. Effective communication within the response team is based on understanding the modes of communication (radios, phones), factors for effective communication (speaking clearly, using correct terminology) and speed of communication. By following the rules and protocols of your region, miscommunication should be kept to a minimum.

Documentation is the final step in providing emergency care. State laws and regulations require that documentation be done as accurately and as soon as possible following the emergency situation. In the midst of the emergency, it is possible to forget instructions or answers to questions, so it is best to take notes when asking questions of patients and bystanders, and also when receiving instructions from medical control.

Always remember to be objective in your reports as these documents may be used for legal purposes or for evaluating procedures. Finally, keep a copy of all records for yourself based on local protocols; this will allow you to have access to the information should it be needed.

YOU ARE THE EMERGENCY MEDICAL RESPONDER

As you assess the elderly patient, you learn that her chief complaint is that she "blacked out" momentarily and fell. The patient is afraid that she has broken her hip. She has pain in her pelvis and is unable to move her left leg. You give a verbal update to the EMS personnel who have just arrived to take over medical care and transport the patient.

Why is it important for communications to be brief and concise? What are some examples of effective interpersonal communication? Why is it important to thoroughly document your call, observations and actions?

UNIT

3

AIRWAY

10 Airway and Ventilation

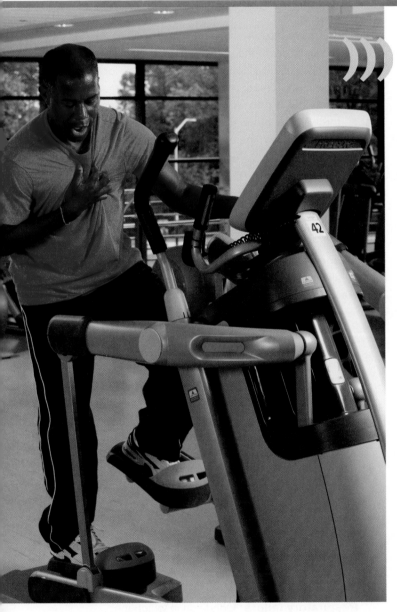

))) **YOU ARE THE EMERGENCY MEDICAL RESPONDER**

Your medical emergency response team has been called to the fitness center by building security, on a report of an employee who complained of having difficulty breathing. You and your partner arrive and find the man conscious. The patient's chief complaint is still difficulty breathing. He says he just "overdid it" on the treadmill. He appears to be out of breath and is having trouble speaking in full sentences. You begin a primary assessment and determine that the patient is in respiratory distress. What should you do? What can you do to assist the patient with his breathing?

Key Terms

Apnea: A condition that causes breathing to stop periodically or be significantly reduced.

Artificial ventilation: A mechanical means used to assist breathing, such as with a *bag-valve-mask resuscitator* (BVM) or resuscitation mask.

Aspiration: To take, suck or inhale blood, vomit, saliva or other foreign material into the lungs.

Asthma: An ongoing condition in which the airways swell; the air passages can become constricted or blocked when affected by various triggers.

Asthma attack: The sudden worsening of asthma signs and symptoms, caused by inflammation of the airways and the tightening of muscles around the airways of a person with asthma, making breathing difficult.

Asthma trigger: Anything that sets off an asthma attack, such as animal dander, dust, smoke, exercise, stress or medications.

Bag-valve-mask resuscitator (BVM): A hand-held breathing device consisting of a self-inflating bag, a one-way valve and a face mask; can be used with or without emergency oxygen.

Breathing emergency: An emergency in which breathing is impaired; can become life threatening; also called a *respiratory emergency*.

Chronic obstructive pulmonary disease (COPD): A progressive lung disease in which the patient has difficulty breathing because of damage to the lungs; airways become obstructed and the alveolar sacs lose their ability to fill with air.

Crackles: An abnormal fine, crackling breath sound on inhalation that may be a sign of fluid in the lungs; also known as *rales*.

Cricoid: A solid ring of cartilage just below and behind the thyroid cartilage.

Cyanosis: A condition in which the patient's skin, nail beds and mucous membranes appear a bluish or greyish color because of insufficient levels of oxygen in the blood.

Deadspace: The areas within the respiratory system between the pharynx and the alveoli that contains a small amount of air that does not reach the alveoli.

Emphysema: A chronic, degenerative lung disease in which there is damage to the alveoli.

Finger sweep: A method of clearing the mouth of foreign material that presents a risk of blocking the airway or being aspirated into the lungs.

Foreign body airway obstruction (FBAO): The presence of foreign matter, such as food, that obstructs the airway.

Head-tilt/chin-lift technique: A common method for opening the airway unless the patient is suspected of having an injury to the head, neck or spine.

Hyperventilation: Rapid, deep or shallow breathing; usually caused by panic or anxiety.

Hypoxia: A condition in which insufficient oxygen is delivered to the body's cells.

Jaw-thrust (without head extension) maneuver: A maneuver for opening the airway in a patient suspected of having an injury to the head, neck or spine.

Midaxillary line: An imaginary line that passes vertically down the body starting at the axilla (armpit); used to locate one of the areas for listening to breath sounds.

Midclavicular line: An imaginary line that passes through the midpoint of the clavicle (collarbone) on the ventral surface of the body; used to locate one of the areas for listening to breath sounds.

Midscapular line: An imaginary line that passes through the midpoint of the scapula (shoulder blade) on the dorsal surface of the body; used to locate one of the areas for listening to breath sounds.

Oxygenation: The addition of oxygen to the body; also, the treatment of a patient with oxygen.

Paradoxical breathing: An abnormal type of breathing that can occur with chest injury; one area of the chest moves in the opposite direction to the rest of the chest.

Pathophysiology: The study of the abnormal changes in mechanical, physical and biochemical functions caused by an injury or illness.

Pneumonia: A lung infection caused by a virus or bacterium that results in a cough, fever and difficulty breathing.

Positive pressure ventilation: An artificial means of forcing air or oxygen into the lungs of a person who has stopped breathing or has inadequate breathing.

Pulmonary embolism: Sudden blockage of an artery in the lung; can be fatal.

Rales: An abnormal breath sound; a popping, clicking, bubbling or rattling sound, also known as *crackles*.

Respiratory failure: Condition in which the respiratory system fails in oxygenation and/or carbon dioxide elimination; the respiratory system is beginning to shut down; the person may alternate between being agitated and sleepy.

Resuscitation mask: A pliable, dome-shaped breathing device that fits over the mouth and nose; used to provide artificial ventilations and administer emergency oxygen.

Rhonchi: An abnormal breath sound when breathing that can often be heard without a stethoscope; a snoring or coarse, dry rale sound.

Stridor: An abnormal, high-pitched breath sound caused by a blockage in the throat or larynx; usually heard on inhalation.

Suctioning: The process of removing foreign matter, such as blood, other liquids or food particles, by means of a mechanical or manual suctioning device.

Tidal volume: The normal amount of air breathed at rest.

Ventilation: The exchange of air between the lungs and the atmosphere; allows for an exchange of oxygen and carbon dioxide in the lungs.

Wheezing: A high-pitched whistling sound heard during inhalation but heard most loudly on exhalation; an abnormal breath sound that can often be heard without a stethoscope.

Learning Objectives

After reading this chapter, and completing the class activities, you will have the information needed to—

- Describe the structure and function of the respiratory system.
- List the signs of inadequate breathing.
- Describe how to care for a patient experiencing respiratory distress.
- Relate the technique used to open the airway to the mechanism of injury.

- Explain why basic airway management and ventilation skills take priority over many other basic life-support skills.
- Describe how to perform mouth-to-mouth, mouth-to-nose and mouth-to-stoma ventilations.
- Describe how to assess for breath sounds (*Enrichment*).

Skill Objectives

After reading this chapter, and completing the class activities, you should be able to—

- Demonstrate how to give ventilations using a resuscitation mask.
- Demonstrate how to give ventilations using a *bag-valve-mask resuscitator* (BVM).
- Demonstrate how to give ventilations if a head, neck or spinal injury is suspected.

- Demonstrate how to perform cricoid pressure (*Sellick's Maneuver*) (*Enrichment skill*).
- Demonstrate how to assist a patient with an asthma inhaler (*Enrichment skill*).

INTRODUCTION

Because oxygen is vital to life, always ensure that the patient has an open airway and is breathing. Ensuring an open airway is the most important step you can take for any patient. Without an open airway, a person cannot breathe and will die. The airway is the pathway from the mouth and nose to the lungs. A person who can speak or cry is conscious, has an open airway, is breathing and has a pulse. It is more difficult to tell if an unconscious person has an open airway. You will have to take into consideration possible injury or illness.

Once you have an open airway, you may need to clear any obstructions, and then assess breathing. If the person is experiencing a **breathing emergency**, you may need to provide **artificial ventilations**.

A breathing emergency is often detected during the primary assessment. In a breathing emergency, a person's breathing can become so impaired that life is threatened. There are two types of respiratory emergencies: respiratory distress, a condition in which breathing becomes difficult, and respiratory arrest, a condition in which breathing stops.

This chapter will address the causes, signs and symptoms of respiratory emergencies. Some of these emergencies are caused by chronic conditions such as **chronic obstructive pulmonary disease** (**COPD**), and others are caused by acute emergencies such as **asthma** and **pulmonary embolism**.

THE RESPIRATORY SYSTEM
Anatomy

The respiratory system is divided into the upper and lower airway tracts. The upper airway tract begins where air enters the respiratory system, through the mouth and nose. Air that is inhaled through the nose is warmed and humidified. Air may also be inhaled through the mouth and over the tongue, within the oral cavity. The mouth provides an airway, especially during an emergency.

Once air is inhaled, it passes through the throat, or pharynx. The pharynx is divided into three parts, from superior to inferior, the nasopharynx, the oropharynx and the laryngopharynx. The nasopharynx lies behind the nasal cavity. The oropharynx lies behind the oral cavity, and is the shared passageway for both food and air.

Below the oropharynx is the laryngopharynx, the lowest part of the throat, which divides into two passageways. In the posterior (back) portion is the entrance to the esophagus, the passageway for food. In the anterior (front) is the larynx, which is the continuation of the respiratory system. Above the larynx is the epiglottis, a flap of cartilage that folds down over the larynx to close off the entrance to the trachea during swallowing, so that food cannot enter. This airway protection does not occur if a person is unconscious.

Once air has traveled through the pharynx, it passes through the larynx. At the top of this structure made mostly of cartilage, muscle and membranes, is the *hyoid bone*—a horseshoe-shaped bone that supports the structures of the larynx below and attaches to the tongue and other oral structures above. Below the hyoid bone are the thyroid and **cricoid** cartilages, which form the larynx. Within the larynx lie the *vocal cords*, narrow muscles that stretch horizontally across from anterior to posterior.

The lower airway tract begins below the level of the vocal cords, and consists of the trachea, bronchi and lungs. The trachea, or windpipe, is a hollow tube, supported by rings of cartilage. It extends downward until it divides into two branches called *bronchi*, one of which travels into each lung. The two bronchi are hollow tubes, also supported by cartilage, that further divide into lower airways called *bronchioles*.

Bronchioles are thin hollow tubes that lead to the alveoli, and that remain open through smooth muscle tone. The millions of alveoli are

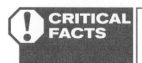

CRITICAL FACTS Ensuring an open airway is the most important step you can take in caring for a patient, because a person cannot breathe without an open airway. A patient who can speak or cry is conscious, has an open airway, is breathing and has a pulse.

small sacs that form the end of the airway. Each one has a thin walled sac that shares a wall with the capillary blood vessels in contact with it. It is at this site, where the one-celled walls of the alveoli and capillaries come into contact, where external respiration—the exchange of oxygen and carbon dioxide between the respiratory and circulatory system—takes place.

The circulatory system then transports the oxygen-rich blood to the brain, organs, muscles and other parts of the body. Some body tissues, such as those in the brain, are very sensitive to oxygen deprivation. Other vital organs can be adversely affected unless oxygen supplies are restored quickly. The brain is the control center for breathing. It adjusts the rate and depth of breaths according to the oxygen and carbon dioxide levels in the body. Breathing requires that the respiratory, circulatory, nervous and musculoskeletal systems work together. Injuries or illnesses that affect any of these systems may cause breathing emergencies.

Pathophysiology

Normal breathing occurs in ambient (surrounding) air, which contains all the necessary gases for normal respiration. Patients may suffer breathing difficulties because of an inadequate amount of oxygen breathed in during respiration. Breathing difficulties may also occur as a result of breathing in a low-oxygen environment or when poisonous gases are in the air. Other causes of breathing difficulties include infection of the lungs; illnesses like asthma, which narrows the airway and causes **wheezing**; excess fluid in the lungs or excess fluid between the lungs and blood vessels; and poor circulation.

Breathing difficulties may also develop due to upper airway problems caused by swelling, obstruction or trauma. Swelling of the upper airway can occur due to anaphylaxis (severe allergic reaction) or asthma. Choking, caused by airway obstruction, is one of the most common causes of breathing emergencies, and can occur due to anatomical or mechanical obstruction. Trauma can occur due to a blow to the upper chest, a puncture or a crush injury.

Breathing problems may develop because of ineffective circulation. This can be the result of *shock*—an acute condition in which the circulatory system fails to adequately circulate oxygen-rich blood to all cells of the body—or *cardiac arrest*, when the heart stops functioning as a pump, often the result of a heart attack.

Sometimes the rate or depth of breathing is inadequate, leading to an insufficient volume of air moving into and out of the lungs. Respiration may be ineffective due to unconsciousness, altered level of consciousness, injury to the chest, poisoning, overdose or diseases such as COPD or **emphysema**.

Oxygenation refers to the amount of oxygen in the bloodstream. Oxygen is exchanged between the alveoli of the lungs and the capillaries, and at the cellular level between the capillaries and the cells. If an insufficient amount of oxygen is delivered to the cells, this is referred to as **hypoxia**, and may result from an obstructed airway, shock, inadequate breathing, drowning, strangulation, choking, suffocation, cardiac arrest, head trauma, carbon monoxide poisoning or complications of general anesthesia.

RESPIRATORY EMERGENCIES

A respiratory emergency occurs when air cannot travel freely and easily into the lungs, and can be life threatening because it greatly cuts down on the oxygen the body receives or because it cuts off the oxygen entirely. This can stop the heart and prevent blood from reaching other vital organs. Unless the brain receives oxygen within 4 to 6

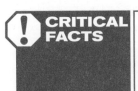
CRITICAL FACTS

There are many reasons why a person may have difficulty breathing. Reasons include an inadequate amount of oxygen being taken in, a low-oxygen environment, the presence of poisonous gases, infection, poor circulation or other health-related issues.

Oxygenation refers to the amount of oxygen in the bloodstream. Hypoxia is the term used to describe an insufficient amount of oxygen delivered to the cells.

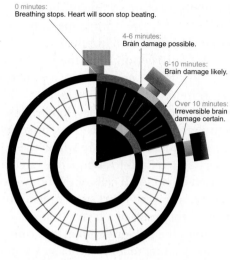

0 minutes:
Breathing stops. Heart will soon stop beating.

4-6 minutes:
Brain damage possible.

6-10 minutes:
Brain damage likely.

Over 10 minutes:
Irreversible brain damage certain.

Fig. 10-1: Time is critical in respiratory emergencies.

minutes, permanent brain damage or death can result (**Fig. 10-1**).

There are two types of respiratory emergencies: respiratory distress, a condition in which breathing becomes difficult, and respiratory arrest, a condition in which breathing stops.

Respiratory distress can be caused by—
- A partially obstructed airway.
- Illness.
- Chronic conditions such as asthma.
- Electrocution, including lightning strikes.
- Heart attack.
- Injury to the head, chest, lungs or abdomen.
- Allergic reactions.
- Drugs.
- Poisoning.
- Emotional distress.

Trouble breathing can be the first sign of a more serious emergency such as a heart problem. Recognizing the signs of breathing problems and providing care are often the keys to preventing these problems from becoming emergencies that are more serious.

If you encounter someone with a breathing problem, the patient will most likely be conscious. Breathing problems can be identified by watching and listening to the patient's breathing and by asking how the patient feels. Although breathing problems have many causes, you do not have to know the exact cause of a breathing emergency to care for it.

Symptoms of respiratory emergencies include—
- Slow or rapid breathing.
- Unusually deep or shallow breathing.

- Gasping for breath.
- Wheezing, gurgling or high-pitched noises.
- Unusually moist or cool skin.
- Flushed, pale, ashen or bluish skin color.
- Shortness of breath.
- Dizziness or light-headedness.
- Pain in the chest or tingling in the hands, feet or lips.
- Apprehensive or fearful feelings.

Chronic Obstructive Pulmonary Disease

COPD is a progressive lung disease in which the patient has difficulty breathing because of damage to the lungs. In a patient with COPD, the airways become partly obstructed and the alveolar sacs lose their ability to fill with air, making it difficult for air to be inhaled and exhaled.

The most common cause of COPD is cigarette smoking but it may also be caused by inhaling other types of lung irritants, pollution, dust or chemicals over a long period of time. It is usually diagnosed when patients are middle aged or older. It is the fourth-ranking cause of death in the United States and a major cause of illness.

Signs and symptoms include the following:
- Coughing up a great deal of mucus
- A tendency to tire easily
- Loss of appetite
- Bent posture with shoulders elevated and lips pursed to make breathing easier
- A fast pulse
- Round, barrel-shaped chest
- Confusion (caused by lack of oxygen to the brain)

Patients with COPD require help focusing on breathing, as deep breaths help fill the lungs with air and maintain flexibility in the chest wall. Patients can learn special breathing exercises to help them relax and breathe slowly, which increases the flow of oxygen to the lungs.

Asthma

Asthma is an ongoing illness in which the airways swell. An **asthma attack** happens when an **asthma trigger**, such as exercise, cold air, allergens or other irritants, affects the airways, causing them to suddenly swell and narrow. This makes breathing difficult, which can be very frightening.

The *Centers for Disease Control and Prevention* (CDC) estimates that more than 30 million

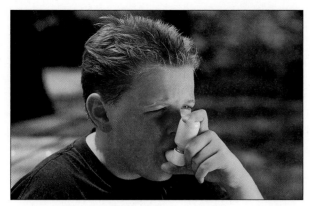

Fig. 10-2: Asthma is more common in children than in adults.

Americans are diagnosed with asthma in their lifetimes. Asthma is more common in children and young adults than in older adults, but its frequency and severity are increasing in all age groups (**Fig. 10-2**). Asthma is the third-ranking cause of hospitalization among those younger than age 15.

You can often tell when a person is having an asthma attack by the hoarse whistling sound the person makes while inhaling and/or exhaling. This sound, known as *wheezing*, occurs because air becomes trapped in the lungs. Coughing that occurs after exercise, crying or laughing is another sign that an asthma attack is taking place.

Sign and symptoms of an asthma attack include—
- Coughing or wheezing noises.
- Difficulty breathing.
- Shortness of breath.
- Rapid, shallow breathing.
- Sweating.
- Tightness in the chest.
- Inability to talk without stopping for breath.
- Bent posture with shoulders elevated and lips pursed to make breathing easier.
- Feelings of fear or confusion.

Usually, people diagnosed with asthma control their attacks by controlling environmental variables and through medication and other forms of treatment. The medications stop the muscle spasms and open the airway, which makes breathing easier. Controlling the environmental variables, whenever possible, helps reduce the triggers that can lead to the start of an asthma attack.

A trigger is anything that sets off or starts an asthma attack. A trigger for one person is not necessarily a trigger for another. Some asthma triggers are—

- Dust, smoke and air pollution.
- Exercise.
- Plants and molds.
- Perfume.
- Medications, such as aspirin.
- Animal dander.
- Temperature extremes and changes in the weather.
- Strong emotions, such as anger, fear or anxiety.
- Infections, such as colds or other respiratory infections.

Some anti-inflammatory medications prescribed for the long-term control of asthma are taken daily. Other medications are prescribed for quick relief and are taken only when a person is experiencing the signs and symptoms of an asthma attack (**Fig. 10-3**). These medications help relieve the sudden swelling and are called *bronchodilators*.

Pneumonia

Pneumonia is an infection that causes inflammation of the lungs. Because of the inflammation, the air sacs in the lungs begin to fill with fluid and oxygen has trouble reaching the bloodstream. Pneumonia can be a serious illness in older adults because of normal age-related changes such as a weakened cough reflex and impaired mobility and can even result in death.

Pneumonia can be caused by viruses (often a complication of the flu), bacteria, fungi or other organisms. Symptoms include high fever, chills, chest pain and shortness of breath. In addition to these symptoms, geriatric patients commonly exhibit additional symptoms including increased respiration rate, breathing difficulty

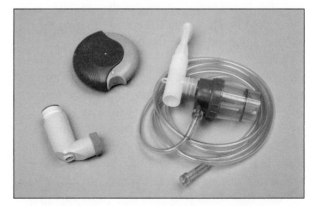

Fig. 10-3: Medications used to treat asthma attacks stop the muscle spasms and open the airway, which makes breathing easier.

and congestion. Altered mental status may also present in elderly patients. Older adults may also develop aspiration pneumonia. Residents who are in a coma or using feeding tubes are especially at risk for developing pneumonia. Bacterial pneumonia is treated with antibiotics. Administering emergency oxygen can help relieve some of the symptoms of pneumonia.

Acute Pulmonary Edema

Pulmonary edema is an abnormal build-up of fluid in the lungs that can result in death if not properly treated. It is usually caused by inadequate heart pumping when the left ventricle starts to eject less blood than the right. This places excessive pressure on the lungs and allows fluid to leak into the alveoli and capillaries. Acute pulmonary edema causes severe respiratory distress, altered mental status and coughing, with some bloody sputum. Signs and symptoms of pulmonary edema include shortness of breath; difficulty breathing, including wheezing or gasping for breath; **cyanosis** (a bluish color of the skin and mucous membranes); frothy (foamy) pink sputum; pale skin; excessive sweating; restlessness, anxiety and a feeling of apprehension; a feeling of suffocating or drowning; and chest pain when the condition is caused by coronary artery disease. Gradual symptoms include difficulty breathing when lying flat, awakening at night with a feeling of breathlessness, unusual shortness of breath during physical activity and significant weight gain when the condition develops because of congestive heart failure. Administering emergency oxygen is the first step in the care of pulmonary edema.

Hyperventilation

Hyperventilation occurs when a person breathes faster and shallower or deeper than normal. When a patient is hyperventilating, carbon dioxide levels in the blood decrease, reducing blood flow to the brain. This causes fear, anxiety and confusion, as well as dizziness and a numb and tingly feeling in the fingers and toes.

Fear or anxiety is often the cause of hyperventilation but it can also result from a head injury, severe bleeding or conditions such as infection, heart failure and lung disease. Asthma and stress can also trigger hyperventilation.

Note that anxiety is only one cause of rapid breathing, and most patients experiencing this symptom are not hyperventilating. If you are certain the patient is not experiencing life-threatening symptoms, the most effective response is to calm the patient. Listen to the patient's concerns and try to reassure and encourage the patient to breathe slower or breathe through pursed lips. If the patient does not respond to this, administer emergency oxygen if it is available.

Pulmonary Embolism

A pulmonary embolism is a blockage in the arteries of the lungs. Symptoms include a sudden onset of dyspnea (difficulty breathing; shortness of breath), chest pain that is localized and does not radiate, coughing, coughing up blood and fainting. The embolism usually has traveled from a blood clot in another part of the circulatory system, and then lodges somewhere in an artery in the lung.

With a pulmonary embolism, there is poor oxygen and carbon dioxide gas exchange in the alveoli, as the clot prevents blood from flowing through the capillaries, and this inadequate exchange results in respiratory distress. The degree of distress depends on the size of the clot. Pulmonary embolism is more common in smokers, cancer patients, fracture patients, surgery patients, patients with cardiovascular disease and those who have been on prolonged bed rest or suffered a trauma. It is also more common in the elderly. Larger clots can cause death very quickly. Therefore, rapid care and transport of the patient to a hospital is crucial.

Emphysema

Emphysema is a chronic disease caused by damage to the air sacs in the lungs. It is also *degenerative*, in that it worsens over time. When the alveoli lose elasticity, they become distended (swollen and expanded) with trapped air and stop working properly. As the number of affected alveoli increases, breathing becomes increasingly difficult. The most common symptom of emphysema is shortness of breath. Exhaling is also extremely difficult. Other signs include cyanosis, barrel-shaped chest, fatigue, loss of appetite and weight loss, mild cough, and breathing through pursed lips. The patient may feel restless, confused and weak. In advanced cases of emphysema, the patient may even go into respiratory or cardiac arrest.

Pediatric Considerations

Respiratory Emergencies

It is very important to recognize breathing emergencies in children and infants and to act before the heart stops beating. When adult hearts stop beating, it is frequently due to disease. Children's and infants' hearts, however, are usually healthy. When a child's or an infant's heart stops, it is usually the result of a breathing emergency.

When attending to a child with respiratory problems, keep in mind that lower airway disease may be caused by birth problems, or infections such as bronchiolitis, bronchospasms, pneumonia or croup.

Several of the illnesses and diseases that affect the respiratory system in children are preventable through vaccines. These include diphtheria; *Haemophilus influenzae* type b (Hib); measles, mumps and rubella (MMR); meningococcal; pertussis (whooping cough); pneumococcal disease; mycoplasma pneumonia (pneumonia-like illnesses); and varicella (chickenpox). Other diseases may not have respiratory symptoms but may be spread through respiratory transmission, such as mumps and rotavirus (severe diarrhea).

Geriatric Considerations

Respiratory Emergencies

It is sometimes less obvious that geriatric patients are suffering symptoms of a respiratory emergency, as they may be less sensitive to pain. You are more likely to encounter elderly patients who suffer from pneumonia or chronic, age-related breathing problems such as emphysema and pulmonary edema. Remember that elderly patients may present with different symptoms from those experienced by younger patients.

AIRWAY

Opening the Airway

As you learned in **Chapter 7**, there are two common methods used to open a patient's airway: the **head-tilt/chin-lift technique** and the **jaw-thrust (without head extension) maneuver**. The first is generally the preferred method *except* in cases where spinal injury is suspected. Both techniques lift the tongue from the back of the throat and allow air to move into

and out of the lungs. Once the airway is open, it is important to maintain an open airway as you continue to provide care.

Head-Tilt/Chin-Lift Technique

Use the head-tilt/chin-lift technique on patients who have no signs of or are not suspected of having an injury to the head, neck or spine. For patients of all ages, tilt the head back and lift the chin to open the airway. Do *not* tilt a child's or an infant's head back as far as an adult's. Tilt a child's head slightly past the neutral position and tilt an infant's head to the neutral position (**Fig. 10-4, A–C**). Keep pressure on the patient's forehead to help maintain the airway in an open position.

Jaw-Thrust (Without Head Extension) Maneuver

To open the airway for someone who has a suspected head, neck or spinal injury, use the jaw-thrust (without head extension) maneuver

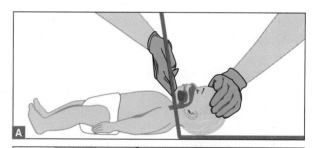
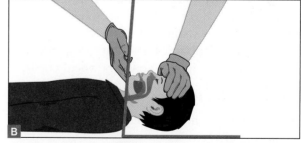
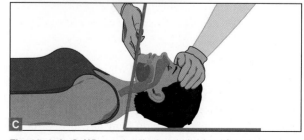

Fig. 10-4, A–C: When using the head-tilt/chin-lift technique to open the airway, **(A)** tilt an infant's head to a neutral position, **(B)** a child's to just past neutral and **(C)** an adult's head even further.

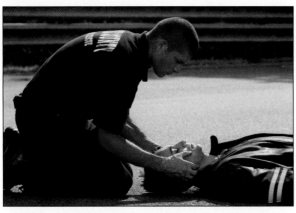

Fig. 10-5: The jaw-thrust (without head extension) maneuver is used to open the airway of a patient whom you suspect has a head, neck or spinal injury.

(Fig. 10-5). Do this while maintaining manual stabilization of the head and neck. For patients of all ages, while using your elbows for support, slide your fingers into position under the angles of the patient's jawbone and without moving the head; lift the jaw to open the airway. You can perform this technique with or without a **resuscitation mask**. Remember, maintaining an open airway is the priority. If the airway cannot be opened with this method, use the head-tilt/chin-lift technique instead.

Signs of an Open Airway

If the airway is open and clear (patent), you will be able to see the rise and fall of the patient's chest, hear air coming out of the patient's mouth and nose and feel air as the patient exhales. If the patient is able to speak in full sentences without distress, the airway is open and adequate. The ability to speak is a sign that air is moving past the vocal cords. The sound of the patient's voice is another indication of airway. A patient who is speaking in normal tones has an adequate airway and is breathing effectively.

Signs of an Inadequate Airway

Patients with an inadequate airway need close attention and monitoring. They may be visibly unable to catch their breath or they may gasp for air and make grunting sounds. Some signs are subtle, but if you are not sure, play it safe and take steps to maintain an open airway at all times. Not every sign is present in every patient who has an inadequate airway.

If you observe any unusual sounds with breathing, take prompt action to open the airway, as they may be signs of an airway obstruction. **Stridor** is a harsh, high-pitched sound the person may make when inhaling possibly due to the larynx being swollen and blocking the upper airway. If the patient is snoring, the tongue or other tissues in the mouth may be relaxed and blocking the upper airway.

A patient who is awake and alert but unable to speak, can only speak a few words or has a hoarse- sounding voice may be having severe difficulty breathing. Inadequate breathing may also be caused by swelling due to trauma, infection or an allergic reaction.

If there is no air movement, the patient is experiencing **apnea**, which is the complete absence of breathing. In this situation, the chest will not rise and fall and you will not be able to hear or feel any air coming out of the patient's mouth and nose. The patient needs artificial ventilation, and if apnea is not corrected in a timely manner there will be significant consequences.

Sometimes there may be no detectable air movement because of an airway obstruction. If efforts to open the airway are unsuccessful and **ventilations** do not make the chest clearly rise, check for an airway obstruction. Look inside the mouth for liquid, food, teeth, dentures, blood, vomit or other foreign objects that may be blocking the airway, such as a small toy.

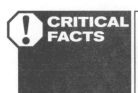

CRITICAL FACTS

A patient who is awake and alert but unable to speak, can only speak a few words or has a hoarse-sounding voice may be having severe difficulty breathing. Inadequate breathing may also be caused by swelling due to trauma, infection or an allergic reaction.

Foreign body airway obstruction (FBAO) is an emergency situation that needs immediate attention. The most common cause of an FBAO is a solid object, such as food.

Causes of Airway Obstruction

There are two types of airway obstruction: mechanical and anatomical. Any foreign body lodged in the airway is a mechanical obstruction and an emergency situation that needs immediate attention. The most common cause of *foreign body airway obstruction* (**FBAO**) in adults is a solid object, such as food. Fluids such as saliva, blood or vomit can also block the airway. Other causes of airway obstruction include loose or broken dentures. In the case of small children under age 4, large chunks of food and small objects such as toy parts and balloons commonly cause airway obstruction.

In an unresponsive patient, the most common cause of airway obstruction is the tongue. This is known as an *anatomical obstruction*. An unconscious patient loses muscle tone, which may cause the tongue to fall back and block the airway. As the patient tries to breathe, the tongue moves further into the throat.

Other conditions that can block the airway anatomically include swelling due to trauma, infection, asthma, emphysema or anaphylaxis. An obstruction may also be caused by trauma to the neck. See **Chapter 11** for more information on airway obstruction.

Clearing the Airway
Techniques to Clear an Airway Obstruction

More than one method exists to clear the airway in conscious and unconscious patients. Protocols may vary but abdominal thrusts, back blows and chest thrusts each have been proven to effectively clear an obstructed airway in conscious patients. Frequently, a combination of more than one technique may be needed to expel an object and clear the airway. Unconscious patients with FBAO should receive a modified form of CPR. See **Chapter 11** for more information on airway obstruction.

Techniques to Remove Foreign Matter From the Upper Airway

Two techniques can be used to remove visible foreign matter and fluids from the upper airway of an unconscious patient: **finger sweeps** and **suctioning**. The particular technique you choose will depend on the patient's condition and the foreign matter, and may require the use of both skills.

- Finger sweeps. Finger sweeps involve removing an object or other foreign matter from a patient's mouth with a finger. They are *only* performed on an unconscious patient and *only* when you can see foreign matter in the patient's mouth. *Always* wear gloves when performing a finger sweep.
- Suctioning. The purpose of suctioning is to remove blood, fluids or food particles from the airway. Some suctioning devices *cannot* remove solid objects such as teeth, foreign bodies or food.

See **Chapter 11** for more information on how to perform a finger sweep and how to use a suctioning device.

Recovery Positions

In some cases, the person may be unconscious but breathing. Generally that person should not be moved from a face-up position, especially if there is a suspected spinal injury. However, there are a few situations when you should move a person into a modified *high arm in endangered spine* (H.A.IN.E.S.) recovery position whether or not a spinal injury is suspected. Examples of these situations include if you are alone and have to leave the person (e.g., to call for help), or you cannot maintain an open and clear airway because of fluids or vomit. Placing a person in a modified H.A.IN.E.S. recovery position will help keep the airway open and clear (**Fig. 10-6**). Refer to **Chapter 5** for the steps for a modified H.A.IN.E.S. recovery position.

ASSESSING BREATHING
Determining the Presence of Breathing

To determine whether or not the patient is breathing, look for the rise and fall of the chest, listen for the sounds of breathing and feel for

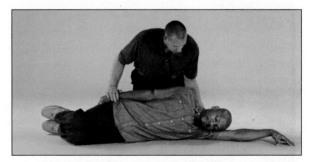

Fig. 10-6: If a head, neck or spinal injury is suspected, use a modified H.A.IN.E.S. recovery position.

movement as air escapes from the patient's mouth and nose. Adequate breathing requires both sufficient rate and depth.

Signs of Adequate Breathing, Oxygenation and Ventilation

Breathing is considered adequate when respiratory rate, depth and effort are normal. The following are normal rates, although some people naturally breathe at slightly slower or faster rates:

- Adults—12 to 20 breaths per minute
- Children—15 to 30 breaths per minute
- Infants—25 to 50 breaths per minute

The depth of respiration is as important as the rate. Breathing must be deep enough to bring oxygen into the lungs and from there to the bloodstream. The normal rise and fall of the patient's chest indicates adequate depth.

A healthy adult should breathe regularly, quietly and effortlessly. No muscles in the neck or shoulders are involved, and there is not excessive use of the abdominal muscles. There are no unusual sounds, such as wheezing or whistling.

Oxygenation

Oxygenation happens naturally with *ventilation*, the mechanical process of moving air in and out of the lungs. A healthy person with adequate oxygenation is clear thinking and calm and has normal skin color.

Signs of Inadequate Breathing

Inadequate breathing needs careful monitoring. You may not notice all of the signs and symptoms at once, and some can be hard to spot. If you see any of them, be prepared to give assisted ventilation.

Ventilation

Any of the following signs suggests that the patient is expending too much effort to breathe and that breathing is inadequate:

- Muscles between the ribs pull in on inhalation: As the patient breathes in, you may notice the muscles pulling inward between the ribs, above the collarbone, around the muscles of the neck and below the rib cage.
- Pursed lips breathing: The patient exhales through pursed lips (much like a whistling); this maneuver helps control the patient's breathing pattern.
- Nasal flaring: Flaring out of the nostrils on inhalation is a sign of inadequate breathing in children and infants.
- Fatigue: Apparent signs of fatigue are also an indication of the work of breathing.
- Excessive use of abdominal muscles to breathe: This means the patient is using the abdominal muscles to force air out of the lungs.
- Sweating: A patient who is sweating and anxious may be in severe respiratory distress.
- Sitting upright and learning forward (tripod position): A patient who is sitting upright and leaning forward with hands on knees is struggling to breathe.
- Deviated trachea: If you observe pendulum motions of the trachea while the patient is breathing in, this may be the result of chest trauma resulting in a lung injury. The trachea will move to the side of the uninjured lung.

Abnormal breath sounds are also a sign of inadequate breathing. Listen for abnormal sounds such as stridor, wheezing or **crackles/rales**. Wheezing or whistling sounds indicate restricted air flow and are common with conditions such as asthma, allergic reactions or emphysema. Crackles/rales have a fine cracking sound on inhalation (much like the sound of Velcro® being pulled apart), and may indicate fluid in the lungs.

Inadequate depth of breathing may also indicate problems with ventilation. Shallow breathing, even if it is rapid, often means that the patient is not getting enough oxygen. Markedly increased breathing that is unusually

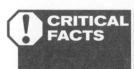

CRITICAL FACTS

The normal rate of breathing for adults is 12 to 20 breaths per minute. For children, it is 15 to 30 breaths per minute. And for infants, it is 25 to 50 per minute. Adequate breathing means that respiratory rate, depth and effort are normal.

Any of the following signs suggests that breathing is inadequate: Muscles between the ribs pull in on inhalation; pursed lips breathing; nasal flaring; fatigue; excessive use of abdominal muscles to breathe; sweating; and deviated trachea.

deep is also a sign of inadequate respiration. If the person is struggling to breathe, the depth is not adequate.

Rate provides additional information about the adequacy of breathing. A very slow breathing rate—less than 8 breaths per minute for adults, less than 10 breaths per minute for children and less than 20 breaths per minute for infants—is a sign of inadequate breathing. Breathing that is too fast is often shallow and inadequate.

Unusual or irregular movement of the chest wall may indicate inadequate breathing. A chest injury needs immediate attention because it can cause rapid and severe deterioration of the person's breathing. Chest wall trauma may cause a few different problems. In **paradoxical breathing**, an area of the chest moves in the opposite direction to the rest of the chest, i.e. moving in while the patient is breathing in (inspiration), and out while the patient is breathing out (expiration). A patient with an injury to the chest wall or ribs will often place an arm over the area to protect and "splint" it. (For further information on chest wall movement, see **Chapter 21**.)

A penetrating wound to the chest can cause rapid deterioration in breathing as well. An injury to one side of the chest wall will cause unequal movement; one side will remain hyper-inflated and not move with the other side during breathing.

Irregular respiratory patterns may also be a sign of inadequate breathing, particularly when associated with a slow or rapid heart rate. These signs typically occur together in children.

Inadequate Oxygenation

Problems with inadequate oxygenation may occur for a variety of reasons and can cause headaches, increased breathing rate, nausea and vomiting, altered mental status and, ultimately, death. The ambient air may be abnormal, for example in an enclosed space or at a high altitude, or there may be poisonous gas or carbon monoxide present. Breathing in poison has an almost immediate impact, destroying lung tissue and causing respiratory distress or failure. Carbon monoxide is a colorless, odorless, tasteless gas whose impact is severe.

A reduction of oxygen in the body causes headaches, increased breathing rate, nausea and vomiting, altered mental status and, ultimately, death.

One of the signs of inadequate oxygenation may be cyanosis, an abnormal blue or grey discoloration of the skin, mucous membranes or nail beds of the fingers and toes. Cyanosis is a serious sign that the body is not receiving enough oxygen. Pale, cool, clammy skin is an early and frequent sign of severe breathing difficulties resulting in falling oxygen levels. *Mottling*, another sign of inadequate oxygenation, is a blotchy

Minute Volume

A patient may appear to be breathing adequately but not be getting enough air to sustain life. One way of determining the adequacy of breathing is by measuring the minute volume. Minute volume is the amount of air breathed in per minute, and it depends on both the rate and depth of breathing. (Both rate and depth must be sufficient for breathing to be considered adequate.) Minute volume is calculated by multiplying these two factors: rate × volume per breath = minute volume.

The amount of air breathed in at each breath, the depth, is also referred to as the **tidal volume**. Normally, a single breath contains approximately 500 milliliters (mL) of air. Tidal volume is best assessed by watching for adequate chest movement (rise and fall), and listening and feeling for air movement from the mouth and nose during inhalation and exhalation.

For example, a patient who is breathing 12 times per minute and taking in 500 mL of air per breath has a minute volume of 6000 mL (500 × 12 = 6000 mL of air per minute). While most of that 6000 mL of air reaches the alveoli, a small amount, approximately 150 mL, remains in the area between the pharynx and the alveoli. This area is referred to as the **deadspace**. This amount must be taken into consideration, as it reduces the volume of each breath. In this example, 150 × 12 breaths = 1800 mL that never reaches the alveoli within a minute. For a patient who is breathing quickly, it may seem that breathing is adequate when it is not. Remember to reduce the calculated minute volume taking deadspace into consideration.

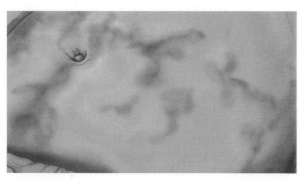

Fig. 10-7: Cyanosis and mottling are some of the visible signs of inadequate oxygenation.

pattern of skin discoloration, often caused by shock (**Fig. 10-7**). Without enough oxygen, patients also experience an altered mental state, becoming restless, agitated, confused or anxious.

ARTIFICIAL VENTILATION

Artificial ventilation refers to the various mechanical ways that can be used to help a patient "breathe." When delivering artificial ventilations, make sure the force of air is consistent and just strong enough to cause the chest to clearly rise during each breath.

Mouth-to-Mask Ventilation
Resuscitation Mask

Using a resuscitation mask allows you to breathe expired air (with or without emergency oxygen) into a patient without making mouth-to-mouth contact (**Fig. 10-8**). Use of the mask reduces the risk of disease transmission while providing enough oxygen (about 16 percent oxygen in your exhaled breath) to sustain life.

Flexible and shaped to fit over the patient's mouth and nose, resuscitation masks—

- Help get air quickly to the patient through both the mouth and nose.

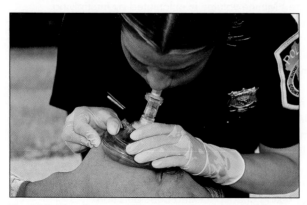

Fig. 10-8: Use of a resuscitation mask reduces the risk of disease transmission.

Mouth-to-Mouth Ventilation

As an *emergency medical responder* (EMR), you should follow standard precautions whenever providing ventilations. However, there may be circumstances when you do not have immediate access to a resuscitation mask or BVM. The risk of contracting a disease from mouth-to-mouth ventilations is low. Although protocols may vary, you may decide to give mouth-to-mouth ventilations without a barrier.

To provide ventilations to a patient *without* a mask—

1. Use the head-tilt/chin-lift technique to open the airway, provided you do not suspect an injury to the head, neck or spine.
2. Gently pinch the patient's nose shut with the thumb and index finger of your hand that is on the patient's forehead.
3. Make a tight seal around the patient's mouth with your mouth. For an infant, seal your mouth over the mouth and nose, instead of pinching the nose shut.
4. Blow into the patient's mouth until you see the chest clearly rise.

Each breath should last about 1 second, with a brief pause between breaths to let the air flow back out. Watch that the patient's chest rises each time you blow in, to ensure that your breaths are effective.

- Create a seal over the patient's mouth and nose.
- Can be connected to emergency oxygen, if equipped with an oxygen inlet.
- Protect against disease transmission.
- Are more effective for delivering ventilations when only one rescuer is present.

Resuscitation masks should be easy to assemble and use, and made of a transparent, pliable material that allows you to make a tight seal over the patient's mouth and nose. They have a one-way valve for releasing exhaled air and a standard 15-mm or 22-mm coupling assembly (the size of the opening for the one-way valve). Resuscitation masks work well under different environmental conditions, such as extreme heat or cold.

To use a resuscitation mask—

- Position yourself at the patient's head.
- Assemble the mask by attaching the one-way valve to the mask.
- Position the mask over the patient's mouth and nose.
- Place the broader end of the mask between the patient's lower lip and chin (**Fig. 10-9, A**). The position of the mask is critical to avoid leaks.
- Using both hands to hold the mask in place, squeeze the mask gently to create a seal that does not allow the air to escape (**Fig. 10-9, B**).
- Tilt the patient's head back, while lifting the jaw (or use the jaw-thrust [without head extension] maneuver for a suspected head, neck or spinal injury).
- Blow into the one-way valve, ensuring that you can see the chest clearly rise (**Fig. 10-9, C**). Each ventilation should last about 1 second, with a brief pause between breaths to let the exhaled breath escape.

A limitation of the resuscitation mask is that, without use of a BVM or emergency oxygen, it only delivers 16 percent oxygen through the responder's exhaled breath (50 percent with emergency oxygen), which is considerably less than is delivered using a BVM or emergency oxygen.

When serious injury or sudden illness occurs, the body does not function properly, and emergency oxygen can help meet the increased demand for oxygen for all body tissues. If the patient requires a higher concentration of oxygen than normal and the resuscitation mask has an oxygen inlet, connect it to emergency oxygen. Normal concentration of oxygen in the air is 21 percent. Your exhaled breath (expired air) contains about 16 percent. A resuscitation mask can deliver approximately 35 to 55 percent oxygen to a person when the oxygen is delivered at 6 to 15 *liters per minute* (LPM). For more information on administration of emergency oxygen, see **Chapter 12**.

Pediatric Considerations

Resuscitation Masks

Pediatric resuscitation masks are available and should be used to care for children and infants (**Fig. 10-10**). Adult resuscitation masks should *not* be used in an emergency

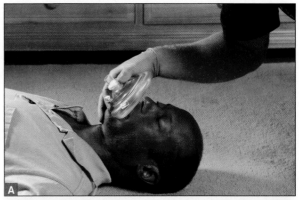
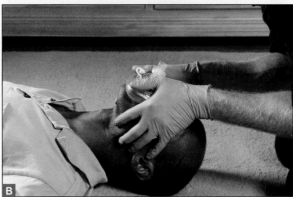
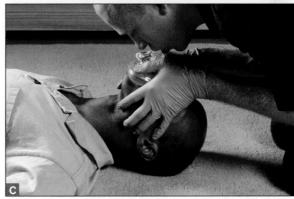

Fig. 10-9, A–C: To perform mouth-to-mask resuscitation: **(A)** Position the mask so that the broad end is between the patient's lower lip and chin, **(B)** make a seal using both hands so that air does not escape, **(C)** while tilting head back, blow into the mask.

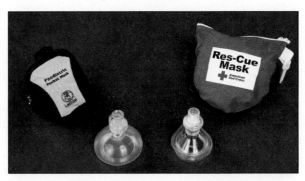

Fig. 10-10: Pediatric masks are available and should be used to care for children and infants.

situation unless a pediatric resuscitation mask is not available *and* medical control advises you to do so. Always use the appropriate equipment matched to the size of the patient.

Special Considerations
Air in the Stomach

When providing ventilations, blow slowly, with just enough air to make the patient's chest clearly rise. If you blow too much air into the patient, it may enter the stomach, causing gastric distention. The patient will then likely vomit, which can obstruct the airway and complicate resuscitation efforts.

Vomiting

When you provide ventilations, the patient may vomit. If this occurs, quickly turn the patient onto the side to keep the vomit from blocking the airway and entering the lungs. Support the head and neck and turn the body as a unit. After vomiting stops, clear the patient's airway by wiping the patient's mouth out using a finger sweep and suction if necessary, turn the patient onto the back and continue with ventilations.

Mask-to-Nose Breathing

If the patient's mouth is injured, you may need to provide ventilations through the nose. To perform mask-to-nose breathing using a resuscitation mask—

- Open the airway using the head-tilt/chin-lift technique.
- Place the resuscitation mask over the patient's mouth and nose.
- Use both hands to keep the patient's mouth closed.
- Seal the resuscitation mask with both hands.
- Provide ventilations.

Mask-to-Stoma Breathing

On rare occasions, you may see an opening in a patient's neck as you tilt the head back to

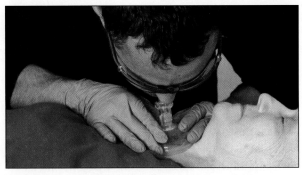

Fig. 10-11: If the patient has a stoma, provide ventilations through a round pediatric resuscitation mask placed over the stoma.

check for breathing. If the patient has a stoma and needs artificial ventilation, follow the same steps for mouth-to-mask breathing, except—

- Look, listen and feel for breathing with your ear over the stoma.
- Maintain the airway in a neutral position. (This ensures the patient's airway is neither flexed nor extended, as the stoma provides access to the lower airway.)
- Use a pediatric resuscitation mask over the patient's stoma.
- If possible, pinch the nose and close the mouth, as some patients with a stoma may still have a passage for air that reaches the mouth and nose in addition to the stoma.
- Provide ventilations (**Fig. 10-11**).

Patients with Dentures

Leave dentures in place unless they become loose and block the airway. Dentures help support the patient's mouth and cheeks, making it easier to seal the resuscitation mask during ventilation.

Patients with Suspected Head, Neck or Spinal injuries

If you suspect a patient has sustained an injury to the head, neck or spine, there are special considerations you must keep in mind. You may not always know if a patient has sustained this kind of injury and may have to rely on bystander information or *mechanism of injury* (MOI). Suspect

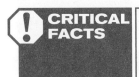
CRITICAL FACTS

Suspect an injury to the head, neck or spine if the patient was involved in a motor-vehicle, motorcycle or bicycle crash as an occupant, rider or pedestrian; was injured as a result of a fall from greater than standing height; complains of neck or back pain, tingling in the extremities or weakness; is not fully alert; appears to be intoxicated; appears frail or over 65 years of age; or has an obvious head or neck injury.

an injury to the head, neck or spine if the patient—

- Was involved in a motor-vehicle, motorcycle or bicycle crash as an occupant, rider or pedestrian.
- Was injured as a result of a fall from greater than standing height.
- Complains of neck or back pain, tingling in the extremities or weakness.
- Is not fully alert.
- Appears to be intoxicated.
- Appears frail or over 65 years of age.
- Has an obvious head or neck injury.

Check for the following signs and symptoms of a possible head, neck or spinal injury before you attempt to provide care:

- Changes in the *level of consciousness* (LOC)
- Severe pain or pressure in the head, neck or back
- Loss of balance
- Partial or complete loss of movement of any body part
- Tingling or loss of sensation in the hands, fingers, feet or toes
- Persistent headache
- Unusual bumps, bruises or depressions on the head, neck or back
- Seizures
- Blood or other fluids in the ears or nose
- External bleeding of the head, neck or back
- Impaired breathing or vision as a result of injury
- Nausea or vomiting
- Bruising of the head, especially around the eyes and behind the ears

If you suspect an unconscious patient may have an injury to the head, neck or spine, remember to take care of the airway and breathing first. Try to open the airway using the jaw-thrust (without head extension) maneuver first. If the jaw-thrust (without head extension) maneuver does not open the airway, use the head-tilt/chin-lift technique.

Bag-Valve-Mask Resuscitator Ventilations

Bag-Valve-Mask Resuscitator

A BVM is a hand-held device used to ventilate patients in respiratory distress or respiratory arrest (**Fig. 10-12, A**). It has three parts: a bag, a valve

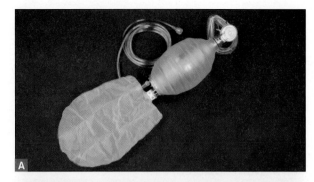

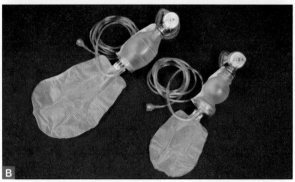

Fig. 10-12, A–B: BVMs come in a variety of sizes for use with **(A)** adults, **(B)** children and infants.

and a mask. By placing the mask on the patient's face and squeezing the bag, you open the one-way valve, forcing air into the patient's lungs. When you release the bag, the valve closes and air from the surrounding environment refills the bag.

BVMs have several advantages. They—

- Increase oxygen levels in the blood by using the air in the surrounding environment instead of the air exhaled by the rescuer.
- Can be connected to emergency oxygen.
- Are more effective for delivering ventilations than using a resuscitation mask, when used correctly by two rescuers.
- Protect against disease transmission and inhalation hazards if the patient has been exposed to a hazardous gas.
- May be utilized with advanced airway adjuncts.

Pediatric Considerations

Pediatric BVMs

Pediatric BVMs are available and should be used for children and infants (**Fig. 10-12, B**). Using an adult BVM on an infant has the potential to cause harm and should **not** be used unless a pediatric BVM is not available *and* medical control advises you to do so. Always use the appropriate equipment matched to the size of the patient.

To use a BVM—

1. Select the correct mask size for the patient (adult, child or infant).
2. Assemble the BVM, if necessary.
3. Position the mask over the patient's mouth and nose.
4. Seal the mask.
5. Open the patient's airway, while maintaining the seal on the mask.
6. Begin ventilations.

Because it is necessary to maintain a tight seal on the mask, two rescuers should operate a BVM. With only a single rescuer, operation of the BVM is difficult and generally does not create an adequate seal to deliver oxygen to the patient. With two rescuers, one rescuer opens and maintains the airway and seals the BVM, while the second rescuer delivers ventilations by squeezing the bag at the correct intervals.

BVMs have some limitations:

- They may not always be available.
- They may interfere with the timing of chest compressions during CPR.
- They require you to monitor the patient to ensure full exhalation.

Providing Controlled Ventilation

Knowing the recommended ventilation rates for use with a BVM will ensure that you provide patients with adequate oxygen without causing harm. For example, too many breaths or too much volume of air can result in air going into the stomach, which can cause vomiting.

Ventilation rates vary with the age of the patient. Adequate ventilation rates are—

- 30–60 ventilations per minute at about 1 second each for a newborn (0 to 1 month).
- 12–20 ventilations per minute at 1 second each for a child or an infant.
- 10–12 ventilations per minute at 1 second each for an adult.

You can determine whether ventilation is adequate by watching the chest rise and fall. Ventilating a patient at rates that are too fast or with too much volume can be dangerous.

Assisted Ventilation During Respiratory Distress

Assisted ventilation improves both oxygenation and ventilation. A patient in respiratory distress cannot breathe easily. Without adequate breathing, not

---

Normal Ventilation Versus Positive Pressure Ventilation

There are several differences between normal ventilation and **positive pressure ventilation**. First, in normal ventilation, the movement of the diaphragm dropping creates negative pressure inside the chest, which causes air to be sucked into the lungs. During positive pressure ventilation using a resuscitation mask or BVM, the movement of air is created by the rescuer pushing the air artificially into the lungs.

A second difference is in how the blood moves within the body during normal versus positive pressure ventilation. In normal ventilation, the blood returns to the heart from the body and is pulled back to the heart as a part of breathing. During positive pressure ventilation, there is a decreased volume of blood returning to the heart when the lungs are inflated. Also, the amount of blood pumped out of the heart is reduced.

Esophageal opening pressure is also different in the two kinds of ventilation. During normal ventilation, the esophagus remains closed, and no air enters the stomach. During positive pressure ventilation, air is pushed into the stomach during ventilation. If there is excess air in the stomach, this may lead to vomiting and **aspiration**.

Finally, positive pressure ventilation has the added risk of harming the patient due to excess rate or depth of ventilation. Ventilating the patient too quickly or too deeply may case low blood pressure, vomiting or a decrease in blood flow when the chest is compressed during CPR.

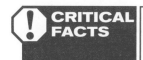

Assisted ventilation is given when the patient shows signs and symptoms of inadequate breathing, including breathing and heart rates that are too fast or too slow, cyanosis, inadequate chest wall motion, changes in consciousness, restlessness and chest pain.

enough oxygen reaches the cells, resulting in hypoxia. The patient becomes agitated and aggressive.

Assisted ventilation is given when the patient shows signs and symptoms of inadequate breathing, including—

- Breathing and heart rates that are too fast or too slow.
- Cyanosis.
- Inadequate chest wall motion.
- Changes in consciousness.
- Restlessness.
- Chest pain.

Procedure

When providing assisted ventilation to a patient during respiratory distress—

- Explain the procedure if the patient is conscious. A patient who is not breathing properly can become anxious or panic. Calming the patient may make him or her more receptive to your assistance.
- Place the mask over the patient's mouth and nose.
- Initially assist at the rate at which the patient has been breathing. Squeeze the bag each time the patient begins or tries to inhale.
- Adjust the rate as the patient's breathing begins to return to normal.

If breathing is slower than usual, provide extra ventilations in between the patient's own breaths. If breathing is rapid and shallow, provide ventilations when the patient inhales. If the patient has adequate breathing, administer emergency oxygen at 15 LPM. Keep checking for signs of inadequate breathing.

Limitations

Patients who are hypoxic may become combative. A patient with this kind of altered mental status may deteriorate quickly and become unable to breathe adequately. Maintain the airway and monitor the patient closely.

Make sure the mask fits tightly around the patient's mouth and nose. If there is not a good seal, an insufficient volume of air will be delivered to the patient.

Ventilation of an Apneic Patient

Absence of breathing (apnea) is a life-threatening condition that requires urgent care. Begin artificial ventilation at once using a resuscitation mask or BVM. Ventilation is provided for an apneic (non-breathing) patient if the chest wall is not moving and there is no air moving in and out of the mouth and nose, or if occasional gasping breathing is noted. Continue to monitor the patient's condition. Ensure you have the proper size equipment for the apneic patient when providing artificial ventilation.

PUTTING IT ALL TOGETHER

Ensuring that a patient's airway is open and clear is an important first step in providing care. A patient whose airway is blocked for any reason may die unless immediate steps are taken to open the airway.

Once the patient's airway is clear, you can begin to assess breathing. Inadequate breathing causes problems with inadequate ventilation and oxygenation. Breathing abnormalities can be assessed by observing physical signs and breath sounds, and by measuring the rate and depth of breathing.

A breathing emergency can become life threatening and should be detected during the primary assessment. Knowing the signs and symptoms of respiratory distress and respiratory arrest will help you determine the appropriate care for each condition.

For a patient who is not breathing, provide artificial ventilation by using a resuscitation mask or BVM. Under specific circumstances, artificial ventilation can be provided mask-to-nose or mask-to-stoma. When using a resuscitation mask, be careful not to breathe too much air into the patient, as this may cause air to enter the stomach and cause vomiting. Also, special considerations must be made for children, patients with dentures and patients suspected of having a head, neck or spinal injury.

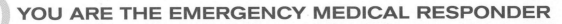

))) YOU ARE THE EMERGENCY MEDICAL RESPONDER

While waiting for emergency medical services (EMS) personnel to arrive, you complete a SAMPLE history and secondary assessment. You have helped the patient into a position of comfort for breathing when he loses consciousness and stops breathing. He has a pulse. What care should you provide now?

SKILLsheet

Giving Ventilations—Adult and Child

NOTE: Always follow standard precautions when providing care. Size-up the scene for safety and then perform a primary assessment. Always select the properly sized mask for the patient.

If there is a pulse but *no* breathing—

STEP 1
Assemble the resuscitation mask as necessary, and position the mask.

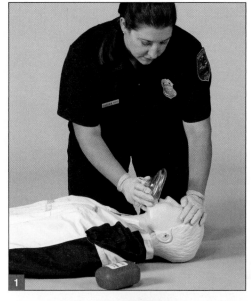

STEP 2
Seal the mask.

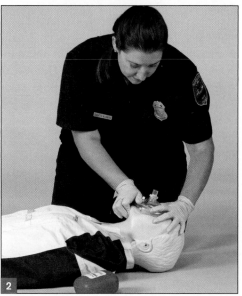

Continued on next page

Giving Ventilations—Adult and Child *continued*

STEP 3

Open the airway by tilting the head back and lifting the chin.

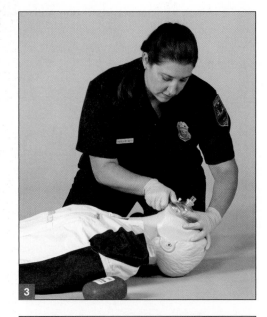

STEP 4

Blow into the mask.
- For an adult, give **1** ventilation about every **5** seconds.
- For a child, give **1** ventilation about every **3** seconds.
- Each ventilation should last about **1** second and make the chest clearly rise. The chest should fall before the next ventilation is given.

NOTE: For a child, tilt the head slightly past a neutral position. Do not tilt the head as far back as for an adult. For a patient with a suspected head, neck or spinal injury, use the jaw-thrust (without head extension) maneuver to open the airway to give ventilations.

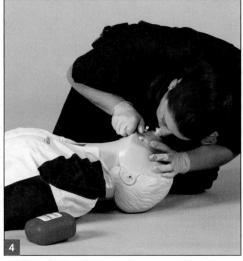

STEP 5

Recheck for breathing and a pulse about every **2** minutes–
- ◆ Remove the mask and look, listen and feel for breathing and a pulse for *no more than **10** seconds.*

If the patient is unconscious but breathing–
- ◆ Leave the patient in a face-up position and maintain an open airway, especially if there is a suspected spinal injury.
- ◆ You are alone and have to leave the person (e.g., to call for help), or you cannot maintain an open and clear airway because of fluids or vomit, place the person in a modified H.A.IN.E.S. recovery position.

If the chest does *not* clearly rise–
- ◆ Retilt the head, and then give another ventilation.
- ◆ Provide care based on the conditions found.

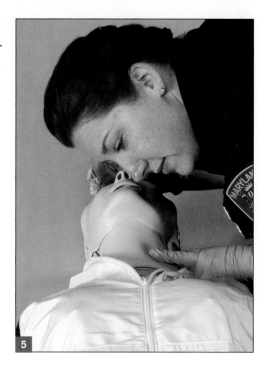

5

SKILLsheet

Giving Ventilations–Infant

NOTE: Always follow standard precautions when providing care. Size-up the scene for safety and then perform a primary assessment. Always select the properly sized mask for the patient.

If there is a pulse but *no* breathing–

STEP 1
Assemble the resuscitation mask as necessary, and position the resuscitation mask.

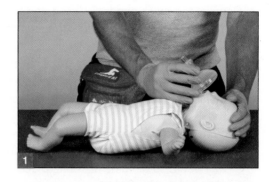

STEP 2
Seal the mask.

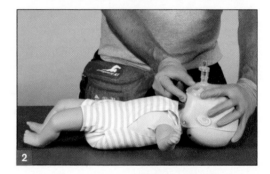

STEP 3
Open the airway by tilting the head to a neutral position and lifting the chin.

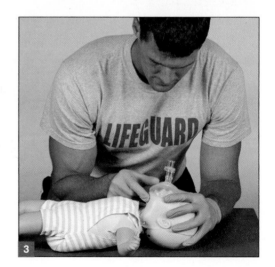

STEP 4

Blow into the mask.

◆ Give **1** ventilation about every **3** seconds.
◆ Each ventilation should last about **1** second and make the chest clearly rise. The chest should fall before the next ventilation is given.

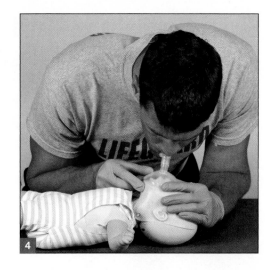

STEP 5

Recheck for breathing and a pulse about every **2** minutes—

◆ Remove the mask and look, listen and feel for breathing and a pulse for *no more than **10** seconds*.

If the infant is unconscious but breathing—

◆ Place the infant in a recovery position as would be done for an older child.
◆ Alternatively hold an infant in a recovery position by—
  • Carefully positioning the infant face-down along your forearm.
  • Supporting the infant's head and neck with your other hand while keeping the infant's mouth and nose clear.

If the chest does *not* clearly rise—

◆ Retilt the head, and then give another ventilation.
◆ Provide care based on the conditions found.

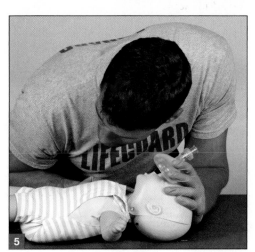

SKILLsheet

Giving Ventilations–Head, Neck or Spinal Injury Suspected Jaw-Thrust (Without Head Extension) Maneuver– Adult and Child

NOTE: Always follow standard precautions when providing care. Size-up the scene for safety and then perform a primary assessment. Always select the properly sized mask for the patient.

If there is a pulse, but *no* breathing and a head, neck or spinal injury *is suspected*–

STEP 1
Assemble the resuscitation mask.

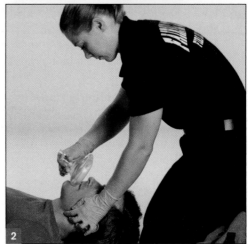

STEP 2
Position the mask.
- Kneel above the patient's head.
- Place the rim of the mask between the lower lip and chin.
- Lower the resuscitation mask until it covers the patient's mouth and nose.

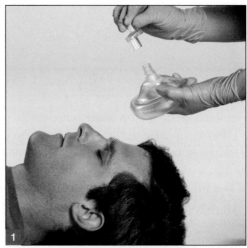

STEP 3

Seal the mask.

◆ Place your thumbs along each side of the resuscitation mask.
◆ Use your elbows for support.
◆ Slide your fingers into position under the angles of the patient's jawbone.
◆ Without moving the patient's head, apply even, downward pressure with your thumbs to seal the mask.

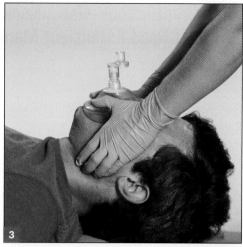

STEP 4

Open the airway.

◆ Without tilting the head back, open the airway by pushing or *thrusting* the lower jaw up with your fingers along the jawbone.

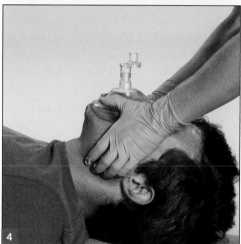

STEP 5

Blow into the mask.

◆ For an adult, give **1** ventilation about every **5** seconds
◆ For a child, give **1** ventilation about every **3** seconds.
◆ Each ventilation should last about **1** second and make the chest clearly rise. The chest should fall before the next ventilation is given.

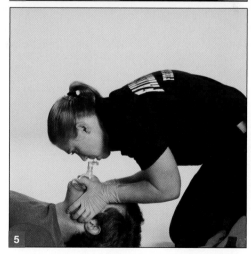

Continued on next page

Giving Ventilations–Head, Neck or Spinal Injury Suspected Jaw-Thrust (Without Head Extension) Maneuver–Adult and Child *continued*

STEP 6

Reassess for breathing and a pulse about every
2 minutes–
◆ Remove the mask and look, listen and feel for breathing and a pulse for *no more than* **10** *seconds.*

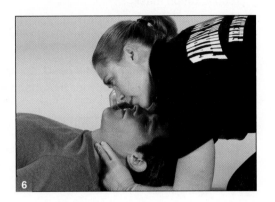

If the patient is unconscious but breathing–
◆ Leave the patient in a face-up position and maintain an open airway, especially if there is a suspected spinal injury.
◆ You are alone and have to leave the person (e.g., to call for help), or you cannot maintain an open and clear airway because of fluids or vomit, place the person in a modified H.A.IN.E.S. recovery position.

If the chest does *not* clearly rise–
◆ Retilt the head, and then give another ventilation.
◆ Provide care based on the conditions found.

SKILLsheet

Giving Ventilations Using a Bag-Valve-Mask Resuscitator– Two Rescuers

NOTE: Always follow standard precautions when providing care. Size-up the scene for safety and then perform a primary assessment. Always select the properly sized mask for the patient. Assemble the BVM if necessary.

If there is a pulse but *no* breathing–

STEP 1
Rescuer 1 positions the mask over the patient's mouth and nose.

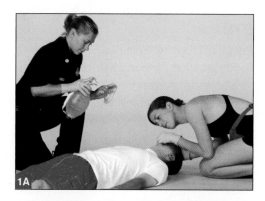

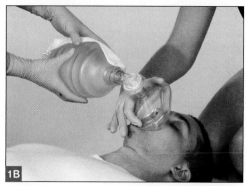

STEP 2
Rescuer 1 seals the mask.

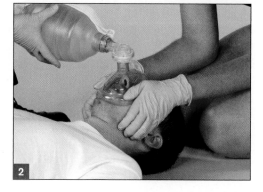

Continued on next page

Giving Ventilations Using a Bag-Valve-Mask Resuscitator– Two Rescuers *continued*

STEP 3

Rescuer 1 opens the airway.

◆ Places thumbs along each side of the mask and uses elbows for support.

◆ Slides fingers behind the angles of the jawbone.

◆ Pushes down on the mask with thumbs, lift the jaw and tilt the head back.

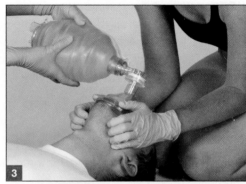

STEP 4

Rescuer 2 begins ventilations.

◆ Squeezes the bag slowly with both hands.

◆ For an adult, give **1** ventilation about every **5** seconds

◆ For a child or an infant, give **1** ventilation about every **3** seconds.

◆ Each ventilation should last about **1** second and make the chest clearly rise. The chest should fall before the next ventilation is given.

NOTE: For a child, tilt the head slightly past a neutral position. Do not tilt the head as far back as for an adult. For an infant, position head in a neutral position.

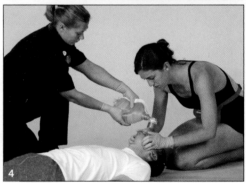

STEP 5
Recheck for breathing and a pulse about every
2 minutes–
◆ Remove the BVM and look, listen and feel for breathing and a pulse for *no more than **10** seconds.*

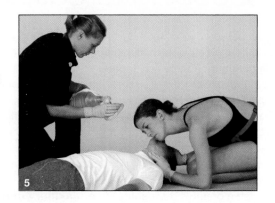

If the patient is unconscious but breathing–
◆ Leave the patient in a face-up position and maintain an open airway, especially if there is a suspected spinal injury.
◆ You are alone and have to leave the person (e.g., to call for help), or you cannot maintain an open and clear airway because of fluids or vomit, place the person in a modified H.A.IN.E.S. recovery position.
◆ Alternatively hold an infant in a recovery position by–
  • Carefully positioning the infant face-down along your forearm.
  • Supporting the infant's head and neck with your other hand while keeping the infant's mouth and nose clear.

If the chest does *not* clearly rise–
◆ Retilt the head, and then give another ventilation.
◆ Provide care based on the conditions found.

Enrichment
Assessing Breath Sounds

Unobstructed airways are easy to identify with a stethoscope. You should hear air moving on inspiration (breathing in) and expiration (breathing out). If there are decreased lung sounds in a particular area of the lungs, you will hear no sound or a reduced sound compared with the other areas in the lungs.

To listen to the lungs in the front, you must identify the **midclavicular lines** and move down the chest. Place your stethoscope at the second intercostal space, usually just above the sternum line **(Fig. 10-13, A)**. Do this on both the left and right sides to compare sounds.

To listen on the side, identify the **midaxillary lines** and place your stethoscope between the fourth and fifth intercostal space, approximately in line with the nipple **(Fig. 10-13, B)**. Again, do this on both sides to be able to compare sounds.

Finally, listen in the back by identifying the **midscapular lines** and moving down the back **(Fig. 10-13, C)**. Do this again on both sides.

When the airway becomes obstructed due to accumulation of fluid in the lungs or a blockage in the airway, you may hear other sounds, such as—

* Wheezing—a high-pitched whistling sound heard during inspiration but heard most loudly on expiration. Wheezing can often be heard without a stethoscope.
* Rales—a popping, clicking, bubbling or rattling sound.
* **Rhonchi**—described as a a snoring or coarse, dry rale sound.
* Stridor—a wheeze-like sound heard on inhalation and exhalation.

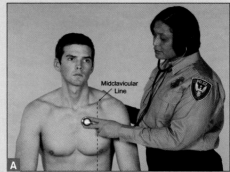

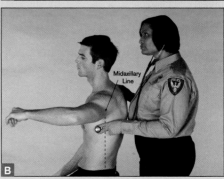

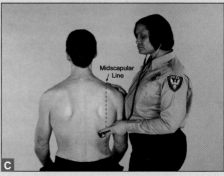

Fig. 10-13, A–C: To assess breath sounds, **(A)** Identify midclavicular lines and place your stethoscope at the second intercostal space, **(B)** place your stethoscope between the fourth and fifth intercostal space, **(C)** identify the midscapular lines and move down below the scapula. Be sure to listen to and compare both sides.

Enrichment
Sellick's Maneuver (Cricoid Pressure)

The Sellick's maneuver should be used during positive pressure ventilation situations when the patient requires **intubation**, which is a skilled procedure performed by more advanced medical personnel. When a patient requires intubation, air may have already entered or can enter the esophagus and go into the stomach. This increases the risk of vomiting. Sellick's maneuver reduces the chance of air entering the esophagus, particularly in patients who are unresponsive and/or have no gag reflex. It also allows the rescuer performing the intubation to have a better view of the vocal cords, allowing for easier insertion of the endotracheal tube. The procedure is performed by one rescuer while another performs the intubation. EMRs may be requested to assist more advanced medical personnel by performing the Sellick's maneuver.

The cricoid cartilage is located just below and behind the thyroid cartilage and makes a circle against the esophagus, which is behind it **(Fig. 10-14)**. Using your thumb and index finger, locate the cartilage and apply pressure on both sides of the cartilage, pressing firmly toward the back of the neck **(Fig. 10-15)**. Continue pressing down until the intubation is complete.

Do *not* use this maneuver if—

* The patient is vomiting or begins to vomit.
* The patient is responsive.
* A breathing tube will be placed by advanced-level providers when they arrive.

If using this procedure on a child, use caution *not* to apply too much pressure on the cartilage and esophagus.

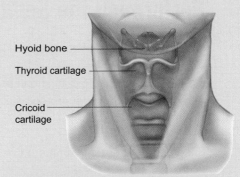

Hyoid bone

Thyroid cartilage

Cricoid cartilage

Fig. 10-14: The cricoid cartilage, located below and behind the thyroid cartilage, makes a circle against the esophagus behind it.

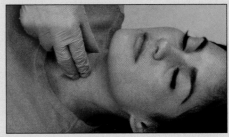

Fig. 10-15: To perform the Sellick's maneuver, apply pressure on both sides of the cricoid cartilage, pressing firmly toward the back of the neck.

Continued on next page

SKILLsheet

Performing the Sellick's Maneuver (Cricoid Pressure)

NOTE: Always follow standard precautions when providing care.

If a patient is unconscious, and your assistance has been requested by more advanced medical personnel and the local protocols allow—

STEP 1

Ensure the patient is in a face-up (supine) position.

STEP 2

Locate the cricoid cartilage.

STEP 3

Apply downward pressure on both sides of the cartilage with your thumb and forefinger.

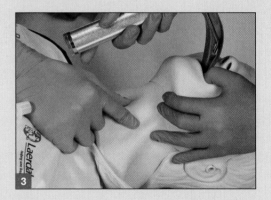

STEP 4

Maintain firm, gentle downward pressure until the intubation is completed and you are instructed to stop by the paramedic or *emergency medical technician* (EMT).

Enrichment
Assisting the Patient with Asthma

As an EMR, you may find yourself in the position of needing to assist a patient with asthma in using an inhaler. Having a basic knowledge of inhalers is of benefit to an EMR and to the patient with asthma to whom you may provide care.

ASTHMA MEDICATION: TYPES, INDICATIONS AND CONTRAINDICATIONS

There are three types of medications used in the management of asthma, each with a different purpose:
- Long-term-control medications are used regularly to control chronic symptoms and prevent attacks.
- Quick-relief medications, also called *rescue medications*, are used as needed for relief of symptoms during an asthma attack.
- Medications for allergy-induced asthma are used to decrease sensitivity to a particular allergen and prevent the immune system from reacting to allergens.

Indications for asthma medication include recurrent wheezing, coughing, trouble breathing and chest tightness. Contraindications include increased risk of skin thinning and bruising. Asthma medication may also affect children's growth.

DELIVERY SYSTEMS FOR ASTHMA MEDICATION

Metered-Dose Inhaler

A *metered-dose inhaler* is a small, hand-held aerosol canister with a mouthpiece. It is designed to allow patients to inhale a specific amount of asthma medication into the lungs in one puff. A *spacer*, a tube attached to an inhaler that serves as a reservoir for the medication, may be present.

Dry Powder Inhaler

A *dry powder inhaler* (DPI) is similar to a metered-dose inhaler. A DPI is a hand-held device that delivers a dry powder form of the medication inside a small capsule, disc or compartment inside the inhaler. Some dry powders may have no taste, while others are mixed with lactose to give them a sweet taste. The DPI is administered by breathing in quickly to activate the inhaler, so there is no depressing of the inhaler.

Small-Volume Nebulizer

A small-volume nebulizer is designed to administer aerosolized medication (mist) over a few minutes, ensuring the efficacy of drug delivery during treatment will not be jeopardized, even if the patient takes a single ineffective breath. Nebulizers are common for children under the age of 5, those who have difficulty using inhalers and those with severe asthma.

Other Delivery Systems for Asthma Medication

Asthma medication can also be taken in pill or liquid form. Most recently, asthma medication can be given through an injection just under the skin.

PEAK FLOW METER

A *peak flow meter* is a hand-held asthma management tool that tracks a person's breathing. It assists in warning the person if their asthma is worsening, and helps show how they are responding to treatment. A peak flow meter measures the person's ability to push air out of the lungs in one quick breath.

Continued on next page

Enrichment
Assisting the Patient with Asthma (continued)

ASSISTING A PATIENT IN THE USE OF AN INHALER

When assisting a patient in the use of an asthma inhaler, *always* obtain consent then follow these general guidelines, if local protocols allow:

1. If the patient has prescribed asthma medication, help the person take it first.
2. Shake the inhaler and then remove the cover from the mouthpiece. Position the spacer if you are using one.
3. Have the patient breathe out fully through the mouth and then place the lips tightly around the inhaler mouthpiece.
4. The patient should inhale deeply and slowly as you or the patient depresses the inhaler canister to release the medication, which is then inhaled into the lungs.
5. The patient should hold the breath for a count of 10. If using a spacer, the patient takes 5 to 6 deep breaths with the spacer still in the mouth, without holding the breath.
6. Once the inhalation is complete, have the patient rinse his or her mouth out with water to reduce side effects.
7. Reassess the patient's breathing.
8. Always wash your hands immediately after providing care.

SIDE EFFECTS

Common side effects of asthma medication include–
- Increased heart rate.
- Palpitations.
- Nausea.
- Vomiting.
- Nervousness.
- Headache.
- Sleeplessness.
- Dry mouth.
- Cough.
- Hoarseness.
- Headache.
- Throat irritation.

DOSE AND ROUTE

The effectiveness of treatment for asthma can vary based on the dose given to the patient, as well as the route by which it is administered. In severe cases, this is tracked by the patient's health care provider in order to find which is the most effective.

MEDICAL CONTROL ROLE

Any time you assist a patient with an inhaler, you need to obtain an order from medical direction. The order can be obtained through radio or phone contact with the medical director or through protocols and standing orders.

Always verify the order by restating the name of the medication. This helps reduce the chance of improper medication or inappropriate dose or route. Know and follow local protocols for administration of inhalers.

SKILLsheet

Assisting with an Asthma Inhaler

REMEMBER: Always obtain consent and wash your hands immediately after providing care. Read and follow all instructions printed on the inhaler prior to administering the medication to the patient.

If the person has medication for asthma, help him or her take it:

STEP 1
Help the patient sit up and rest in a position comfortable for breathing.

STEP 2
Ensure that the prescription is in the patient's name and is prescribed for "quick relief" or "acute" attacks.
◆ Ensure that the expiration date of the medication has *not* passed.

STEP 3
Shake the inhaler.

STEP 4
Remove the cover from the inhaler mouthpiece.
◆ If an extension tube (spacer) is available, attach and use it.

STEP 5
Tell the patient to breathe out as much as possible through the mouth.

STEP 6
Have the patient place his or her lips tightly around the mouthpiece and take a long, slow breath.
◆ As the patient breathes in slowly, administer the medication by quickly pressing down on the inhaler canister, or the patient may self-administer the medication.
◆ The patient should continue a full, deep breath.
◆ Tell the patient to try to hold his or her breath for a count of **10**.
◆ When using an extension tube (spacer) have the patient take **5** to **6** deep breaths through the tube *without* holding his or her breath.

NOTE: The patient may use different techniques, such as holding the inhaler two-finger lengths away from the mouth.

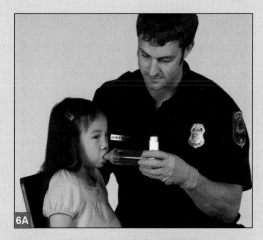
6A

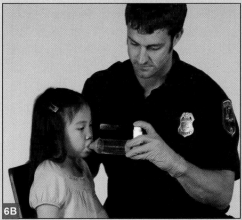
6B

Continued on next page

Assisting with an Asthma Inhaler *continued*

STEP 7

Note the time of administration and any change in the patient's condition.
◆ The medication may be repeated once after
  1 to **2** minutes.

NOTE: The medication may be repeated every **5** to
10 minutes thereafter, as needed, for emergency calls
in areas with long EMS response times such as
rural locations.

STEP 8

Have the patient rinse his or her mouth out with water to
reduce side effects.
◆ Stay with the patient and monitor his or her condition.
  Provide care for any other injuries.

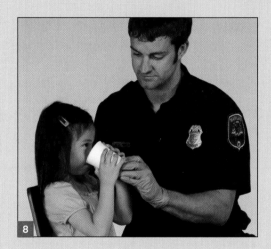

STEP 9

Care for shock. Keep the patient from getting chilled or overheated. Call for more advanced medical
care if difficulty breathing does not improve quickly.

NOTE: These medications might take **5** to **15** minutes to reach full effectiveness.

11
Airway Management

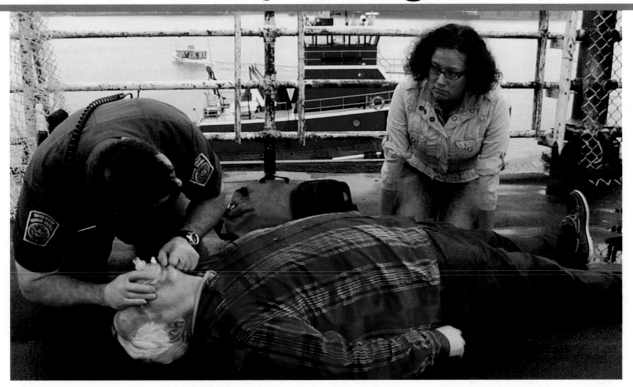

))) YOU ARE THE EMERGENCY MEDICAL RESPONDER

As border security in the immediate vicinity and trained as an emergency medical responder (EMR), you respond to a call at one of the docks for an unconscious adult who collapsed for no apparent reason. You size-up the scene and notice that a middle-age male is lying face-up on the floor and not moving. You discover that the patient's chest does not rise when you attempt ventilations. What would you do next? What do you think the problem is?

Key Terms

Airway adjunct: A mechanical device used to help keep the tongue from obstructing the airway; can be either nasal or oral.

Nasal (nasopharyngeal) airway (NPA): An airway adjunct inserted through the nostril and into the throat to help keep the tongue from obstructing the airway; may be used on a conscious or an unconscious patient.

Oral (oropharyngeal) airway (OPA): An airway adjunct inserted through the mouth and into the throat to help keep the tongue from obstructing the airway; used *only* with unconscious patients.

Learning Objectives

After reading this chapter, and completing the class activities, you will have the information needed to—

- Explain the purposes and use of airway adjuncts.
- Describe the two types of suctioning devices and their use.
- List the circumstances when airway adjuncts should *not* be used.
- List some common causes of airway obstruction and describe appropriate care.
- Describe how to provide care for an unconscious choking adult, child and infant.

Skill Objectives

After reading this chapter, and completing the class activities, you should be able to—

- Demonstrate how to insert an oral airway.
- Demonstrate the techniques of suctioning.
- Demonstrate how to provide care for a conscious choking adult, child and infant.
- Demonstrate how to insert a nasal airway *(Enrichment skill).*

INTRODUCTION

Although most of the care you provide will not require the use of breathing devices or **airway adjuncts**, in some situations they can be used effectively as part of your care. Breathing devices and airway adjuncts can assist with—

- Helping maintain an open airway.
- Ventilating a patient.
- Supplying emergency oxygen.

In this chapter, you will learn the purpose and use of airway adjuncts, suctioning and how to handle situations involving *foreign body airway obstructions* (FBAOs).

SUCTIONING

Sometimes injury or sudden illness results in foreign matter, such as mucus, fluids or blood, collecting in a patient's airway. One method of clearing the airway is to roll the patient onto the side and sweep the mouth with a gloved finger. However, finger sweeps *only* should be performed on an *unconscious* patient and *only* when material is visible in the mouth. Another method of keeping the airway clear is to place an unconscious patient who is breathing in a recovery position. But a more effective method is to suction the airway clear. Suctioning is the process of removing foreign matter from the upper airway by means of a mechanical or manual device.

Suctioning is an important step, when fluids or foreign matter are present or suspected, because the airway must be open and clear in order for the patient to breathe or for any CPR breathing barrier to be effective.

Suctioning Equipment

There are two types of suction devices: mechanical and manual **(Fig. 11-1, A–B)**. A variety of mechanical and manual devices are used to suction the airway. Not all suction units are able to remove solid objects like teeth, foreign bodies and food. Always follow standard precautions when using a suctioning device.

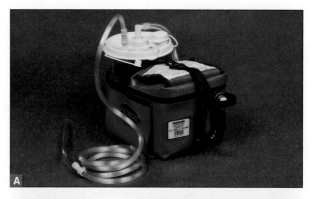

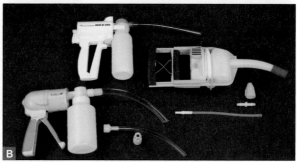

Fig. 11-1, A–B: **(A)** Mechanical suctioning equipment; **(B)** Manual suctioning equipment

Mechanical suction units are electrically powered. They produce a vacuum that is powerful enough to suction substances from the throat. Mechanical units operate on batteries, which must be checked to ensure they are fully charged, unless the units are of a type with batteries that can be constantly charged. Otherwise, there may be insufficient vacuum to operate the unit effectively and for a sufficient amount of time. Mechanical suction devices are normally found on ambulances or other transport vehicles and use either battery-powered pumps or oxygen-powered aspirators.

Manual suction units, as the term implies, are operated by hand. They are lightweight, compact and relatively inexpensive. Because they do not require an energy source, they avoid some of the problems associated with mechanical units.

For either type of unit, several sizes of sterile suction catheters should be kept on hand for use, depending on the size of the patient. An installed suction unit should be powerful enough to provide an airflow of >40 *liters per minute* (LPM) at

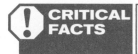

CRITICAL FACTS Suctioning is the process of removing foreign matter, such as mucus, fluids or blood, from a patient's upper airway. Suctioning can be done through mechanical or manual devices.

the end of the delivery tube and, when clamped, a vacuum of >300 mmHg.

How to Suction

To use a *mechanical* suctioning device—

1. Position the patient on the side with the mouth open. If a spinal injury is suspected, be sure to manually stabilize the spine and log roll the patient to the side.
2. Remove any visible large debris from the mouth with a gloved finger if the patient is unconscious.
3. Measure and check the suction tip.
4. Turn on the machine and test.
5. Suction the mouth of an adult for *no more than 15 seconds at a time*. Suctioning for longer periods can starve the patient of air. This can create an environment that is too low in oxygen to sustain life.

To use a *manual* suctioning device—

1. Position the patient on the side with the mouth open.
2. Remove any visible large debris from the mouth with a gloved finger if the patient is unconscious.
3. Measure and check the suction tip.
4. Suction the mouth of an adult for *no more than 15 seconds at a time*.

> ### Pediatric Considerations
> When using mechanical or manual suction on a child or an infant, suction for *no more than 10 seconds for a child* and *5 seconds for an infant at a time*.

BREATHING DEVICES

Breathing devices allow the *emergency medical responder* (EMR) to provide positive pressure ventilations to patients in need of CPR, emergency oxygen and/or artificial ventilations. These devices include CPR breathing barriers such as face shields and resuscitation masks, *bag-valve-mask resuscitators* (BVM) and emergency oxygen equipment. CPR breathing barriers

should have certain standard features such as a one-way valve to reduce the possibility of direct contact with, or exposure to, body fluids and a patient's exhaled breath. Such devices can help to deliver life-sustaining ventilations when a patient is unable to breathe on his or her own. See **Chapter 10** for more information and how to use these devices.

AIRWAY ADJUNCTS

The tongue is the most common cause of airway obstruction in an unconscious person. Keeping the tongue from blocking the air passage is a high priority. Mechanical airway adjuncts known as *oral (oropharyngeal) airways* (**OPAs**) and *nasal (nasopharyngeal) airways* (**NPAs**) can help you accomplish this task. (For more information on NPAs, refer to the **Enrichment** at the end of this chapter.)

Airway adjuncts come in a variety of sizes (**Fig. 11-2, A–B**). The curved design fits the

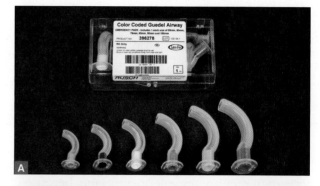

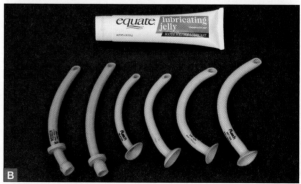

Fig. 11-2, A–B: (A) Oropharyngeal (OPA) airways; **(B)** Nasopharyngeal (NPA) airways

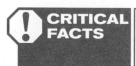 **CRITICAL FACTS** The tongue is the most common cause of airway obstruction in an unconscious person. Keeping the tongue from blocking the air passage is a high priority. Mechanical airway adjuncts known as *OPAs* and *NPAs* can help you accomplish this task.

natural contour of the mouth and throat. Once you have positioned the device, you can use a resuscitation mask or BVM to ventilate a nonbreathing patient.

Oropharyngeal Airway

As the name implies, this type of airway is inserted into the mouth. When properly positioned, the OPA keeps the tongue away from the back of the throat, thereby helping to maintain an open airway. An improperly placed airway device can compress the tongue into the back of the throat, further blocking the airway.

When preparing to insert an OPA, first be sure the patient is unconscious. OPAs are used *only* on unconscious, unresponsive patients with *no* gag reflex. If a patient begins to gag, remove the airway immediately. OPAs should not be used if the patient has suffered oral trauma, such as broken teeth, or has recently undergone oral surgery. Follow local protocols for the use of OPAs.

Next, select the proper size of airway. Measure the device on the patient to see that it extends from the patient's earlobe to the corner of the mouth (**Fig. 11-3**). To insert the airway, grasp the patient's lower jaw and tongue and lift upward. With the patient's jaw raised, insert the OPA with the curved end (tip) along the roof of the mouth (**Fig. 11-4, A**). As the tip of the device approaches the back of the throat, you will feel resistance. Rotate it a *half turn* to drop it into the back of the patient's throat (**Fig. 11-4, B**). The OPA should drop into the throat without resistance. The flange end should rest on the patient's lips (**Fig. 11-4, C**).

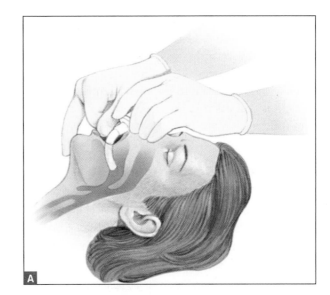

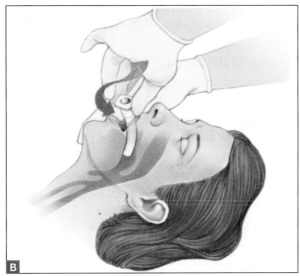

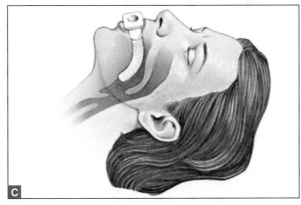

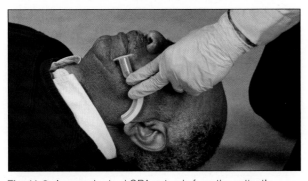

Fig. 11-3: A properly sized OPA extends from the patient's earlobe to the corner of the mouth.

Fig. 11-4, A–C: **(A)** Insert an OPA with the curved tip along the roof of the mouth. **(B)** Rotate it to drop it into the back of the throat. **(C)** If inserted properly, the flange end should rest on the lips.

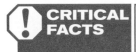 **CRITICAL FACTS** When preparing to insert an OPA, first be sure the patient is unconscious. OPAs are used *only* on unconscious, unresponsive patients with *no* gag reflex.

If the patient begins gagging as the device is positioned in the back of the throat, remove the device. Suction the airway, ensuring all debris is removed from the airway. Thoroughly clean the device and reinsert into the airway only if the patient is still unconscious and does *not* have a gag reflex.

Pediatric Considerations

The airway of a child or infant is smaller than an adult's. The size can also vary according to the age of the child or infant, so it is important to use an appropriately sized OPA for pediatric patients. Additionally, the palate of a child and an infant is softer than that of an adult. It can be injured if an OPA is inserted with the tip pointing upward toward the roof of the mouth and rotated 180 degrees as is performed on an adult. Because of this risk of injury, when inserting an OPA in a child or an infant, the airway is inserted with the tip of the device either *sideways* then rotated *90 degrees* into position or, using a tongue depressor, inserted with the tip of the device pointing toward the back of the tongue and throat in the position it will rest after insertion **(Fig. 11-5, A–B)**.

AIRWAY OBSTRUCTION
Types of Airway Obstruction

There are two types of airway obstruction, *anatomical* and *mechanical*:

Anatomical obstruction occurs when an airway is blocked by an anatomical structure, such as the tongue or swollen tissues of the mouth, tongue or throat. The tongue is a common cause of airway obstruction in an unconscious patient because the tongue relaxes when the body is deprived of oxygen, causing the tongue to rest on the back of the throat, blocking the flow of air to the lungs.

Mechanical obstruction, also known as *FBAO*, occurs when foreign objects, such as food or toys, or fluids, such as vomit, block the airway.

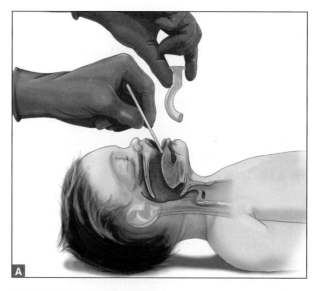

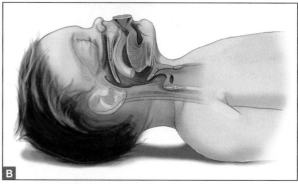

Fig. 11-5, A–B: To insert an OPA in a pediatric patient: **(A)** Use a tongue depressor and insert the OPA, with the device pointing toward the back of the tongue, **(B)** ensure that the OPA rests in proper position.

Foreign Body Airway Obstruction

Foreign body airway obstruction (FBAO) causes choking and commonly occurs because of poorly chewed food, eating too fast or laughing, talking, running or walking while eating. A conscious person who is clutching the throat is showing what is commonly called the "universal" sign of choking **(Fig. 11-6)**. A person with a mild FBAO, or partial airway obstruction, can still move some air to and from the lungs, often while wheezing.

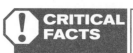 **CRITICAL FACTS** There are two types of airway obstruction: anatomical (e.g., swollen tongue) and mechanical (e.g., food, toys).

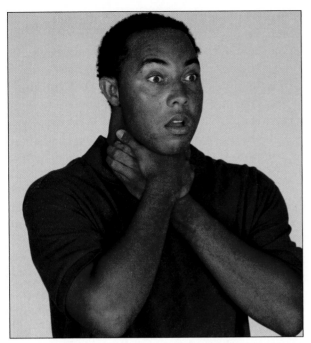

Fig. 11-6: A conscious person who is clutching the throat is showing what is commonly called the "universal" sign of choking.

As long as the person can cough forcefully, encourage continued coughing but do not provide first aid care for choking. Severe airway obstruction is apparent when the person cannot cough, speak, cry or breathe and requires *immediate* action.

FBAO in an Adult

As an EMR, you must get consent before helping a conscious choking adult. Unlike the conscious patient suffering FBAO, consent is implied when a patient is unconscious.

When caring for a conscious choking adult, perform a combination of back blows followed

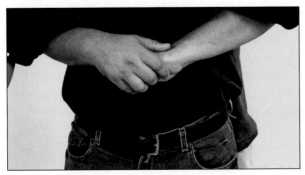

Fig. 11-7: Proper hand placement for abdominal thrusts

by abdominal thrusts **(Fig. 11-7)**. Each back blow and abdominal thrust should be a distinct attempt to dislodge the object. Using more than one technique is often necessary to dislodge an object and clear a patient's airway. Continue back blows and abdominal thrusts until the object is dislodged and the patient can cough forcefully, speak or breathe or until the patient becomes unconscious.

Abdominal thrusts may not be an effective method of care for conscious choking adults in cases where you cannot reach far enough around the patient to give effective abdominal thrusts or if the patient is obviously pregnant or known to be pregnant. In these situations, you should give back blows followed by chest thrusts **(Fig. 11-8, A–B)**.

To perform chest thrusts—

1. Stand behind the patient and make a fist with one hand.
2. Place the thumb side against the center of the patient's chest, or slightly higher on the patient's chest if she is pregnant.

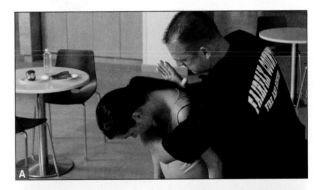

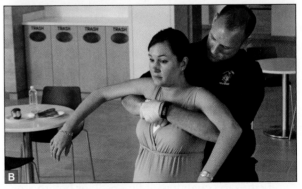

Fig. 11-8, A–B: If you cannot reach around the patient to give effective abdominal thrusts, or if the patient is pregnant, give **(A)** back blows followed by **(B)** chest thrusts.

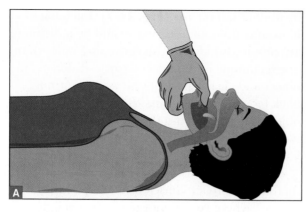

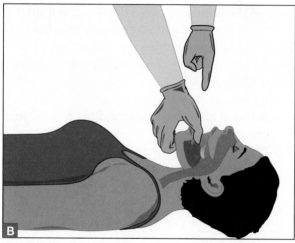

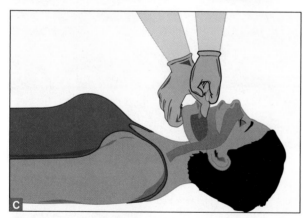

Fig. 11-9, A–C: If a conscious choking patient becomes unconscious, carefully lower the person to the ground, open the mouth and look for an object. If an object is seen, remove it with a finger sweep using the index finger.

3. Grab your fist with your other hand and give quick, inward thrusts.
4. Repeat until the object is forced out; the patient begins to cough forcefully, speak or breathe; or until the patient becomes unconscious.

If a conscious patient becomes unconscious, carefully lower the person to the ground, open the mouth and look for an object. If an object is seen, remove it with a finger sweep using the index finger (**Fig. 11-9, A–C**). If no object is seen, reopen the airway and try to give a ventilation. If the chest does not clearly rise, retilt the head, and then give another ventilation. If the chest still does not clearly rise, begin chest compressions.

If an unconscious adult's chest does not clearly rise after giving a ventilation, retilt the head, and then try another ventilation. If the ventilation still does not make the chest clearly rise, assume the airway is blocked by a foreign object and position yourself to give chest compressions as you would when performing CPR chest compressions. Use two hands in the center of the chest. Compress the chest then check the mouth for an object and, if one is seen, remove it out with a gloved finger. Reattempt two ventilations. Repeat cycles of chest compressions, foreign object check/removal and ventilations until the chest clearly rises. If the chest clearly rises, look, listen and feel for breathing and a pulse for *no more than 10 seconds*. Provide care based on the conditions found.

Pediatric Considerations

Children are prone to choking on small objects as well as food. Choking hazards among children include small objects such as coins, buttons, small toys and parts of toys and balloons, as well as certain food items. While hazardous for all children, these objects generally pose a larger threat to children under 4 years of age. Children under 4 do not have a full set of teeth and cannot chew as well as older children, so large chunks of foods may lodge in the throat and cause choking.

The *American Academy of Pediatrics* (AAP) recommends that children younger than 4 not be fed any round, firm food unless it is cut into small pieces no larger than one-half inch. It further recommends keeping the following foods away from children younger than 4:

• Hot dogs
• Nuts and seeds

- Chunks of meat or cheese
- Whole grapes
- Hard, gooey or sticky candy
- Popcorn
- Chunks of peanut butter
- Raw vegetables
- Raisins
- Chewing gum

While food items cause the most choking injuries in children, toys and household items can also be hazardous. Balloons, when not inflated or when broken, can choke or suffocate young children who try to swallow them. According to the *Consumer Product Safety Commission* (CPSC), more children have suffocated on non-inflated balloons and pieces of broken balloons than any other type of toy.

As an EMR, you must get consent from a parent or guardian, if present, before helping a conscious or unconscious choking child or infant.

For a *conscious* child or infant, use less force when giving back blows and abdominal thrusts or chest thrusts. Using too much force may cause internal injuries. Use a combination of back blows and abdominal thrusts for a child and a combination of back blows and chest thrusts for an infant. Continue back blows and abdominal thrusts or chest thrusts until the object is dislodged and the child or infant can cough forcefully, speak, cry or breathe or until the child or infant becomes unconscious. If a child or infant becomes unconscious before the airway obstruction is cleared, follow the same general steps as you would for an adult.

For an *unconscious* child or infant, if the ventilation does not make the chest clearly rise, retilt the head, and then try another ventilation. If the ventilation still does not make the chest clearly rise, position yourself to give chest compressions as you would when performing CPR chest compressions. Compress the child's or infant's chest then check the mouth for an object and, if one is seen, remove it with a gloved finger **(Fig. 11-10, A–C)**.

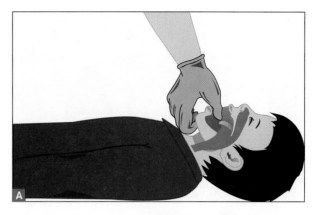
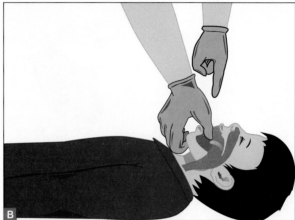
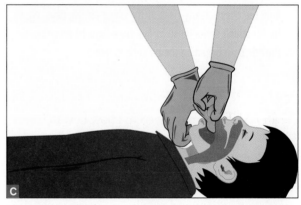

Fig. 11-10, A–C: A finger sweep in a child is similar to that of an adult.

For a smaller child or infant, you should use your little finger to remove the object. Reattempt two ventilations **(Fig. 11-11, A–C)**.

For an *unconscious* child or infant, repeat cycles of chest compressions, foreign object check/removal and ventilations

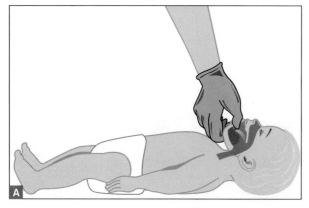

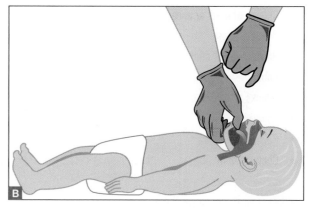

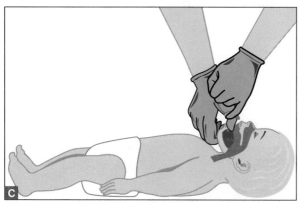

Fig. 11-11, A–C: A finger sweep in an infant is similar to that of an adult or child. However, for an infant it should always be performed using the small finger.

until the chest clearly rises. If the chest clearly rises, check for breathing and a pulse for no more than 10 seconds. Provide care based on the conditions found.

PUTTING IT ALL TOGETHER

As an EMR, you may need to know how to insert OPAs, oral airways, use a suctioning device and care for a conscious or an unconscious patient who is choking. Breathing devices and airway adjuncts allow the EMR to help maintain an open airway, ventilate a patient and supply emergency oxygen.

OPAs can help maintain an open airway by keeping the tongue away from the back of the throat. An OPA can be used on an unconscious patient who does *not* have a gag reflex and requires an airway adjunct. Suction equipment helps clear the upper airway of substances, such as fluids, blood, saliva or vomit. You should also know the difference between a mechanical and anatomical obstruction and the actions required to assist a patient who is choking as a result.

Special considerations must be given when caring for a child or an infant, including the size of equipment used. Remember that a child's and an infant's chest does not need to be compressed as deeply as an adult's chest. The situation also may require the use of the little finger when sweeping the mouth.

YOU ARE THE EMERGENCY MEDICAL RESPONDER

You reposition the patient's airway and attempt 2 ventilations, but the chest still does not rise. How would you respond? After a few minutes of care, the patient's chest begins to rise and fall with the ventilations, but he is not breathing on his own. How would you continue to provide care for this patient?

SKILLsheet

Using a Mechanical Suctioning Device

NOTE: Size-up the scene for safety, follow standard precautions. If needed, assemble the device according to manufacturer's instructions.

STEP 1

Position the patient.
◆ Roll the body as a unit onto one side.
◆ Open the mouth.

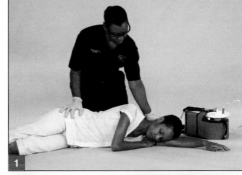

STEP 2

Remove any visible large debris from the mouth with a gloved finger.

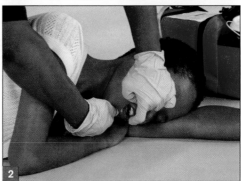

STEP 3

Measure and check the suction tip.
◆ Measure from the patient's earlobe to the corner of the mouth.
◆ Note the distance to prevent inserting the suction tip too deeply.

Continued on next page

Using a Mechanical Suctioning Device *continued*

STEP 4

Turn on the machine and check that the suction is working according to the manufacturer's instructions.

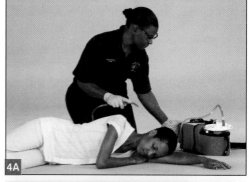

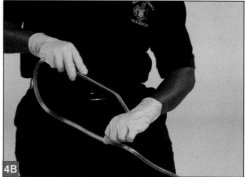

STEP 5

Suction the mouth.

◆ Insert the suction tip into the back of the mouth.
◆ Apply suction as you withdraw the tip using a sweeping motion, if possible.
◆ Suction for *no more than* **15** *seconds at a time for an adult*, **10** *seconds for a child* and **5** *seconds for an infant*.

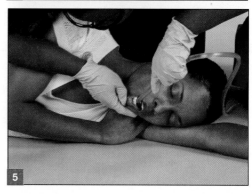

SKILLsheet

Using a Manual Suctioning Device

NOTE: Size-up the scene for safety, follow standard precautions. If needed, assemble the device according to manufacturer's instructions.

STEP 1

Position the patient.
- ◆ Roll the body as a unit onto one side.
- ◆ Open the mouth.

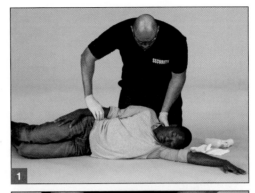

STEP 2

Remove any visible large debris from the mouth with a gloved finger.

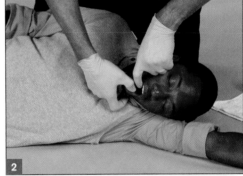

STEP 3

Measure and check the suction tip.
- ◆ Measure from the patient's earlobe to the corner of the mouth.
- ◆ Note the distance to prevent inserting the suction tip too deeply.
- ◆ Check that the suction is working by placing your finger over the end of the suction tip as you squeeze the handle of the device.

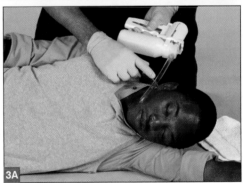

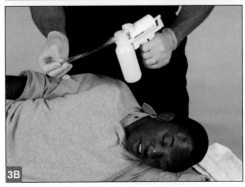

Continued on next page

Using a Manual Suctioning Device *continued*

STEP 4

Suction the mouth.

◆ Insert the suction tip into the back of the mouth.

◆ Squeeze the handle of the suction device repeatedly to provide suction.

◆ Apply suction as you withdraw the tip using a sweeping motion, if possible.

◆ Suction for *no more than* **15** *seconds at a time for an adult,* **10** *seconds for a child and* **5** *seconds for an infant.*

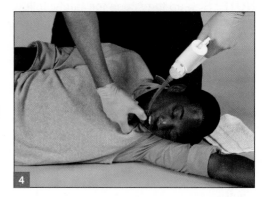

SKILLsheet

Inserting an Oral Airway

NOTE: Size-up the scene for safety, follow standard precautions and then perform a primary assessment. Before inserting an oral airway (OPA), be sure the patient is unresponsive, has no oral trauma such as broken teeth, and has not had recent oral surgery. If the patient gags, remove the airway immediately.

STEP 1

Select the proper size.
- Measure the OPA from the patient's earlobe to the corner of the mouth.

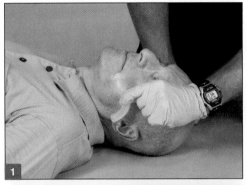

STEP 2

Open the patient's mouth.
- Use the cross-finger technique to open the patient's mouth.

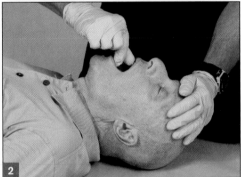

STEP 3

Insert the OPA.

NOTE: When inserting an OPA in a child or an infant, the OPA is inserted using a tongue blade or a tongue depressor, then inserted with the tip of the device pointing toward the back of the tongue and throat in the position it will rest in after insertion.

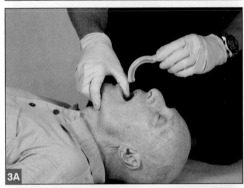

- To insert the OPA, grasp the patient's lower jaw and tongue and lift upward.
- Insert the OPA with the curved end along the roof of the mouth.

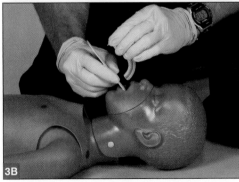

Continued on next page

Inserting an Oral Airway *continued*

◆ As the tip approaches the back of the mouth, rotate it one-half turn (**180** degrees).
◆ Slide the OPA into the back of the throat.

NOTE: The alternative procedure for a child or an infant is to insert the OPA sideways and then rotate it **90** degrees.

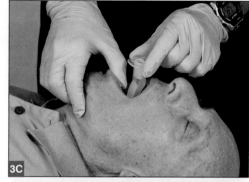

STEP 4

Ensure correct placement.
◆ The flange should rest on the patient's lips.
◆ If the patient begins to gag, *immediately* remove the OPA.
◆ If the patient vomits, remove and suction the airway, ensuring all debris is removed from the airway. Thoroughly clean the device and reinsert into the airway *only* if the patient is still unconscious and does *not* have a gag reflex.

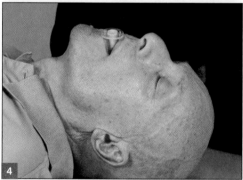

SKILLsheet

Conscious Choking—Adult and Child

NOTE: Obtain consent from a choking adult. If a child is choking, obtain consent from the parent or guardian if present. Tell the child's parent or guardian your level of training and the care you are going to provide. If the parent or guardian is not available, consent is implied.

STEP 1

Ask the patient "Are you choking?"
◆ Identify yourself and ask if you can help.
◆ If the patient is coughing forcefully, encourage continued coughing.

STEP 2

If the patient cannot cough, speak or breathe, have someone else summon more advanced medical personnel.

STEP 3

Bend the patient forward and give **5** back blows with the heel of your hand.
◆ Position yourself slightly behind the patient.
◆ Provide support by placing one arm diagonally across the chest and bend the patient forward. The patient's upper airway should be at least parallel to the ground.
◆ Firmly strike the patient between the shoulder blades with the heel of your hand.
◆ Each blow is a distinct attempt to dislodge the object.

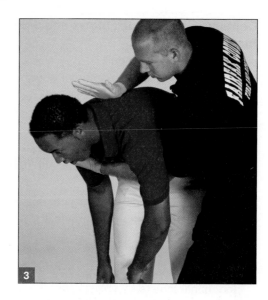

Continued on next page

Conscious Choking—Adult and Child *continued*

STEP 4

Give **5** abdominal thrusts.

◆ Stand behind the patient.
  • For a child, stand or kneel behind the child, depending on the child's size. Use *less force* on a child than you would on an adult.
◆ Use one or two fingers of one hand to find the navel.
◆ Make a fist with your other hand and place the thumb side of your fist against the middle of the patient's abdomen, just above the navel.
◆ Grab the fist with your other hand.
◆ Give quick, upward thrusts. Each thrust should be a distinct attempt to dislodge the object.

Continue giving 5 back blows and 5 abdominal thrusts until–

◆ The object is forced out.
◆ The patient begins to breathe or cough forcefully on his or her own.
◆ The patient becomes unconscious.

If the patient becomes unconscious–

◆ Provide care for an unconscious choking patient.

NOTE: Some conscious choking patients may need chest thrusts instead of abdominal thrusts.

Use chest thrusts if–

◆ You cannot reach far enough around the patient to give abdominal thrusts.
◆ The patient is obviously pregnant or known to be pregnant.

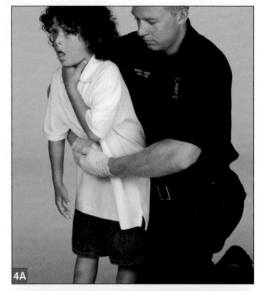

4A

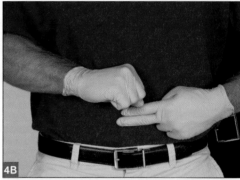

4B

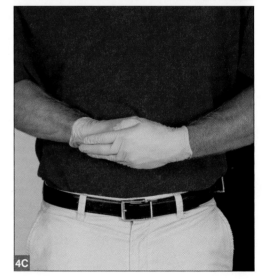

4C

SKILLsheet

Conscious Choking—Infant

NOTE: If an infant is choking, obtain consent from the parent or guardian if present. Tell the infant's parent or guardian your level of training and the care you are going to provide. If the parent or guardian is not available, consent is implied.

STEP 1

If the infant cannot cough, cry or breathe, carefully position the infant face-down along your forearm.
◆ Support the infant's head and neck with your hand.
◆ Lower the infant onto your thigh, keeping the infant's head lower than his or her chest.

STEP 2

Give **5** back blows.
◆ Use the heel of your hand.
◆ Give back blows between the infant's shoulder blades.
◆ Each back blow should be a distinct attempt to dislodge the object.

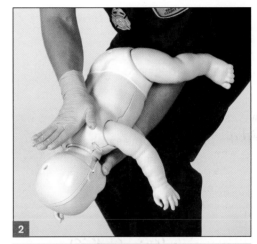

STEP 3

Position the infant face-up along your forearm.
◆ Position the infant between both of your forearms, supporting the infant's head and neck.
◆ Turn the infant face-up.
◆ Lower the infant onto your thigh with the infant's head lower than his or her chest.

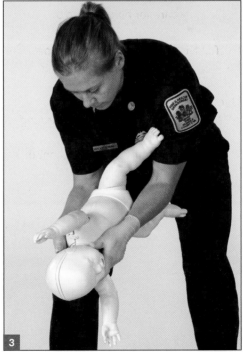

Continued on next page

Conscious Choking—Infant *continued*

STEP 4

Give **5** chest thrusts.
◆ Put two or three fingers on the center of the chest just below the nipple line.
◆ Compress the chest **5** times about **1½** inches.
◆ Each chest thrust should be a distinct attempt to dislodge the object.

Continue giving 5 back blows and 5 chest thrusts until–
◆ The object is forced out.
◆ The infant begins to cough or breathe on his or her own.
◆ The infant becomes unconscious.

If the infant becomes unconscious–
◆ Provide care for an unconscious choking infant.

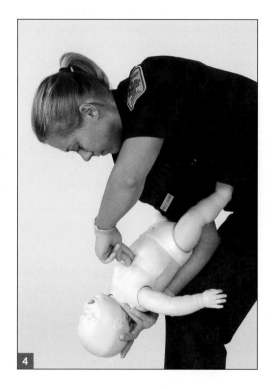

SKILLsheet

Unconscious Choking—Adult and Child

NOTE: Always follow standard precautions when providing care. Size-up the scene for safety and then perform a primary assessment.

NOTE: Ensure patient is on a firm, flat surface.

STEP 1
If at any time a ventilation does not make the chest clearly rise, retilt the head, and then give another ventilation.

STEP 2
If ventilation attempts still do not make the chest clearly rise, give **30** chest compressions.
◆ Place the heel of one hand on the center of the chest.
◆ Place the other hand on top of the first hand and compress the chest **30** times.
◆ For an adult, compress the chest at least **2** inches.
◆ For a child, compress the chest about **2** inches.
◆ Each chest compression should be a distinct attempt to dislodge the object.
◆ Compress at a rate of at least **100** compressions per minute.

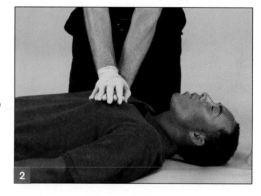

NOTES:
◆ *Keep your fingers off the chest when giving chest compressions.*
◆ *Use your body weight, not your arms, to compress the chest.*
◆ *Position your shoulders over your hands with your arms as straight as possible.*

STEP 3
Look inside the patient's mouth.
◆ Grasp the tongue and lower jaw between your thumb and fingers and lift the jaw.

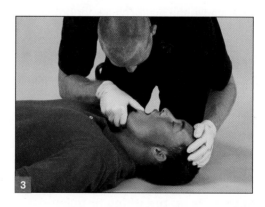

Continued on next page

Unconscious Choking—Adult and Child *continued*

STEP 4

If you see the object, take it out.

◆ Remove the object with your finger by sliding the finger along the inside of the cheek, using a hooking motion to sweep the object out.

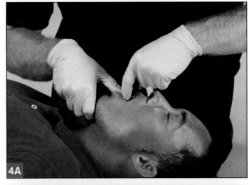

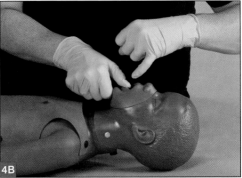

STEP 5

Replace the resuscitation mask and give **2** ventilations.

If the ventilations still do not make the chest clearly rise–

◆ Repeat Steps 2–5.

If the ventilations make the chest clearly rise–

◆ Remove the mask, check for breathing and a pulse for *no more than **10** seconds*.

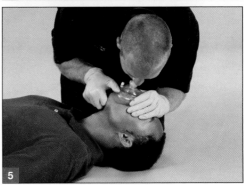

If there is breathing and a pulse–

◆ Leave the patient face-up and continue to monitor the patient's condition.
◆ Administer emergency oxygen, if available and you are trained to do so.

If there is a pulse, but *no* breathing–

◆ Give ventilations.

If there is *no* breathing or pulse–

◆ Perform CPR.

SKILLsheet

Unconscious Choking–Infant

NOTE: Always follow standard precautions when providing care. Size-up the scene for safety and then perform a primary assessment.

NOTE: Ensure infant is on a firm, flat surface.

STEP 1

If at any time a ventilation does not make the chest clearly rise, retilt the head, and then give another ventilation.

STEP 2

If ventilation attempts still do not make the chest clearly rise, remove the resuscitation mask and give **30** chest compressions.

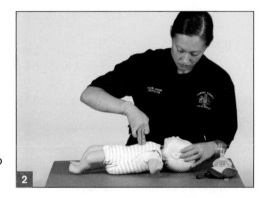

- ◆ Keep one hand on the infant's forehead to maintain an open airway.
- ◆ Put two or three fingers on the center of the chest just below the nipple line.
- ◆ Compress the chest about **1½** inches.
- ◆ Each chest compression should be a distinct attempt to dislodge the object.
- ◆ Compress at a rate of at least **100** compressions per minute.

STEP 3

Look for an object.

- ◆ Grasp the tongue and lower jaw between your thumb and fingers and lift the jaw.

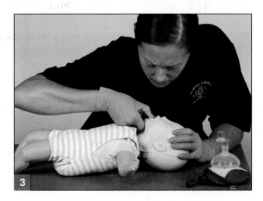

Continued on next page

Unconscious Choking–Infant *continued*

STEP 4

If you see the object, take it out.
- ◆ If you see an object, remove it with your little finger by sliding it along the inside of the cheek, using a hooking motion to sweep the object out.

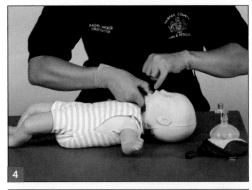

STEP 5

Replace the resuscitation mask and give **2** ventilations.

If the ventilations still do not make the chest clearly rise–
- ◆ Repeat Steps 2–5.

If the ventilations make the chest clearly rise–
- ◆ Check for breathing and a pulse for *no more than **10** seconds*.

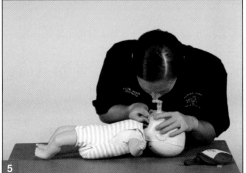

If there is breathing and a pulse–
- ◆ Maintain an open airway and continue to monitor the infant's condition.
- ◆ Administer emergency oxygen, if available and you are trained to do so.

If there is a pulse, but *no* breathing–
- ◆ Give ventilations.

If there is *no* breathing or a pulse–
- ◆ Perform CPR.

Enrichment
Nasopharyngeal Airway

When properly positioned, the **nasal (nasopharyngeal) airway** (NPA) keeps the tongue out of the back of the throat, thereby keeping the airway open. An NPA may be used on a conscious, responsive patient *or* an unconscious patient. Unlike an oral airway, the NPA does not cause the patient to gag. NPAs *must not be used* on a patient with suspected head trauma or a suspected skull fracture.

When using an NPA, select the proper size. Measure the device on the patient to see that it extends from the earlobe to the tip of the nose. Also, make sure the diameter of the NPA is not larger than the diameter of the nostril. To insert the NPA, lubricate the airway with a water-soluble lubricant. Insert the NPA into a nostril, with the bevel *toward* the septum (the wall of tissue that separates the nostrils). Advance the NPA gently, straight in, not upward, until the flange rests on the nose. If you feel even minor resistance, do not force the NPA. If you cannot get the NPA to pass easily, remove it and try the other nostril.

SKILLsheet

Inserting a Nasal Airway

NOTE: Size-up the scene for safety, follow standard precautions and then perform a primary assessment. NPAs must not be used on a patient with suspected head trauma or a suspected skull fracture.

STEP 1

Select the proper size.
- ◆ Measure the NPA from the patient's earlobe to the tip of the nostril. Ensure that the diameter of the NPA is not larger than the nostril.

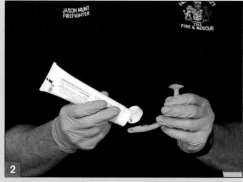

STEP 2

Lubricate the NPA.
- ◆ Use a water-soluble lubricant to lubricate the NPA prior to insertion.

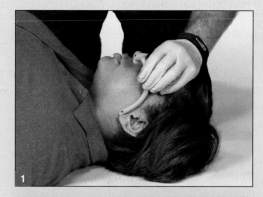

Continued on next page

Inserting a Nasal Airway *continued*

STEP 3

Insert the NPA.
◆ Insert the NPA into the nostril, with the bevel toward the septum (center of the nose).
◆ Advance the NPA gently, straight in, following the floor of the nose.
◆ If resistance is felt, do *not* force.
◆ If you are experiencing problems, try the other nostril.

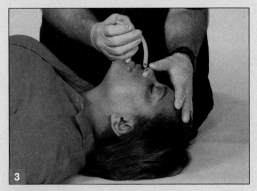

STEP 4

Ensure correct placement.
◆ The flange should rest on the nostril.

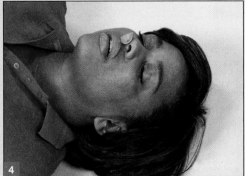

12 Emergency Oxygen

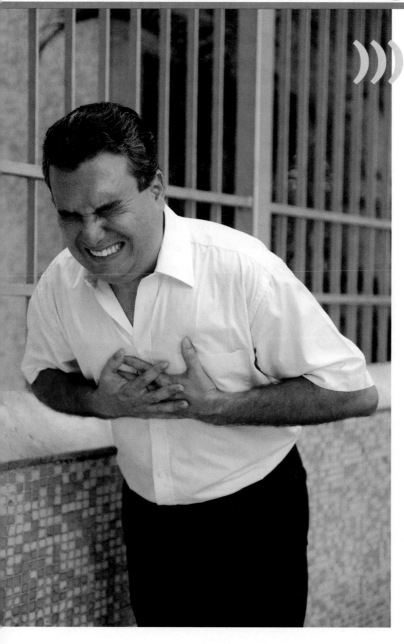

))) **YOU ARE THE EMERGENCY MEDICAL RESPONDER**

A 45-year-old man is experiencing chest pain. When he finally calls for assistance, he states that the pain started about 30 minutes ago as a mild, squeezing sensation. Now the pain is severe and he is gasping for breath. You, as the responding member of your company's emergency response team, recognize that these signs and symptoms suggest a serious cardiac condition. You complete a primary assessment, physical exam and SAMPLE history. The patient has no known history of hypertension or heart disease. While waiting for an ambulance or other transport vehicle to arrive, you help the patient get into the most comfortable position for breathing, keep him from getting chilled or overheated and ask him to remain still. You open a nearby window to circulate fresh air into the stuffy room. What else can you do to help?

Key Terms

Emergency oxygen: Oxygen delivered to a patient from an oxygen cylinder through a delivery device; can be given to a nonbreathing or breathing patient who is not receiving adequate oxygen from the environment.

Flowmeter: A device used to regulate, in *liters per minute* (LPM), the amount of oxygen administered to a patient.

Hyperoxia: A condition in which an excess of oxygen reaches the body's cells.

Hypoxia: A condition in which insufficient oxygen reaches the body's cells.

Nasal cannula: A device used to administer emergency oxygen through the nostrils to a breathing person.

Non-rebreather mask: A type of oxygen mask used to administer high concentrations of oxygen to a breathing person.

"O-ring" gasket: Plastic, O-shaped ring that makes the seal of the pressure regulator on an oxygen cylinder tight; can be a built-in or an attachable piece.

Oxygen cylinder: A steel or alloy cylinder that contains 100 percent oxygen under high pressure.

Pressure regulator: A device on an oxygen cylinder that reduces the delivery pressure of the oxygen to a safe level.

Learning Objectives

After reading this chapter, and completing the class activities, you will have the information needed to—

- Identify when it is appropriate to administer emergency oxygen.
- List the delivery devices for use in administering emergency oxygen.
- Describe the steps required to administer emergency oxygen.
- List precautions to take when using emergency oxygen.

Skill Objectives

After reading this chapter, and completing the class activities, you should be able to—

- Demonstrate how to prepare the equipment and administer emergency oxygen to breathing and nonbreathing patients using a nasal cannula, non-rebreather mask, resuscitation mask and *bag-valve-mask resuscitator* (BVM).

INTRODUCTION

When someone has a breathing or cardiac emergency, supplying **emergency oxygen** can be critical. During such an emergency, the amount of oxygen carried by the blood cells to the brain, heart and body is reduced, resulting in **hypoxia**. If breathing stops (respiratory arrest), the brain and heart will soon be starved of oxygen, resulting in cardiac arrest and ultimately death if not managed quickly and appropriately.

The air you normally breathe contains about 21 percent oxygen. When you provide ventilations using a *bag-valve-mask resuscitator* (BVM), you deliver that 21 percent oxygen to the patient. The expired air in your exhaled breath, however, contains about 16 percent oxygen, and this is the concentration delivered when using a resuscitation mask. Neither of these percentages of oxygen alone may be adequate for the patient. By administering emergency oxygen, you can deliver a higher percentage of oxygen that an injured or ill person may need.

Emergency oxygen can be given for many breathing and cardiac emergencies. Emergency oxygen can be given to nonbreathing patients, sometimes in conjunction with an airway adjunct. If a patient is breathing but has no obvious signs or symptoms of injury or illness, emergency oxygen should be considered for—

- An adult breathing fewer than 12 breaths or more than 20 breaths per minute.
- A child breathing fewer than 15 breaths or more than 30 breaths per minute.
- An infant breathing fewer than 25 breaths or more than 50 breaths per minute.

Administer emergency oxygen to all patients with respiratory distress or respiratory failure, as these conditions are usually caused by abnormal oxygen levels to the tissues. In most cases, short-term **hyperoxia** as a result of emergency oxygen intake should not cause problems. In fact, hyperoxia is desirable while caring for patients with carbon monoxide (CO) poisoning. Always administer emergency oxygen for suspected CO poisoning and all smoke-inhalation cases.

Oxygen should be delivered with properly-sized equipment for the patient and appropriate flow rates for the delivery device.

ADMINISTERING EMERGENCY OXYGEN

To deliver emergency oxygen, you must have—
- An **oxygen cylinder**.
- A **pressure regulator** with **flowmeter**.
- A delivery device.

According to the U.S. *Food and Drug Administration* (FDA), emergency oxygen units are available without prescription for first aid use, provided they contain at least a 15-minute supply of oxygen, and that they are designed to deliver a preset flow rate of at least 6 *liters per minute* (LPM). Filling and refilling of empty or spent oxygen cylinders is strictly controlled by state and local regulations. Local protocols must always be followed.

Variable-Flow-Rate Oxygen

Variable-flow-rate oxygen systems allow the rescuer to vary the flow of oxygen. Because of the large amount of oxygen *emergency medical services* (EMS) systems deliver and the variety of equipment and emergency situations they respond to, variable-flow-rate oxygen is practical. To deliver emergency oxygen using a variable-flow-rate system, you must assemble the equipment.

Fixed-Flow-Rate Oxygen

Some emergency oxygen systems have the regulator set at a fixed-flow rate. Most fixed-flow-rate tanks are set at 15 LPM; however, an *emergency medical responder* (EMR) may come across tanks set at 6 LPM, 12 LPM or another rate. In some cases, the fixed-flow-rate systems may have a dual (high/low) flow setting. Fixed-flow-rate oxygen systems typically come with the delivery device,

---

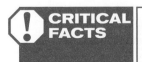
CRITICAL FACTS Emergency oxygen may be needed for nonbreathing patients in many breathing and cardiac emergencies. The use of oxygen in breathing adults, children and infants depends on the number of breaths per minute.

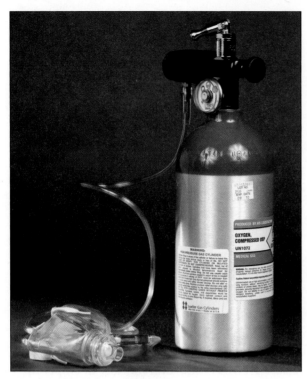
Fig. 12-1: A fixed-flow-rate oxygen system

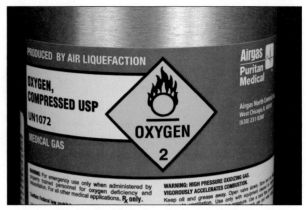
Fig. 12-2: Oxygen cylinders are marked with a yellow diamond that says "Oxygen" and, in the United States, typically have green markings.

regulator and cylinder already connected to each other (**Fig. 12-1**). This eliminates the need to assemble the equipment, which makes it quick and very simple to deliver emergency oxygen. A drawback to using fixed-flow-rate oxygen systems is that you cannot adjust the flow rate to different levels. This limits both the type of delivery device you can use and the concentration of oxygen you can deliver. For example, a fixed-flow-rate unit with a preset flow of 6 LPM can only be used with a **nasal cannula** or resuscitation mask, while a preset flow rate of 12 LPM only allows the use of a resuscitation mask or **non-rebreather mask.**

Because of the simplicity of the preconnected fixed-flow-rate systems and the lifesaving benefits of oxygen, these systems are becoming increasingly popular in the workplace, schools and other places where EMRs may have to respond to on-site emergencies.

Oxygen Cylinders

Oxygen cylinders are made to be easily recognizable. These cylinders, made of steel or alloy, can hold between 350 and 625 liters

of oxygen, and have internal pressures of approximately 2000 *pounds per square inch* (psi). Oxygen cylinders are labeled "U.S.P." and are marked with a yellow diamond that says "Oxygen" (**Fig. 12-2**). The U.S.P. stands for *United States Pharmacopeia*, which indicates the oxygen is medical grade. In the United States, oxygen cylinders typically have green markings, such as a green top; however, the color scheme is not regulated. Different manufacturers and other countries may use different color markings. Oxygen cylinders are under high pressure and must be handled carefully; **do not drop**. Ensure oxygen cylinders have proper hydrostatic testing and are marked appropriately.

Pressure Regulator and Flowmeter

The pressure inside an oxygen cylinder is far too great to allow you to open the cylinder and

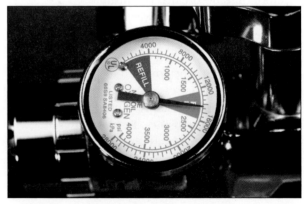
Fig. 12-3: A pressure regulator is attached to an oxygen cylinder to reduce the pressure of oxygen to a safe level.

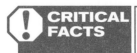
CRITICAL FACTS Oxygen cylinders have U.S.P. and yellow diamond labels that make them easy to recognize. In the United States, oxygen cylinders typically have green markings.

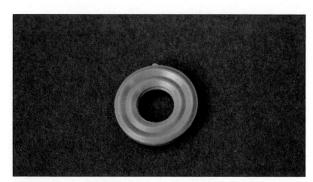

Fig. 12-4: An O-ring gasket

administer the oxygen. Therefore, a device called a pressure regulator is attached to the cylinder to reduce the delivery pressure of the oxygen to a safe level (**Fig. 12-3**). The pressure regulator reduces the pressure from approximately 2000 psi inside the cylinder to a safe pressure range of 30 to 70 psi. The amount of pressure inside the cylinder is indicated on a gauge. By checking the gauge, you can determine how full a cylinder is. A full cylinder will show 2000 psi, while a nearly empty cylinder will show about 200 psi. Always monitor the pressure in the oxygen cylinder to make sure it is above 200 psi. When the cylinder reaches 200 psi, replace the oxygen cylinder with a new tank.

A pressure regulator typically has two metal prongs that fit into the valve at the top of the oxygen cylinder. This is called the *pin index safety system*. It is standard on any type of tank that has these pins; a different pin placement depending on the type of tank prevents unintentional use. To ensure a tight seal between the regulator and the tank, a gasket, commonly called an **"O-ring" gasket**, must be used (**Fig. 12-4**). Never lubricate any part of an oxygen system.

A flowmeter controls the amount of oxygen administered in LPM, with a normal delivery rate from 1–25 LPM.

Oxygen Delivery Devices

An oxygen delivery device is the piece of equipment a patient breathes through when receiving emergency oxygen. Tubing carries the oxygen from the regulator to the delivery device. When delivering emergency oxygen, make sure the tubing does not get tangled or kinked so as to stop the flow of oxygen to the mask. These devices can include nasal cannulas, non-rebreather masks, BVMs and resuscitation masks. Various sizes of these devices are available for adults, children and infants. Appropriate sizing is important to ensure adequate airway management.

Nasal Cannula

The nasal cannula is used *only* on breathing patients and delivers oxygen through the patient's nostrils (**Fig. 12-5**). A plastic tube is held in place over the patient's ears, and oxygen is delivered through two small prongs inserted into the nostrils. Nasal cannula use is limited, as it normally delivers oxygen at a flow rate of 1-6 LPM, which provides a peak oxygen concentration of approximately 44 percent. Flow rates above 6 LPM are not commonly used because of the tendency to quickly dry out mucous membranes and cause nosebleeds and headaches.

Because of these limitations, the nasal cannula is commonly used for patients with only minor breathing difficulty or for those who have a history of respiratory medical conditions. Patients

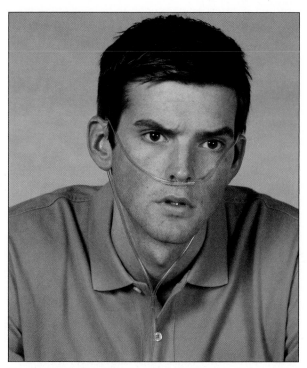

Fig. 12-5: A nasal cannula

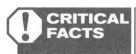

Oxygen devices, such as nasal cannulas, non-rebreather masks, BVMs and resuscitation masks, allow the patient to effectively receive emergency oxygen.

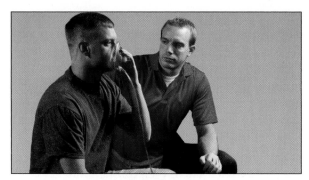

Fig. 12-6: A resuscitation mask with oxygen inlet

experiencing a serious breathing emergency generally breathe through the mouth and need a device that can supply a greater concentration of oxygen. The nasal cannula can be ineffective for patients who have a nasal airway obstruction, nasal injury or a bad cold causing blocked sinus passages. It is useful for patients who cannot tolerate a mask over their face.

Resuscitation Mask with Oxygen Inlet

The resuscitation mask with oxygen inlet can be used with emergency oxygen to deliver oxygen to a nonbreathing patient. It also can be used to deliver emergency oxygen to someone who is breathing but still requires oxygen. Some resuscitation masks come with elastic straps to place over the patient's head to keep the mask in place (**Fig. 12-6**). If the mask does not have a strap, you or the patient can hold it in place.

With a resuscitation mask, set the oxygen flow rate at 6–15 LPM. A resuscitation mask can deliver up to 55 percent oxygen to a breathing person, when delivered at 6 LPM or more. When used on a nonbreathing patient while you perform ventilations, it will deliver an oxygen concentration of approximately 35 percent. The oxygen concentration is reduced because oxygen mixes with your exhaled breath as you perform mouth-to-mask ventilations.

Non-Rebreather Mask

A non-rebreather mask is used to deliver high concentrations of oxygen to breathing patients (**Fig. 12-7, A-B**). It consists of a face mask with an attached oxygen reservoir bag and a one-way valve between the mask and bag to prevent the patient's exhaled air from mixing with the oxygen in the reservoir bag. The patient inhales oxygen

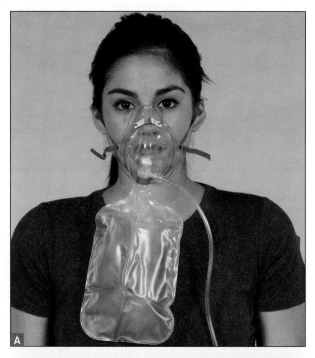

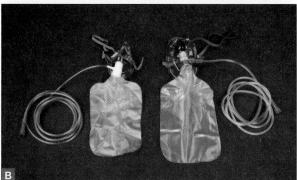

Fig. 12-7, A–B: A non-rebreather mask

from the bag and exhaled air escapes through flutter valves on the side of the mask. To inflate the reservoir bag, cover the one-way valve with your thumb before placing it on the patient's face. The oxygen reservoir bag should be sufficiently inflated (about two-thirds full) so as not to deflate when the patient inhales. If this happens, increase the flow rate of the oxygen to refill the reservoir bag. The flow rate should be set at 10–15 LPM. When using a non-rebreather mask with a high flow rate of oxygen, up to 90 percent or more oxygen concentration can be delivered to the patient.

BVM

A BVM can be used on a breathing or nonbreathing patient. With a BVM, the oxygen flow rate should be set at 15 LPM or more. The BVM with an oxygen reservoir bag is

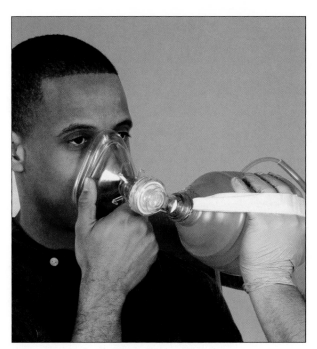

Fig. 12-8: A bag valve mask

capable of supplying 90 percent or more oxygen concentration when used at 15 LPM or more (**Fig. 12-8**). The conscious patient can hold the BVM to inhale the oxygen or you can squeeze the bag as the patient inhales to deliver more oxygen. Squeeze the bag between each breath for patients breathing less than 10 times per minute. To assist a person breathing more than 30 times per minute, squeeze the bag on every second breath.

Assembly for a Variable-Flow-Rate System

Begin by examining the cylinder to be certain that it is labeled "Oxygen." The cylinders come

with a protective covering over the tank opening. Remove this covering. If it is not built into the tank, remove the O-ring gasket. While pointing the cylinder away from you, open the cylinder for 1 second. This will remove any dirt or debris from the cylinder valve. If necessary, reposition the O-ring gasket.

Next, examine the pressure regulator to be sure it is labeled "Oxygen." Check to see that the pin index corresponds to an oxygen tank. Attach the pressure regulator to the cylinder, seating the prongs inside the holes in the valve. Hand-tighten the screw until the regulator is snug. Open the cylinder one-full turn and listen for leaks.

Check the pressure gauge to determine how much pressure is in the cylinder. A full cylinder should have approximately 2000 psi. Attach the chosen delivery device to the oxygen port near the flowmeter, using the appropriate tubing.

Oxygen Administration

To administer emergency oxygen using a variable-flow-rate system, follow the steps described earlier, then turn on the flowmeter and adjust it to the desired flow rate. Listen and feel to make sure that oxygen is flowing into your delivery device. If you are using a non-rebreather mask, ensure that the reservoir bag is two-thirds full before placing the device on the patient. Finally, place the delivery device on the patient.

If young children and infants are frightened by a mask being placed on their face, use a "blow-by" technique. To perform this technique, you, a parent or guardian holds the mask about 2 inches from the child's or infant's face waving it slowly from side-to-side as if you are playing a game,

Table 12-1:

Oxygen Delivery Devices

DELIVERY DEVICE	COMMON FLOW RATE	OXYGEN CONCENTRATIONS	FUNCTION
Nasal Cannula	1–6 LPM	24 to 44 percent	Breathing patients only
Resuscitation Mask	6–15 LPM	25 to 55 percent	Breathing and nonbreathing patients
Non-rebreather Mask	10–15 LPM	up to 90 percent	Breathing patients only
BVM	15+ LPM	90+ percent	Breathing and nonbreathing patients

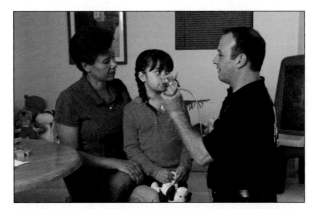

Fig. 12-9: Use the blow-by technique for children and infants who are frightened by having oxygen masks on their faces.

thus allowing the oxygen to pass over the face and be inhaled (**Fig. 12-9**).

You should monitor the effectiveness of the oxygen delivery; a pulse oximeter can be used to do so.

Assembly and Administration for a Fixed-Flow-Rate System

To operate a fixed-flow-rate system, simply turn it on according to the manufacturer's instructions, check that oxygen is flowing and place the delivery device on the patient. You can also use the "blow-by" technique using a fixed-flow-rate system by following the same procedure outlined above.

Securing and Handling Cylinders

Never attempt to refill an oxygen cylinder; only an appropriately licensed professional should do this. When high-pressure oxygen cylinders have been emptied, close the cylinder valve, replace the valve protection cap or outlet plug where provided and mark or tag the cylinder as EMPTY. Then return the cylinder promptly, to be refilled according to state and local regulations.

Specific attention should be given to the following areas concerning oxygen cylinders:

- Check for cylinder leaks, abnormal bulging, defective or inoperative valves or safety devices.
- Check for the physical presence of rust or corrosion on a cylinder or cylinder neck (**Fig. 12-10, A**).

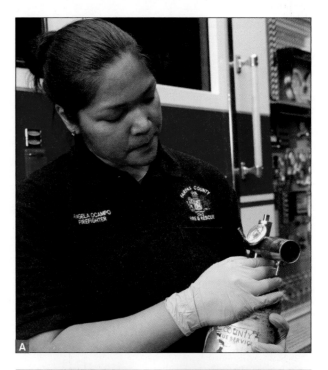

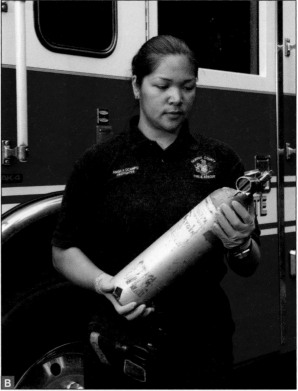

Fig. 12-10, A–B: Because they are highly pressurized, special care should be taken when handling oxygen cylinders. Be sure to (A) check for defects before use and (B) carry them appropriately by the body of the cylinder, not the valve.

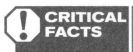 **CRITICAL FACTS** Use emergency oxygen equipment according to the manufacturer's instructions and in a manner consistent with federal and local regulations.

- Any foreign substances or residues, such as adhesive tape around the cylinder neck, oxygen valve or regulator assembly, can hamper oxygen delivery and in some cases may have the potential to cause a fire or explosion.
- Ensure that all oxygen cylinders have proper hydrostatic testing and are marked appropriately.
- Be aware of the specific testing requirements of steel and aluminum tanks (e.g., 10 years initial testing for steel cylinders and 5 years for aluminum cylinders).

- Do not deface, alter or remove any labeling or markings on the oxygen cylinder.
- Do not attempt to mix gases in an oxygen cylinder or transfer oxygen from one cylinder to another.

If defibrillating using an *automated external defibrillator* (AED), make sure that no one is touching or is in contact with the patient or the resuscitation equipment. Do not defibrillate someone when around flammable materials, such as free-flowing oxygen or gasoline.

SAFETY PRECAUTIONS

When preparing and administering emergency oxygen, safety is a major concern. Use emergency oxygen equipment according to the manufacturer's instructions and in a manner consistent with federal and local regulations.

Also, follow these recommended guidelines:
- Be sure that oxygen is flowing before putting the delivery device over the patient's face.
- Do not use oxygen around flames or sparks including smoking materials, such as cigarettes, cigars and pipes. Oxygen causes fire to burn more rapidly and intensely.
- Do not use grease, oil or petroleum products to lubricate or clean the regulator. This could cause an explosion.
- Do not stand oxygen cylinders upright unless they are well secured. If a cylinder falls, the regulator or valve could become damaged or cause injury due to the intense pressure in the tank.
- Do not drag or roll cylinders.
- Do not carry a cylinder by the valve or regulator (**Fig. 12-10, B**).
- Do not hold on to protective valve caps or guards when moving or lifting cylinders.

PUTTING IT ALL TOGETHER

Administering emergency oxygen to someone experiencing a breathing emergency can help improve hypoxia. It can also help reduce pain and breathing discomfort. When using emergency oxygen, follow safety precautions and use the equipment according to the manufacturer's instructions.

An oxygen delivery device is the piece of equipment a patient breathes through when receiving emergency oxygen. These delivery devices include nasal cannulas, resuscitation masks, non-rebreather masks and BVMs. The resuscitation mask and BVM are the most appropriate devices for EMRs, as they can be used with breathing and nonbreathing patients. These devices can significantly increase the oxygen concentration that an injured or ill person needs, help ventilate a nonbreathing patient and reduce the likelihood of disease transmission.

Be familiar with the unique features and benefits of these devices as well as their appropriate flow rates and situations in which they should be used.

))) YOU ARE THE EMERGENCY MEDICAL RESPONDER

The 45-year-old man who was experiencing chest pain and difficulty breathing is now slightly cyanotic (skin has a bluish color), is gasping for air and is breathing 26 times per minute. What breathing devices could you use to help this patient? After a couple of minutes, the man complains of having a mask on his face but is still gasping for air. How would you change your care for this patient?

SKILLsheet

Oxygen Delivery

STEP 1

Make sure the oxygen cylinder is labeled "U.S.P." (United States Pharmacopeia) and marked with a yellow diamond that says: "Oxygen."

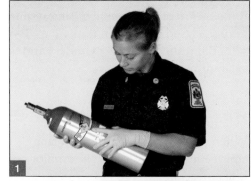

STEP 2

Clear the valve.
- ◆ Remove the protective covering.
- ◆ Remove and save the O-ring gasket, if necessary.
- ◆ Turn the cylinder away from you and others before opening.
- ◆ Open the cylinder valve for **1** second to clear the valve of any debris.

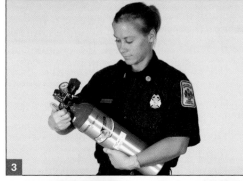

STEP 3

Attach the regulator.
- ◆ Put the O-ring gasket into the valve on top of the cylinder, if necessary.
- ◆ Make sure that it is marked "Oxygen Regulator" and that the O-ring gasket is in place.
- ◆ Check to see that the pin index corresponds to an oxygen tank.
- ◆ Secure the regulator on the cylinder by placing the two metal prongs into the valve.
- ◆ Hand-tighten the screw until the regulator is snug.

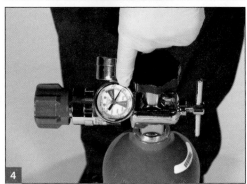

STEP 4

Open the cylinder counterclockwise one full turn.
- ◆ Check the pressure gauge.
- ◆ Determine that the cylinder has enough pressure (more than **200** psi). If the pressure is lower than **200** psi, **DO NOT** use.

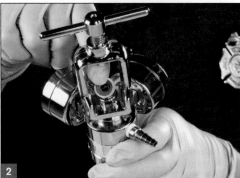

STEP 5

Attach the delivery device.

◆ Attach the plastic tubing between the flowmeter and the delivery device.

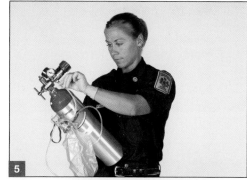

STEP 6

Adjust the flowmeter.

◆ Turn the flowmeter to the desired flow rate.
- With a nasal cannula, set the rate at **1–6** LPM.
- With a resuscitation mask, set the rate at **6–15** LPM.
- With a non-rebreather mask, set the rate at **10–15** LPM.
  - ○ Ensure that the oxygen reservoir bag is two-thirds inflated by placing your thumb over the one-way valve in the bottom of the mask until the bag is sufficiently inflated.
- With a BVM, set the rate at **15** LPM or more.

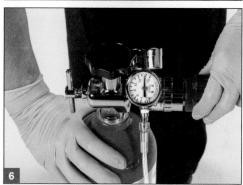

STEP 7

Verify the oxygen flow.

◆ Listen for a hissing sound and feel for oxygen flow through the delivery device.

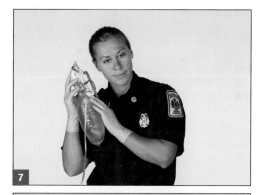

STEP 8

Place the delivery device on the patient and continue care until more advanced medical personnel take over.

STEP 9

Break down the oxygen equipment.

◆ To break down the tank reverse the steps from above, being sure to bleed the pressure regulator by turning on the flowmeter after the tank has been turned off.

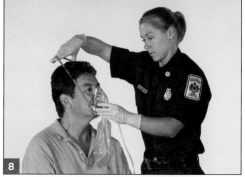

UNIT

4

CIRCULATION

13 Circulation and Cardiac Emergencies

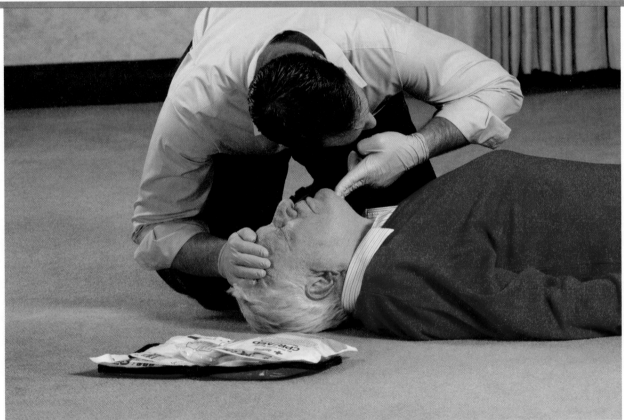

))) YOU ARE THE EMERGENCY MEDICAL RESPONDER

An elderly man suddenly collapses while working in the office. He is lying on the floor and does not appear to be moving. You, as a member of the medical emergency response team (MERT), recognize the emergency, activate the emergency response plan and perform a primary assessment. The emergency medical services (EMS) system has been activated. You determine that the man is unconscious, not breathing and does not have a pulse. The office building has an automated external defibrillator (AED). How would you respond?

Key Terms

Acute coronary syndrome (ACS): Term that describes a range of clinical conditions, including unstable angina, that are due to insufficient blood supply to the heart muscle resulting from *coronary heart disease* (CHD).

Acute myocardial ischemia: An episode of chest pain due to reduced blood flow to the heart muscle.

Angina pectoris: Pain in the chest that comes and goes at different times; caused by a lack of oxygen reaching the heart; can be stable (occurring under exertion or stress) or unstable (occurring at rest, without reason).

Arrhythmia: Disturbance in the regular rhythmic beating of the heart.

Asystole: A condition where the heart has stopped generating electrical activity.

Atherosclerosis: A condition in which deposits of plaque, including cholesterol (a fatty substance made by the liver and found in foods containing animal or animal products) build up on the inner walls of the arteries, causing them to harden and narrow, reducing the amount of blood that can flow through; develops gradually and can go undetected for many years.

Atrial fibrillation: Irregular and fast electrical discharges of the heart that lead to an irregular heartbeat; the most common type of abnormal cardiac rhythm.

Atrioventricular (AV) node: A cluster of cells in the center of the heart, between the atria and ventricles; serves as a relay to slow down the signal received from the *sinoatrial* (SA) node before it passes through to the ventricles.

Automated external defibrillator (AED): A portable electronic device that analyzes the heart's electrical rhythm and, if necessary, can deliver an electrical shock to a person in cardiac arrest.

Cardiac arrest: A condition in which the heart has stopped or beats too irregularly or weakly to pump blood effectively.

Cardiac chain of survival: A set of four critical steps in responding to a cardiac emergency: early recognition and access to the EMS system, early *cardiopulmonary resuscitation* (CPR), early defibrillation and early advanced medical care.

Cardiopulmonary resuscitation (CPR): A technique that combines chest compressions and ventilations to circulate blood containing oxygen to the brain and other vital organs for a person whose heart and breathing have stopped.

Cardiovascular disease: A disease affecting the heart and blood vessels.

Chest compressions: A technique used in CPR, in which external pressure is placed on the chest to increase the level of pressure in the chest cavity and cause the blood to circulate through the arteries.

Cholesterol: A fatty substance made by the liver and found in foods containing animal or animal products; diets high in cholesterol contribute to the risk of heart disease.

Commotio cordis: Sudden cardiac arrest from a blunt, non-penetrating blow to the chest, of which the basis is *ventricular fibrillation* (V-fib) triggered by chest wall impact immediately over the heart.

Congestive heart failure: A chronic condition in which the heart no longer pumps blood effectively throughout the body.

Coronary heart disease (CHD): A disease in which cholesterol and plaque build up on the inner walls of the arteries that supply blood to the heart; also called *coronary artery disease* (CAD).

Defibrillation: An electrical shock that disrupts the electrical activity of the heart long enough to allow the heart to spontaneously develop an effective rhythm on its own.

Electrocardiogram (ECG or EKG): A test that measures and records the electrical activity of the heart.

Heart: A fist-sized muscular organ that pumps blood throughout the body.

Hypertension: Another term for high blood pressure.

Implantable cardioverter-defibrillator (ICD): A miniature version of an AED, implanted under the skin, that acts to automatically recognize and help correct abnormal heart rhythms.

Myocardial infarction (MI): The death of cardiac muscle tissue due to a sudden deprivation of circulating blood; also called a heart attack.

Normal sinus rhythm (NSR): The normal, regular rhythm of the heart, set by the SA node in the right atrium of the heart.

Pacemaker: A device implanted under the skin, sometimes below the right collarbone, to help regulate heartbeat in someone with a weak heart, a heart that skips beats or one that beats too fast or too slow.

Risk factors: Conditions or behaviors that increase the chance that a person will develop a disease.

Silent heart attack: A heart attack during which the patient has either no symptoms or very mild symptoms that the person does not associate with heart attacks; mild symptoms include indigestion or sweating.

Sinoatrial (SA) node: A cluster of cells in the right atrium that generates the electrical impulses that set the pace of the heart's natural rhythm.

Sudden cardiac arrest: A condition where the heart's pumping action stops abruptly, usually due to abnormal heart rhythms called arrhythmias, most commonly V-fib; unless an effective heart rhythm is restored, death follows within a matter of minutes.

Transdermal medication patch: A patch on the skin that delivers medication; commonly contains nitroglycerin, nicotine or other medications; should be removed prior to defibrillation.

Ventricular fibrillation (V-fib): A life-threatening heart rhythm in which the heart is in a state of totally disorganized electrical activity.

Ventricular tachycardia (V-tach): A life-threatening heart rhythm in which there is very rapid contraction of the ventricles.

Learning Objectives

After reading this chapter, and completing the class activities, you will have the information needed to—

- Describe how to recognize and care for a victim who may be experiencing a heart attack.
- Describe how to care for a patient who may be experiencing cardiac arrest.
- List the reasons for the heart to stop beating.
- Describe the skill components of CPR.
- List the steps of one-rescuer CPR for an adult, a child and an infant.
- Explain when it is appropriate to stop performing CPR.
- Describe how to perform two-rescuer CPR for an adult, a child and an infant.

- Define defibrillation and describe how it works.
- Identify the abnormal heart rhythms commonly present during cardiac arrest.
- Describe the role and importance of early defibrillation in cardiac arrest.
- List the general steps for using an *automated external defibrillator* (AED).
- Identify precautions for using an AED.
- Identify special situations that may arise when using an AED.
- Identify controllable risk factors for cardiovascular disease (*Enrichment*).

Skill Objectives

After reading this chapter, and completing the class activities, you should be able to—

- Demonstrate one-rescuer CPR for an adult, a child and an infant.
- Demonstrate two-rescuer CPR for an adult, a child and an infant.

- Demonstrate how to use an AED for adult and pediatric patients in cardiac arrest.

INTRODUCTION

In this chapter, you will learn how to recognize and provide care for a patient who is experiencing signs and symptoms of a heart attack or whose **heart** stops beating. A heart attack occurs when blood vessels supplying the heart become blocked and fail to provide the heart enough blood and oxygen necessary to function properly. The condition in which the heart stops functioning is known as **cardiac arrest**. It can sometimes result from a heart attack but cardiac arrest can also be caused by sudden, irregular electrical activity of the heart. To provide care for a patient in cardiac arrest, you need to know how to perform *cardiopulmonary resuscitation* (**CPR**) and use an *automated external defibrillator* (**AED**). CPR can keep a patient's vital organs supplied with blood containing oxygen until more highly trained personnel arrive to provide advanced care. In many cases, however, CPR by itself cannot correct the underlying problem. An AED can analyze the heart's electrical rhythm and deliver a shock to help the heart to restore an effective rhythm. **Sudden cardiac arrest** can happen to anyone at anytime, and although rare, can occur in children and infants.

As an *emergency medical responder* (EMR), you must assess patients quickly and be prepared to perform quality CPR and use an AED in cases of cardiac arrest. This chapter covers the basic principles of how to recognize cardiac emergencies and provide the appropriate care.

THE CIRCULATORY SYSTEM

Anatomy of the Circulatory System

The heart is a muscular organ, which functions like a pump. About the size of one's fist, it lies between the lungs, in the middle of the chest, behind the lower half of the sternum (breastbone) (**Fig. 13-1**). The heart is protected by the ribs and sternum in front and by the spine in back. It has four chambers and is separated into right and left halves. The right side of the heart has two chambers known as the *right atrium*, which receives oxygen-depleted blood from the veins of the body, and the *right ventricle*, which pumps the oxygen-depleted blood

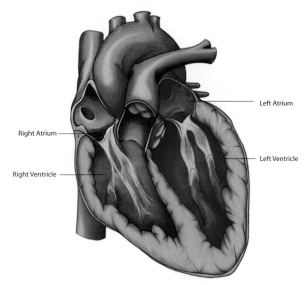

Fig. 13-1: The heart

to the lungs where waste products are removed and oxygen is absorbed.

The now oxygen-rich blood returns to the left side of the heart, where it enters the *left atrium* and goes on to the *left ventricle*, where it is pumped to all parts of the body. One-way valves direct the flow of blood as it moves through each of the heart's four chambers. For the circulatory system to be effective, the respiratory system must also be working so that the blood can pick up oxygen in the lungs.

Physiology of the Circulatory System
The Heart's Electrical System

An electrical system in the heart triggers the contraction or pumping action of the heart muscle. In a healthy heart, an electrical impulse comes from a point near the top of the heart called the

---

How the Heart Functions

Too often we take our hearts for granted. The heart is extremely reliable. The heart beats about 70 times each minute or more than 100,000 times a day. During the average lifetime, the heart will beat nearly 3 billion times. The heart moves about a gallon of blood per minute through the body. This is about 40 million gallons in an average lifetime. The heart moves blood through about 60,000 miles of blood vessels.

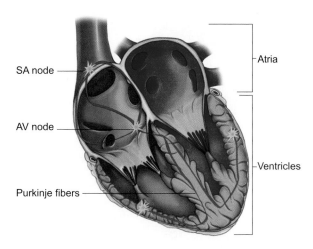

Fig. 13-2: The heart's electrical system

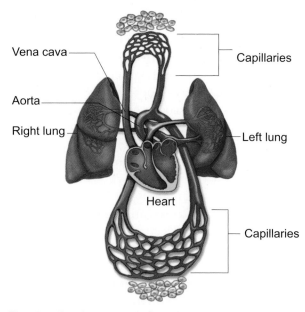

Fig. 13-3: Blood continuously flows through the arteries delivering oxygen and other nutrients to the body's cells. It also flows through the veins, taking away carbon dioxide and other wastes. The process is called perfusion.

sinoatrial (**SA**) **node**. The impulse travels through the atria, the upper chambers of the heart, down to the *atrioventricular* (**AV**) **node**, near the bottom of the right atrium (**Fig. 13-2**).

From the AV node, the impulse divides into two branches, then into the right and left ventricles. These right and left branches become a network of fibers, called *Purkinje fibers*, which spread electrical impulses across the heart. Under normal circumstances, these impulses reach the muscular walls of the ventricles causing the muscles to contract and force blood out of the heart to circulate throughout the body. The contraction of the left ventricle results in a pulse. The pauses between the pulse beats are the periods between contractions. As the left ventricle relaxes, or is at rest, blood refills the chamber and there is a pause between pulse beats.

An *electrocardiogram* (**ECG or EKG**) is a graphic measure of the electrical activity and rhythm of the heart. Electrodes attached to an electrocardiograph pick up electrical impulses and transmit them to a monitor. The peaks and valleys of each wave, the size, shape and frequency, show the heart's rhythm and how the electrical system is functioning. The normal conduction of electrical impulses without any disturbances is known as *normal sinus rhythm* (**NSR**).

Perfusion

As the blood flows through the arteries, oxygen and nutrients such as glucose are delivered to cells throughout the body, and as blood flows through the veins, carbon dioxide and other wastes are taken away. This continuous process is called perfusion (**Fig. 13-3**).

The primary gases exchanged are oxygen and carbon dioxide. All cells require oxygen to function. Cells also require energy to function. Glucose, a simple sugar molecule, is the main source of energy inside the cell.

Pathophysiology of the Circulatory System

Cardiovascular disease is an abnormal condition that affects the heart and blood vessels. An estimated 80 million Americans suffer from some form of the disease. It remains the number-one killer in the United States, and a major cause of disability. The most common conditions caused by cardiovascular disease include ***coronary heart disease*** (**CHD**), also known as *coronary artery disease* (CAD), and stroke, also called a *brain attack*. (See **Chapter 14** for more information on stroke.)

CHD occurs when the arteries that supply blood to the heart muscle become hardened and narrowed, a process called **atherosclerosis**. This damage occurs gradually, as **cholesterol**

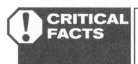 **CRITICAL FACTS** Cardiovascular disease afflicts approximately 80 million Americans and is the number-one killer in the United States. Common conditions caused by this disease include CHD and stroke.

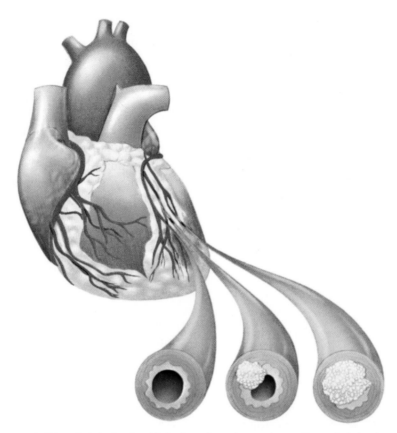

Fig. 13-4: In atherosclerosis, a buildup of cholesterol and fatty deposits on inner artery walls results in hardened, narrowed arteries.

and fatty deposits called *plaque* build up on the inner artery walls. As this buildup worsens, the arteries become narrower, reducing the amount of blood that can flow through them and preventing the heart from getting the blood or oxygen it needs (**Fig. 13-4**).

Patients who suffer from **acute myocardial ischemia** (reduced blood flow to the cardiac muscle) suffer chest pain, which usually results from CHD and is referred to as *acute coronary syndrome* (**ACS**). This reduced blood and oxygen supply to the heart can cause symptoms of **angina pectoris** or a heart attack.

A heart attack, or *myocardial infarction* (**MI**), occurs when coronary blood vessels become blocked by plaque buildup or a blood clot blocks one of the arteries supplying the heart. This may lead to an irregular heartbeat (**arrhythmia**) which then causes the pumping action of the heart to work less efficiently. A heart attack can also lead to a cardiac arrest where the heart ceases to function as a pump. As the reduction of blood flow or blockage progresses, some people experience symptoms such as chest pain, pressure or discomfort, an early warning sign that the heart is not receiving enough oxygen-rich blood. Others may suffer a heart attack or even cardiac arrest without any warning signs or symptoms. If a blockage in a coronary artery of the heart is not treated quickly, the affected heart muscle tissue will die.

Pediatric Considerations

Cardiac Pathophysiology

Heart problems in children and infants are almost always secondary to airway and respiratory problems, but can also be related to congenital heart conditions. When cardiac arrest occurs in children and infants, it is often caused by—
- Airway and breathing problems.
- Traumatic injuries or an accident (e.g., motor-vehicle collision, drowning, electrocution or poisoning).

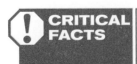 **CRITICAL FACTS** A heart attack is caused by blockages from plaque buildup or blood clots, which affect the ability of the heart to pump effectively. A heart attack can lead to cardiac arrest—where the heart ceases to function as a pump.

- A hard blow to the chest (e.g., **Commotio cordis**).
- Congenital heart disease.
- *Sudden infant death syndrome* (SIDS).

Geriatric Considerations

Cardiac Pathophysiology

In geriatric patients, a general decrease in pain perception may cause a different reaction to a heart attack. Elderly patients often suffer what is known as a **"silent heart attack,"** meaning that there is an absence of chest pain. The symptoms of a heart attack most commonly shown by a geriatric patient include general weakness or fatigue, aching shoulders and abdominal pain or indigestion.

Other Specific Cardiovascular Emergencies

Angina Pectoris

A medical term for "pain in the chest," angina pectoris develops when the heart needs more oxygen than it gets, because the arteries leading to it are too narrow. Angina pectoris is normally a transient condition. When a person with angina exercises, gets excited or is emotionally upset, the heart might not get enough oxygen. This lack of oxygen can cause chest discomfort or pain. People with angina usually have medicine they can take to stop the pain. Stopping physical activity or easing the distress and taking the medicine usually end the discomfort or pain.

Arrhythmias

Arrhythmias are disturbances in the regular rhythmic beating of the heart. Some people have heart arrhythmias that do not cause problems. In others, they can indicate a more serious problem that leads to heart disease, stroke or sudden cardiac death.

Atrial Fibrillation

Atrial fibrillation is the most common type of abnormal cardiac rhythm. When someone experiences atrial fibrillation, the two upper chambers of the heart (the atria) beat out of coordination with the two lower chambers (the ventricles). This causes an irregular and often rapid heart rate, thus leading to the inability to adequately deliver blood to the ventricles. Atrial fibrillation can be controlled with medication and treatment. Although not usually life threatening, atrial fibrillation is a risk factor for stroke and heart attack.

Congestive Heart Failure

Also called *heart failure*, **congestive heart failure** is a chronic condition in which the heart no longer pumps blood effectively throughout the body. This may cause high blood pressure and a buildup of fluid throughout the body, resulting in difficulty breathing and weight gain. Fluid buildup and swelling usually occur in the face, hands, legs, ankles and feet.

Hypertension

Also known as *high blood pressure*, **hypertension** is one of the main **risk factors** for heart attack. A patient is considered to have hypertension when blood pressure is higher than 140/90 mmHg. The causes of hypertension are not clear; however, certain medications, salt intake and stress can contribute to a rise in blood pressure. Secondary hypertension is caused by an underlying condition such as a kidney abnormality or tumor of the adrenal gland.

Diabetes

Diabetes can affect the nerves; therefore, people with diabetes may not experience chest pain and may suffer a "silent heart attack." People who experience silent heart attacks may have no warning signs or they may have very mild signs. When this occurs, the diagnosis of a heart attack may have to be confirmed by special tests. (See **Chapter 14** for more information on diabetes.)

Women and Heart Attacks

Although women may experience chest pain or discomfort during a heart attack, they are more likely to experience some of the other warning signals, particularly shortness of breath; nausea or vomiting; stomach, back or jaw pain; or unexplained fatigue or malaise. When they do experience chest pain, women may have a greater tendency to have atypical chest pain: sudden, sharp but short-lived pain outside the breastbone. As a result, women often will delay telling others about their symptoms to avoid bothering or worrying them.

Assessment of Cardiac Emergencies

The sooner you recognize the signs and symptoms of a heart attack and act, the better chance you have to save a life. Many people will deny they are having a heart attack. Summon more advanced medical personnel if the patient shows some or all of the following signs and symptoms:

- Discomfort, pressure or pain. The major sign is persistent discomfort, pressure or pain in the chest that does not go away. Unfortunately, it is not always easy to distinguish heart attack pain from the pain of indigestion, muscle spasms or other conditions. This often causes people to delay getting medical care. Brief, stabbing pain or pain that gets worse when you bend or breathe deeply is not usually caused by a heart problem.

- The pain associated with a heart attack can range from discomfort to an unbearable crushing sensation in the chest. The patient may describe it as pressure, squeezing, tightness, aching or heaviness in the chest. Many heart attacks start slowly, as mild discomfort, pressure or pain often felt in the center of the chest (**Fig. 13-5**). It may spread to the shoulder, arm, neck, jaw, stomach or back. The discomfort or pain becomes constant. It is usually not relieved by resting, changing position or taking medicine. When interviewing the patient, ask open-ended questions, such as "Can you describe how you feel for me?" so you can hear the symptoms described in the patient's own words.

- Any chest discomfort or pain that is severe, lasts longer than a few minutes (about 3–5 minutes), goes away and comes back or persists even during rest requires medical care at once. Even people who have had a previous heart attack may not recognize the signs and symptoms, because each heart attack can have entirely different signs and symptoms.

- Pain that comes and goes, such as with angina pectoris. Some people with CHD may have chest pain or pressure that comes and goes and

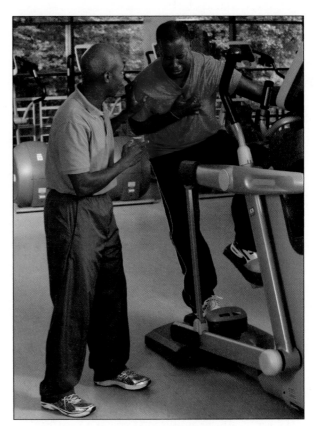

Fig. 13-5: Some people experience symptoms such as chest pain, pressure or discomfort during a heart attack.

is usually treated with a nitroglycerin pill or patches. This medication reduces the workload of the heart by dilating the coronary arteries.

- Difficulty breathing is another sign of a heart attack. The patient may be breathing faster than normal because the body tries to get much-needed oxygen to the heart. A patient who is sitting upright and learning forward with hands on knees in the tripod position is struggling to breathe. Difficulty breathing also includes noisy breathing and shortness of breath.

- Other signs and symptoms include pale or ashen skin, especially around the face. The face also may be damp with sweat. Some people suffering from a heart attack sweat heavily, feel dizzy or lightheaded and/or may lose consciousness. Nausea is also a sign and symptom of a heart attack.

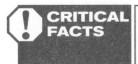

CRITICAL FACTS The key to saving a heart attack victim's life is early recognition of signs and symptoms, including chest discomfort, pressure or pain that does not go away or comes and goes, and difficulty breathing.

Providing Care for Cardiac Emergencies

If you think someone is having a heart attack—

- Take immediate action and summon more advanced medical personnel.
- Have the patient stop any activity and rest (**Fig. 13-6**).
- Loosen any tight or uncomfortable clothing.
- Closely monitor the patient until more advanced medical personnel take over. Notice any changes in the patient's appearance or behavior.
- Comfort the patient.
- If medically appropriate and local protocols or medical direction permit, give aspirin if the patient can swallow and has no known contraindications. Be sure the patient has *not* been told by his or her physician to *not* take aspirin.
- Assist the patient with prescribed medication and administer emergency oxygen, if it is available.
- Be prepared to perform CPR and use an AED.

Aspirin Can Lessen Heart Attack Damage

You may be able to help a conscious patient who is showing early signs of a heart attack by offering an appropriate dose of aspirin when the signs first begin. Local protocols regarding administration of medicines, such as aspirin, may vary for EMRs and should be followed. Aspirin should never take the place of more advanced medical care. If the patient is conscious and able to take medicine by mouth, ask if he or she—

- Is allergic to aspirin.
- Has a stomach ulcer or stomach disease.

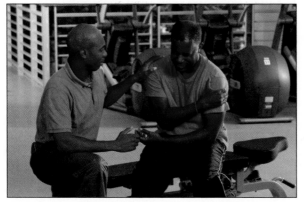

Fig. 13-6: If you think someone is having a heart attack, call for help and have the patient stop any activity and rest.

- Is taking any blood thinners, such as warfarin (Coumadin®).
- Has been told by a physician to *not* take aspirin.

If the patient answers **no** to **all** of these questions, administration of two chewable (162 mg) baby aspirins, or one 5-grain (325 mg) adult aspirin tablet with a small amount of water should be considered.

Be sure that *only* aspirin is given and *not* acetaminophen (e.g., Tylenol®) or *nonsteroidal anti-inflammatory drugs* (NSAIDs) such as ibuprofen (e.g., Motrin® or Advil®) and naproxen (e.g., Aleve®). Likewise, coated aspirin products or products meant for multiple symptoms/uses such as cold, fever and headache, should not be used. Coated aspirin takes too long to dissolve to be effective.

CARDIAC ARREST

When the heart stops beating, or beats too ineffectively to circulate blood to the brain and other vital organs, this is called cardiac arrest. The beats or contractions of the heart become ineffective if they are weak, irregular or uncoordinated, because, at that point, the blood no longer flows through the arteries to the rest of the body.

When the heart stops beating properly, the body cannot survive. Breathing will stop soon after, and the body's organs will no longer receive the oxygen they need to function. Without oxygen, brain damage can begin in about 4–6 minutes, and the damage can become irreversible after about 10 minutes.

A person in cardiac arrest is not breathing and has no pulse. The heart has either stopped beating or is beating weakly and irregularly so that a pulse cannot be detected.

Cardiovascular disease is the primary cause of cardiac arrest. About 900,000 people in the United States die each year from all forms of the disease. Other causes of cardiac arrest include drowning, choking, drugs, severe injury, brain damage and electrocution.

Cardiac arrest can happen suddenly, without any of the warning signs usually seen in a heart attack. This is known as *sudden cardiac arrest* or *sudden cardiac death* and accounts for more than 300,000 deaths annually in the United States. Sudden cardiac arrest is caused by abnormal, chaotic electrical activity of the heart (known as *arrhythmias*). The most common life-threatening abnormal arrhythmia is ***ventricular fibrillation*** (V-fib).

Cardiac Chain of Survival

During the primary assessment, you learned to identify and care for life-threatening conditions. As an EMR, you must learn how to provide care for cardiac emergencies, such as heart attack and cardiac arrest. To effectively respond to cardiac emergencies, it helps to understand the importance of the **Cardiac Chain of Survival (Fig. 13-7)**.

The four links in the Cardiac Chain of Survival are—

1. *Early recognition of the emergency and early access to the emergency medical services (EMS) system.* The sooner more advanced medical personnel or the local emergency number are called, the sooner EMS personnel will take over.
2. *Early CPR.* CPR helps supply blood containing oxygen to the brain and other vital organs to keep the patient alive until an AED is used or advanced medical care is provided.
3. *Early **defibrillation**.* An electrical shock called defibrillation may help the heart restore an effective rhythm.
4. *Early advanced medical care.* EMS personnel provide more advanced medical care and transport the patient to a hospital.

For each minute CPR and defibrillation are delayed, the patient's chance for survival is reduced by about 10 percent.

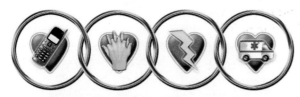

Fig. 13-7: The Cardiac Chain of Survival

In the Cardiac Chain of Survival, each link of the chain depends on and is connected to the other links. The layperson or bystander is the first link in the cardiac chain of survival. But for this four-step sequence to work and ensure the greatest chance of survival, it is very important to quickly recognize the emergency and call for help, start CPR promptly and continue until an AED is ready to use or more advanced medical personnel take over.

Laypersons should be informed through community outreach programs and public awareness campaigns that by taking quick action, including calling 9-1-1 or the local emergency number, starting CPR immediately and using an AED if one is available, it is more likely a person in cardiac arrest will survive.

CPR

A patient who is unconscious, not breathing and has no pulse is in cardiac arrest and needs CPR. CPR is a combination of **chest compressions** and ventilations which circulate blood containing oxygen to the brain and other vital organs for a person whose heart and breathing have stopped. Summoning more advanced medical personnel immediately is critical for the patient's survival. If an AED is available, use it in combination with CPR and according to your local protocols until more advanced medical personnel take over.

Artificial Ventilation

Artificial ventilation is a way of forcing air into the lungs of a patient who is not breathing. The oxygen in the air will be absorbed by blood flowing through the lungs and carried to tissues and the body's vital organs.

There are several different methods of artificial ventilation, including—

- Mouth-to-mask ventilations.
- Resuscitation using a *bag-valve-mask resuscitator* (BVM).

> **CRITICAL FACTS**
>
> The four links in the Cardiac Chain of Survival are early recognition and early access to the EMS system; early CPR; early defibrillation; and early advanced medical care.
>
> ———
>
> A patient who is unconscious, not breathing and has no pulse is in cardiac arrest and needs CPR. CPR is a combination of chest compressions and ventilations which circulate blood containing oxygen to the brain and other vital organs for a person whose heart and breathing have stopped.

- Fixed- and variable-flow oxygen when used in conjunction with delivery devices.

Artificial ventilation can save a patient's life, but over-ventilation can be potentially harmful, especially for a patient in cardiac arrest. For example, if the ventilation is given too forcefully, or at too fast a rate, the pressure in the patient's chest will remain too high even between breaths. This stops the blood from returning to the right side of the heart, and means that less blood is available to be pumped to other vital organs and tissues as CPR continues.

External Chest Compressions

Effective chest compressions are essential for high-quality CPR. While not fully understood, it is believed the compressions increase the level of pressure in the chest cavity, which squeezes the heart and stimulates a contraction, causing oxygenated blood to circulate through the arteries to the brain and other vital organs (**Fig. 13-8, A–B**). Chest compressions can also increase the likelihood that a successful shock can be delivered to a patient suffering a sudden cardiac arrest, especially if more than several minutes have elapsed since the patient's collapse.

The effectiveness of compressions can be reduced if—
- Compressions are too shallow.
- Compression rate is too slow.
- There is sub-maximum recoil (not letting the chest come all the way back up).
- There are frequent interruptions.
- The patient is not on a firm, flat surface.

Correct Hand Position

Keeping your hands in the correct position allows you to give the most effective compressions. The correct position for your hands is over the lower half of the sternum (breastbone) in the middle of the chest (**Fig. 13-9**). At the lowest point of the sternum is an arrow-shaped piece of hard tissue called the *xiphoid process*. Avoid pressing directly on the xiphoid process, which can break off and puncture underlying organs and tissues causing potentially serious injury.

To find the correct hand position, place the heel of one hand on the center of the chest, along the sternum, and then place the other hand on top. Use only the *heel* of your hand to apply pressure on the sternum when compressing the chest. Try to keep your fingers off the chest by interlacing

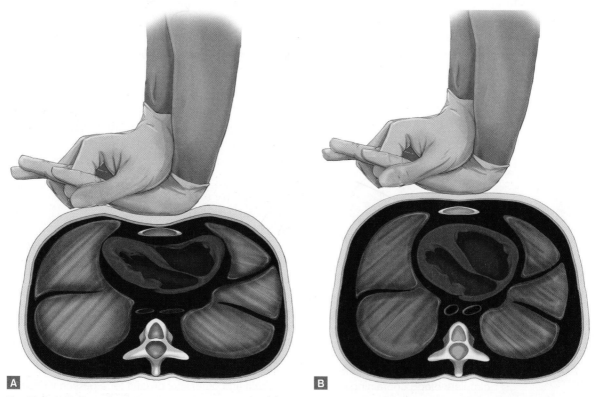

Fig. 13-8, A–B: To perform chest compressions correctly: **(A)** Push straight down at least 2 inches with a smooth movement, and **(B)** after each compression, completely release the pressure on the chest, allowing it to fully return to its normal position.

them or holding them upward. Applying pressure with your fingers can cause inefficient chest compressions or unnecessary injury to the chest. Positioning the hands correctly allows for the most effective compressions and decreases the chance of causing injury.

If you have arthritis or a similar condition in your hands or wrists, you may use an alternative hand position. Find the correct hand position, as above, and then grasp the wrist of the hand on the chest with the other hand (**Fig. 13-10**).

The patient's clothing will not necessarily interfere with your ability to position your hands correctly. If you can find the correct position without removing thin clothing, such as a T-shirt, do so. Sometimes a layer of thin clothing will help keep your hands from slipping, since the patient's chest may be moist with sweat. However, if you are not sure you can find the correct hand position, bare the patient's chest. Fat does not accumulate over the sternum; therefore, finding the correct hand position is the same regardless of patient size.

Position of the Rescuer

Your body position is important when giving chest compressions. Compressing the chest straight down provides the best blood flow. The correct body position is also less tiring for you.

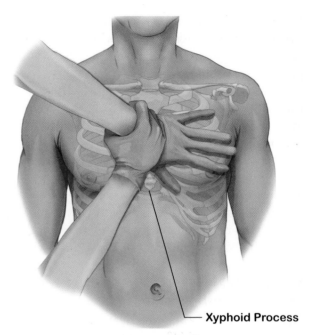

Xyphoid Process

Fig. 13-10: If you have arthritis or another condition that weakens your hands or wrists, you may use this alternative position.

Kneel at the patient's side opposite the chest with your hands in the correct position. Keep your elbows as straight as possible, with your shoulders directly over your hands (**Fig. 13-11**).

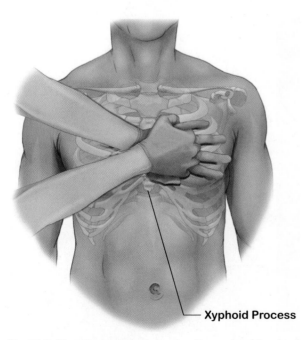

Xyphoid Process

Fig. 13-9: Place the heel of one hand on the center of the chest, along the sternum, and then place the other hand on top. Try to keep your fingers off the chest by interlacing them or holding them upward.

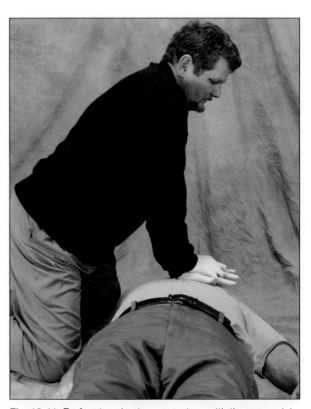

Fig. 13-11: Performing chest compressions with the appropriate body position ensures their effectiveness and prevents you from tiring quickly.

When you press down in this position, you are pushing straight down onto the patient's sternum. Keeping your arms as straight as possible prevents you from tiring quickly.

Compressing the chest requires less effort in this position. When you press down, the weight of your upper body creates the force needed to compress the chest. Push with the weight of your upper body, not with the muscles of your arms. Push straight down. Do not rock back and forth. Rocking results in less effective compressions and wastes energy. If your arms and shoulders tire quickly, you are not using the correct body position.

Compression Technique

Rate of Compression

Give compressions at a rate of at least 100 per minute. You can help yourself maintain the right pace by counting either aloud or in your head: *one* (as you press down) *and* (as you release the pressure) *two* (pressing down again) *and* (release again) and so on. When you get into the twenties, you can drop the "and" as it may be tiring and may alter the timing of compressions. Count the number of compressions, then give ventilations, before starting another cycle of compressions.

Depth of Compressions

Each time you push down, the breastbone of an adult should move at least 2 inches. The downward movement should be smooth, not jerky. Maintain a steady down-and-up rhythm and do not pause in between. If your hands slip out of position, follow the steps listed earlier to quickly reposition them.

Recoil

After each compression, completely release the pressure on the chest. Do not break contact with the chest; simply allow the chest to fully return to its normal position (full recoil) before you start the next compression. It is during this phase of CPR that the chambers of the heart will refill with blood, ready to be circulated throughout the body with the next compression. Chest compressions are more effective when the patient is on a firm, flat surface. If the patient is on a softer surface such as a bed, couch or pressure relieving mattress, carefully position the patient face up on the floor or a backboard.

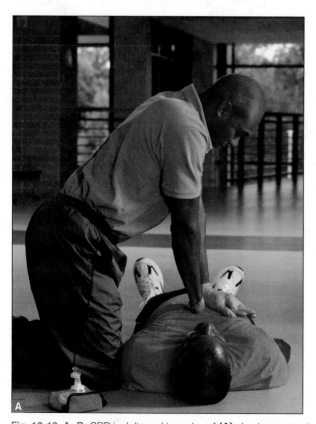 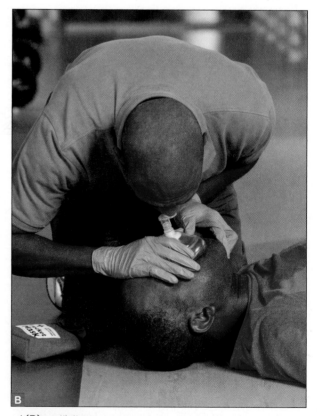

Fig. 13-12, A–B: CPR is delivered in cycles of **(A)** chest compressions and **(B)** ventilations.

Compression and Breathing Cycles

When performing CPR on an adult, child or infant, it is delivered in cycles of chest compressions followed by ventilations (**Fig. 13-12, A–B**). Complete the compressions, then re-establish an open airway by tilting the patient's head and lifting the chin and then provide ventilations. When you are finished giving ventilations, quickly reposition your hands on the center of the chest and start another cycle of compressions and ventilations. See **Table 13-1** regarding the compression-to-ventilation ratios for adult, child and infant one- and two-rescuer CPR. Note that these ratios can change every 5 years due to updates in scientific research and evidence that result from the Consensus on Science with Treatment Recommendations (CoSTR) by international experts in the field of emergency medicine.

Interruptions

Minimize interruptions in giving chest compressions. If compressions must be interrupted, do so for no more than a few seconds. For example, you may need to move the patient to a location where CPR can be more effectively administered, such as if the patient is on a bed or couch, moving the patient to lie flat on the floor. CPR may also be interrupted briefly for defibrillation, insertion of an advanced airway or when two rescuers change positions between compressions and ventilations. Continue CPR while the patient

Table 13-1:

Summary of Techniques for Adult, Child and Infant CPR

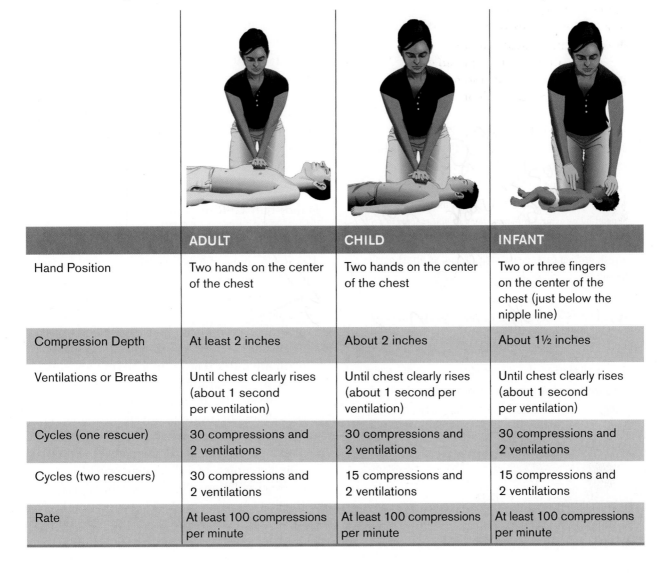

	ADULT	CHILD	INFANT
Hand Position	Two hands on the center of the chest	Two hands on the center of the chest	Two or three fingers on the center of the chest (just below the nipple line)
Compression Depth	At least 2 inches	About 2 inches	About 1½ inches
Ventilations or Breaths	Until chest clearly rises (about 1 second per ventilation)	Until chest clearly rises (about 1 second per ventilation)	Until chest clearly rises (about 1 second per ventilation)
Cycles (one rescuer)	30 compressions and 2 ventilations	30 compressions and 2 ventilations	30 compressions and 2 ventilations
Cycles (two rescuers)	30 compressions and 2 ventilations	15 compressions and 2 ventilations	15 compressions and 2 ventilations
Rate	At least 100 compressions per minute	At least 100 compressions per minute	At least 100 compressions per minute

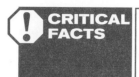

Once you begin CPR, do not stop. If you must, do so for no more than a few seconds. Reasons to discontinue CPR include more advanced medical personnel taking over for you, seeing obvious signs of life, an AED being available and ready to use or being too exhausted to continue.

is being moved into an ambulance or other transport vehicle or from the ambulance into a hospital emergency department.

When to Stop CPR

Once you begin CPR, do not stop. Do not stop CPR except in one of these situations:

- You see an obvious sign of life, such as breathing.
- An AED is ready to use.
- Another trained responder takes over.
- More advanced medical personnel take over.
- You are presented with a valid *Do Not Resuscitate* (DNR) order.
- You are too exhausted to continue.
- The scene becomes unsafe.

Pediatric Considerations

CPR

The principles of CPR (compressing the chest and providing ventilations) are the same for children and infants as for adults, but the techniques are modified because children's and infants' bodies are smaller and weaker. Cardiac arrest in children and infants is usually caused by a respiratory emergency. If you recognize that a child or an infant is in respiratory distress or arrest, provide care immediately. If cardiac arrest occurs, begin CPR.

To perform CPR on a child or an infant, also perform cycles of chest compressions and ventilations at the rate of at least 100 compressions per minute. As with an adult, let the chest fully recoil to its normal position after each compression. For a child, use two hands on the center of the chest and compress about 2 inches. For an infant, use two or three fingers on the center of the chest, just below the nipple line, and compress about 1½ inches.

Two-Rescuer CPR

When an additional rescuer is available, perform two-rescuer CPR. One rescuer gives ventilations and the other rescuer gives chest compressions. Rescuers should change positions (alternate turns performing compressions and ventilations) about every 2 minutes to reduce the possibility of rescuer fatigue. Changing positions should take less than 5 seconds.

Perform two-rescuer CPR in the following situations:

- Two rescuers arrive on the scene at the same time and begin CPR together.
- One rescuer is performing CPR and a second rescuer becomes available.

When CPR is in progress by one rescuer and a second rescuer arrives, the second rescuer should confirm whether more advanced medical personnel have been summoned. If they have not, the second rescuer should do so before getting the AED or assisting with care. If more advanced medical personnel have been summoned, the second rescuer should get the AED, or if an AED is not available, the second rescuer should help perform two-rescuer CPR.

Hands-Only CPR

Hands-only CPR or *continuous chest compressions*, is a simplified form of CPR that eliminates ventilations or rescue breaths. It has its roots in dispatcher-assisted cardiac emergency situations where the caller is untrained, unwilling, unsure or otherwise unable to perform full CPR (chest compressions with ventilations or rescue breaths). Providing instruction on how to give chest compressions alone is less complex than trying to explain full CPR. The main focus of hands-only CPR is on the untrained layperson or a bystander who witnesses the sudden collapse of an adult. EMRs should be aware that if they come upon a bystander giving chest compressions only, that person is performing CPR correctly.

Chest compressions alone may provide effective circulation of blood containing oxygen in the first few minutes of an out-of-hospital cardiac arrest. The same quality compression techniques of full CPR apply to compression-only CPR, including hand position, compression depth, speed, full recoil and minimal interruptions. Hands-only CPR does not affect the use of an AED.

AUTOMATED EXTERNAL DEFIBRILLATION

Each year, more than 300,000 Americans die suddenly of cardiac arrest. CPR can help by supplying blood containing oxygen to the brain and other vital organs. In many cases, however, an AED is needed to correct an abnormal electrical problem and allow the heart to restore an effective rhythm. Sudden cardiac arrest can happen to anyone at any time and, although rare, can occur in children and infants.

History of Defibrillation

The presence of cardiac arrhythmias or disturbances of the heart's electrical system, and the ability to correct fibrillation with electrical shock, has been known since the mid-19th century.[1] Electrical-shocking devices, or *defibrillators*, were first developed during the 1920s. A portable version was introduced onto mobile coronary units in Belfast, Northern Ireland in 1966.[2] Defibrillation by *emergency medical technicians* (EMTs) without the presence of a physician was first performed in Portland, Oregon in 1969.

As technology improved over the years, newer generations of more compact, simple to operate, semi-automatic defibrillators known as AEDs evolved allowing EMTs and EMRs, as well as trained citizen responders, to provide this life-saving technology. With these newer devices, a computer analyzes the heart's rhythm and advises whether a shock is needed. Typically, the responder is guided through the steps of providing defibrillation by voice instructions and visual prompts from the AED. This includes placing the electrode (defibrillation) pads on the

person's chest, analyzing the heart' delivering a shock if needed and r perform CPR when appropriate. can be configured to deliver low considered appropriate for chil

When EMRs and other res[to use AEDs, they can significa.... amount of time it takes to administer a first in a sudden cardiac arrest, researchers say. In Eugene and Springfield, Oregon, AEDs were placed on every fire truck, and all firefighters were trained to use them. Researchers saw these communities' survival rates for cardiac arrest increase by 18 percent in the first year.[3]

The vast majority of states recognize defibrillator training for EMTs, EMRs and other responders. All states and the District of Columbia have enacted AED Good Samaritan protection for lay responders.[4] Today, AEDs are widely dispersed and can be found in areas where large groups of people gather, such as convention centers, airports, stadiums, shopping malls, large businesses, schools and industrial complexes.

The most common abnormal heart rhythm that causes sudden cardiac arrest occurs when the ventricles simply quiver, or *fibrillate*, without any organized rhythm. This condition is called *ventricular fibrillation* (V-fib). In V-fib, the electrical impulses fire at random, creating chaos and preventing the heart from pumping and circulating blood.

Another less common life-threatening heart rhythm, called ***ventricular tachycardia (V-tach)***, occurs when the heart beats too fast. In V-tach, an abnormal electrical impulse controls the heart, originating in the ventricles instead of in the SA node. This abnormal impulse fires so fast that the heart's chambers do not have time to fill, and the heart is unable to pump blood effectively. With little or no blood circulating, there may be no pulse. As with V-fib, there is no breathing or pulse.

---

[1]Bocka, Joseph J., MD: *Automatic External Defibrillation*, eMedicine, April 3, 2006.
[2]Pantridge JF, Geddes JS: A mobile intensive care unit in the treatment of myocardial infarction, *Lancet* 2:271, 1967.

[3]Graves JR, Austin D Jr, Cummins RO: *Rapid zap: automated defibrillation*, Englewood Cliffs, NJ, 1989, Prentice-Hall.
[4]American Heart Association–*AED Legislation/Good Samaritan Laws by State* reviewed/updated 07/16/2008.

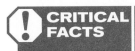
CRITICAL FACTS V-fib is the most common cause of sudden cardiac arrest. In V-fib, heart ventricles quiver instead of beating properly, due to erratic electrical impulses.

AUTOMATED EXTERNAL DEFIBRILLATORS

AEDs are portable electronic devices that analyze the heart's rhythm and can deliver an electrical shock, known as defibrillation, which helps the heart to re-establish an effective rhythm (**Fig. 13-13**). They can greatly increase the likelihood of survival if the shock is administered soon enough. For every minute lifesaving care, including CPR and defibrillation is delayed, it is estimated that survival declines by about 10 percent. There are different types of AEDs available but all are similar in operation and have some common features, such as electrode (AED or defibrillation) pads, voice prompts, visual displays and/or lighted buttons that help guide the responder through the steps of the AED operation.

AEDs monitor the heart's electrical activity through two electrodes (i.e., AED pads) placed on the chest. The computer determines the need for a shock by looking at the pattern, size and frequency of EKG waves. If the EKG waves resemble a shockable rhythm, such as V-fib or V-tach, the machine readies an electrical charge. When the electrical charge disrupts the irregular heartbeat, it is called defibrillation. This allows the heart's natural electrical system to correct itself and begin to fire off electrical impulses that will cause the heart to beat effectively.

Delivering an electrical shock with an AED disrupts all electrical activity long enough to allow the heart to spontaneously develop an effective rhythm on its own. If V-fib or V-tach is not corrected, all electrical activity will eventually cease, a condition called **asystole**. Asystole cannot be corrected by defibrillation.

You cannot tell what, if any, rhythm the heart has by feeling for a pulse. CPR, started immediately and continued until defibrillation, helps maintain a low level of circulation in

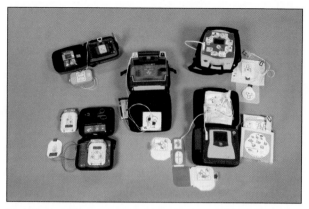

Fig. 13-13: AEDs

the body until defibrillation and increases the likelihood that the defibrillation shock will allow the heart to correct the abnormal rhythm.

Use an AED when the following conditions are present:
- The patient is unresponsive.
- There is *no* breathing.
- You do *not* detect a pulse.

Using an AED

When a cardiac arrest occurs, an AED should be used as soon as it is available and ready to use. If the AED advises that a shock is needed, follow protocols to give 1 shock followed by about 2 minutes of CPR. If CPR is in progress, chest compressions should not be interrupted until the AED is turned on, the defibrillation pads are applied and the AED is ready to analyze the heart rhythm.

Chest compressions can increase the likelihood that a defibrillation shock will be successful, especially if more than 4 minutes have elapsed since the patient's collapse. Always follow local protocols and medical direction when using an AED and performing CPR. Be thoroughly familiar with the manufacturer's operating instructions and maintenance guidelines for the device that you will be operating.

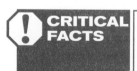

CRITICAL FACTS

AEDs are portable electronic devices that analyze the heart's rhythm and can deliver an electrical shock, known as defibrillation, which helps the heart to re-establish an effective rhythm.

When a cardiac arrest occurs, an AED should be used as soon as it is available and ready to use. If the AED advises that a shock is needed, follow protocols to give 1 shock followed by about 2 minutes of CPR.

The general steps of operating an AED include—

1. Turning on the AED and preparing it for use. Once the AED is turned on, it will guide the responder through all the steps of operation with voice and visual prompts. Some models have a power button that must be pressed, while others will activate upon opening the case or lid.

2. Exposing the patient's chest and wiping the chest dry. The AED pads must be applied to the patient's *bare, dry* chest. If the patient's chest is moist or wet, it should be wiped with a small towel or gauze pads to ensure the best adhesion of the AED pads.

3. Attaching the AED pads to the patient's bare, dry chest. Remove the AED pads from their sealed packaging. Peel the backing off from each pad, one at a time, to expose the adhesive, conductive surface of the pad before it is applied to the patient's bare chest. Many AED pads have illustrations on them that show correct pad placement. Some AED pads are preconnected to the device, and some must be plugged into the device before rhythm analysis can begin. The pads should be appropriate to the patient. For example, *pediatric* AED pads must not be used on an adult patient because the lower energy levels may not be enough to defibrillate the patient.

4. Analyzing the heart rhythm. Some AEDs will automatically begin analysis when the pads are attached to the patient and connected to the device, while others have an "analyze" button that must be pushed. *No one* should touch or bump into the patient during the rhythm analysis as this could produce faulty readings.

5. Delivering a defibrillation shock. Once the analysis of the rhythm is complete, the AED will advise either to shock or not to shock the patient. If a shockable rhythm is detected, the AED will cycle up an electrical energy charge which will supply the shock to the patient. Some models can deliver the shock automatically while others have a "shock" button that must be manually pushed to deliver the shock. *No one* should be in contact with the patient when the shock is delivered, because they could also receive a shock and thereby reduce the effectiveness of the

defibrillation shock by absorbing some of the electrical energy. After a shock is delivered, or if no shock is advised, a period of time is programmed to allow for CPR until the next rhythm analysis begins. If the AED prompts to troubleshoot a problem such as "check electrodes" or "check pads," check to see that the AED pads are connected properly to the device and placed on the patient's chest with good adhesion, according to the manufacturer's instructions and local protocols. Spare batteries should be available in case of a "low battery" warning, but shocks can still be delivered with a low battery warning on some models.

After a shock is delivered, or if no shock is indicated, perform about 2 minutes of CPR before the AED begins rhythm analysis again. If at any time you notice an obvious sign of life, such as breathing, stop CPR and monitor the patient's condition.

Pediatric Considerations

AED Use

While the incidence of cardiac arrest in children and infants is relatively low compared with that for adults, cardiac arrest resulting from V-fib does happen in young children. Most cardiac arrests in children and infants are not sudden and may be caused by–

- Airway and breathing problems.
- Traumatic injuries or accidents (e.g., motor-vehicle collision, drowning, electrocution or poisoning).
- A hard blow to the chest.
- Congenital heart disease.
- *Sudden infant death syndrome* (SIDS).

AEDs equipped with pediatric defibrillation pads are capable of delivering lower levels of energy considered appropriate for children and infants up to 8 years old or weighing less than 55 pounds. Use pediatric AED pads and/or equipment, if available. If pediatric-specific equipment is not available, an AED designed for adults can be used on children and infants. In any event, always follow local protocols and medical direction and the manufacturer's instructions. For a child or an infant in cardiac arrest, follow the same general steps and precautions that you would when using an AED on an adult. If the pads risk touching each other because of the smaller chest size, use the anterior/posterior method of pad placement (**Fig. 13-14**).

After a shock is delivered or if no shock is indicated, perform about 2 minutes of CPR before the AED begins analyzing the heart rhythm again. This pause is automatically programmed into the device and will be preceded by a voice prompt to resume CPR. If at any time you notice an obvious sign of life, such as breathing, stop CPR and monitor the patient's condition.

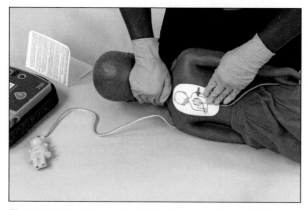

Fig. 13-14: Posterior method of pad placement on a child

Special AED Situations

Some situations require responders to pay special attention when using an AED. These include using AEDs around water, on patients with implantable devices, on patients with transdermal patches and on patients with jewelry or body piercings, as well as what to do when confronted with other AED protocols. Be familiar with these situations and know how to respond appropriately. Always use common sense when using an AED and follow manufacturer's recommendations.

Pacemakers and Implantable Cardioverter-Defibrillators

Sometimes patients may have had a **pacemaker** implanted if they have a weak heart or a heart that skips beats or beats too slow or fast. These small implantable devices are sometimes located in the area below the right collarbone. There may be a small lump that can be felt under the skin.

Other patients may have an ***implantable cardioverter-defibrillator*** (**ICD**), a miniature version of an AED, which acts to automatically recognize and restore abnormal heart rhythms. Sometimes, a patient's heart beats irregularly, even if the patient has a pacemaker or an ICD.

If the implanted device is visible, or you know that the patient has one, do *not* place the defibrillation pad directly over the device (**Fig. 13-15**). This may interfere with the delivery of the shock. Adjust pad placement if necessary and continue to follow established protocols. If you are not sure, use the AED as needed. It will not harm the patient or rescuer.

Rescuers should be aware that it is possible to receive a mild shock if an implantable ICD delivers a shock to the patient while CPR is performed. This risk of injury to rescuers is minimal and the amount of electrical energy involved is low. Much of the electrical energy is absorbed by the patient's own body tissues. Some protocols may include temporarily deactivating the shock capability of an ICD with a donut magnet or other precautions. EMRs should be aware of and follow any special precautions associated with ICDs, but delays in delivering CPR and defibrillation shocks from an AED should *not* occur.

AEDs Around Water

If the patient is in freestanding water, remove the patient before defibrillation. A shock delivered in water could conduct to rescuers or bystanders. Once you have removed the patient from the water, be sure there are no puddles of water around you, the patient or the AED. Remove wet clothing for proper pad placement, if necessary. Dry the patient's chest and attach the AED pads.

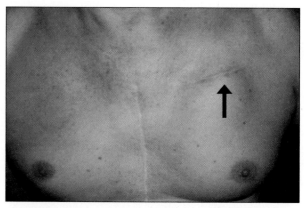

Fig. 13-15: Scars and/or a small lump may indicate that the patient has had some sort of device implanted. *Courtesy of Ted Crites.*

If it is raining, ensure that the patient is as dry as possible and sheltered from the rain. Wipe the patient's chest dry. Minimize delaying defibrillation when taking steps to provide for a dry environment. The electrical current of an AED is very directional between the pads. AEDs are quite safe, even in rain and snow, when all precautions and manufacturer's operating instructions are followed.

Transdermal Medication Patches

Some patients may use a **transdermal medication patch**. The most common of these patches is the nitroglycerin patch, used by those with a history of cardiac problems. Since nitroglycerin or other medications can be absorbed by a rescuer, remove the patch from the patient's chest with a gloved hand before defibrillation. Nicotine patches used to stop smoking look similar to nitroglycerin patches. To avoid wasting time trying to identify patches, remove any patch you see on the patient's chest with a gloved hand (**Fig. 13-16**). *Never* place AED electrode pads directly on top of medication patches.

Hypothermia

Some patients who have experienced hypothermia have been resuscitated successfully even after prolonged exposure. If you do not feel a pulse, begin CPR until an AED becomes available. Follow local protocols as to whether an AED should be used. If the patient is wet, dry his or her chest and attach the AED pads. If a shock is indicated, deliver a shock and follow the instructions of the AED. If there are no obvious signs of life, continue CPR. Continue CPR and protect the patient from further heat loss.

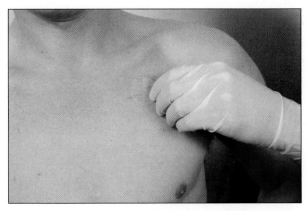

Fig. 13-16: Remove any type of transdermal medication patch from the patient's chest with a gloved hand before defibrillation.

Wet garments should be removed, if possible. The patient should *not* be defibrillated in water. CPR or defibrillation should *not* be withheld to rewarm the patient. EMRs should handle hypothermia patients gently, as shaking them could result in V-fib.

Trauma

If a patient is in cardiac arrest resulting from traumatic injuries, an AED may still be used. Defibrillation should be administered according to local protocols.

Chest Hair

Some men have excessive chest hair that may cause difficulty with pad-to-skin contact. Since time to first shock is critical, and chest hair *rarely* interferes with pad adhesion, attach the pads and analyze the heart's rhythm as soon as possible. Press firmly on the pads to attach them to the patient's chest. If you get a "check pads" or similar message from the AED, remove the pads and replace with new ones. The pad adhesive may pull out some of the chest hair, which may solve the problem. If you continue to get the "check pads" message, remove the pads, shave the patient's chest and attach new pads to the patient's chest. Spare defibrillation pads and a safety razor should be included in the AED kit. Be careful not to cut the patient while shaving, as cuts and scrapes can interfere with rhythm analysis.

Jewelry and Body Piercings

Jewelry and body piercings do *not* need to be removed when using an AED. These are simply distractions that do no harm to the patient, but taking time to remove them delays delivery of the first shock. Do *not* delay the use of an AED to remove jewelry or body piercings. Do *not* place the defibrillation pad directly over metallic jewelry or body piercings. Adjust pad placement if necessary and continue to follow established protocols.

Other AED Protocols

Other AED protocols are not incorrect, nor harmful. For example, delivering three shocks and then performing CPR. However, improved methods, based on new scientific evidence, make it easier to coordinate performing CPR and using the AED. Follow the instructions of the AED you are using, whether it is to give one shock and then perform CPR or to give three shocks followed by CPR.

AED PRECAUTIONS

When operating an AED, follow these general precautions:

- Do *not* use alcohol to wipe the patient's chest dry; alcohol is flammable.
- Do *not* use an AED and/or pads designed for adults on a child or an infant under age 8 or weighing less than 55 pounds, unless pediatric pads specific to the device are not available. Local protocols may differ on this and should be followed.
- Do *not* use pediatric AED pads on an adult, as they may not deliver enough energy for defibrillation.
- Do *not* touch the patient while the AED is analyzing. Touching or moving the patient may affect the analysis.
- Before shocking a patient with an AED, make sure that *no one* is touching or is in contact with the patient or the resuscitation equipment.
- Do *not* touch the patient while defibrillating. You or someone else could be shocked.
- Do *not* defibrillate someone when around flammable or combustible materials such as gasoline or free-flowing oxygen.
- Do *not* use an AED in a moving vehicle. Movement may affect the analysis.
- Do *not* use an AED on a patient who is in contact with water. Move the patient away from puddles of water or swimming pools, or out of the rain, before defibrillating.
- Do *not* use an AED on a patient wearing a nitroglycerin patch or other patch on the chest. With a gloved hand, remove any patches from the chest before attaching the device.
- Do *not* use a mobile phone or radio within 6 feet of the AED. *Radio frequency interference* (RFI) and *electromagnetic interference* (EMI), as well as infrared interference, generated by radio signals can disrupt analysis.

AED MAINTENANCE

For defibrillators to function optimally, they must be maintained like any other machine. AEDs require minimal maintenance. These devices have various self-testing features. However, it is important that operators be familiar with any visual or audible prompts the AED may have to warn of malfunction or a low battery. It is important that you read the operator's manual thoroughly and check with the manufacturer to obtain all necessary information regarding maintenance.

In most instances, if the machine detects any malfunction, you should contact the manufacturer. The device may need to be returned to the manufacturer for service. While AEDs require minimal maintenance, it is important to remember the following:

- Follow the manufacturer's specific recommendations for periodic equipment checks.
- Make sure that the batteries have enough energy for one complete rescue. (A fully charged backup battery should be readily available.)
- Make sure that the correct defibrillation pads are in the package and are properly sealed.
- Check any expiration dates on defibrillation pads and batteries and replace as necessary.
- After use, make sure that all accessories are replaced and that the machine is in proper working order before placing it back in service.
- If at any time the machine fails to work properly or warning indicators are recognized, discontinue use, place it out-of-service and contact the manufacturer immediately.

PUTTING IT ALL TOGETHER

When the heart stops beating, or beats too ineffectively to circulate blood to the brain and other vital organs, this is called cardiac arrest. Irreversible brain damage is likely to occur after about 10 minutes from lack of oxygen. By starting CPR immediately, and using an AED, you can help keep the patient's brain and other vital organs supplied with oxygen and help the heart restore an effective, pumping rhythm. By summoning more advanced medical personnel, you can increase the cardiac arrest patient's chances for survival.

A patient who is unconscious, not breathing and has no pulse is in cardiac arrest and needs immediate CPR. When performing CPR, always remember the following points regarding the quality and maximum effectiveness of CPR:

- Chest compressions should be given fast, smooth and deep.
- Let the chest fully recoil or return to its normal position after each compression before starting the downstroke of the next compression.
- Minimize any interruptions of chest compressions.

If two rescuers are available, begin two-rescuer CPR as soon as possible. Change positions about every 2 minutes and continue CPR. Once you start CPR, do not stop unnecessarily.

The heart's electrical system controls the pumping action of the heart. Damage to the heart from disease or injury can disrupt the heart's electrical system, resulting in an abnormal heart rhythm that can stop circulation. The two most common treatable abnormal rhythms initially present in patients suffering sudden cardiac arrest are V-fib and V-tach.

An AED is a portable electronic device that analyzes the heart's rhythm and delivers an electrical shock to the heart, called defibrillation. Defibrillation disrupts the electrical activity of V-fib and V-tach long enough to allow the heart to develop an effective rhythm on its own. AEDs are used in conjunction with CPR.

Use an AED as soon as one becomes available. The sooner the shock is administered, the greater the likelihood of the patient's survival. AEDs are appropriate for use on adults, children and infants in cardiac arrest. When using an AED, follow your local protocols and the manufacturer's operating instructions and be aware of AED precautions and special situations.

YOU ARE THE EMERGENCY MEDICAL RESPONDER

The man who collapsed is unconscious, is not breathing and does not have a pulse. You send another MERT member to summon more advanced medical personnel and to bring the AED from inside the building. You begin CPR. Once the AED arrives, the other MERT prepares the AED for use. How would you respond? When can you stop performing CPR?

SKILLsheet

CPR–Adult and Child

NOTE: Ensure patient is on a firm, flat surface.

NOTE: Always follow standard precautions when providing care. Size-up the scene for safety and then perform a primary assessment. If the patient is not breathing and has no pulse–

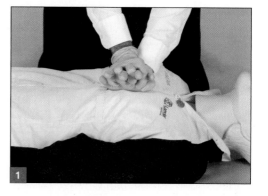

STEP 1

Find the correct hand position to give chest compressions.
- ◆ Place the heel of one hand on the center of the chest.
- ◆ Place the other hand on top.
- ◆ Keep the arms as straight as possible and the shoulders directly over the hands.

STEP 2

Give **30** chest compressions.
- ◆ Push hard, push fast.
  - Compress the chest at least **2** inches for an adult and about **2** inches for a child.
  - Compress at a rate of at least **100** times per minute.
  - Let the chest rise completely before pushing down again.

NOTES:

◆ Keep your fingers off the chest when giving compressions.

◆ Use your body weight, not your arms, to compress the chest.

◆ Counting out loud helps keep an even pace.

STEP 3

Replace the resuscitation mask and give **2** ventilations.

◆ Each ventilation should last about **1** second.

◆ Give ventilations that make the chest clearly rise.

◆ The chest should fall before the next ventilation is given.

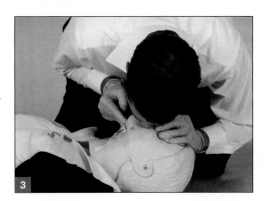

STEP 4

Perform cycles of **30** chest compressions and **2** ventilations.

Do not stop CPR except in one of these situations:

◆ You see an obvious sign of life, such as breathing.

◆ An AED is ready to use.

◆ Another trained responder takes over.

◆ More advanced medical personnel take over.

◆ You are presented with a valid DNR order.

◆ You are too exhausted to continue.

◆ The scene becomes unsafe.

SKILLsheet

CPR–Infant

NOTE: Place the infant on his or her back on a firm, flat surface, such as the floor or a table.

NOTE: Always follow standard precautions when providing care. Size-up the scene for safety and then perform a primary assessment. If the patient is not breathing and has no pulse–

STEP 1

Find the correct hand position to give chest compressions.

◆ Put two or three fingers on the center of the chest just below the nipple line.

◆ Keep one hand on the infant's forehead to maintain an open airway.

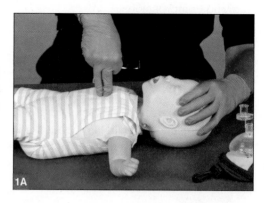

STEP 2

Give **30** chest compressions.

◆ Push hard, push fast.

- Compress the chest about **1½** inches for an infant.
- Compress at a rate of at least **100** times per minute.
- Let the chest rise completely before pushing down again.

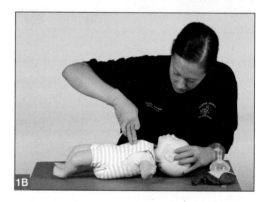

STEP 3

Replace the resuscitation mask and give **2** ventilations.

◆ Each ventilation should last about **1** second.

◆ Provide ventilations that make the chest clearly rise.

◆ The chest should fall before the next ventilation is given.

STEP 4

Perform cycles of **30** chest compressions and **2** ventilations.

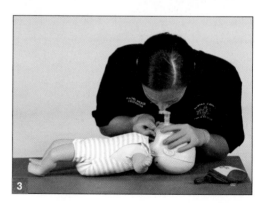

Do not stop CPR except in one of these situations:

◆ You see an obvious sign of life, such as breathing.

◆ An AED is ready to use.

◆ Another trained responder takes over.

◆ More advanced medical personnel take over.

◆ You are presented with a valid DNR order.

◆ You are too exhausted to continue.

◆ The scene becomes unsafe.

SKILLsheet

Two-Rescuer CPR—Adult and Child

NOTE: Ensure the patient is on a firm, flat surface.

NOTE: Always follow standard precautions when providing care. Size-up the scene for safety. Rescuer 1 then performs a primary assessment. If the patient is not breathing and has no pulse—

STEP 1

Rescuer 2 finds the correct hand position to give chest compressions.
◆ Place the heel of one hand on the center of the chest.
◆ Place the other hand on top.
◆ Keep the arms as straight as possible and the shoulders directly over the hands.

STEP 2

Rescuer 2 gives chest compressions.
◆ Give compressions when Rescuer 1 says "Patient has no pulse. Begin CPR."
◆ Push hard, push fast.
  • Compress the chest at least **2** inches for an adult and about **2** inches for a child.
  • For an adult, give **30** chest compressions. For a child, give **15** chest compressions.
  • Compress at a rate of at least **100** times per minute.
  • Let the chest rise completely before pushing down again.

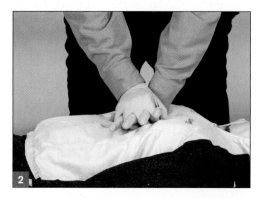

STEP 3

Rescuer 1 replaces the resuscitation mask and gives **2** ventilations.
◆ Each ventilation should last about **1** second.
◆ Give ventilations that make the chest clearly rise.
◆ The chest should fall before the next ventilation is given.

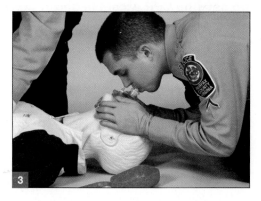

Continued on next page

Two-Rescuer CPR—Adult and Child *continued*

STEP 4

Give about **2** minutes of compressions and ventilations.
- ◆ **Adult:** cycles of **30** compressions and **2** ventilations
- ◆ **Child:** cycles of **15** compressions and **2** ventilations

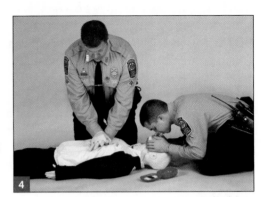

STEP 5

Change positions.
- ◆ Rescuer 2 calls for a position change by using the word "change" at the end of the last compression cycle.
  - • For an adult, by using the word "change" in place of the word "**30**" in the last compression cycle.
  - • For a child, by using the word "change" in place of the word "**15**" in the last compression cycle.
- ◆ Rescuer 1 gives **2** ventilations.
- ◆ Rescuer 2 quickly moves to the patient's head with his or her own mask.
- ◆ Rescuer 1 quickly moves into position at the patient's chest and locates correct hand position on the chest.
- ◆ Changing positions should take less than **5** seconds.

STEP 6

Rescuer 1 gives chest compressions.
- ◆ Continue cycles of compressions and ventilations.

Do not stop CPR except in one of these situations:
- ◆ You see an obvious sign of life, such as breathing.
- ◆ An AED is ready to use.
- ◆ Another trained responder takes over.
- ◆ More advanced medical personnel take over.
- ◆ You are presented with a valid DNR order.
- ◆ You are too exhausted to continue.
- ◆ The scene becomes unsafe.

NOTES:
- ◆ Keep your fingers off the chest when performing compressions.
- ◆ Use your body weight, not your arms, to compress the chest.
- ◆ Position your shoulders over your hands with your elbows as straight as possible.
- ◆ Counting out loud helps keep an even pace.

SKILLsheet

Two-Rescuer CPR–Infant

NOTE: Place the infant on his or her back on a firm, flat surface, such as the floor or a table.

NOTE: Always follow standard precautions when providing care. Size-up the scene for safety and then perform a primary assessment. If the infant is not breathing and has no pulse—

STEP 1

Rescuer 2 finds the correct hand position to give compressions.
- ◆ Place thumbs next to each other on the center of the chest just below the nipple line.
- ◆ Place both hands underneath the infant's back and support the infant's back with your fingers.
- ◆ Ensure that your hands do not compress or squeeze the side of the ribs.
- ◆ If available, a towel or padding can be placed underneath the infant's shoulders to help maintain the head in the neutral position.

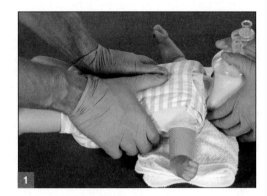

STEP 2

Rescuer 2 gives **15** chest compressions.
- ◆ Give compressions when Rescuer 1 says "Patient has no pulse, begin CPR."
- ◆ Push hard, push fast.
  - • Compress the chest about **1½** inches for an infant.
  - • Compress at a rate of at least **100** times per minute.
  - • Let the chest rise completely before pushing down again.

STEP 3

Rescuer 1 replaces the mask and gives **2** ventilations.
- ◆ Each ventilation should last about **1** second.
- ◆ Give ventilations that make the chest clearly rise.
- ◆ The chest should fall before the next ventilation is given.

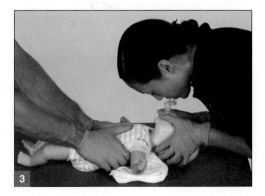

Continued on next page

Two-Rescuer CPR–Infant *continued*

STEP 4

Perform cycles of **15** chest compressions and
2 ventilations.

STEP 5

Change positions.
- ◆ Rescuer 2 calls for a position change by using the word "change" in place of the word "**15**" in the last compression cycle.
- ◆ Rescuer 1 gives **2** ventilations.
- ◆ Rescuer 2 moves to the infant's head with his or her own mask.
- ◆ Rescuer 1 moves into position and locates correct finger placement on the infant's chest.
- ◆ Changing positions should take less than **5** seconds.

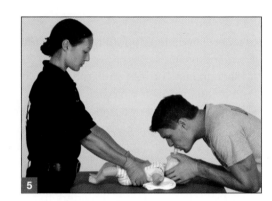

STEP 6

Rescuer 1 gives chest compressions.
- ◆ Continue cycles of **15** compressions and **2** ventilations.

Do not stop CPR except in one of these situations:
- ◆ You see an obvious sign of life, such as breathing.
- ◆ An AED is ready to use.
- ◆ Another trained responder takes over.
- ◆ More advanced medical personnel take over.
- ◆ You are presented with a valid DNR order.
- ◆ You are too exhausted to continue.
- ◆ The scene becomes unsafe.

NOTE: Counting out loud or to yourself helps keep an even pace.

SKILLsheet

AED—Adult, Child and Infant

NOTE: Always follow standard precautions when providing care. Size-up the scene for safety and then perform a primary assessment. If the patient is not breathing and has no pulse—

STEP 1

Turn on the AED and follow the voice and/or visual prompts.

STEP 2

Wipe the patient's bare chest dry.

NOTE: Remove any medication patches with a gloved hand.

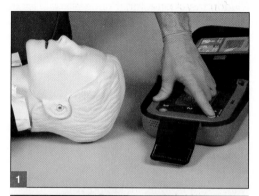

STEP 3

Attach the AED pads to the patient's bare chest.
◆ Place one pad on the patient's upper right chest and other pad on the left side of the chest.
  • **For a child or an infant:** Use pediatric AED pads if available.

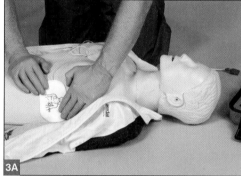

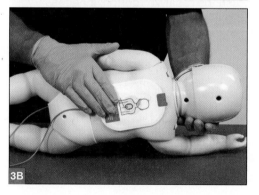

NOTE: If the pads risk touching, use anterior/posterior pad placement. Place one pad in the middle of the child's chest and the other pad on the child's back, between the shoulder blades.

Continued on next page

AED–Adult, Child and Infant *continued*

STEP 4

Plug in the connector, if necessary.

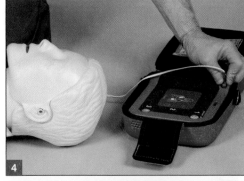

STEP 5

Make sure *no one*, including you, is touching the patient.

◆ Say, "EVERYONE, STAND CLEAR!"

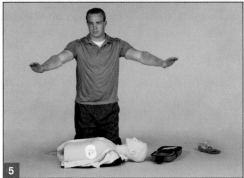

STEP 6

Push the "analyze" button, if necessary.

◆ Let the AED analyze the heart rhythm.

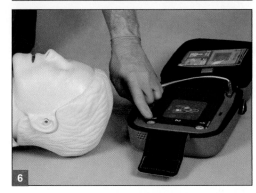

STEP 7

Deliver a shock or perform CPR based on the AED recommendation.

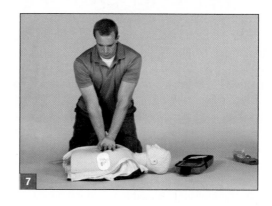

- ◆ If a shock is advised—
  - Make sure *no one*, including you, is touching the patient.
  - Say, "EVERYONE, STAND CLEAR."
  - Deliver the shock by pushing the "shock" button, if necessary.
  - After delivering the shock, perform about 2 minutes of CPR.
- ◆ If no shock is advised—
  - Perform about **2** minutes of CPR.

NOTE: If at any time you notice an obvious sign of life (e.g., breathing), stop CPR and monitor the patient's condition.

Enrichment
Preventing Coronary Heart Disease

Recognizing a heart attack and getting the necessary care at once may prevent a patient from going into cardiac arrest. However, preventing a heart attack in the first place is even more effective—there is no substitute for prevention. Heart attacks are usually the result of disease of the heart and blood vessels. *Coronary heart disease* (CHD) is the leading cause of death for adults in the United States. It accounts for nearly 500,000 deaths each year.

CHD develops slowly. Deposits of *cholesterol*, a fatty substance made by the body and present in certain foods, build up on the inner walls of the arteries. As the arteries that carry blood to the heart get narrower, less oxygen-rich blood flows to the heart. This reduced oxygen supply to the heart can eventually cause a heart attack.

Although a heart attack may seem to strike suddenly, many people gradually put their hearts in danger from cardiovascular disease. Because cardiovascular disease develops slowly, people may not be aware of it for many years. Fortunately, it is possible to slow the progress of cardiovascular disease by making lifestyle changes.

Behavior that can harm the heart and blood vessels may begin in early childhood. Junk food, which is high in cholesterol and saturated fats but has little real nutritional value, can contribute to cardiovascular disease. Cigarette smoking also greatly contributes to cardiovascular disease and to other diseases.

There are many factors that increase a person's chances of developing cardiovascular disease. These are called risk factors. Some of them you cannot change. For instance, although more women than men die each year from cardiovascular disease in the United States, heart disease generally affects men at younger ages than it does women.

Besides gender, ethnicity also plays an important role in determining the risk for heart disease. African Americans and Native Americans in the United States have higher rates of heart disease than do other populations. A history of heart disease in your family also increases your risk.

ALTERING RISK FACTORS

Many risk factors can be altered, however. Cigarette smoking; uncontrolled diabetes, high blood cholesterol or high blood pressure; obesity; and lack of regular exercise all increase the risk of heart disease. When you combine one risk factor, such as smoking, with others, such as high blood pressure and lack of regular exercise, the risk of heart attack is much greater.

It is never too late to take steps to control risk factors, thereby improving your chances for living a long and healthy life. It is important to know how to perform CPR and use an AED. However, since the chances of surviving cardiac arrest are poor, the best way to deal with cardiac arrest is to be aware of risk factors and take steps to help prevent it, including exercise and quitting smoking.

UNIT
5
MEDICAL EMERGENCIES

14

Medical Emergencies

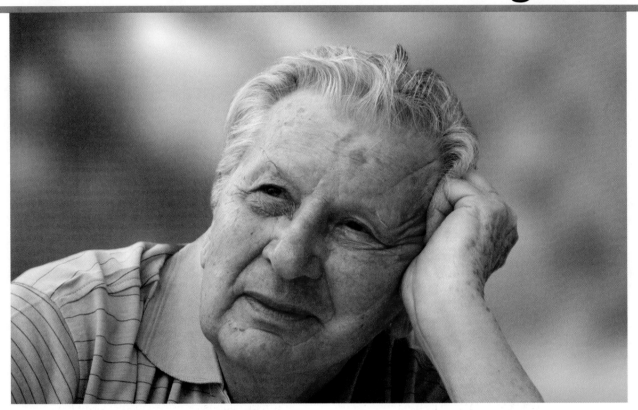

))) **YOU ARE THE EMERGENCY MEDICAL RESPONDER**

You are the *emergency medical responder* (EMR) responding to a scene on a downtown street involving a male who appears to be about 60 years old. He is confused and appears agitated. Several bystanders state that they saw the man wandering aimlessly and that he appeared to be lost. Upon interviewing the patient all you can learn is that his name is Earl. He does not seem to know where he is or where he is going. During your physical exam you note that the patient is sweating profusely but, other than his diminished *level of consciousness* (LOC), his vital signs are normal. More advanced medical personnel have been called. As an EMR, you want to provide proper care for the patient. What other information would help you to provide proper care? What should you do while waiting for advanced medical personnel?

Key Terms

Absence seizures: A type of generalized seizure in which there are minimal or no movements; patient may appear to have a blank stare; also known as petit mal or non-convulsive seizures.

Acute abdomen: The sudden onset of severe abdominal pain that may be related to one of many medical conditions or a specific injury to the abdomen.

Altered mental status: A disturbance in a patient's *level of consciousness* (LOC) including confusion and delirium; causes include injury, infection, poison, drug abuse and fluid/electrolyte imbalance.

Aneurysm: An abnormal bulging of an artery due to weakness in the blood vessel; may occur in the aorta (main artery of the heart), brain, leg or other location.

Aphasia: A disorder characterized by difficulty or inability to produce or understand language, caused by injury to the areas of the brain that control language.

Aura phase: The first stage of a generalized seizure, during which the patient experiences perceptual disturbances, often visual or olfactory in nature.

Blood glucose level (BGL): The level of glucose circulating in the blood; measured using a glucometer.

Clonic phase: The third phase of a generalized seizure, during which the patient experiences the seizure itself.

Complex partial seizures: A type of partial seizure in which the patient may experience an altered mental status or be unresponsive.

Diabetes: A disease in which there are high levels of blood glucose due to defects in insulin production, insulin action or both.

Diabetic coma: A life-threatening complication of diabetes in which very high blood sugar causes the patient to become unconscious.

Diabetic emergency: A situation in which a person becomes ill because of an imbalance of insulin and sugar in the bloodstream.

Diabetic ketoacidosis (DKA): An accumulation of organic acids and ketones (waste products) in the blood; occurs when there is inadequate insulin and high blood sugar levels.

Embolism: A blockage in an artery or a vein caused by a blood clot or fragment of plaque that travels through the blood vessels until it gets stuck, preventing blood flow.

Epilepsy: A brain disorder characterized by recurrent seizures.

Fainting: Temporary loss of consciousness; usually related to temporary insufficient blood flow to the brain; also known as *syncope,* "blacking out" or "passing out."

FAST: An acronym to help remember the symptoms of stroke; stands for **F**ace, **A**rm, **S**peech and **T**ime.

Febrile seizures: Seizure activity brought on by an excessively high fever in a young child or an infant.

Generalized tonic clonic seizures: Seizures that affect most or all of the brain; types include petit mal and grand mal seizures.

Gestational diabetes: A type of diabetes that occurs only during pregnancy.

Glucose: A simple sugar that is the primary source of energy for the body's tissues.

Grand mal seizures: A type of generalized seizure; involves whole body contractions with loss of consciousness.

Hemodialysis: A common method of treating advanced kidney failure in which blood is filtered outside the body to remove wastes and extra fluids.

Hyperglycemia: A condition in which too much sugar is in the bloodstream, resulting in higher than normal BGLs; also known as *high blood glucose.*

Hyperkalemia: Abnormally high levels of potassium in the blood; if extremely high, can cause cardiac arrest and death.

Hypervolemia: A condition in which there is an abnormal increase of fluid in the blood.

Hypoglycemia: A condition in which too little sugar is in the bloodstream, resulting in lower than normal BGLs; also known as *low blood glucose.*

Hypovolemia: A condition in which there is an abnormal decrease of fluid in the blood.

Hypoxemia: A condition in which there are decreased levels of oxygen in the blood; can disrupt the body's functioning and harm tissues; may be life threatening.

Insulin: A hormone produced by the pancreas to help glucose move into the cells; in patients with diabetes, it may not be produced at all or may not be produced in sufficient amounts.

Partial seizures: Seizures that affect only part of the brain; may be simple or complex.

Peritoneal dialysis: A method of treatment for kidney failure in which waste products and extra fluid are drawn into a solution which has been injected into the abdominal cavity and are withdrawn through a catheter.

Post-ictal phase: The final phase of a generalized seizure, during which the patient becomes extremely fatigued.

Seizure: A disorder in the brain's electrical activity, sometimes marked by loss of consciousness and often by uncontrollable muscle movement; also called a *convulsion*.

Sepsis: A life-threatening illness in which the body is overwhelmed by its response to infection; commonly referred to as *blood poisoning*.

Shunt: A surgically created passage between two natural body channels, such as an artery and a vein, to allow the flow of fluid.

Simple partial seizures: Seizures in which a specific body part experiences muscle contractions; does not affect memory or awareness.

Status epilepticus: An epileptic seizure (or repeated seizures) that lasts longer than 5 minutes without any sign of slowing down; should be considered life threatening and requires prompt advanced medical care.

Stroke: A disruption of blood flow to a part of the brain, which may cause permanent damage to brain tissue.

Syncope: A term used to describe the loss of consciousness; also known as fainting.

Thrombus: A blood clot that forms in a blood vessel and remains there, slowing the flow of blood and depriving tissues of normal blood flow and oxygen.

Tonic phase: The second phase of a generalized seizure, during which the patient becomes unconscious and muscles become rigid.

Transient ischemic attack (TIA): A condition that produces stroke-like symptoms but causes no permanent damage; may be a precursor to a stroke.

Type 1 diabetes: A type of diabetes in which the pancreas does not produce insulin; formerly known as *insulin-dependent diabetes* or *juvenile diabetes*.

Type 2 diabetes: A type of diabetes in which insufficient insulin is produced or the insulin is not used efficiently; formerly known as *non-insulin-dependent diabetes* or *adult-onset diabetes*.

Learning Objectives

After reading this chapter, and completing the class activities, you will have the information needed to—

- Identify a patient who has a general medical complaint.
- Describe the general care for a patient with a general medical complaint.
- Identify the signs and symptoms of an altered mental state.
- Describe the care for a patient who has an altered mental status.
- Describe the different types of seizures.
- Identify the signs and symptoms of seizures.
- Describe the care for a patient who has a seizure.
- Identify the signs and symptoms of a diabetic emergency.
- Describe the care for a patient who has a diabetic emergency.

- Identify the different causes of a stroke.
- Identify the signs and symptoms of stroke.
- Describe the care for a patient who has a stroke.
- Identify the signs and symptoms of abdominal pain.
- Describe the care for a patient who has abdominal pain.
- Describe the special considerations for a patient on hemodialysis.
- Identify various types of medications (*Enrichment skill*).
- Explain how to use a blood glucose meter (*Enrichment skill*).

INTRODUCTION

As an *emergency medical responder* (EMR), you could someday face a situation involving an unidentifiable medical emergency. Therefore, you may feel uncertain about how to provide care.

When you face an emergency that is unclear, it is normal to feel indecisive. Yet, like any EMR, you will still want to provide care to the best of your ability. You do not have to "diagnose" or choose among possible problems to provide appropriate care. By following a few basic guidelines for care, you can provide appropriate care until more advanced medical personnel arrive. Because you know these guidelines for care, you can approach any medical emergency with confidence.

Medical emergencies can develop rapidly (acute conditions) or gradually (chronic conditions) and may persist for a long time. Sometimes, there are no warning signs or symptoms to alert you or the patient that something is about to happen. At other times, the only symptoms the patient complains of are feeling "ill" or feeling that "something is wrong." Symptoms may also be atypical; older adults or those with **diabetes**, for example, may have a heart attack without experiencing chest pain.

Medical emergencies have a wide range of causes, including chronic problems from diseases such as heart disease and diabetes, allergies, **seizures** from illnesses such as **epilepsy** or overexposure to heat or cold. There can be a variety of signs and symptoms, including sudden, unexplained **altered mental status**. A patient may complain of feeling lightheaded, dizzy or weak. Or, the patient may feel nauseated or may vomit. Breathing, pulse and skin characteristics may change. Ultimately, if a person looks and feels ill, there could be a medical emergency that requires immediate care.

GENERAL MEDICAL COMPLAINTS
Making the Assessment and Providing Care

The assessment and care of general medical complaints follow the same general guidelines:
- Size-up the scene to ensure your own safety and the safety of others.
- Conduct your primary assessment to identify and correct any immediately life-threatening conditions.
- Conduct a SAMPLE history and secondary assessment to gather additional information, whenever possible.
- Summon more advanced medical personnel.
- Help the patient rest comfortably.
- Keep the patient from getting chilled or overheated.
- Provide reassurance.
- Prevent further harm.
- Administer emergency oxygen if it is available and indicated.

ALTERED MENTAL STATUS
Causes

Altered mental status can result from many causes. Some of these include the following:
- Fever
- Infection
- Poisoning or overdose, including substance abuse or misuse
- Blood sugar/endocrine emergencies
- Head injury
- Inadequate oxygenation or ventilation
- Any condition resulting in decreased blood flow or oxygen to the brain
- Cardiac emergencies
- Diabetic emergencies
- Shock
- **Stroke**
- Behavioral illness
- Seizures

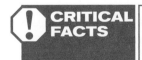 **CRITICAL FACTS** Medical emergencies have a wide range of causes, including chronic problems from diseases such as heart disease and diabetes, allergies, seizures from illnesses such as epilepsy or overexposure to heat or cold.

Signs and Symptoms of Altered Mental Status

Altered mental status is one of the most common medical emergencies. It is often characterized by a sudden or gradual change in a person's *level of consciousness* (LOC), including drowsiness, confusion and partial or complete loss of consciousness. Sometimes altered mental status is caused by a temporary reduction of blood flow to the brain, such as occurs when blood collects or pools in the legs and lower body. When the brain is suddenly deprived of its normal blood flow, it momentarily shuts down. This condition is called **fainting**, or **syncope**.

Fainting can be triggered by an emotional shock, such as the sight of blood. It may be caused by pain, specific medical conditions like heart disease, standing for a long time or overexertion. Some people, such as pregnant women or the elderly, are more likely to faint when suddenly changing positions, for example when moving from lying down to standing up. Whenever changes inside the body momentarily reduce the blood flow to the brain, fainting may occur.

A person may faint with or without warning. Often, the person may first feel lightheaded or dizzy. There may be signs of shock, such as pale or ashen, cool, moist skin. The person may feel nauseated and complain of numbness or tingling in the fingers and toes. The person's breathing and pulse may become faster.

Providing Care for Altered Mental Status

To care for patients with altered mental status, complete primary and secondary assessments and history as needed. Perform ongoing assessments as you provide care. Make sure the airway is open, and place an unconscious patient in the supine (face-up) position. Have suction equipment available if needed. If the patient is conscious or becomes conscious, do *not* give anything to eat or drink. Eating or drinking can increase the chance of vomiting. If possible, attempt to get information from the patient, family members or bystanders. This is important, as a patient's

condition may deteriorate rapidly in these situations, making conversation impossible. Any information you can obtain may help with the patient's treatment upon arrival at the hospital.

Sometimes a person may briefly faint and slowly begin to regain consciousness. Fainting often resolves itself when the patient moves from a standing or sitting position to a lying down position, as normal circulation to the brain often resumes. The patient usually regains consciousness within a minute.

Fainting itself does not usually harm the patient, but injury may occur from falling. Take spinal precautions if trauma is suspected. If you can reach a person who is starting to collapse, lower the patient to the ground or another flat surface and position the patient on his or her back, lying flat. Monitor the patient's breathing and pulse. Loosen any restrictive clothing, such as a tie or collar. Do not splash water on the patient's face. Doing so does little to stimulate the patient, and the patient could aspirate the water. Administer emergency oxygen if it is available.

Although a fainting patient usually recovers quickly, you may not be able to determine if the fainting is associated with a more serious medical condition. For this reason, more advanced medical care is indicated and the EMS system should be activated.

Pediatric Considerations

Altered Mental Status in Pediatrics

Children who are experiencing altered mental status may exhibit a change in behavior, personality or responsiveness beyond what is expected at their age. These children may exhibit anxiety, agitation, aggression and/or combativeness. Alternatively, they may be difficult to rouse, sleepy or even unresponsive. It is not unusual for altered mental status to result in decreased muscle tone.

Common causes of altered mental status requiring immediate medical attention include respiratory failure, deficiency in oxygen concentration in arterial blood (**hypoxemia**), shock, **hypoglycemia**, brain injury (including shaken baby syndrome), seizures, poisoning,

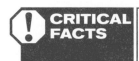 **CRITICAL FACTS** Altered mental status is a common medical emergency often characterized by a sudden or gradual change in a person's LOC, including drowsiness, confusion and partial or complete loss of consciousness.

intentional overdose, **sepsis**, meningitis, hyperthermia and hypothermia.

Left untreated, altered mental status can lead to life-threatening problems, including inefficient respiration, hypoxemia, airway obstruction and respiratory failure. For care of children with altered mental status, take spinal precautions if the cause is not clear or trauma is suspected. Treat any breathing emergency and care for any other injuries or conditions found. Obtain more advanced medical care and provide ongoing assessment and care.

SEIZURES

When the normal functions of the brain are disrupted by injury, disease, fever, infection, metabolic disturbances or conditions causing a decreased oxygen level, a seizure may occur. The seizure is a result of abnormal electrical activity in the brain and causes temporary involuntary changes in body movement, function, sensation, awareness or behavior.

Types of Seizures
Generalized Seizures

Generalized tonic clonic seizures, also called **grand mal seizures**, are the most well-known type of seizure. They involve both hemispheres (halves) of the brain and usually result in loss of consciousness. The seizure activity is known as tonic-clonic, which refers to the initial rigidity (tonic phase) followed by rhythmic muscle contractions (clonic phase), or *convulsions*. This type of seizure rarely lasts for more than a few minutes.

Signs and Symptoms of Generalized Seizures

Before a generalized seizure occurs, the patient may experience an unusual sensation or feeling called an aura. An aura can include a strange sound, taste, smell or an urgent need to get to safety. If the patient recognizes the aura, there may be time to warn bystanders and to sit or lie down before the seizure occurs.

Generalized seizures usually last 1 to 3 minutes and can produce a wide range of signs and symptoms. When a seizure occurs, the patient loses consciousness and can fall, causing injury. The patient may become rigid, and then experience sudden, uncontrollable muscular contractions (convulsions), lasting several minutes. Breathing may become irregular and even stop temporarily. The patient may drool and the eyes may roll upward. As the seizure subsides and the muscles relax the patient may have a loss of bladder or bowel control. The patient experiences sudden, uncontrollable muscular contractions (convulsions), lasting several minutes.

The stages of most generalized seizures are as follows:

1. **Aura phase**—patient may sense something unusual (not all patients will experience an aura)
2. **Tonic phase**—unconsciousness then muscle rigidity
3. **Clonic phase**—uncontrollable muscular contractions (convulsions)
4. **Post-ictal phase**—diminished responsiveness with gradual recovery and confusion (patient may feel confused and want to sleep)

Partial Seizures

Partial seizures may be simple or complex. They usually involve only a very small area of one hemisphere of the brain. Partial seizures are the most common type of seizure experienced by people with epilepsy. Partial seizures can spread and become a generalized seizure. In **simple partial seizures**, the patient usually remains aware. **Complex partial seizures** usually last for 1 to 2 minutes, though they may last longer and awareness is either impaired or lost while the patient remains conscious.

Signs and Symptoms of Partial Seizures

With simple partial seizures, the patient usually remains aware, but someone experiencing a complex partial seizure

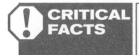

CRITICAL FACTS

A seizure is temporary abnormal electrical activity in the brain caused by injury, disease, fever, infection, metabolic disturbances or conditions that decrease oxygen levels.

Generalized seizures, also called grand mal seizures or tonic-clonic seizures, are the most easily recognized type of seizure.

experiences altered mental status or unresponsiveness.

In simple partial seizures, there may be involuntary, muscular contractions in one area of the body, for example the arm, leg or face. Some people cannot speak or move during a simple partial seizure, although they may remember everything that occurred. Simple partial seizures may produce a feeling of fear or a sense that something bad is about to happen. Simple partial seizures can also produce odd sensations such as strange smells or hearing voices. Rarely, feelings of anger and rage or joy and happiness can be brought on by the seizure. Auras are a form of simple partial seizure.

Complex partial seizures often begin with a blank stare followed by random movements such as smacking the lips or chewing. The patient appears dazed, the movements are clumsy and the patient's activities lack direction. They may be unable to follow directions or answer questions. This type of seizure usually lasts for only a few minutes but it may last longer. The patient cannot remember what happened after the seizure is over, and may be confused. This is called the post-ictal phase.

Absence (Petit Mal) Seizures

Individuals may also experience an **absence seizure**, also known as a petit mal seizure. These are most common in children. During an absence seizure, there is brief, sudden loss of awareness or conscious activity. There may be minimal or no movement and the person may appear to have a blank stare. Most often these seizures last only a few seconds.

Signs and Symptoms of Absence Seizures

Absence seizures cause the person to experience loss of awareness for short periods that may be mistaken for daydreaming. This type of seizure may also be referred to as a non-convulsive seizure, because the body remains relatively still during the episode, though eye fluttering and chewing movements may be seen.

Febrile Seizures

Young children and infants may be at risk for **febrile seizures**, which are seizures brought on by a rapid increase in body temperature. They are most common in children under the age of 5.

Febrile seizures are often caused by ear, throat or digestive system infections and are most likely to occur when a child or an infant runs a rectal temperature of over 102° F. An individual experiencing a febrile seizure may experience some or all of the following symptoms:

- Sudden rise in body temperature
- Change in LOC
- Rhythmic jerking of the head and limbs
- Loss of bladder or bowel control
- Confusion
- Drowsiness
- Crying out
- Becoming rigid
- Holding the breath
- Rolling the eyes upward

Epilepsy

Epilepsy is a common neurological disorder, estimated to affect approximately 3 million people in the United States alone. Epilepsy is not a specific disease but a term used to describe a group of disorders in which the individual experiences recurrent seizures as the main symptom. In about one third of all cases, seizures occur as a result of a brain abnormality or neurological disorder but, in two thirds, there is no known cause.

The risk of having epilepsy for young people (up to the age of 20) is approximately 1 percent, with the greatest likelihood occurring during the first year of life. People aged 20 to 55 may also develop epilepsy, but have a somewhat lower risk. The risk increases again after the age of 65, and in fact, the highest rate of new epilepsy diagnoses are in this age group. The prevalence of epilepsy, or the number of individuals suffering with it at any time, is estimated to be approximately 5 to 8 in every 1000 people. By age 75, approximately 3 percent of people will have been diagnosed with epilepsy.

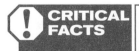 **CRITICAL FACTS** Young children and infants may be at risk for febrile seizures, which are seizures brought on by a rapid increase in body temperature.

People of any age can be affected by epilepsy. Patients who have epilepsy often can control the seizures with medication. Those with difficult to control seizures may also be treated with surgical resection which can be curative, or with implanted devices, such as the vagus nerve stimulator, that help reduce their seizure frequency. While some patients require life-long medical therapy, sometimes medication may be reduced or even eliminated over time. Some childhood epilepsies may resolve with age.

Providing Care for Seizures

Seeing someone have a seizure may be intimidating, but you can easily care for the patient. The patient cannot control any muscular contractions that may occur and it is important to allow the seizure to run its course, because attempting to stop it or restrain the patient can cause musculoskeletal injuries.

Protecting the patient from injury and managing the airway are your priorities when caring for a patient having a seizure. To help avoid injury, you should move nearby objects, such as furniture, away from the patient. People having seizures rarely bite the tongue or cheeks with enough force to cause any significant bleeding. Do *not* place anything in the mouth to prevent this type of injury. Foreign bodies in the mouth may cause airway obstruction. Do *not* put fingers into the mouth of an actively seizing patient to clear the airway. After the seizure passes, position the patient on his or her side, if possible, so that fluids (saliva, blood, vomit) can drain from the mouth.

In many cases, the seizure will be over by the time you arrive. In this case, the patient may be drowsy and disoriented; this is the post-ictal phase. Check to see if the patient was injured during the seizure. Offer comfort and reassurance, especially if the seizure occurred in public, as the patient may feel embarrassed and self-conscious. If this is the case, keep bystanders well back to provide maximum privacy and stay with the patient until he or she is fully conscious and aware of the surroundings.

Care for a child or an infant who experiences a febrile seizure is similar to the care for any other patient experiencing a seizure. Immediately after a febrile seizure, cool the body by removing excess clothing and giving the patient a sponge bath in *lukewarm* water. Ensure the water is lukewarm; cold water could lead to a rapid drop in body temperature, which could cause shivering and/or could cause stimulation of the nervous system, which could bring on another seizure. Rapid cooling with cold water could bring on other complications as well. Contact a health care provider before administering any medication, such as acetaminophen, to control fever. Do *not* give aspirin to a feverish child under 18 years of age or infant, as this has been linked to Reye's syndrome, an illness that affects the brain and other internal organs.

When to Call for More Advanced Medical Personnel

The patient will usually recover from a seizure in a few minutes. If you discover the patient has a medical history of seizures that is medically controlled, there may be no further need for medical attention. However, in the following cases, more advanced medical care should be provided:

- The seizure lasts more than 5 minutes or the patient has repeated seizures with no sign of slowing down (**status epilepticus**).
- The patient appears to be injured.
- You are uncertain about the cause of the seizure.
- The patient is pregnant.
- The patient is known to have diabetes.
- The patient is a child or an infant.
- The seizure takes place in water.
- The patient fails to regain consciousness after the seizure.
- The patient is a young child or an infant who experienced a febrile seizure brought on by a high fever.
- The patient is elderly and could have suffered a stroke.
- This is the patient's first seizure.

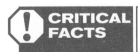 **CRITICAL FACTS** Protecting the patient from injury and managing the airway are your priorities when caring for a patient having a seizure.

Status epilepticus is an epileptic seizure (or repeated seizures) that lasts longer than 5 minutes without any sign of slowing down. A status epilepticus seizure is a true medical emergency that may be fatal. If you suspect the patient is experiencing this type of seizure, call for more advanced medical personnel immediately. If the seizure passes, place the patient on the side and suction, if possible. If the patient is having difficulty breathing, administer ventilations with a *bag-valve-mask resuscitator* (BVM), along with emergency oxygen.

DIABETIC EMERGENCIES
Incidence

Diabetes mellitus is one of the leading causes of death and disability in the United States today. As of 2005, 20.8 million Americans—7 percent of the population—currently had diabetes, and 1.5 million new cases were diagnosed in people ages 20 years or older in 2005. It is estimated that another 6.2 million people with the disease are undiagnosed.

Diabetes contributes to other conditions, including blindness, kidney disease, heart disease, periodontal (gum) disease and stroke.

Definition of Terms
Diabetes

There are two major types of diabetes. **Type 1 diabetes**, formerly known as *insulin-dependent diabetes* or *juvenile diabetes,* causes the body to produce little or no **insulin**. Most people who have Type 1 diabetes have to inject insulin into their bodies daily.

In **Type 2 diabetes**, formerly known as *non-insulin-dependent diabetes* or *adult-onset diabetes,* the body produces insulin, but either the cells do not use the insulin effectively or not enough insulin is produced. This type of diabetes is more common than Type 1 diabetes. Most people with Type 2 diabetes can regulate their ***blood glucose level*** (**BGL**) sufficiently through

diet, and sometimes through oral medications, without insulin injections.

People with diabetes must carefully monitor their BGL, diet and amount of exercise. People with diabetes must also regulate their use of insulin. When diet and exercise are not controlled, either of two problems can occur: too much or too little sugar in the body. This imbalance of sugar and insulin in the blood causes illness.

Some women develop diabetes in the late stages of pregnancy; this form usually goes away after the baby is born. This type is called **gestational diabetes** and is caused by the hormones of pregnancy or a shortage of insulin. Women who have had this condition have an increased likelihood of developing Type 2 diabetes later in life.

High Blood Glucose

When the insulin level in the body is too low, the sugar level in the blood is high. This condition is called **hyperglycemia (Fig. 14-1)**. Sugar is present in the blood but cannot be transported from the blood into the cells without insulin, causing body cells to become starved for sugar. The body attempts to meet its need for energy by using other stored food and energy sources, such as fats. However, converting fat to energy is less efficient, produces waste products and

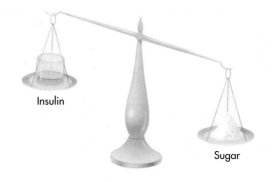

Insulin

Sugar

HYPERGLYCEMIA
>200 mg/dL

Fig. 14-1: A low insulin level results in high blood sugar, called hyperglycemia;. It can be life threatening if not quickly treated.

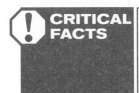
CRITICAL FACTS

Type 1 diabetes is characterized by the body's inability to produce insulin. Type 2 diabetes is characterized by the body's inability to use insulin effectively. Type 2 diabetes is more common.

Hypoglycemia and hyperglycemia have similar signs and symptoms, including changes in LOC, irregular breathing, abnormal pulse, feeling and looking ill and abnormal skin characteristics.

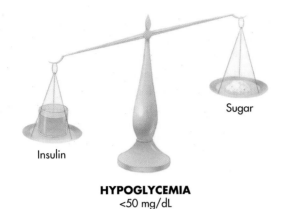

HYPOGLYCEMIA
<50 mg/dL

Fig. 14-2: A high insulin level results in low blood sugar, called hypoglycemia. Like hyperglycemia, it can be life threatening if not quickly treated.

increases the acidity level in the blood, causing a condition known as ***diabetic ketoacidosis*** (**DKA**). As this occurs, the person becomes ill. The patient may have flushed, hot, dry skin and a sweet breath odor that can be mistaken for the smell of alcohol. The patient may also appear restless or agitated, have abdominal pain or be thirsty. If this condition is not treated promptly, **diabetic coma**, a life-threatening emergency in which very high blood sugar causes the patient to become unconscious, can occur.

Low Blood Glucose

When the insulin level in the body is too high, the patient has a low sugar level, known as hypoglycemia (**Fig. 14-2**). The blood sugar level can become too low if the person with diabetes—

- Takes too much insulin.
- Fails to eat adequately.
- Over-exercises and burns off sugar faster than normal.
- Experiences great emotional stress.

In this situation, the small amount of sugar is used up rapidly, so not enough sugar is available for the brain to function properly. If left untreated, even for a short time, hypoglycemia from an insulin reaction can cause brain damage or death. Call for more advanced medical care immediately. This condition is also known as **insulin shock**.

Role of Glucose

To function normally, body cells need sugar as an energy source. Through the digestive process, the body breaks down food into simple sugars, such as **glucose**, which are absorbed into the bloodstream. However, sugar cannot pass freely from the blood into the body cells. Insulin, a hormone produced in the pancreas, is needed for sugar to pass into the cells. Without a proper balance of sugar and insulin in the blood, the cells will starve and the body will not function properly (**Fig. 14-3**).

Maintaining normal BGLs reduces the risk of eye, kidney, heart and nerve problems. Many people with diabetes have blood glucose monitors that can be used to check their BGL at home. Many hypoglycemic and hyperglycemic episodes are now managed at home because of the rapid information these monitors provide.

Signs and Symptoms of Diabetic Emergencies

Although hypoglycemia and hyperglycemia are different conditions, the major signs and symptoms are similar. These include—

- Changes in the LOC, including dizziness, drowsiness and confusion.
- Irregular breathing.
- Abnormal pulse (rapid or weak).
- Feeling and looking ill.
- Abnormal skin characteristics.

NORMAL

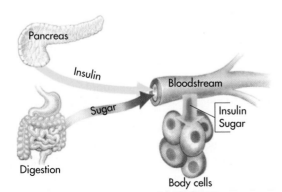

DIABETIC

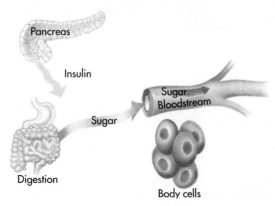

Fig. 14-3: The hormone insulin enables sugar in the bloodstream or stored forms of sugar to be used by the body cells for energy.

Providing Care for Diabetic Emergencies

To care for **diabetic emergencies**, first perform a primary assessment and care for any life-threatening conditions. If the patient is conscious, conduct a physical exam and SAMPLE history, looking for anything visibly wrong. Ask if the patient has diabetes, and look for a medical *identification* (ID) tag or bracelet. If the patient is known to have diabetes and exhibits the signs and symptoms previously stated, then suspect a **diabetic emergency**.

If the conscious patient can take food or fluids, give sugar preferably in the form of glucose tablets. Glucose paste, milk and most fruit juices (e.g., about 12 ounces of orange juice) and nondiet soft drinks have enough sugar to be effective. Common table sugar, either dry or dissolved in a glass of water, can restore the patient to a normal condition (**Fig. 14-4**).

Sometimes, patients with diabetes will be able to tell you what is wrong and will ask for something with sugar in it. If the patient's problem is low sugar (hypoglycemia), the sugar you give will help quickly. If the patient already has too much sugar (hyperglycemia), the excess sugar will do no further harm.

Do not try to assist the patient by administering insulin. Only give something by mouth if the patient is fully conscious. If the patient is unconscious, monitor the patient's condition, keep the patient from getting chilled or overheated, summon more advanced medical personnel and administer emergency oxygen if it is available. If the patient is conscious but does not feel better within approximately 5 minutes after taking sugar, summon more advanced medical personnel.

STROKE

A stroke, also called a *cerebrovascular accident* (CVA) or a *brain attack*, is a disruption of blood flow to a part of the brain, which may cause permanent damage to brain tissue if not appropriately treated within several hours.

Causes

Most commonly, a stroke is caused by a blood clot, called a **thrombus** or **embolism**, that forms or lodges in the arteries supplying blood to the brain (**Fig. 14-5**). Fat deposits lining an artery (atherosclerosis) may also cause a stroke known as an *ischemic stroke*.

Another less common cause of stroke is bleeding from a ruptured artery in the brain. Known as a *hemorrhagic stroke*, this condition is brought on by high blood pressure or an **aneurysm**—a weak area in an artery wall that balloons out and can rupture (**Fig. 14-6**). Less commonly, a tumor or swelling from a head injury may cause a stroke by compressing an artery.

A **transient ischemic attack (TIA)**, often referred to as a "mini-stroke," is a temporary episode that, like a stroke, is caused by reduced blood flow to a part of the brain. Unlike a stroke, the signs and symptoms of a TIA disappear within a few minutes or hours of its onset. If symptoms persist after 24 hours, the event is not considered a TIA but a stroke.

Although the indicators of TIA disappear quickly, the patient is not out of danger. In fact,

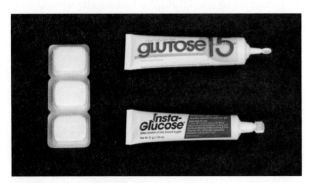

Fig. 14-4: Commercial oral glucose is available for fast administration of glucose to a diabetic.

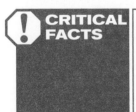

CRITICAL FACTS

Two causes of stroke are blood clots that form or lodge in arteries supplying blood to the brain and arteries in the brain that rupture and bleed. Blood clots are the most common cause of stroke.

A TIA, sometimes called a "mini-stroke," is caused by reduced blood flow to a part of the brain, but unlike a stroke its signs and symptoms disappear within a few minutes or hours of onset.

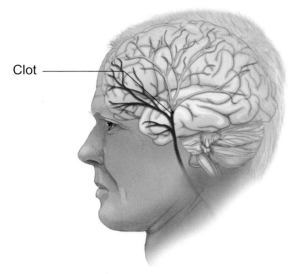

Fig. 14-5: Strokes are most commonly caused by a blood clot in the arteries that supply blood to the brain.

someone who experiences a TIA has a nearly 10 times greater chance of having a stroke in the future than does someone who has not experienced a TIA.

The risk factors for stroke and TIA are similar to those for heart disease. Some risk factors are beyond the patient's control, such as age, gender or family history of stroke, TIA, diabetes or heart disease. Others can be controlled, such as blood pressure, smoking, diet and exercise. Stroke is common in the geriatric population.

The Sudden Signs and Symptoms of Stroke

As with other sudden illnesses, looking or feeling ill or displaying abnormal behavior are common signs of a stroke or TIA. Other specific signs and symptoms of stroke come on *suddenly*, including—

- Weakness or numbness of the face, arm or leg, often on one side of the body (**Fig. 14-7, A**).
- Facial droop or drooling (**Fig. 14-7, B**).
- Difficulty with speech. The patient may have trouble talking, getting words out or being understood when speaking and may have trouble understanding (**aphasia**).
- Loss of vision or disturbed (blurred or dim) vision in one or both eyes; pupils of the eyes may be of unequal size.
- Sudden severe headache (unexplained and often described as the worst headache ever).
- Dizziness, confusion, agitation, loss of consciousness or other severe altered mental status.
- Loss of balance or coordination, trouble walking or ringing in the ears.
- Incontinence.

Stroke Alert Criteria

Two common stroke assessment scales used in the prehospital setting are the Cincinnati Prehospital

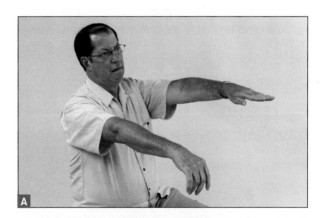

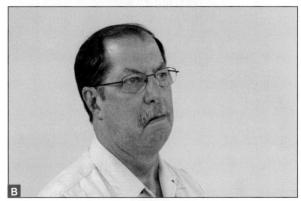

Fig. 14-7, A–B: **(A)** Weakness or numbness of an arm or leg and **(B)** sudden facial droop or drooling, often on one side of the body, are signs and symptoms of a stroke.

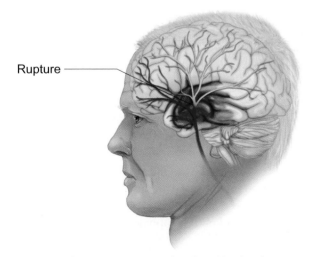

Fig. 14-6: A less common cause of stroke is bleeding from a ruptured artery in the brain.

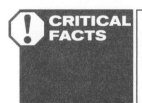
As the common mnemonic for stroke identification, FAST stands for **F**ace, **A**rm, **S**peech and **T**ime. Facial drooping, arm weakness and slurred speech are distinctive symptoms, and timely advanced medical care is critical.

Modern stroke medication and medical procedures can limit the damage caused by stroke, but timely administration is crucial to reduce the effects of stroke to the brain.

Stroke Scale and the *Los Angeles Prehospital Stroke Screen* (LAPSS), which assess facial droop, arm drift and speech. Both scales should be included in your assessment of the stroke patient and reported to the medical facility. A *Glasgow Coma Score* (GCS) also should be obtained on the patient (see **Chapter 7** for further information). Collecting and reporting this information will help ensure the required management of the stroke patient.

FAST

The **FAST** mnemonic is based on the Cincinnati Prehospital Stroke Scale, which was originally developed for EMS workers in 1997. The scale was designed to help paramedics identify strokes in the field, so that the emergency room can be prepared before the paramedics arrive. The FAST method for public awareness has been in use in the community of Cincinnati, Ohio since 1999, and has since been used in several other variations of the message. It was validated by researchers at the University of North Carolina in 2003.

FAST stands for the following:

- Face: Ask the person to smile. Does one side of the face droop?
- Arm: Ask the person to raise both arms. Does one arm drift downward?
- Speech: Ask the person to repeat a simple sentence. Are the words slurred? Can the person repeat the sentence correctly?
- Time: Try to determine the time of onset of symptoms. If the person shows any signs or symptoms of stroke, time is critical. Immediate transport by more advanced medical care is necessary.

LAPSS

The LAPSS mnemonic is another common one-page tool designed to help prehospital personnel rapidly identify strokes in the field.

Providing Care for Stroke

If the patient is unconscious, ensure that the airway is open, and care for any life-threatening conditions. If fluid or vomit is in the unresponsive patient's mouth, position the patient on one side to allow any fluids to drain out of the mouth. You may have to remove some fluids or vomit from the patient's mouth using a finger or suctioning equipment.

Stay with the patient and monitor his or her condition. If the patient is conscious, check for non-life-threatening conditions. A stroke can make the patient fearful and anxious due to not understanding what has happened. Offer comfort and reassurance and have the patient rest in a comfortable position. Do *not* give anything to eat or drink. Although a stroke patient may find it difficult to speak, the patient may understand what you say. If the patient is unable to speak, you may have to use nonverbal forms of communication, such as hand squeezing or eye blinking (once for yes, twice for no) and communicate in ways that require a yes-or-no response.

In the past, a stroke almost always caused irreversible brain damage. Today, new medications and medical procedures can limit or reduce the damage caused by stroke. Many of these new treatments are time-sensitive; therefore, you should immediately call for more advanced medical personnel to get the best care for the patient. It is very important to interview the patient, family members and bystanders to determine the time of the onset of symptoms and to transport the patient to an appropriate receiving facility immediately.

ABDOMINAL PAIN

Abdominal pain is felt between the chest and groin, which is commonly referred to as the stomach region or belly. There are many organs in the abdomen, so when a patient is suffering from abdominal pain it can originate from any one of them. These include digestive organs such as the inferior end of the esophagus, stomach, small and large intestines, liver, gallbladder, pancreas, aorta, appendix, kidneys and spleen. Abdominal emergencies can be life threatening and require

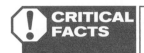
immediate care to prevent shock, so they should always be treated seriously. A sudden onset of abdominal pain is called **acute abdomen**.

Causes

Abdominal pain can be difficult to pinpoint, as the pain may start from somewhere else and could be a result of any number of generalized infections including the flu or strep throat.

The intensity of the pain does not always reflect the seriousness of the condition. Severe abdominal pain can be from mild conditions, such as intestinal gas, whereas relatively mild pain or no pain may be present with life-threatening conditions such as early appendicitis.

Signs and Symptoms of Abdominal Pain

If you are called to see a patient who is experiencing abdominal pain, assume the pain is serious, as the patient or family members were concerned enough to seek emergency medical attention. Patients suffering from abdominal pain may show the following signs and symptoms:

- Colicky pain or cramps that come in waves
- Abdominal tenderness, local or diffuse (spread out)
- Guarded position
- Anxiety
- A reluctance to move, for fear of pain
- Loss of appetite
- Nausea or vomiting
- Fever
- Rigid, tense or distended stomach
- Signs of shock
- Vomiting blood with a red or brownish appearance
- Blood in the stool, appearing red or black
- Rapid pulse
- Blood pressure changes

When conducting an assessment, monitor the patient's movements. Take note if the patient is restless or quiet and if the patient feels pain when moving. Check to see if the abdomen is distended and, if possible, confirm with the patient whether

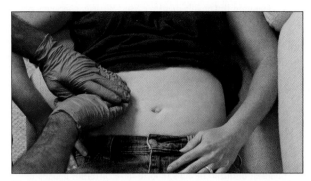

Fig. 14-8: When assessing abdominal pain in a patient, palpate the stomach to determine if it is rigid or soft.

the appearance of the stomach is normal. See if the patient is able to relax the abdomen, and palpate the stomach to determine if it is rigid or soft (**Fig. 14-8**). Examine the area the patient indicates as the location of the pain *last*. Do *not* overpalpate, as this can aggravate the condition as well as cause more pain.

Providing Care for Abdominal Pain

First, ensure the patient has an open airway. Call for transport to a medical facility. In the case of abdominal pain, it is important to watch for signs of potential aspiration due to vomiting. In cases in which the patient is experiencing nausea, place the patient on the side if it is not too painful. Do *not* give the patient food, water or medication. Watch for signs of shock. If vital signs and other observations indicate the patient is in shock, place the patient on the back, maintain normal body temperature and administer emergency oxygen if available.

Pediatric Considerations

Abdominal Pain

Abdominal pain in children can indicate a vast range of conditions. A sudden or progressive onset of pain, excessive vomiting or diarrhea, blood noted in vomit or stool, abdominal distention, high blood sugar, altered mental status and abnormal vital signs are all signs the child could be suffering from a serious condition or illness. Vomiting and diarrhea in children are significant symptoms as they may cause dehydration and shock.

To assess a child complaining of abdominal pain, take the following steps:

- Obtain a first impression of the child's appearance, breathing and circulation to determine urgency.
- Evaluate the child's mental status, airway, adequacy of breathing and circulation.
- Take the child's history and perform a hands-on physical examination noting any injury, hemorrhage, discoloration, distention, rigidity, guarding or tenderness within the four abdominal quadrants.
- If a life-threatening condition is noted, provide immediate treatment before continuing.

Children of different ages tend to have different causes of pain. Causes in an infant can include colic, allergy to cow's milk, reflux esophagitis, volvulus (bowel obstruction) or Hirschsprung's Disease (congenital disease affecting the large intestine). In school-age children, the most frequent cause of abdominal pain is gastroenteritis or "stomach flu," which may result in significant fluid loss. Also common is the ingestion of toxic substances or food poisoning.

In adolescents, growth, development and fertility issues can cause problems such as testicular torsion (twisting of the testicles), ovarian cysts, pelvic inflammatory disease, ectopic pregnancy (pregnancy that occurs outside the womb), inflammatory bowel disease, ulcerative colitis, Crohn's disease, DKA, pneumonia and sickle cell anemia.

Geriatric Considerations

Abdominal Pain

Understanding that elderly patients may experience vague symptoms and have non-specific findings on examination is important. Keep in mind that abdominal pain may actually be caused by a heart attack or other medical conditions. Many elderly patients may have much less severe pain than expected for a particular illness or disease, which can lead to elderly patients with serious conditions being misdiagnosed with less serious conditions such as gastroenteritis or constipation. Vomiting and diarrhea are significant symptoms in geriatric patients, as they can cause dehydration and shock.

Causes of abdominal pain in elderly patients may include biliary tract disease, appendicitis, diverticulitis, mesenteric ischemia (reduced blood flow to the small intestines), bowel obstruction, abdominal aortic aneurysm, peptic ulcer disease, malignancy and gastroenteritis.

Common Abdominal Emergencies

Many different conditions can cause abdominal pain, including inflammation of the appendix (appendicitis), bowel obstruction, inflammation of the gallbladder, abdominal aortic aneurysm, diverticular disease, shingles, food allergies, food poisoning, gastroenteritis and others. Consider the situation an emergency when the abdominal pain restricts activity.

HEMODIALYSIS

People with advanced renal failure, or kidney failure, often need dialysis to filter waste products from the blood using a special filtering solution. There are two types of dialysis: **peritoneal dialysis**, which injects a solution through the abdominal wall and then withdraws it after a period of time, and **hemodialysis**, which uses a machine to clean waste products from the blood. Dialysis is often used on patients with renal disease while they are waiting for a kidney transplant.

Complications of dialysis include hypotension (abnormally low blood pressure), disequilibrium syndrome (a reduction of the blood urea level relative to the levels found in brain tissues), hemorrhage (abdominal, *gastrointestinal* [GI] and intracranial bleeding), introduction of an air embolus or other foreign body into the patient's circulatory system due to equipment malfunction, and complications caused by temporarily stopping a patient's medications during the dialysis process.

Special Considerations for Hemodialysis Patients

The following details should be considered when taking a history and physical exam with a patient who has renal failure:

- A comprehensive history should include information about past dialysis and complications; recent salt, potassium and fluid

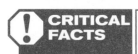
CRITICAL FACTS People with advanced renal failure, or kidney failure, often need dialysis to filter waste products from the blood using a special filtering solution.

intake; information about the current dialysis session and the patient's dry weight and how much fluid was removed before the session was terminated.

- The general physical assessment should include fluid status, mental status, cardiac rhythm and **shunt** location.

Note: Shunts in the arm are common in long-term hemodialysis patients. If an active shunt is located in the patient's arm, *do not* take blood pressure using that arm. Old, nonfunctional shunts are not uncommon, and blood pressure can be taken on an arm with a nonfunctional shunt. Ask the patient about active and nonfunctional shunt locations when taking a history. Shunts can also be potential sites of infection and/or blockage.

- Pay attention for associated medical problems such as arrhythmias, internal bleeding, hypoglycemia, altered mental status and seizures.
- Be aware that, after dialysis, patients may have **hypovolemia** (reduced blood volume) and exhibit cold, clammy skin; poor skin turgor (elasticity); tachycardia; and hypotension. Delayed dialysis patients will have **hypervolemia** (increased blood volume) and may have abnormal lung sounds such as crackles, generalized edema, hypertension or jugular venous distension.
- Be alert for altered mental status.
- Be sure to assess cardiac rhythm.

Life-Threatening Emergencies Associated With Dialysis Patients

Patients on dialysis can experience several types of complications, for example uremia (accumulation of urinary waste products in the blood), fluid overload (reduction in the body's ability to excrete fluid through urine), anemia (hemoglobin deficiency), hypertension, **hyperkalemia** (excess potassium in the blood) and coronary artery disease. Emergencies also can occur as complications of the dialysis itself, including hypotension, disequilibrium syndrome, hemorrhage, equipment malfunction (e.g. introducing an air embolus or other foreign body into the circulatory system) or complications from being temporarily removed from medications.

PUTTING IT ALL TOGETHER

As is true of all emergencies, a medical emergency can strike anyone, at any time. The signs and symptoms for each of the medical emergencies described in this chapter, such as changes in LOC, sweating, confusion, weakness and appearing ill, will indicate the necessary initial care you should provide.

In most cases involving a medical emergency, your biggest challenge is that you may not know the cause. In the case of a diabetic emergency, seizure, stroke and fainting, the causes may be easier to ascertain. However, you can provide proper care without knowing the exact cause, allowing the patient to remain as comfortable and safe as possible until arrival at a medical facility. You can also recognize the dangers and complications of dealing with those with diabetes or renal failure. And you have learned the importance of age considerations in many conditions, such as abdominal pain and seizure.

Performing a proper assessment and following the general guidelines of care for any emergency will help prevent the condition from becoming worse. While it is not your role to diagnose the problem, it is your job to provide initial care to the patient until a proper diagnosis can be made.

))) YOU ARE THE EMERGENCY MEDICAL RESPONDER

As you continue monitoring the patient, he becomes even more confused and agitated. You begin to notice signs of shock. As an EMR, what should you do while awaiting EMS personnel?

Enrichment
Basic Pharmacology

COMMON FORMS OF MEDICATION

Emergency medical responders (EMRs) are often called upon to help give or administer medications. These medications come in several types and forms, including tablets, capsules, powders, liquids, creams and aerosol sprays. They also have a range of options regarding how they are administered and the doses used in a given circumstance.

BASIC MEDICATION TERMINOLOGY

Drug Name

Upon initial discovery, a drug is given a chemical name based on its chemical properties. It is then given a generic, or non-proprietary name, usually a shorter version of the chemical name. This is the name used for the *Food and Drug Administration* (FDA) approval application. Drugs are also given a brand or trade name, which is used in marketing. It may or may not sound like the generic name, depending on the complexity of the generic name and the drug's purpose. For example, with a chemical name of N-acetyl-*p*-aminophenol, the generic name of this drug is acetaminophen and the trade name is Tylenol®.

Drug Profile

A drug's profile is a description of what it does, what it is or is not given for and any issues that may develop as a result of taking it.

* Actions: The action of a medication is what it does. If you are administering a drug, you should know how the drug works. For example, does the medication dilate the blood vessels (vasodilator) to lower blood pressure?
* Indications: The indication of a drug is the intended use for a specific condition. Why is the drug given? What are you trying to achieve? For example, the indication for nitroglycerin would be for chest pain or angina.
* Contraindications: Not everyone can take every medication. Contraindications are the conditions in which you would not administer a drug to a patient. This could be because the patient has a medical condition that would be worsened by administration of the drug, because of adverse interactions with other medications or because the patient may be allergic to the medication. For example, it would be contraindicated to give morphine to a patient who is allergic to it, or to give a medication with a known effect of hypotension (lowering blood pressure) to a patient whose blood pressure is already low.
* Side effects: Side effects are reactions caused by the drug that were not intended. Side effects may or may not cause problems. If they do cause problems, these are called adverse effects, adverse reactions or untoward effects. These are the effects you must watch for when administering medications such as nitroglycerin. Nitroglycerin works by dilating the blood vessels, but it can cause the sudden and possibly harmful side effect of lowering blood pressure.
* Dose: The usual dose is a range of an acceptable amount of the medication, given the patient's age, weight and reason for giving the drug. There are also times when the patient's gender must be taken into account. Administering an overdose, or too much of a drug, can result in severe, sometimes fatal, consequences. Administering too little of a drug may cause the problem to worsen, because the drug will not have the desired effect on the patient.
* Route: You must know by which route a drug is to be given. Some medications can be given in different ways; for example, by injection or intravenously. However, there is a significant difference in the dose given by each route. If a patient receives a dose intravenously that was intended to be delivered by injection, this could result in death.

Prescribing Information

Medication prescriptions must contain the following information:
* Pharmacy's name and address
* Prescription's serial number

- Date of the prescription (initial filling or refill date)
- Prescriber's name
- Patient's name
- Directions for use, including any precautions
- Medication name and strength
- Federal law inscription on transfer of drugs

Medication prescriptions also commonly contain the following additional information:
- Patient's address
- Pharmacist's initials or name
- Pharmacy's telephone number
- Manufacturer's lot number
- Drug's expiration date
- Manufacturer's or distributor's name
- Quantity of medication dispensed
- Number of refills remaining

Routes of Administration

Medications can be given in many ways, including the following:
- By mouth: Many medications, such as tablets, capsules, powders and liquids may be given by mouth to be absorbed by the stomach and intestines. The amount of time it takes for them to become effective can vary considerably. The patient must be responsive enough to follow directions to swallow and able to swallow.
- Sublingually: These medications dissolve under the tongue and are absorbed into the bloodstream through the mucous membrane.
- By inhalation: Some medications are inhaled (i.e., through mouth, nose or tracheotomy) directly into the lungs. These are usually medications for respiratory illnesses like asthma. Oxygen, which is inhaled, is also considered a medication.
- By injection: These medications are usually administered by a licensed health-care professional or by a caregiver. They can be given straight into the muscle or under the skin, depending on the product.
- Topically: Topical medications are given by patch or gel and absorbed by the skin. EMRs must be careful when encountering a patch on a patient's skin, as the medication could be absorbed by the responder when trying to remove the patch.
- Intravenously: Medications given intravenously must be administered by a licensed health-care professional. It is one of the quickest ways to deliver fluids and medications, as substances are directly transmitted to the veins.
- Vaginally: Some creams and suppositories must be given vaginally.
- Rectally: Many medications are available in rectal suppository format.

ADMINISTERING MEDICATIONS OVERVIEW

The "Rights" of Drug Administration

Health care personnel who administer medication follow a concept called the "Five Rights." These help ensure the medication is being given correctly.
- Right patient: If administering a patient's own medication, you must ensure it truly is the patient's medication. Check the label for the correct name. An exception may be if medical direction calls for a medication that is available but does not belong to the patient. If you are administering a stock medication (one that is kept on hand until needed), you must understand the action and effects to be sure that it is right for this patient.
- Right medication: When reaching for a medication, read the label properly and ensure that the medication in the bottle is what the label says it is. If in doubt, do not give it. If you are reaching for a stock medication, read the label as you remove it from your stock, while you remove the medication from the container and again as you give it to the patient.

Continued on next page

Enrichment
Basic Pharmacology (continued)

- Right route: Be sure you are administering the drug as prescribed. You may find a prescription for a drug given by a route with which you are not familiar. When in doubt, double check.
- Right dose: Double check the dosage of the drugs you give to patients. Some medications vary considerably in dose between patients.
- Right date: Medications have expiration dates. This is the first day of the month listed, unless otherwise specified. Do not give expired drugs.

Administration of Versus Assistance with Medication

Administering a medication means you are physically giving the medication to the patient. In some situations, the patient is able to take medication alone, such as by a metered-dose inhaler (MDI) for a respiratory emergency **(Fig. 14-9, A–B)**. In this case, you may assist by helping get the medication ready and perhaps holding the inhaler while the patient presses the pump. Always follow medical direction, regulations and local protocols regarding your role in assisting patients with medications.

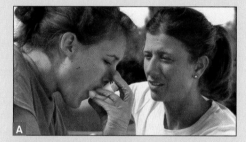

Administration Routes

You may only administer medications by routes you have been licensed or authorized to administer. Generally, for EMRs, this is by inhalation, orally or sublingually (under the tongue). There may be regulatory exceptions regarding EMR use of auto-injectors for anaphylaxis and inhalers for asthma. Check local protocols and medical direction to know the medications that you can deliver.

Reassessment

After administering a drug, you must always assess the effect. You will need to watch for—
- Signs and symptoms of the original problem.
- Improvement or deterioration in the patient's condition, including the following:
  - Mental status
  - Respiratory status
  - Pulse rate and quality
  - Blood pressure
  - Skin color, temperature and condition
  - Adverse effects

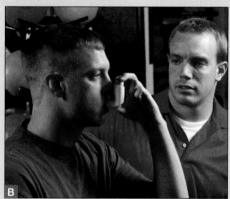

Fig. 14-9, A–B: To administer medication, **(A)** physically give it to the patient. **(B)** When assisting, help get the medication ready and assist the patient in taking it, but do not physically administer it.

Documentation

Any time a drug is administered, from a patient's supply or from your stock, this must be documented thoroughly. You must document: 1) the reason for administration, 2) drug name, 3) dose, 4) route of administration, 5) time(s) of administration, 6) any side effects noted, 7) how often administered and 8) any improvement noted and any changes in the patient's status.

Role of Medical Oversight in Medical Administration

Medical direction, the oversight provided by a physician who assumes responsibility for care, provides direction on what medication to give, as well as the dose, route of administration and how often it is given. When receiving medical direction, you must repeat back the order for confirmation even if you are sure you understood correctly **(Fig. 14-10)**.

ADMINISTERING ASPIRIN

Generic and Trade Names

Aspirin was the original trade name of acetylsalicylic acid (ASA). It is now marketed under several trade names, such as Ecotrin® Enteric Coated Aspirin, Excedrin® (which also contains acetaminophen), Pravigard® and St. Joseph® **(Fig. 14-11)**. In countries where aspirin is trademarked (owned by Bayer), the term ASA is the generic name.

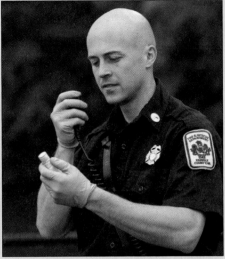

Fig. 14-10: When receiving medical direction from a physician, always repeat back the order for confirmation.

Indications

Aspirin, or ASA, was originally an analgesic, which is a type of pain reliever. However, today health care providers often use it for its blood-thinning capability to prevent blood clots. Aspirin is used to provide relief for mild-to-moderate pain, including headache, menstrual pain, muscle pain, minor pain of arthritis and toothache. It also reduces fever and inflammation. Aspirin may also be given for angina and heart attack (see **Chapter 13** for more information on aspirin and heart attacks). A health care provider should be consulted before using aspirin to treat or prevent any cardiovascular condition.

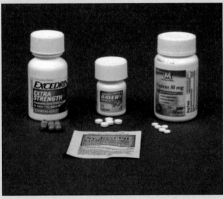

Fig. 14-11: Aspirin

Contraindications

Patients already on blood thinners should not take aspirin. It should not be given to patients who have a known allergy to non-steroidal anti-inflammatory drugs (NSAIDs). Because of the rare complication of Reye's Syndrome, children and adolescents who show flu-like symptoms or who may have a viral illness such as chicken pox should not be given aspirin or products that contain aspirin. Women who are pregnant or nursing should avoid taking aspirin unless they are instructed to by their health care provider. Patients with asthma, ulcer or ulcer symptoms; a recent history of stomach or intestinal bleeding; or a bleeding disorder, such as hemophilia, should not take aspirin. Aspirin will not prevent hemorrhagic strokes and should not be given to someone showing signs and symptoms of a stroke.

Actions

Aspirin acts to thin the blood by reducing the platelets' ability to produce a chemical that helps form blood clots. To relieve pain, aspirin reduces inflammation at the source, thereby reducing the pain.

Side Effects

The majority of side effects and complications associated with aspirin are due to taking too much of the medication or from taking it for too long a period. However, side effects can occur with just a few doses in some people. The most common side effects include heartburn, nausea, vomiting and gastrointestinal bleeding. Some people are allergic to aspirin, so it is important to watch for an allergic reaction to the medication.

Continued on next page

Enrichment
Basic Pharmacology (continued)

Expiration Date

It is important not to administer aspirin past its expiration date. The effect of the drug decreases if it is too old. Therefore, by giving a dose of expired aspirin, you will not know how much of the drug the patient will actually receive. Do not use the aspirin if there is a strong smell of vinegar as this may indicate the medication is expired.

Dosage

The dosages for pain relief and for blood thinning differ. The average adult dose for minor pain and fever relief is one to two 325 milligram (mg) tablets about every 3 to 4 hours, not to exceed 6 doses a day. For the prevention of a heart attack, the average adult dose is one 81 mg/low dose tablet daily.

A health care provider may recommend a stronger dosage of aspirin. Follow local protocols and medical direction before giving aspirin to treat or prevent cardiovascular conditions.

Administration

Aspirin is most commonly available in oral form; however, it is also available as a rectal suppository and in a liquid form for children.

ADMINISTERING NITROGLYCERIN
Generic and Trade Names

Nitroglycerin is the generic name for Nitrolingual® Pump Spray, Nitrostat® Tablets and the Minitran® Transdermal Delivery System. It is also available by the generic name.

Indications

Nitroglycerin is given to patients with angina pectoris, a condition in which the blood vessels in the heart constrict and do not allow enough blood and oxygen to circulate. This, in turn, causes chest pain.

Contraindications

Nitroglycerin should not be given to patients whose systolic blood pressure is below 90 mm/Hg. Also, it should not be given more often than prescribed (usually one to three times is indicated, with 5 minutes spaced between doses). Do not give nitroglycerin to patients taking sildenafil (Viagra®), as this could lead to life-threatening complications such as a dangerous drop in blood pressure. Nitroglycerin should not be given to individuals who have severe anemia or a brain injury, hemorrhage or tumor. Nitroglycerin may be harmful to an unborn baby.

Actions

Nitroglycerin dilates the blood vessels, allowing blood to flow more freely, thus providing more oxygen to the heart tissue.

Side Effects

Rapid dilation of the blood vessels can cause a severe and sudden headache. The headaches may become gradually less severe as the individual continues to take nitroglycerin. Other side effects may include dizziness, flushed skin of the neck and face, lightheadedness and worsened angina pain.

Precautions

Nitroglycerin tablets are reactive to light and should be stored in a dry area in a dark-colored container to maintain their potency.

Expiration Date

Check expiration dates for all types of nitroglycerin. Failure to do so may result in administering medication that is no longer active, thereby delaying proper treatment.

Dosage and Administration

Nitroglycerin sprays and tablets are usually administered as one spray or pill under the tongue, and can be taken by the patient up to three times, with 5 minutes between each dose, if there is no change in his or her condition. Have the patient sit while taking nitroglycerin as it can cause dizziness or fainting. Nitroglycerin is a very potent medication. It should never be given without a health care provider's order.

ADMINISTERING ORAL GLUCOSE

Action

Oral glucose acts by increasing the amount of blood glucose (sugar) in the bloodstream.

Indication

Oral glucose is administered to patients who have diabetes and whose blood sugar level has dropped below tolerable levels **(Fig. 14-12)**. At this point, the insulin has no glucose to metabolize.

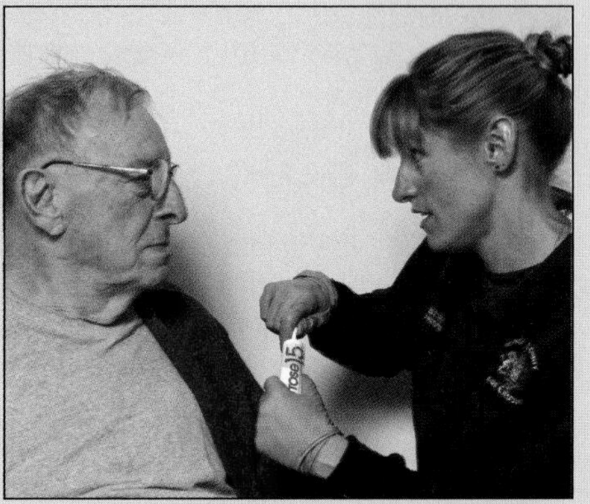

Contraindications

Oral glucose should not be given to patients with diabetes whose blood sugar is within normal range or above normal range. It also should not be given to patients who are unresponsive and unable to follow instructions to swallow safely.

Fig. 14-12: Administer oral glucose to patients with diabetes whose blood sugar has dropped below tolerable levels.

Side Effects

Side effects may include nausea, heartburn and bloating.

Dose

The product comes as glucose tablets and in 15-gram, single-use tubes.

Route

Oral glucose is given by mouth.

Enrichment
Blood Glucose Monitoring

Blood glucose monitoring refers to the measurement of blood sugar (glucose). Everyone's blood has some glucose in it because our bodies turn the food we eat into this form of sugar, which is transported throughout the body. Insulin, a hormone from the pancreas, helps get the glucose into our cells to be used for energy. Without insulin (e.g., in patients with Type 2 diabetes), the BGL rises, leading to long-term health complications if untreated. In patients taking insulin, low blood glucose creates critical health risks and must be treated immediately.

TESTING BGL WITH A GLUCOSE METER

Patients with diabetes check their BGLs regularly, often using a portable device called a *glucometer* **(Fig. 14-13)**. Monitoring can be done at any time using a glucometer. The test requires a drop of blood on a test strip containing a chemical substance, which is then inserted into the glucometer. The drop of blood is obtained by piercing the skin of a finger pad with a sharp sterile device such as a lancet or needle.

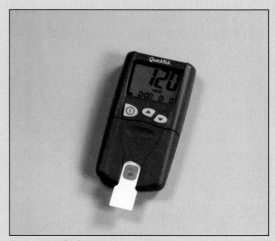

Fig. 14-13: A glucometer

USING A GLUCOMETER

- Ensure your hands are clean and the glucometer is in good working order.
- Wipe the pad of the patient's finger with an alcohol swab, or clean the finger with soap and water. Allow the skin to dry completely.
- Using a sterile lancet, prick the pad of the finger and allow a blood drop to form.
- Collect a drop of blood on the test strip.
- Insert the test strip into the glucometer, read and record the numerical result.

Read the owner's manual for the blood glucose meter carefully, and *only use the test strips specified for that meter.* Otherwise, the device may fail to give results or may generate an inaccurate reading.

What the Numbers Mean

Although the result may vary depending upon the patient and the testing device used, it is generally accepted that the normal range before meals is 90–130 *milligrams per deciliter* (mg/dL) and after meals is less than 180 mg/dL.

Low blood glucose, also called hypoglycemia, occurs when the BGL drops below 70 mg/dL. This requires immediate treatment. If the patient is conscious, provide 4 ounces of fruit juice or regular soft drink or 2–5 glucose tablets, and recheck glucose in 15 minutes. If the patient is unconscious, seek medical attention immediately.

Pediatric Considerations

Blood Glucose Monitoring

The *American Diabetes Association* (ADA) warns of the problems that could be caused by blood sugar levels that are too low in children under 7 years of age. Young children require higher blood sugar levels than do adults for brain development. Also, children's food intake and activity level tend to vary quite a bit from day to day, causing blood sugar levels to fluctuate, so they are more at risk of blood sugar levels falling too low. Further, it may be difficult for very young children to report and describe symptoms of low blood sugar, so this may go undetected.

Also keep in mind that, before reaching puberty, children seem to be at lower risk of the complications of diabetes even when blood sugar levels are abnormally high. The ADA recommends aiming for the safe adult range of BGL only when children grow older and can recognize the early symptoms of BGLs dropping too low.

15 Poisoning

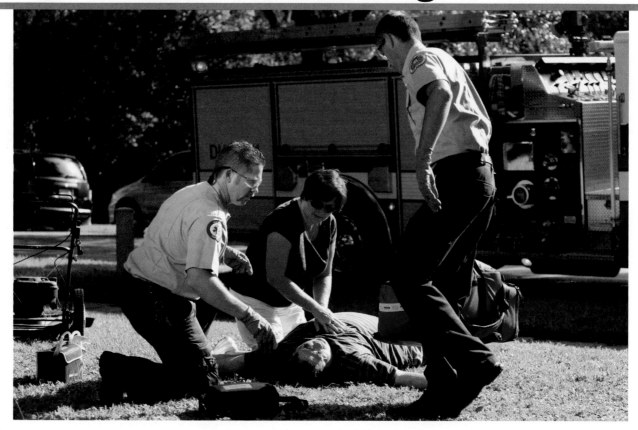

))) YOU ARE THE EMERGENCY MEDICAL RESPONDER

Your *emergency medical services* (EMS) unit is summoned to a residence on a report of an unconscious person. When you arrive and size-up the scene, you discover an older couple. The wife is distraught and says that her husband had been drinking alcoholic beverages heavily earlier in the day. Shortly after taking his prescribed Valium®, she says he became drowsy and incoherent, and then collapsed. Unable to get him to respond, she called 9-1-1. On assessing the patient, you find that he is unresponsive, his breathing is shallow and slow, his heart rate is slow and his pulse is weak. How would you respond?

Key Terms

Absorbed poison: A poison that enters the body through the skin.

Addiction: The compulsive need to use a substance; stopping use would cause the user to suffer mental, physical and emotional distress.

Anabolic steroid: A drug sometimes used by athletes to enhance performance and increase muscle mass; also has medical use in stimulating weight gain for people unable to gain weight naturally.

Antidote: A substance that counteracts and neutralizes the effects of a poison.

Antihistamine: A type of drug taken to treat allergic reactions.

Anti-inflammatory drug: A type of drug taken to reduce inflammation or swelling.

Cannabis products: Substances such as marijuana and hashish that are derived from the *Cannabis sativa* plant; can produce feelings of elation, distorted perceptions of time and space, and impaired motor coordination and judgment.

Carbon monoxide (CO): An odorless, colorless, toxic gas produced as a byproduct of combustion.

Dependency: The desire or need to continually use a substance.

Depressant: A substance that affects the central nervous system and slows down physical and mental activity; can be used to treat anxiety, tension and high blood pressure.

Designer drugs: Potent and illegal street drugs formed from a medicinal substance whose drug composition has been modified (designed).

Drug: Any substance, other than food, intended to affect the functions of the body.

Hallucinogen: A substance that affects mood, sensation, thinking, emotion and self-awareness; alters perceptions of time and space; and produces hallucinations or delusions.

Ingested poison: A poison that is swallowed.

Inhalant: A substance, such as a medication, that a person inhales to counteract or prevent a specific condition; also a substance inhaled to produce mood-altering effects.

Inhaled poison: A poison breathed into the lungs.

Injected poison: A poison that enters the body through a bite, sting or syringe.

Narcotic: A drug derived from opium or opium-like compounds; used to reduce pain and can alter mood and behavior.

Overdose: The use of an excessive amount of a substance, resulting in adverse reactions ranging from mania (mental and physical hyperactivity) and hysteria, to coma and death.

Poison: Any substance that can cause injury, illness or death when introduced into the body, especially by chemical means.

Poison Control Center (PCC): A specialized health center that provides information on poisons and suspected poisoning emergencies.

Stimulant: A substance that affects the central nervous system and speeds up physical and mental activity.

Substance abuse: The deliberate, persistent, excessive use of a substance without regard to health concerns or accepted medical practices.

Substance misuse: The use of a substance for unintended purposes or for intended purposes but in improper amounts or doses.

Synergistic effect: The outcome created when two or more drugs are combined; the effects of each may enhance those of the other.

Tolerance: A condition in which the effects of a substance on the body decrease as a result of continued use.

Toxin: A poisonous substance produced by microorganisms that can cause certain diseases but is also capable of inducing neutralizing antibodies or antitoxins.

Toxicology: The study of the adverse effects of chemical, physical or biological agents on the body.

Withdrawal: The condition of mental and physical discomfort produced when a person stops using or abusing a substance to which the person is addicted.

Learning Objectives

After reading this chapter, and completing the class activities, you will have the information needed to—

- List the four ways poisons enter the body.
- Identify the signs and symptoms of poisoning.
- Describe general care guidelines for a poisoning emergency.
- Describe specific care for different types of poisoning emergencies.
- Have a basic understanding of drug interactions.

- Define substance abuse and misuse.
- Identify factors related to substance abuse and misuse and list prevention strategies.
- List information resources available to responders and the general public from *Poison Control Centers* (PCCs).

INTRODUCTION

A **poison** is any substance that causes injury, illness or death if it enters the body. A person can be poisoned by ingesting or swallowing poison, breathing it, absorbing it through the skin or by injecting it into the body.

In 2007, ***Poison Control Centers* (PCCs)** received more than 2.4 million calls about people who had come into contact with a poison. About 90 percent (2.1 million) of these poisonings took place in the home and 50 percent (1.1 million) involved children under 6 years of age. Poisoning deaths in children under age 6 represented less than 3 percent of the total deaths from poisoning, while the 20- to 59-year-old age group represented about 73 percent of all deaths from poisoning. Due in part to child-resistant packaging for medications and to preventive actions by parents and others who care for children, there has been a decline in child poisonings. At the same time, there has been an increase in adult poisoning deaths, which is linked to an increase in both suicides and drug-related poisonings.

A **toxin** is a poisonous substance produced by microorganisms that can cause certain diseases but is also capable of inducing neutralizing antibodies or antitoxins. **Toxicology** is the scientific study of poisons and **antidotes** and how they affect people. Some poisons—including many medications—are not deadly or harmful in small doses, but become dangerous if taken into the body in larger amounts. When a dangerously large amount of a **drug** is taken, this is called an **overdose**.

Poisons can be solid, liquid, spray or fumes (gases and vapors). A solid or liquid substance may turn into a gas if heated or under pressure. Poisonings can be accidental or intentional, and intentional poisoning can be self-inflicted—in the case of a suicide—or caused by another person intending to harm or kill the person. The severity of a poisoning depends on the type and amount of the substance, the time that has elapsed since the poison entered the body and the patient's age, size (build), weight and medical conditions. Many substances that are not poisonous in small amounts are poisonous in larger amounts. Medications (prescription or *over-the-counter* [OTC]) can be poisonous if they are not taken as prescribed or directed.

In a manufacturing facility, *Material Safety Data Sheets* (MSDS) are required on site for every product/chemical in use **(Fig. 15-1)**. In the case of a poisoning, the MSDS should go with the patient to the hospital, as it will give *emergency medical services* (EMS) personnel and hospital staff more detailed information as to the treatment of the exposed worker. There is also a 24-hour chemical hotline (CHEMTEC) to answer questions about the chemical.

In this chapter, you will learn about the four ways in which poisons can enter the body—ingestion, inhalation, absorption and injection. You will also learn about the types of poisons that fall into each of these categories, how to recognize the signs and symptoms of each type of poisoning and how to provide care for each. You will learn about how and when to contact the National PCC Hotline or summon more advanced medical personnel. This chapter also provides an overview of **substance abuse** and **substance misuse**: the types of substances that can be abused or misused, how they enter the body and how to provide care for someone who has been exposed to, inhaled or has ingested a poisonous substance.

POISON CONTROL CENTERS

PCCs are specialized health care centers that provide information on poisons and suspected poisoning emergencies. A network of PCCs exists throughout the United States. Some PCCs are located in the emergency departments of large hospitals. Medical professionals in these centers have access to information about virtually all

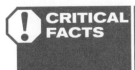

CRITICAL FACTS

A poison is any substance that causes injury, illness or death if it enters the body. A person can be poisoned by ingesting or swallowing poison, breathing it, absorbing it through the skin or by injecting it into the body.

A toxin is a poisonous substance produced by microorganisms that can cause certain diseases but is also capable of inducing neutralizing antibodies or antitoxins.

PCCs are specialized health care centers that provide information on poisons and suspected poisoning emergencies.

The Clorox Company
1221 Broadway
Oakland, CA 94612
Tel. (510) 271-7000

Material Safety Data Sheet

I Product:	CLOROX REGULAR-BLEACH
Description:	CLEAR, LIGHT YELLOW LIQUID WITH A CHARACTERISTIC CHLORINE ODOR

Other Designations	Distributor	Emergency Telephone Nos.
Clorox Bleach EPA Reg. No. 5813-50	Clorox Sales Company 1221 Broadway Oakland, CA 94612	For Medical Emergencies call: (800) 446-1014 For Transportation Emergencies Chemtrec (800) 424-9300

II Health Hazard Data

DANGER: CORROSIVE. May cause severe irritation or damage to eyes and skin. Vapor or mist may irritate. Harmful if swallowed. Keep out of reach of children.

Some clinical reports suggest a low potential for sensitization upon exaggerated exposure to sodium hypochlorite if skin damage (e.g., irritation) occurs during exposure. Under normal consumer use conditions the likelihood of any adverse health effects are low.

Medical conditions that may be aggravated by exposure to high concentrations of vapor or mist: heart conditions or chronic respiratory problems such as asthma, emphysema, chronic bronchitis or obstructive lung disease.

FIRST AID:

Eye Contact: Hold eye open and rinse with water for 15-20 minutes. Remove contact lenses, after first 5 minutes. Continue rinsing eye. Call a physician.

Skin Contact: Wash skin with water for 15-20 minutes. If irritation develops, call a physician.

Ingestion: Do not induce vomiting. Drink a glassful of water. If irritation develops, call a physician. Do not give anything by mouth to an unconscious person.

Inhalation: Remove to fresh air. If breathing is affected, call a physician.

III Hazardous Ingredients

Ingredient	Concentration	Exposure Limit
Sodium hypochlorite CAS# 7681-52-9	6.15%	Not established
Sodium hydroxide CAS# 1310-73-2	<1%	2 mg/m$^{3; 1}$ 2 mg/m$^{3; 2}$

[1]ACGIH Threshold Limit Value (TLV) - Ceiling

[2]OHSA Permissible Exposure Limit (PEL) – Time Weighted Average (TWA)

None of the ingredients in this product are on the IARC, NTP or OSHA carcinogen lists.

IV Special Protection and Precautions

No special protection or precautions have been identified for using this product under directed consumer use conditions. The following recommendations are given for production facilities and for other conditions and situations where there is increased potential for accidental, large-scale or prolonged exposure.

Hygienic Practices: Avoid contact with eyes, skin and clothing. Wash hands after direct contact. Do not wear product-contaminated clothing for prolonged periods.

Engineering Controls: Use general ventilation to minimize exposure to vapor or mist.

Personal Protective Equipment: Wear safety glasses. Use rubber or nitrile gloves if in contact liquid, especially for prolonged periods.

KEEP OUT OF REACH OF CHILDREN

V Transportation and Regulatory Data

DOT/IMDG/IATA - Not restricted.

EPA - SARA TITLE III/CERCLA: Bottled product is not reportable under Sections 311/312 and contains no chemicals reportable under Section 313. This product does contain chemicals (sodium hydroxide <0.2% and sodium hypochlorite <7.35%) that are regulated under Section 304/CERCLA.

TSCA/DSL STATUS: All components of this product are on the U.S. TSCA Inventory and Canadian DSL.

VI Spill Procedures/Waste Disposal

Spill Procedures: Control spill. Containerize liquid and use absorbents on residual liquid; dispose appropriately. Wash area and let dry. For spills of multiple products, responders should evaluate the MSDS's of the products for incompatibility with sodium hypochlorite. Breathing protection should be worn in enclosed, and/or poorly ventilated areas until hazard assessment is complete.

Waste Disposal: Dispose of in accordance with all applicable federal, state, and local regulations.

VII Reactivity Data

Stable under normal use and storage conditions. Strong oxidizing agent. Reacts with other household chemicals such as toilet bowl cleaners, rust removers, vinegar, acids or ammonia containing products to produce hazardous gases, such as chlorine and other chlorinated species. Prolonged contact with metal may cause pitting or discoloration.

VIII Fire and Explosion Data

Flash Point: None

Special Firefighting Procedures: None

Unusual Fire/Explosion Hazards: None. Not flammable or explosive. Product does not ignite when exposed to open flame.

IX Physical Data

Boiling point..approx. 212°F/100°C
Specific Gravity (H$_2$0=1) .... ~ 1.1 at 70°F
Solubility in Water .... complete
pH ....~11.4

©1963, 1991 THE CLOROX COMPANY
DATA SUPPLIED IS FOR USE ONLY IN CONNECTION WITH OCCUPATIONAL SAFETY AND HEALTH   DATE PREPARED 05/05

Fig. 15-1: An MSDS

poisonous substances, and can tell you how to care for someone who has been poisoned.

You can obtain the phone number of your local center from your telephone directory,

your health care provider, a local hospital or your local EMS system. PCCs answer over 2 million calls about poisoning each year. Since many poisonings can be treated without the help of EMS personnel, PCCs help prevent overburdening of the EMS system.

The American Association of Poison Control Centers (AAPCC) also has a 24-Hour Poison Help Hotline, which is staffed by pharmacists, physicians, nurses and toxicology specialists and can be reached at **1-800-222-1222**. More than 70 percent of poison exposure cases can be managed over the phone. For more information, visit the American Association of Poison Control Centers website at *www.aapcc.org*.

Call for more advanced medical personnel if you are unsure about what to do, you are unsure about the severity of the problem or if it is a life-threatening condition. Otherwise, call the PCC for assistance.

In general, call for more advanced medical personnel if the patient—

- Is unconscious, confused or seems to be losing consciousness.
- Has trouble breathing or is breathing irregularly.
- Has persistent chest pain or pressure.
- Has pressure or pain in the abdomen that does not go away.
- Is vomiting blood or passing blood.
- Has a seizure, severe headache or slurred speech.
- Acts violently.

HOW POISON ENTERS THE BODY

Poisons are generally placed in four categories, based on how they enter the body: ingestion, inhalation, absorption and injection.

Ingested Poison
Types of Ingested Poisons

Ingested poisons are poisons that are swallowed and include items such as foods (e.g., certain mushrooms and shellfish), drugs (e.g., alcohol), medications (e.g., aspirin) and household items (e.g., cleaning products, pesticides and even household plants).

Young children tend to put almost everything in their mouths, so they are at a higher risk of ingesting poisons, including household cleaners and medications (**Fig. 15-2**). Seniors may make medication errors if they are prone to forgetfulness or have difficulty reading the small print on medicine container labels.

In 2007, the *Centers for Disease Control and Prevention* (CDC) estimated that 76 million people contract food-borne illnesses each year in the United States. Approximately 325,000 people are hospitalized and more than 5000 die from food-borne illness.

Two of the most common categories of food poisoning are bacterial and chemical food poisoning. *Bacterial* food poisoning typically occurs when bacteria grow on food that is allowed to stand at room temperature after being cooked, which releases toxins into the food. Foods most likely to cause bacterial food poisoning are meats, fish and dairy or dairy-based foods.

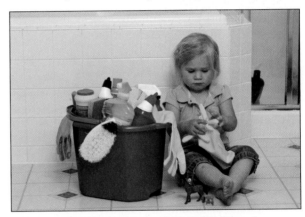

Fig. 15-2: Young children are at a higher risk of ingesting poisons because they tend to put almost everything into their mouths.

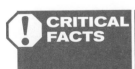
CRITICAL FACTS

The American Association of Poison Control Centers also has a 24-Hour Poison Help Hotline, which is staffed by pharmacists, physicians, nurses and toxicology specialists and can be reached at **1-800-222-1222**.

Call for more advanced medical personnel if you are unsure about what to do, you are unsure about the severity of the problem or if it is a life-threatening condition. Otherwise, call the PCC for assistance. There are several reasons that warrant calling for more advanced medical personnel, including unconsciousness, breathing problems, chest or abdominal pain or pressure, vomiting blood or passing blood, seizures or violent behavior.

Poisons are generally placed in four categories, based on how they enter the body: ingestion, inhalation, absorption and injection.

Chemical food poisoning typically occurs when foods with high acid content, such as fruit juices or sauerkraut, are stored in containers lined with zinc, cadmium or copper or in enameled metal pans. Another primary source of chemical food poisoning is lead, which is sometimes found in pipes that supply drinking and cooking water. Mercury can also be a source of food poisoning. Fish, such as shark and swordfish, are a major dietary source of mercury. However, mercury can also come from diet, dental fillings, pharmaceuticals and contact with mercury metal or its compounds.

Two of the most common causes of food poisoning are *Salmonella* bacteria (most often found in poultry and raw eggs) and *Escherichia coli* (E. coli) (most often found in raw meats and unpasteurized milk and juices). The most deadly type of food poisoning is botulism, which is caused by a bacterial toxin usually associated with home canning.

Signs and Symptoms of Ingested Poisons

A person who has ingested poison generally looks ill and displays symptoms common to other sudden illnesses. If you have even a slight suspicion that a patient has been poisoned, seek immediate medical assistance. Signs and symptoms to look for include—

- Nausea, vomiting or diarrhea.
- Chest or abdominal pain.
- Difficulty breathing.
- Sweating.
- Changes in *level of consciousness* (LOC).
- Seizures.
- Headache or dizziness.
- Weakness.
- Irregular pupil size.
- Burning or tearing eyes.
- Abnormal skin color.
- Burn injuries around the lips or tongue or on the skin around the mouth.

The symptoms of food poisoning, which can begin between 1–48 hours after eating contaminated food, include nausea, vomiting, abdominal pain, diarrhea, fever and dehydration. Severe cases of food poisoning can result in shock or death, particularly in children, the elderly and those with an impaired immune system.

Providing Care for Ingested Poisons

If the patient is fully conscious and alert, immediately call the PCC and follow the directions given. *DO NOT* give the patient anything to eat or drink unless you are told to do so. If you do not know what the poison was and the patient vomits, save some of the vomit. The hospital may analyze it later to identify the poison.

In some cases of ingested poisoning, the PCC may instruct you to induce vomiting. Vomiting may prevent the poison from moving to the small intestine, where most absorption takes place. However, vomiting should be induced only if advised by a medical professional. The PCC or a medical professional will advise you exactly how to induce vomiting. In some instances, vomiting should *not* be induced. This includes when the patient—

- Is unconscious.
- Is having a seizure.
- Is pregnant (in the last trimester).
- Has ingested a corrosive substance (such as drain or oven cleaner) or a petroleum product (such as kerosene or gasoline).
- Is known to have heart disease.

Examples of such poisons are caustic or corrosive chemicals, such as acids, that can eat away or destroy tissues. Vomiting these corrosives could burn the esophagus, throat and mouth. Diluting the corrosive substance decreases the potential for burning and damaging tissues. *DO NOT* give the patient anything to eat or drink unless medical professionals tell you to do so.

Some people who have contracted food poisoning may require antibiotic or antitoxin therapy. Fortunately, most cases of food poisoning can be prevented by proper food handling and preparation.

Inhaled Poison
Types of Inhaled Poisons

Poisoning by inhalation occurs when a person breathes in poisonous gases or fumes. A commonly **inhaled poison** is *carbon monoxide* (**CO**), which is present in substances such as car exhaust and tobacco smoke. CO can also be produced by fires (gas and natural), defective gas cooking equipment, defective gas furnaces, gas water heaters and kerosene heaters. CO, which is colorless, odorless and tasteless is highly lethal and can cause death after only a few minutes of exposure.

Other common inhaled poisons include carbon dioxide, chlorine gas, ammonia, sulfur dioxide, nitrous oxide, chloroform, dry cleaning solvents, fire extinguisher gases, industrial gases and hydrogen sulfide. Paints and solvents produce fumes that some people deliberately inhale to get high, as do certain drugs, such as crack cocaine.

Signs and Symptoms of Inhaled Poisons

Look for paint or solvent around the mouth and nose of the patient if you suspect deliberate inhalation. A pale or bluish skin color, which indicates a lack of oxygen, may signal CO poisoning. Other signs and symptoms of inhaled poisons include—

- Difficulty breathing or respiratory rate faster or slower than normal.
- Chest pain or tightness.
- Nausea or vomiting.
- Cyanosis.
- Headaches, dizziness, confusion.
- Coughing, possibly with excessive secretions.
- Seizures.
- Altered mental status with possible unresponsiveness.

Providing Care for Inhaled Poisons

When providing care to a patient who may have inhaled poison, follow appropriate safety precautions to ensure that you do not also become poisoned. Toxic fumes may or may not have an odor. If you notice clues at an emergency scene that lead you to suspect toxic fumes are present—such as a strong smell of fuel (sulfur or skunk smell) or a hissing sound (which could indicate gas escaping from a pipe or valve)—you may not be able to reach the patient without risking your own safety. In cases like this, call for specialized services instead of entering the scene. Let EMS professionals know what you discovered, and only enter the scene if you are told it is safe to do so or if you are trained to do so.

All patients who have inhaled poison need emergency oxygen as soon as possible. If you can remove the patient from the source of the poison without endangering yourself, then do so. You can help a conscious patient by getting him or her to fresh air and then calling for more advanced care personnel. If you find an unconscious patient, remove the patient from the scene if it is safe to do so, and call for more advanced medical personnel. Then provide care for any life-threatening conditions.

Absorbed Poison
Types of Absorbed Poisons

An **absorbed poison** enters through the skin or the mucous membranes in the eyes, nose and mouth. Absorbed poisons come from plants, as well as from chemicals and medications. Millions of people each year suffer irritating effects after touching or brushing against poisonous plants such as poison ivy, poison oak and poison sumac (**Fig. 15-3, A–C**). Other poisons absorbed through the skin include dry and wet chemicals, such as those used in flea collars for dogs and in

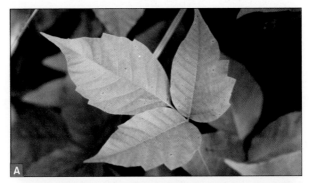

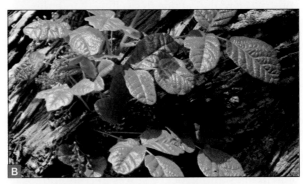

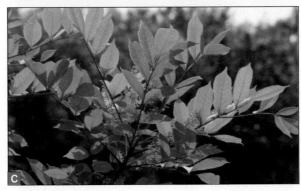

Fig. 15-3, A–C: (A) Poison ivy, *Shutterstock.com/Tim Mainiero;* (B) Poison oak, *Shutterstock.com/Dwight Smith;* (C) Poison sumac, *www.poison-ivy.org.*

yard and garden maintenance products, which may also burn the skin. Some medications, such as topical medications or transdermal patches, can also be absorbed through the skin.

Signs and Symptoms of Absorbed Poisons

Some of the signs and symptoms of absorbed poisons include—
- Traces of the liquid, powder or chemical on the patient's skin.
- Skin that looks burned, irritated, red or swollen.
- Blisters that may ooze fluid, or a rash.
- Itchy skin.

Providing Care for Absorbed Poisons

To care for a patient who has come into contact with a poisonous plant, follow standard precautions and then immediately rinse the affected area thoroughly with water. Using soap cannot hurt, but soap may not do much to remove the poisonous plant oil that causes the allergic reaction. Before washing the affected area, you may need to have the patient remove any jewelry. This is only necessary if the jewelry is contaminated or if it constricts circulation due to swelling. Rinse the affected areas for *at least 20 minutes*, using a shower or garden hose if possible. If a rash or weeping lesion (an oozing sore) develops, advise the patient to seek the opinion of a pharmacist or health care provider about possible treatment. Medicated lotions may help soothe the area.

Antihistamines may also help dry up the lesions and help stop or reduce itching. OTC antihistamines are available at pharmacies and grocery stores and should be used according to the manufacturer's directions. If the condition worsens or if large areas of the body or the face are affected, the patient should see a health care provider, who may administer **anti-inflammatory drugs**, such as corticosteroids, or other medications to relieve discomfort.

If the poisoning involves dry chemicals, brush off the chemicals using gloved hands before flushing with tap water (under pressure). Take care not to inhale any of the chemical or get any of the dry chemical on you, your eyes or the eyes of the patient or any bystanders. Many

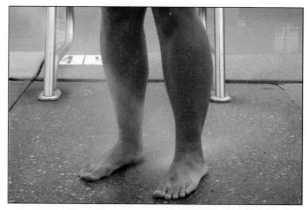

Fig. 15-4: If the poisoning involves chemicals, flush the exposed area continuously with cool, running water for at least 20 minutes.

dry chemicals are activated by contact with water. However, if continuous running water is available, it will flush the chemical from the skin before the activated chemical can do harm. If wet chemicals contact the skin, flush the area continuously with large amounts of cool, running water. Running water reduces the threat to you and quickly and easily removes the substance from the patient. Continue flushing for *at least 20 minutes* or until more advanced medical personnel arrive (**Fig. 15-4**).

If poison has been in contact with the patient's eye or eyes, irrigate the affected eye or eyes, from the nose side of the eye, *not* directly onto the middle of the cornea of the eye, with clean water for *at least 20 minutes*. If only one eye is affected, make sure you do not let the water run into the unaffected eye by tilting the head so the water runs from the nose side of the eye downward to the ear side (**Fig. 15-5**). Continue care while transporting the patient if you can.

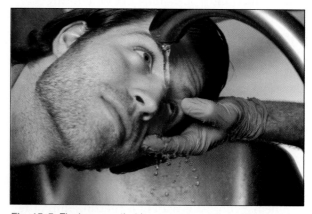

Fig. 15-5: Flush an eye that has come in contact with poison with clean water from the nose side toward the ear side, being sure not to contaminate the unaffected eye.

Injected Poison

Types of Injected Poisons

Injected poisons enter the body through the bites or stings of certain insects, spiders, aquatic life, animals and snakes or as drugs or misused medications injected with a hypodermic needle. Insect and animal bites and stings are among the most common sources of injected poisons. See **Chapter 16** for more information about the signs of these bites and how to provide care for them.

Signs and Symptoms of Injected Poisons

Some of the signs and symptoms of injected poisons include—

- Bite or sting mark at the point of entry.
- A stinger, tentacle or venom sac in or near the entry site.
- Redness, pain, tenderness or swelling around the entry site.
- Signs of allergic reaction, including localized itching, hives or rash.
- Signs of a severe allergic reaction (anaphylaxis), including weakness, nausea, dizziness, swelling of the throat or tongue, constricted airway or difficulty breathing.

Providing Care for Injected Poisons

Size up the scene and follow standard precautions. Perform a primary assessment and care for conditions found. Applying an ice pack or cold pack can reduce pain and swelling of the bitten area. To provide specific care for certain bites and stings, see **Chapter 16**. Call for more advanced medical personnel if there are signs and symptoms of anaphylaxis and assist the patient with his or her prescribed epinephrine auto-injector if protocols allow and you are trained to do so.

SUBSTANCE ABUSE AND MISUSE

A *drug* is any substance, other than food, taken to affect body functions. A drug given therapeutically to prevent or treat a disease or otherwise enhance mental or physical well-being is a *medication*. *Substance abuse* is the deliberate, persistent and excessive use of a substance without regard to health concerns or accepted medical practices. *Substance misuse* refers to the use of a substance for unintended purposes or for appropriate purposes but in improper amounts or doses.

Because of the publicity they receive, we tend to think of illegal (also known as *illicit* or *controlled*) drugs when we hear of substance abuse. However, legal substances (also called *licit* or *non-controlled substances*) are among those most often abused or misused. These include nicotine (found in tobacco products), alcohol and OTC medications such as sleeping pills and diet pills.

In the United States, substance abuse costs tens of billions of dollars each year in medical care, insurance and lost productivity. Even more important, however, are the lives lost or permanently impaired each year from injuries or medical emergencies related to substance abuse or misuse. For example, experts estimate that as many as two-thirds of all homicides and serious assaults occurring annually involve alcohol. Other problems directly or indirectly related to substance abuse include dropping out of school, adolescent pregnancy, suicide, involvement in crime and transmission of HIV.

If you think someone has taken an overdose or has another substance abuse problem requiring medical attention or other professional help, size up the scene for safety, then check the person. If you have good reason to suspect a substance was taken, call the National PCC Hotline and follow the directions given.

Forms of Substance Abuse and Misuse

Many substances that are abused or misused are legal. Other substances are legal only when prescribed by a health care provider. Some are illegal only for those under a certain age, such as alcohol.

Any drug can cause **dependency**, or the desire to continually use the substance. Those

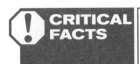 **CRITICAL FACTS** Substance abuse is the deliberate, persistent and excessive use of a substance without regard to health concerns or accepted medical practices. Substance misuse refers to the use of a substance for unintended purposes or for appropriate purposes but in improper amounts or doses.

with drug dependency issues feel that they need the drug to function normally. Those with a compulsive need for a substance and those who would suffer mental, physical and emotional distress if they stopped taking it are said to have an **addiction** to that substance.

The term **withdrawal** describes the condition produced when people stop using or abusing a substance to which they are addicted. Stopping the use of a substance may occur as a deliberate decision or because the person is unable to obtain the specific drug. Withdrawal from certain substances, such as alcohol, can cause severe mental and physical distress. Because withdrawal may become a serious medical condition, medical professionals often oversee the process.

When someone continually uses a substance, its effects on the body often decrease—a condition called **tolerance**. The person then has to increase the amount and frequency of use to obtain the desired effect.

An overdose occurs when someone uses an excessive amount of a substance. Symptoms can vary but may range from mania and hysteria to coma and death. Specific reactions include changes in blood pressure and heartbeat, sweating, vomiting and liver failure. An overdose may occur unintentionally if a person takes too much medication at one time. For example, an elderly person might forget about taking one dose of a medication and thus takes an additional dose. An overdose may also be intentional, as in a suicide attempt. Sometimes the patient takes a sufficiently high dose of a substance to be certain to cause death. In other cases, the patient may take enough of a substance to need medical attention but not enough to cause death.

Abused and Misused Substances

Substances are categorized according to their effects on the body (**Table 15-1**). The six major categories are **stimulants**, **hallucinogens**, **depressants**, **narcotics**, **inhalants** and **cannabis products**. The category to which a substance belongs depends mostly on the effects it has on the central nervous system or the way the substance is taken. Some substances depress the nervous system, whereas others speed up its activity. Some are not easily categorized because they have various effects or may be taken in a

variety of ways. A heightened or exaggerated effect may be produced when two or more substances are used at the same time. This is called a **synergistic effect**, which can be deadly.

Stimulants

Stimulants are drugs that affect the central nervous system by increasing physical and mental activity. They produce temporary feelings of alertness and prevent fatigue. They are sometimes used for weight reduction because they also suppress appetite, or to enhance exercise routines because they provide bursts of energy.

Many stimulants are ingested as pills, but some can be absorbed or inhaled. Amphetamine, dextroamphetamine and methamphetamine are stimulants. On the street, an extremely addictive, dangerous and smokeable form of methamphetamine is often called "crystal meth" or "ice." The street term "speed" usually refers to amphetamine or methamphetamine. Other street terms for amphetamines are "uppers," "bennies," "black beauties," "crystal," "meth" and "crank."

Cocaine is one of the most publicized and powerful stimulants. It can be taken into the body in different ways. The most common way is sniffing it in powder form, known as "snorting." In this method, the drug is absorbed into the blood through capillaries in the nose. Street names for cocaine include "coke," "snow," "blow," "flake," "foot" and "nose candy." A purer and more potent form of cocaine is crack, which is smoked. The vapors inhaled into the lungs reach the brain and cause almost immediate effects. Crack is highly addictive. Street names for crack include "rock" and "freebase rocks."

Ephedra, also known as "ma huang," is a stimulant plant that has been used in China and India for over 5000 years. Until it was banned by the *Food and Drug Administration* (FDA) in 2004, it was a common ingredient in dietary supplements sold in the United States. The dried stems and leaves are put into capsules, tablets, extracts, tinctures or teas, and then ingested. It is used for weight loss, increased energy and to enhance athletic performance.

The FDA banned ephedra because it appears to have little effectiveness, along with some substantial health risks. Taking ephedra can cause nausea, anxiety, headache, psychosis, kidney stones, tremors, dry mouth, irregular heart rhythms, high blood pressure, restlessness

Table 15-1:
Commonly Abused and Misused Substances

CATEGORY	SUBSTANCES	COMMON NAMES	POSSIBLE EFFECTS
Stimulants	Caffeine Cocaine, crack cocaine Amphetamines Methamphetamine Dextroamphetamine Nicotine Ephedra OTC diet aids Asthma treatments Decongestants	Coke, snow, nose candy, blow, flake, Big C, lady, white, snowbirds, powder, foot, crack, rock, cookies, freebase rocks, speed, uppers, ups, bennies, black beauties, crystal, meth, crank, crystal meth, ice, ma huang	Increase mental and physical activity. Produce temporary feelings of alertness. Prevent fatigue. Suppress appetite.
Hallucinogens	Diethyltryptamine (DET) Dimethyltryptamine (DMT) LSD PCP Mescaline Peyote Psilocybin 4-Methyl-2,5-Dimethoxyamphetamine (DOM)	Psychedelics, acid, white lightning, sugar cubes, angel dust, hog, loveboat, peyote, buttons, cactus, mesc, mushrooms, magic mushrooms, 'shrooms, STP (serenity, tranquility and peace)	Cause changes in mood, sensation, thought, emotion and self-awareness. Alter perceptions of time and space. Can produce profound depression, tension and anxiety, as well as visual, auditory or tactile hallucinations.
Depressants	Barbiturates Benzodiazepines Narcotics Alcohol Antihistamines Sedatives Tranquilizers OTC sleep aids Ketamine Rohypnol® GHB	Valium®, Xanax®, downers, barbs, goofballs, yellow jackets, reds, Quaaludes, ludes, club drugs, date rape drugs, special K, vitamin K, roofies, roach, rope, liquid ecstasy, soap, vita-G	Decrease mental and physical activity. Alter consciousness. Relieve anxiety and pain. Promote sleep. Depress respiration. Relax muscles. Impair coordination and judgment.
Narcotics	Morphine Codeine Heroin Oxycodone Methadone Opium	Pectoral syrup, Oxycontin®, Percodan®, smack, horse, mud, brown sugar, junk, black tar, big H	Relieve pain. Produce stupor or euphoria. Can cause coma or death. Highly addictive.

(continued)

Table 15-1:
Commonly Abused and Misused Substances *(continued)*

CATEGORY	SUBSTANCES	COMMON NAMES	POSSIBLE EFFECTS
Inhalants	Medical anesthetics Lacquer and varnish thinners Propane Toluene Butane Acetone Fuel Propellants	Laughing gas, whippets, glue, lighter fluid, nail polish remover, gasoline, kerosene, aerosol sprays	Alter moods. Produce a partial or complete loss of feeling. Produce effects similar to drunkenness, such as slurred speech, lack of inhibitions and impaired motor coordination. Can cause damage to the heart, lungs, brain and liver.
Cannabis Products	Hashish Marijuana THC	Hash, pot, grass, weed, reefer, ganja, mary jane, dope	Produce feelings of elation. Increase appetite. Distort perceptions of time and space. Impair motor coordination and judgment. Irritate throat. Redden eyes. Increase pulse. Cause dizziness.
Other	MDMA	Ecstasy, E, XTC, Adam, essence	Elevate blood pressure. Produce euphoria or erratic mood swings, rapid heartbeat, profuse sweating, agitation and sensory distortions.
	Anabolic steroids	Androgens, hormones, juice, roids, vitamins	Enhance physical performance. Increase muscle mass. Stimulate appetite and weight gain. Chronic use can cause sterility, disruption of normal growth, liver cancer, personality changes and aggressive behavior.

(continued)

Table 15-1:
Commonly Abused and Misused Substances *(continued)*

CATEGORY	SUBSTANCES	COMMON NAMES	POSSIBLE EFFECTS
Other *(continued)*	Aspirin		Relieves minor pain. Reduces fever. Impairs normal blood clotting. Can cause inflammation of the stomach and small intestine.
	Laxatives and emetics	Ipecac syrup	Relieve constipation or induce vomiting. Can cause dehydration, uncontrolled diarrhea and other serious health problems.
	Decongestant nasal sprays		Relieve congestion and swelling of nasal passages. Chronic use can cause nosebleeds and changes in the lining of the nose, making it difficult to breathe without sprays.

and sleep problems. It has been found to increase the risk of heart problems, stroke and even death.

Interestingly, the most common stimulants in America are legal. Leading the list is caffeine, present in coffee, tea, high energy drinks, many kinds of sodas, chocolate, diet pills and pills used to combat fatigue. The next most common stimulant is nicotine, found in tobacco products. Other stimulants used for medical purposes are asthma medications or decongestants that can be taken by mouth or inhaled.

Hallucinogens

Hallucinogens, also known as *psychedelics*, are substances that cause changes in mood, sensation, thought, emotion and self-awareness. They alter one's perception of time and space and produce visual, auditory and tactile (relating to the sense of touch) delusions.

Among the most widely abused hallucinogens are *lysergic acid diethylamide* (LSD), called "acid"; psilocybin, called "mushrooms"; *phencyclidine*

(PCP), called "angel dust"; and mescaline, called "peyote," "buttons" or "mesc." These substances are usually ingested, but PCP is also often inhaled.

Hallucinogens often have physical effects similar to stimulants but are classified differently because of the other effects they produce. Hallucinogens sometimes cause what is called a "bad trip." A bad trip can involve intense fear, panic, paranoid delusions, vivid hallucinations, profound depression, tension and anxiety. The patient may be irrational and feel threatened by any attempt others make to help.

Depressants

Depressants are substances that affect the central nervous system by decreasing physical and mental activity. Depressants are commonly used for medical purposes. All depressants alter consciousness to some degree. They relieve anxiety, promote sleep, depress respiration, relieve pain, relax muscles and impair coordination and judgment. Like other substances, the larger the dose or the stronger the substance, the greater its effects.

Common depressants are barbiturates, benzodiazepines (e.g., Valium®, Xanax®), narcotics and alcohol. Most depressants are ingested or injected. Their street names include "downers," "barbs," "goofballs," "yellow jackets," "reds" or "ludes."

Three depressants that have gained popularity as club drugs (so-called because they are used at all-night dance parties) include ketamine (also referred to as "special K," "vitamin K"), an anesthetic approved for use in animals and humans; Rohypnol® (also referred to as "roofies," "roach," "rope"), a benzodiazepine that is illegal in the United States; and *gamma-hydroxybutyrate* (GHB) (also referred to as "liquid ecstasy," "soap," "vita-G"), an illicit drug that has depressant, euphoric and body-building effects. These drugs are particularly dangerous because they are often used in combination or with other depressants (including alcohol), which can have deadly effects, and because they are "date rape drugs" of choice. As such, they are sometimes slipped to others unnoticed.

Alcohol is the most widely used and abused substance in the United States. In small amounts, its effects may be fairly mild. In higher doses, its effects can be toxic. Alcohol is like other depressants in its effects and risks for overdose. Frequent drinkers may become dependent on the effects of alcohol and increasingly tolerant of those effects. Alcohol poisoning occurs when a large amount of alcohol is consumed in a short period of time and can result in unconsciousness and, if untreated, death.

Drinking alcohol in large or frequent amounts can have many unhealthy consequences. Alcohol can irritate the digestive system and even cause the esophagus to rupture, or it can injure the stomach lining. Chronic drinking can also affect the brain and cause memory loss, apathy and a lack of coordination. Other problems include liver disease, such as cirrhosis. In addition, many psychological, family, social and work problems are related to chronic drinking.

Narcotics

While they have a depressant effect, narcotics (which are derived from opium) are used mainly to relieve pain. Narcotics are so powerful and highly addictive that all are illegal without a prescription, and some are not prescribed at all. When taken in large doses, narcotics can produce euphoria, stupor, coma or death. The most common natural narcotics are morphine and codeine. Most other narcotics, including heroin, are synthetic or semi-synthetic. Oxycodone, also known by the trade names Oxycontin® or Percodan®, is a powerful semi-synthetic narcotic that has recently gained popularity as a street drug.

Inhalants

Substances inhaled to produce mood-altering effects are called inhalants. Inhalants also depress the central nervous system. In addition, inhalant use can damage the heart, lungs, brain and liver. Inhalants include medical anesthetics, such as amyl nitrite and nitrous oxide (also known as "laughing gas"), as well as hydrocarbons, known as *solvents*. The effects of solvents are similar to those of alcohol. People who use solvents may appear to be drunk. Other effects of inhalant use include swollen mucous membranes in the nose and mouth, hallucinations, erratic blood pressure and pulse and seizures. Solvents include toluene, found in glues; butane, found in lighter fluids; acetone, found in nail polish removers; fuels, such as gasoline and kerosene; and propellants, found in aerosol sprays.

Cannabis Products

Cannabis products, including hash oil, *tetrahydrocannabinol* (THC) and hashish, are all derived from the plant *Cannabis sativa*. Street names for marijuana include "marijuana," "pot," "grass," "weed," "reefer," "ganja" and "dope." Marijuana is the most widely used illicit drug in the United States. It is typically smoked in cigarette form or in a pipe, but it can also be ingested. The effects include feelings of elation, distorted perceptions of time and space and impaired judgment and motor coordination. Marijuana irritates the throat, reddens the eyes and causes a rapid pulse, dizziness and often an increased appetite. Depending on the dose, the person and many other factors, cannabis products can produce effects similar to those of substances in any of the other major substance categories.

Marijuana, although illegal, has been legalized in some states for limited medical use to help alleviate symptoms of certain conditions, such as multiple sclerosis. Marijuana and its legal synthetic versions are used as an anti-nausea medication for people undergoing chemotherapy for cancer, for treating glaucoma, for treating muscular weakness caused by multiple sclerosis and to combat the weight loss caused by cancer and AIDS.

Other Substances

Some other substances do not fit neatly into these categories. These substances include **designer drugs**, steroids and OTC substances, which can be purchased without a prescription.

Designer Drugs

Designer drugs are variations of other substances, such as narcotics and amphetamines. Through simple and inexpensive methods, the molecular structure of substances produced for medicinal purposes can be modified into extremely potent and dangerous street drugs; hence the term "designer drug." When the chemical makeup of a drug is altered, the user can experience a variety of unpredictable and dangerous effects. The people who modify these drugs may have no knowledge of the effects a new designer drug might produce.

One of the more commonly used designer drugs is *methylenedioxymethamphetamine* (MDMA). Another popular club drug, it is often called "ecstasy" or "E." Although ecstasy is structurally related to stimulants and hallucinogens, its effects are somewhat different from either category. Ecstasy can evoke a euphoric high that makes it popular. Other signs and symptoms of ecstasy use range from the stimulant-like effects of high blood pressure, rapid heartbeat, profuse sweating and agitation to the hallucinogenic-like effects of paranoia, sensory distortion and erratic mood swings.

Anabolic Steroids

Anabolic steroids are drugs sometimes used by athletes to enhance performance and increase muscle mass. Their medical uses include stimulating weight gain for persons unable to gain weight naturally. They should not be confused with corticosteroids, which are used to counteract toxic effects and allergic reactions. Chronic use of anabolic steroids can lead to sterility, liver cancer and personality changes, such as aggressive behavior. Steroid use by younger people may also disrupt normal growth. Street names for anabolic steroids include "androgens," "hormones," "juice," "roids" and "vitamins."

OTC Substances

Aspirin, nasal sprays, laxatives and emetics are among the most commonly abused or misused OTC substances (**Fig. 15-6**). Aspirin is an effective minor pain reliever and fever reducer that is found in a variety of medicines. People use aspirin for many reasons and conditions. In recent years, cardiologists have praised the benefits of low-dose aspirin for the treatment of heart disease and stroke prevention. As useful as aspirin is, misuse can have toxic effects on the body. Typically, aspirin can cause inflammation of the stomach and small intestine that can result in bleeding ulcers. Aspirin can also impair normal blood clotting.

Decongestant nasal sprays can help relieve the congestion of colds or hay fever. If misused, they can cause physical dependency. Using the spray over a long period can cause nosebleeds and changes in the lining of the nose that make it difficult to breathe without the spray.

Laxatives are used to relieve constipation. They come in a variety of forms and strengths. If used improperly, laxatives can cause uncontrolled diarrhea that may result in dehydration, the excessive loss of water from the body tissues. The very young and the elderly are particularly susceptible to dehydration.

Emetics are drugs that induce vomiting. A popular OTC emetic is ipecac syrup. It has been used in the past to induce vomiting following the ingestion of some toxic substances.

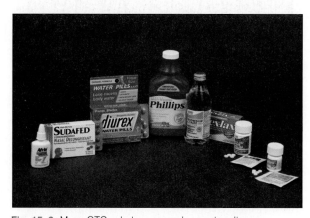

Fig. 15-6: Many OTC substances, such as pain relievers, decongestants, laxatives and emetics, can be abused or misused.

The routine administration of ipecac syrup for ingested poisons is *not* recommended. Improper use can be quite dangerous and may cause recurrent vomiting, diarrhea, dehydration, pain and weakness in the muscles, abdominal pain and heart problems. Over time, the recurrent vomiting can erode tooth enamel, causing dental problems.

The abuse of laxatives and emetics is frequently associated with attempted weight loss and eating disorders, such as anorexia nervosa or bulimia. *Anorexia nervosa* is a disorder that most often affects young women and is characterized by a long-term refusal to eat food with sufficient nutrients and calories. People with anorexia typically use laxatives and emetics to keep from gaining weight. *Bulimia* is a condition in which people gorge themselves with food, then purge by vomiting (sometimes with the aid of emetics) or using laxatives. For this reason, the behavior associated with bulimia is often referred to as "binging and purging." Anorexia nervosa and bulimia have underlying psychological factors that contribute to their onset. The effect of both of these eating disorders can be severe malnutrition, which can result in death.

The American Academy of Pediatrics (AAP) and the American Association of Poison Control Centers do *not* recommend that ipecac syrup be stocked at home.

ADOLESCENTS AND SUBSTANCE ABUSE

Adolescents and young adults are more likely to be involved in substance abuse and misuse. According to a 2005 survey by the CDC, 17 percent of those aged 16–17, and 20 percent of those aged 18–25, had used an illicit drug in the previous month. More alarmingly, 30 percent of those aged 16–17 and over 60 percent of those aged 18–25 had used alcohol in the previous month.

Males are somewhat more likely to use illicit drugs and alcohol than females, although they are almost equally likely to use psychotherapeutic drugs for non-medical purposes. Middle and high school students are also likely to abuse or misuse prescription drugs such as narcotic pain killers, sedatives or stimulants because they can access them easily at home, from people they know, or on the Internet.

Geriatric Considerations

Substance Abuse and Misuse Among Older Adults

Substance abuse and misuse does occur in older populations. Older adults are likely to suffer from chronic diseases or conditions that require multiple prescription medications. These medications can interact with each other or with alcohol, and cause adverse reactions. The slower metabolisms of older adults can cause alcohol and medications to remain in the body longer, increasing the chance of an overdose. Sometimes, because of failing eyesight, an elderly person may unintentionally take a drug at the wrong time or consume the wrong dosage and experience an overdose. Mixing medications or mixing drugs with alcohol and failing to follow directions are also factors in substance abuse and misuse among older people.

Signs and Symptoms of Substance Abuse and Misuse

Many of the signs and symptoms of substance abuse and misuse are similar to those of other medical emergencies. Do not necessarily assume that individuals who are stumbling, disoriented or have a fruity, alcohol-like odor on the breath are intoxicated by alcohol or other drugs, as this may also be a sign of a diabetic emergency.

As in other medical emergencies, you do not have to diagnose substance abuse or misuse to provide care. It can be helpful, however, if you detect clues that suggest the nature of the problem. Such clues help you provide more complete information to more advanced medical personnel so that they can provide prompt and appropriate care.

Often these clues will come from the patient, bystanders or the scene. Look for containers, pill bottles, drug paraphernalia and signs of other medical problems. If the patient is incoherent or unconscious, try to get information from any bystanders or family members. Since many of the physical signs of substance abuse mimic other conditions, you may not be able to determine that a patient has overdosed on a substance. To provide care, you only need to recognize abnormalities in breathing, skin color and moisture, body temperature and behavior, any of which may indicate a condition requiring professional help.

The abuse or misuse of stimulants can have many unhealthy effects on the body that mimic other conditions. For example, a stimulant overdose can cause moist or flushed skin, sweating, chills, nausea, vomiting, fever, headache, dizziness, rapid pulse, rapid breathing, high blood pressure and chest pain. In some instances, it can cause respiratory distress, disrupt normal heart rhythms or cause death. The patient may appear very excited, restless, talkative or irritable or may suddenly lose consciousness. Stimulant abuse can lead to addiction and can cause heart attack or stroke.

Specific signs and symptoms of hallucinogen abuse, as well as abuse of some designer drugs, may include sudden mood changes and a flushed face. The patient may claim to see or hear something not present or may be anxious and frightened.

Specific signs and symptoms of depressant abuse may include drowsiness, confusion, slurred speech, slow heart and breathing rates and poor coordination. A person who abuses alcohol may smell of alcohol. A person who has consumed a great deal of alcohol in a short time may become unconscious or hard to arouse. The person may vomit violently. Specific signs and symptoms of alcohol withdrawal, a potentially dangerous condition that can be life threatening, include confusion and restlessness, trembling, hallucinations and seizures.

A telltale sign of *cannabis* use is red, bloodshot eyes, while those abusing inhalants may appear drunk or disoriented in a similar manner to a person abusing hallucinogens.

Providing Care for Substance Abuse and Misuse

Always summon more advanced medical personnel if you suspect a patient is suffering from alcohol withdrawal or from any form of substance abuse. Since substance abuse and misuse are forms of poisoning, care follows the same general principles as for other types of poisoning. As in other medical emergencies, however, people who abuse or misuse substances may become aggressive or uncooperative when you try to help. If the person becomes agitated or makes the scene unsafe in any way, retreat until the scene can be secured. Provide care only if you feel the patient is not a danger to you and others.

Your initial care for substance abuse or misuse does not require that you know the specific substance taken. Follow these general principles as you would for any poisoning:

- Size up the scene to be sure it is safe.
- Perform a primary assessment to check for any life-threatening conditions.
- Summon more advanced medical personnel.
- Perform a physical exam.
- Take a SAMPLE history (signs and symptoms, allergies, medications, pertinent past history, last oral intake and events leading up to the incident) to try to find out what substance was taken, how much was taken and when it was taken.
- Calm and reassure the patient.
- Keep the patient from getting chilled or overheated.
- Keep the patient's airway clear.
- If the patient is having difficulty breathing, administer emergency oxygen if it is available.

Preventing Substance Abuse and Misuse

Experts in the field of substance abuse generally agree that prevention efforts are far more cost-effective than treatment. Yet preventing substance abuse is a complex process that involves many underlying factors. Various approaches, including educating people about substances and their effects on health and attempting to instil fear of penalties, have not by themselves proved particularly effective. It is becoming clearer that, to be effective, prevention efforts must address the various underlying issues of substance abuse and ways to approach it.

Recognizing and understanding the factors below may help prevent and treat substance abuse. The following factors may contribute to substance abuse:

- A lack of parental supervision
- The breakdown of traditional family structure
- A wish to escape unpleasant surroundings and stressful situations
- The widespread availability of substances
- Peer pressure and the basic need to belong
- Low self-esteem, including feelings of guilt or shame
- Media glamorization, especially of alcohol and tobacco, promoting the idea that using substances enhances fun and popularity

- A history of substance abuse in the home or community environments

Some poisonings from medications occur when patients knowingly increase the dosage beyond what is directed. Medications should be taken only as directed. On the other hand, many poisonings from medications are not intentional.

The following guidelines can help prevent unintentional misuse or overdose:
- Read the product information and use only as directed.
- Ask your health care provider or pharmacist about the intended use and side effects of prescription and OTC medication. If you are taking more than one medication, check for possible interaction effects.
- Never use another person's prescribed medications; what is right for one person is seldom right for another.
- Always keep medications in their original, marked containers.
- Discard all out-of-date medications. Time can alter the chemical composition of medications, causing them to be less effective and possibly even toxic.
- Always keep medications out of the reach of children.

PUTTING IT ALL TOGETHER

Poisonings can occur in four ways: ingestion, inhalation, absorption and injection. Substance abuse and misuse are types of poisoning that can occur in any of these ways. Substance abuse and misuse can produce a variety of signs and symptoms, most of which are common to other types of poisoning. You do not need to determine the cause of a poisoning to provide appropriate initial care.

If you see any of the signs and symptoms of sudden illness, follow the basic guidelines of care for any medical emergency. For suspected poisonings, contact the National PCC Hotline or summon more advanced medical personnel. Beyond following the general guidelines for providing care for a suspected poisoning, medical professionals may advise you to provide some specific care, such as neutralizing the poison.

Six major categories of substances, when abused or misused, can produce a variety of signs and symptoms, some of which are indistinguishable from those of other medical emergencies. Remember, you do not have to know the specific condition to provide care. If you suspect that the patient's condition is caused by substance abuse or misuse, provide care for a poisoning emergency.

YOU ARE THE EMERGENCY MEDICAL RESPONDER

Based on your findings, you suspect that the patient ingested a combination of drugs and alcohol. What initial care can you provide? What else should you do and why? Is this a case of substance misuse? Why or why not?

Enrichment
Administering Activated Charcoal

If a patient has ingested poison, activated charcoal may be recommended by the PCC or medical control. Ideally, this will be administered within 1 hour of the patient swallowing the poison **(Fig. 15-7)**.

Activated charcoal should only administered if the patient is fully conscious and alert and you have been directed by medical control or the PCC. A patient who is not able to swallow should *not* be given activated charcoal, nor should it be given to a patient who has overdosed on cyanide, swallowed acids or swallowed alkalis (including hydrochloric acid, bleach and ammonia).

Many patients experience black stools after taking activated charcoal. Vomiting is another common side effect, especially if the patient is already feeling nauseated. If the patient does vomit, ask medical control or PCC for permission to give a second dose of the activated charcoal, and arrange to take the patient to the hospital immediately.

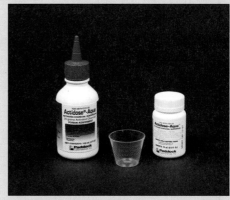

Fig. 15-7: Activated charcoal

The PCC or local medical authority will give you instructions on how to administer the activated charcoal. The container should also list instructions. Generally, you will be told to shake the bottle to mix the activated charcoal with water. Give it to the patient to drink. Using a straw or opaque container may make it easier for the patient to tolerate the mixture's less-than-appetizing appearance. If the charcoal settles, shake it again to mix it thoroughly; then let the patient finish drinking.

Medical control or PCC may give you directions about the dose. In general, the dosage is calculated at 1 gram of activated charcoal per kilogram of the patient's weight or 1 g/kg. An adult dose is usually between 30-100 grams; for a child or an infant, the dose is between 12-25 grams. Follow the correct dosage that is given by the PCC or by local protocols.

Enrichment
Carbon Monoxide and Cyanide Poisoning

Carbon monoxide (CO) and cyanide poisoning can result from disasters such as fires and industrial accidents, terrorist attacks and the use of weapons of mass destruction. As with all emergency responses, in cases of inhaled poison, it is essential that responders ensure their own safety before performing rescues.

CARBON MONOXIDE

Thousands of individuals die each year in the United States, and thousands more are hospitalized, due to CO poisoning. People often think about CO as related to car exhaust. However, CO is the byproduct of many combustible types of machinery, several of which people have in their homes, including wood stoves and barbecues. It is also the byproduct of larger fires, such as industrial or building fires. CO, which is present in substances such as tobacco smoke, can also be produced by defective cooking equipment, defective furnaces and kerosene heaters. CO is also found in indoor skating rinks and when charcoal is used indoors.

Everyday items that emit CO include—

- Heating systems, large or small (including portable types), that burn coal, gasoline, kerosene, oil, propane and wood; this includes camping stoves.
- Barbecues or grills, both propane and charcoal.
- Natural gas water heaters.
- Gas lawn mowers or any gas-powered vehicle.
- Portable generators, often used during power outages.
- Kitchen stoves, when used for heating homes or house trailers.

CO poisoning is the leading cause of death by poisoning in the United States. Its colorless and odorless presentation increases its danger, as patients may never be aware of its presence before succumbing to its poisonous effects. CO is highly lethal and can cause death after only a few minutes of exposure. CO detectors, which work much like smoke detectors, are widely available for use in homes and businesses **(Fig. 15-8)**. CO is lighter than air, which is why detectors should be placed in homes near sleeping areas at as high an elevation as possible, consistent with the manufacturer's operating instructions.

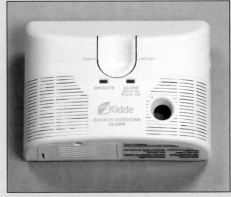

Fig. 15-8: A CO detector

Signs and Symptoms of CO Poisoning

The initial symptoms of CO poisoning, such as a dull or throbbing headache, nausea and vomiting, can easily be mistaken for something benign. Other signs and symptoms of CO poisoning include—

- Bluish skin color.
- Chest pain.
- Confusion.
- Convulsions.
- Dizziness.
- Drowsiness.
- Fainting.
- Hyperactivity.
- Impaired judgment.
- Irritability.

- Loss of consciousness.
- Low blood pressure.
- Muscle weakness.
- Rapid or abnormal heartbeat.
- Shock.
- Shortness of breath.

Providing Care for CO Poisoning

Because of the danger of CO, it is essential that responders are properly outfitted for safety and that the patient is removed from the situation as quickly as possible. If a patient experiences symptoms of CO poisoning, get the patient to fresh air immediately by opening doors and windows, turning off combustion appliances and leaving the building.

If CO poisoning is suspected, make sure emergency room staff and physicians are aware. Questions to ask the patient should include:
- Where the symptoms occurred.
- Whether symptoms disappear or decrease away from that location (e.g., home).
- Whether anyone else in the building is complaining of similar symptoms and whether those symptoms appeared at about the same time.
- Whether there are any fuel-burning appliances in the location.
- Whether these appliances have been inspected recently to ensure they are working properly.

If CO poisoning has occurred, the patient may be asked to undergo a blood test, which is done soon after exposure to confirm the diagnosis.

Everyone present in the area of the poisoning, even if they do not display any signs or symptoms, should be monitored or treated. The only treatment for CO poisoning that can be administered on the scene is providing emergency oxygen.

CYANIDE POISONING

Cyanide poisoning makes your body unable to utilize oxygen, and can quickly cause death. It can occur through the digestive and respiratory tracts and through the skin. It can also be injected.

Cyanide poisoning is generally thought of as a weapon used in terrorism or wartime. However, cyanide is found naturally in some everyday foods, such as apricot pits; in other products, such as cigarettes; and as byproducts of production such as plastic manufacturing. Cyanide is also used in some production processes such as making paper and textiles, developing photographs, cleaning metal and in rodent poisons.

Signs and Symptoms of Cyanide Poisoning

The signs and symptoms of cyanide poisoning depend on the extent of the exposure and the route by which it enters the body. If exposure is through eating products that have naturally occurring cyanide or by absorbing it through the skin, symptoms may include sudden onset of—
- Dizziness.
- Headache.
- Nausea and vomiting.
- Rapid breathing.
- Rapid heart rate.
- Restlessness.
- Weakness.

Patients who were subjected to larger, concentrated or more intense exposure to cyanide, such as from an industrial accident or a terrorist attack, could display symptoms such as—

Continued on next page

Enrichment
Carbon Monoxide and Cyanide Poisoning (continued)

- Convulsions.
- Loss of consciousness.
- Low blood pressure.
- Lung injury.
- Respiratory failure leading to death.
- Slow heart rate.

Exams and Tests for Cyanide Poisoning

There is no quick, simple blood test that will confirm cyanide poisoning at the scene of an accident or at a fire, the two most common places where this type of poisoning is likely to occur. Cyanide poisoning must therefore be assumed when it is likely based on circumstances, so that life-saving care may be started quickly. You should suspect cyanide poisoning at the scene of a fire if the patient has been exposed to smoke in a confined space, whether or not the patient has been burned. If the patient has soot around the mouth and nose and an altered LOC, the probability of cyanide toxicity is greater. The most likely set of symptoms in someone who has suffered cyanide toxicity is altered mental status, abnormal pupil dilation (widening), low respiratory rate, low systolic blood pressure with increased heart rate, metabolic acidosis (increased plasma acidity) and a large increase in lactate levels in the plasma.

Providing Care for Cyanide Poisoning

Hydrogen cyanide can enter the body through inhalation or ingestion, or by being absorbed into the skin or eyes. Avoid all contact. If you or someone else is exposed, seek medical attention immediately.

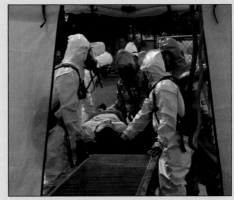

Fig. 15-9: Patients from an industrial accident or terrorist attack can be subjected to larger, concentrated or more intense exposure to cyanide. *Courtesy of Captain Phil Kleinberg, EMT-P, Lake-Sumter EMS.*

If there is a risk of inhalation, seek ventilation or local exhaust, or use breathing protection with a gas mask that has a *hydrogen cyanide* (HC) canister (escape). The use of positive-pressure *self-contained breathing apparatus* (SCBA) or SCBA CBRN (*chemical, biological, radiological and nuclear*), if available, is recommended when responding to nonroutine emergency situations **(Fig. 15-9)**. Use a CBRN, full face-piece *air purifying respirator* (APR), when available, in nonroutine, emergency situations, environments less than immediately dangerous to life or health concentrations, but above recommended exposure limit or permissible exposure limit levels. If you or someone else is exposed to hydrogen cyanide via inhalation, seek fresh air and rest in a half-upright position. Avoid mouth-to-mouth resuscitation, and administer emergency oxygen if it is available.

If there is risk of absorption into the skin, use butyl rubber gloves and Teflon® or Tychem® protective clothing as appropriate. If you or someone else has been exposed through absorption into the skin, remove the contaminated clothing and rinse the skin with plenty of water or use a shower to rinse. Wear protective gloves when administering first aid, and seek medical attention immediately.

Hydrogen cyanide vapor can be absorbed through the eyes. For prevention, wear safety goggles, a face shield or eye protection in combination with breathing protection. If the eyes are exposed, rinse with plenty of water for several minutes. If you or the patient exposed is wearing contact lenses, remove them if easily possible. Seek medical attention immediately.

Hydrogen cyanide can also be ingested. To prevent such an exposure, do not eat, drink or smoke during work, and wash your hands before eating. If you are exposed by ingestion, rinse your mouth and follow the same steps as for inhalation. Do *not* induce vomiting. Seek medical attention immediately.

Hydrogen cyanide poses several hazards associated with fire. It is extremely flammable and the fire emits toxic or irritating gases. To prevent fire around this gas, ensure that there is *no* smoking, and there are *no* open flames or sparks. If fire does break out, shut off the gas supply. If this is not possible and there are no risks to the surrounding environment, let the fire burn out on its own. If you can extinguish it, use powder, water spray, foam or carbon dioxide.

When mixed with air, hydrogen cyanide also poses a risk of explosion. Keep the area closed and well ventilated, and use explosion-proof electrical equipment and lighting. To prevent an explosion, if there is a fire, keep the cylinder cool by spraying it with water. If you do have to fight the fire, do so from a sheltered position.

If a patient is suspected of exposure to hydrogen cyanide, the SAMPLE history and scene size-up will be vital. The hospital will administer blood tests, X-rays, other diagnostic tests and IV lines. It is important to accurately convey details about the scene to health care providers, as they will use this information, along the patient's presentation and the test results, to determine if the patient has indeed suffered from cyanide poisoning. Also, because cyanide poisoning is rare, health care providers may not consider the possibility unless you report it, and treatment may come too late.

16 Environmental Emergencies

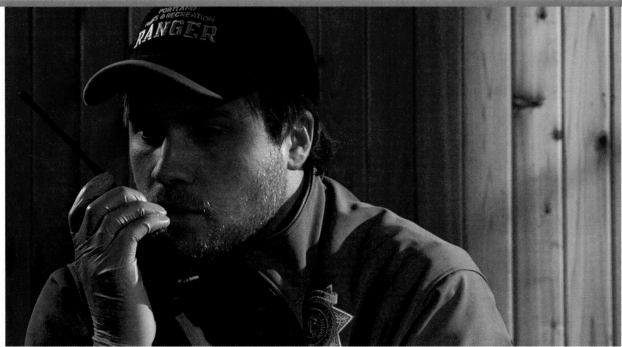

))) **YOU ARE THE EMERGENCY MEDICAL RESPONDER**

As the nearest park ranger in the area, you are summoned to a campsite for an incident involving a possible venomous snakebite. When you arrive and size-up the scene, you find several campers assisting one of the others, a young adult male. As you begin your primary assessment and investigate the patient's chief complaint, you see two puncture wounds and swelling on his right hand. The patient described the snake as having a triangular shaped head and distinct diamond-shaped patterns on its body. It struck him like "a bolt of lightning" when he bent down to move some rocks beside the stream. He says the pain is about an 8 or a 9, on a scale of 1 to 10. There is a medical facility at the park headquarters and a regional medical center with antivenin nearby. How would you respond?

Key Terms

Anaphylaxis: A form of distributive shock caused by an often sudden severe allergic reaction, in which air passages may swell and restrict breathing; also referred to as *anaphylactic shock*.

Antivenin: A substance used to counteract the poisonous effects of venom.

Arterial gas embolism: A condition in which air bubbles enter the bloodstream and subsequently travel to the brain; results from a rapid ascent from deep water, which expands air in the lungs too quickly.

Barotrauma: Injury sustained because of pressure differences between areas of the body and the surrounding environment; most commonly occurs in air travel and scuba diving.

Conduction: One of the ways the body loses or gains heat; occurs when the skin is in contact with something with a lower or higher temperature.

Convection: One of the ways the body loses or gains heat; occurs when air moves over the skin and carries away or increases heat.

Core temperature: The temperature inside the body.

Decompression sickness: A sometimes fatal disorder caused by the release of gas bubbles into body tissue; also known as "*the bends*"; occurs when scuba divers ascend too rapidly, without allowing sufficient time for gases to exit body tissues and be removed through exhalation.

Dehydration: Inadequate fluids in the body's tissues.

Drowning: An event in which a victim experiences respiratory impairment due to submersion in water. Drowning may or may not result in death.

Electrolytes: Substances that are electrically conductive in solution and are essential to the regulation of nerve and muscle function and fluid balance throughout the body; include sodium, potassium, chloride, calcium and phosphate.

Evaporation: One of the ways the body loses heat; occurs when the body is wet and the moisture evaporates, cooling the skin.

Free diving: An extreme sport in which divers compete under water without any underwater breathing apparatus.

Frostbite: A condition in which body tissues freeze; most commonly occurs in the fingers, toes, ears and nose.

Heat cramps: A form of heat-related illness; painful involuntary muscle spasms that occur during or after physical exertion in high heat, caused by loss of electrolytes and water from perspiration; may be a sign that a more serious heat-related illness is developing; usually affects the legs and abdomen.

Heat exhaustion: More severe form of heat-related illness; results when fluid and electrolytes are lost through perspiration and are not replaced by other fluids; often results from strenuous work or wearing too much clothing in a hot, humid environment.

Heat index: An index that combines the air temperature and relative humidity to determine the perceived, human-felt temperature; a measure of how hot it feels.

Heat stroke: The most serious form of heat-related illness; life threatening and develops when the body's cooling mechanisms are overwhelmed and body systems begin to fail.

Hyperthermia: Overheating of the body; includes heat cramps, heat exhaustion and heat stroke.

Hypothalamus: Control center of the body's temperature; located in the brain.

Hypothermia: The state of the body being colder than the usual core temperature, caused by either excessive loss of body heat and/or the body's inability to produce heat.

Metabolism: The physical and chemical processes of converting oxygen and food into energy within the body.

Rabies: An infectious viral disease that affects the nervous system of humans and other mammals; has a high fatality rate if left untreated.

Radiation: One of the ways the body loses heat; heat radiates out of the body, especially from the head and neck.

Tetanus: An acute infectious disease caused by a bacterium that produces a powerful poison; can occur in puncture wounds, such as human and animal bites; also called *lockjaw*.

Learning Objectives

After reading this chapter, and completing the class activities, you will have the information needed to—

- Identify the signs and symptoms of a heat-related illness.
- Describe how to care for a patient who has a heat-related illness.
- Identify the signs and symptoms of a cold-related emergency.
- Describe how to care for a patient who has a cold-related emergency.
- Identify the signs and symptoms of the most common types of bites and stings.
- Describe how to provide general care for various bites and stings.
- Describe various methods of rescuing a victim in the water.
- Identify the signs and symptoms of anaphylaxis (*Enrichment*).
- Describe the care provided to a patient experiencing anaphylactic shock (*Enrichment*).
- Explain how to stay safe during lightning (*Enrichment*).
- Identify SCUBA and free diving emergencies (*Enrichment*).

Skill Objectives

After reading this chapter, and completing the class activities, you should be able to—

- Demonstrate the use of an epinephrine auto-injector *(Enrichment skill)*
- Demonstrate appropriate handling and disposal of an epinephrine auto-injector *(Enrichment skill)*

INTRODUCTION

Environmental emergencies include a wide range of situations—from **heat stroke** and **frostbite**, to snakebites and **drowning**. They range from minor to life threatening. In some cases, the same problem—such as a bee sting—can result in minor pain and discomfort in one patient while causing a life-threatening condition in another, such as **anaphylaxis**.

Environmental emergencies often occur during the course of everyday events. For example, a teenager may get caught without shelter and proper clothing during a sudden downpour while on a hike, a senior may collapse from **dehydration** during a heat spell or a bathtub may be the cause of a drowning for a small child.

In this chapter, you will learn how to recognize and care for heat-related illnesses and cold-related emergencies, bites and stings, and drowning incidents.

BODY TEMPERATURE

The human body usually keeps itself at a constant **core temperature** (internal temperature) of 98.6° F, or 37° C. The control center of body temperature is in the brain and is called the **hypothalamus**. The hypothalamus receives information and adjusts the body's function accordingly. The body needs to be kept within a specific range of temperatures for the cells to stay alive and healthy (97.8° F to 99° F, or 36.5° C to 37.2° C). It is vital the body responds properly to temperature signals.

How the Body Stays Warm

Heat is a byproduct of **metabolism**, the conversion of food and drink into energy. The

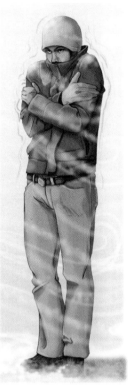

Skin surface

Constricted blood vessel

Fig. 16-1: The body stays warm by constricting blood vessels close to the skin. If this does not work, it begins to shiver.

body also gains heat with any kind of physical activity. If the body starts to become too cold, it responds by *constricting* (closing up) the blood vessels close to the skin so it can keep the warmer blood near the center of the body (**Fig. 16-1**). This helps keep the organs warm. If this does not work, the body then begins to shiver. The shivering motion increases body heat because it is a form of movement.

How the Body Stays Cool

In a warm or hot environment, the hypothalamus detects an increase in blood temperature. Blood vessels near the skin *dilate* (widen), to bring more

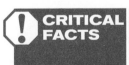

CRITICAL FACTS

The human body usually keeps itself at a constant core temperature (internal temperature) of 98.6° F, or 37° C.

In a warm or hot environment, the hypothalamus detects an increase in blood temperature. Blood vessels near the skin dilate (widen), to bring more blood to the surface, which allows heat to escape.

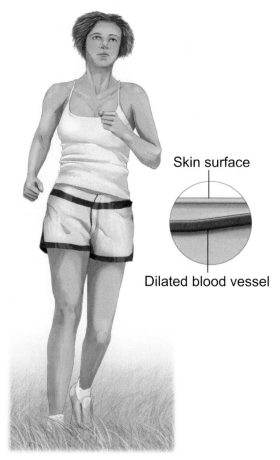

Fig. 16-2: The body stays cool by dilating blood vessels near the skin so heat can escape.

blood to the surface, which allows heat to escape (**Fig. 16-2**).

There are five general ways in which the body can be cooled:

- **Radiation**: This process involves the transfer of heat from one object to another without physical contact. The body loses the majority of heat through radiation, mostly from the head, hands and feet.
- **Convection**: This process occurs when cold air moves over the skin and carries the skin's heat away. The faster the air is moving, the faster the body will be cooled. Convection is what makes warm skin feel cooler in a breeze. Convection also assists in the **evaporation** process.
- **Conduction**: This occurs when the body is in direct contact with a substance that is cooler than the body's temperature. Through conduction, the body's heat is transferred to the cooler substance (e.g., if you are swimming in cold water or sitting on a cool rock in the shade).
- Evaporation: This is the process by which a liquid or solid becomes a vapor. When body heat causes one to perspire and the perspiration evaporates, the heat that was absorbed into sweat dissipates into the air which cools off the skin.
- Respiration: Heat is also lost through respiration, another term for breathing. Before air is exhaled, it is warmed by the lungs and airway. Respiration normally accounts for approximately 10 to 20 percent of heat loss.

PEOPLE AT RISK FOR HEAT-RELATED ILLNESSES AND COLD-RELATED EMERGENCIES

Although anyone can be at risk for heat-related illnesses and cold-related emergencies, some people are at even greater risk than others. People who are susceptible to a heat-related illness or cold-related emergency include those who—

- Work or exercise strenuously in a warm or hot and humid environment or a cold environment.
- Have a pre-existing health problem, such as diabetes or heart disease. Pre-existing health problems can increase susceptibility to a heat-related illness. Medications taken for these conditions can also cause dehydration.
- Have had a previous heat-related illness or cold-related emergency.
- Take medications to eliminate water from the body (*diuretics*). Diuretics increase the risk of dehydration which, in turn, causes an increase in core body temperature by preventing adequate blood flow to remove excess heat.
- Consume other substances that have a diuretic effect, such as fluids containing caffeine, alcohol or carbonation.
- Live in a situation or environment that does not provide them with enough heating or cooling, depending on the season.
- Do not maintain adequate hydration by drinking enough water to counteract the loss

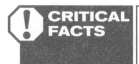

CRITICAL FACTS

Heat-related illnesses and cold-related emergencies occur more frequently among elderly, especially those exposed to poor living conditions. The young and those with health problems are also considered high-risk groups.

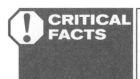

CRITICAL FACTS

There are several types of illness related to overheating of the body, or hyperthermia: heat cramps, heat exhaustion and heat stroke.

Dehydration can be a serious and even life-threatening situation. The people at highest risk of dying from dehydration are the very young and the very old.

of fluids through perspiration, exertion or exposure to heat and humidity.
- Wear clothing inappropriate for the weather.

Heat-related illnesses and cold-related emergencies occur more frequently among the elderly, especially those living in poorly ventilated or poorly insulated buildings or buildings with poor heating or cooling systems. Young children and people with health problems are also at greater risk because their bodies do not respond as effectively to temperature extremes.

HEAT-RELATED ILLNESSES

There are several types of illness related to overheating of the body, or **hyperthermia**, including **heat cramps**, **heat exhaustion** and heat stroke. Heat-related illnesses can happen to anyone, but several predisposing factors can put some people at higher risk. These factors include—
- Climate. In very warm or hot and humid weather, the body may not be able to cool off sufficiently. If the temperature is high, the body is not as able to lower its temperature through radiation. The more humid the air, the less the body is able to cool down through sweating. Evaporation decreases as the relative humidity increases because the air contains excessive moisture (**Fig. 16-3**).

- Exercise and activity. Exercise or strenuous labor in the heat does not allow the body to cool off, particularly since exercise itself increases body temperature. When combined with a high **heat index**, there is a much greater risk of increasing the core temperature as it becomes more difficult to cool the body.
- Age. The very young and very old are not as able to regulate body temperature as others are. Infants and young children, for example, may not be able to get the fluids they need, move away from the heated area or speak up and tell someone they are too warm.
- Pre-existing illness and/or conditions. Certain illnesses and conditions can make someone feel the heat more than others. Examples include people with diabetes, infections (which can cause fever, increasing the body temperature even more), obesity and heart disease.
- Drugs and/or medications. Medications or substances, such as alcohol and diuretics, cause an increase in blood vessel constriction, increase urination, increase the risk of dehydration and increase core temperature.

Dehydration

Dehydration refers to inadequate fluids in the body's tissues. Dehydration can be a serious and even life-threatening situation. The people at

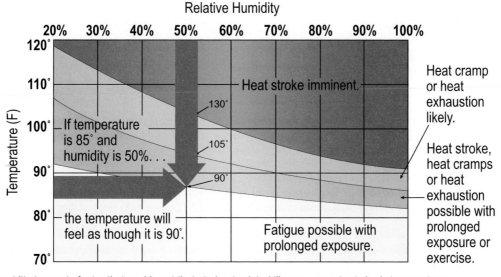

Fig. 16-3: Humidity is a main factor that could contribute to heat-related illnesses or a rise in body temperature.

highest risk of dying from dehydration are the very young and the very old.

Signs and Symptoms of Dehydration

The signs and symptoms of dehydration worsen as the body becomes dryer. The first signs of dehydration include—

- Fatigue.
- Weakness.
- Headache.
- Irritability.
- Nausea.
- Dizziness.
- Excessive thirst.
- Dry lips and mouth.

As dehydration worsens, symptoms can include—

- Disorientation or delirium.
- Loss of appetite.
- Severe thirst.
- Dry mucous membranes.
- Sunken eyes.
- Lowered blood pressure.
- Rapid pulse.
- Dry skin that does not spring back if pinched, creating a "tenting" effect.
- Lack of tears (particularly important among young children).
- Decrease in perspiration.
- Dark, amber urine or complete lack of urine output.
- Unconsciousness.

Providing Care for Dehydration

To care for dehydration, replace the lost fluid. If the patient is still conscious and able to swallow, encourage the patient to drink small amounts of a carbohydrate/electrolyte-containing liquid, such as a commercial sports drink or milk. Juice or water also can be given. Do not let the patient gulp the fluid down; instead, have the patient sip it at a slow pace. If the patient drinks too quickly, vomiting may occur. If dehydration is severe, the patient will likely need more advanced medical care to receive fluids intravenously.

Heat Cramps
Signs and Symptoms of Heat Cramps

Heat cramps are painful, involuntary muscle spasms that occur during or after physical exertion in high heat, and are caused by loss of fluids and associated **electrolytes** from perspiration. Heat cramps usually develop fairly quickly and are most often in the legs and abdomen. People who perspire excessively during strenuous activity are often at an increased risk for heat cramps. Although the patient's body temperature may be normal and the skin moist, heat cramps could be an indication that a more severe heat-related illness is developing. It does *not* have to be very hot for heat cramps to occur.

Providing Care for Heat Cramps

Heat cramps must be taken seriously, particularly if there is a history of heart disease or the patient is on a low-sodium diet. To care for heat cramps, the most important initial action is to reduce the cramps. Have the patient rest, then gently massage and lightly stretch the cramped muscles to ease the discomfort. Encourage the patient to drink fluid (carbohydrate/electrolyte solution [e.g., commercial sports drinks or milk] or water) to replace what was lost to perspiration.

While the patient should rest as long as possible, if the cramping has gone away and the patient feels better, activity can be resumed with caution. Advise the patient to rest frequently and drink fluids to prevent further dehydration and cramping.

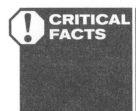
CRITICAL FACTS

To care for dehydration, replace the lost fluid by having him or her slowly drink small amounts of a carbohydrate/electrolyte-containing liquid, such as a commercial sports drink or milk, juice or water.

Heat cramps are painful, involuntary muscle spasms, most often in the legs and abdomen, caused by loss of fluids and electrolytes after physical exertion, especially (but not always) in high heat. Heat cramps may indicate severe heat-related illness.

To care for heat cramps, have the patient rest, then gently massage and lightly stretch the cramped muscles. Encourage the patient to drink a commercial sports drink, milk or water.

Heat Exhaustion

Heat exhaustion is a more severe form of heat-related illness. Heat exhaustion results when fluid lost through perspiration is not replaced by other fluids. This results in the body pulling the blood away from the surface areas of the body to protect the vital organs, like the heart and brain.

Anyone can be at risk of developing heat exhaustion from exposure to a hot or humid environment. However, it happens most often to those engaged in intense physical activity—like firefighters, construction or factory workers and athletes. Simply being in a hot and humid environment while overdressed with heavy clothes can cause heat exhaustion.

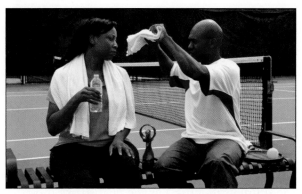

Fig. 16-4: Applying cool, wet cloths to the skin, fanning and encouraging rehydration are all effective ways to help a patient with heat exhaustion.

Signs and Symptoms of Heat Exhaustion

The signs and symptoms of heat exhaustion include—

- Cool, moist, pale, ashen (grayish) or flushed skin.
- Weakness.
- Dizziness.
- Rapid, weak pulse.
- Shallow breathing.
- Low blood pressure.
- Exhaustion.
- Light-headedness.
- Decreasing *level of consciousness* (LOC).
- Heavy sweating.
- Headache.
- Nausea.
- Fainting.
- Muscle cramps (heat cramps).

Providing Care for Heat Exhaustion

Care for heat exhaustion includes—

- Moving the patient out of the hot environment to a cooler area.
- If the problem is due to overdressing, helping the patient remove coats, sweaters or other layers of clothing.
- Cooling the patient's body by spraying with cool water or applying cool, wet cloths or towels to the skin. Some respond well to fanning, as this increases evaporative cooling (**Fig. 16-4**).
- Encouraging rehydration with a carbohydrate/electrolyte solution, such as a commercial sports drink or milk, or water if the patient is fully conscious and able to swallow.
- Applying ice packs or cold packs wrapped in a thin towel to the wrists, ankles, armpits, groin and back of the neck to cool the blood in major blood vessels, if further cooling down is required.
- Calling for more advanced medical personnel and providing care for heat stroke, when the patient does not improve in a few minutes, refuses to drink water, vomits, shows other signs of heat stroke or begins to lose consciousness.

Low blood pressure and rapid, weak pulse are signs of shock, so take steps to prevent or minimize shock. Refer to **Chapter 18** for more information on how to care for shock.

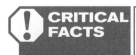

CRITICAL FACTS

Heat exhaustion is a more severe form of heat-related illness. Heat exhaustion results when fluid lost through perspiration is not replaced by other fluids.

To provide care for heat exhaustion, move the patient out of the heat to a cooler area and loosen or remove as much clothing as possible. Spray the person with cool water, apply cool wet cloths or towels to the skin and fan the person. Encourage drinking small amounts of a commercial sports drink, milk or water if the patient is fully conscious and able to swallow.

Heat Stroke

The most serious of heat-related illnesses is heat stroke. Heat stroke is a life-threatening condition that occurs when the body has become overheated and is no longer able to cool itself down. Two types of heat stroke are typically reported—classic heat stroke and exertional heat stroke.

Classic heat stroke is normally caused by environmental changes and often occurs during the summer months. Classic heat stroke most often occurs in infants, children, the elderly, those with chronic medical illnesses and in those individuals who suffer from inefficient body heat-regulation mechanisms—such as those in poor socioeconomic settings with limited access to air conditioning and those on certain medications (e.g., antihistamines, amphetamines, diuretics, and blood pressure and heart medicines). Typically, classic heat stroke develops slowly, over a period of several days, with patients presenting with minimally elevated core temperatures.

Exertional heat stroke, however, is the opposite of classic heat stroke. Exertional heat stroke— which primarily affects younger, active individuals, such as athletes (recreational and competitive), military recruits and heavy laborers—occurs when excess heat is generated through exercise and exceeds the body's ability to cool off. Exposure to factors such as high air temperature, high relative humidity and dehydration increases the risk for developing exertional heat stroke.

Signs and Symptoms of Heat Stroke

Tell-tale signs of heat stroke are cessation of sweating and high body temperature. When the body no longer sweats, the chance of cooling off decreases significantly. Be aware that the skin may still be wet from prior physical exertion.

Other signs and symptoms of heat stroke can include—
- Extremely high body temperature (above 104° F, or 40° C).
- Flushed or red skin that can be either dry, or moist from recent exercise.
- Rapid, weak pulse or shallow breathing.
- Low blood pressure.
- Throbbing headache.
- Dizziness, nausea or vomiting.
- Decreasing LOC.
- Altered mental status.
- Confusion, disorientation, irrational behavior or attention deficit.
- Unconsciousness or coma.
- Convulsions or seizure.

Providing Care for Heat Stroke

Since heat stroke is life threatening, you should immediately call for more advanced medical personnel. Your next priority is to begin rapid cooling of the patient's body, to bring the core temperature down. The quicker you can get the body temperature down, the better the outcome. Bring down the patient's body temperature quickly, to reduce the possibility of brain damage, organ failure or death.

Perform a primary assessment and then provide care by using any of the following techniques to cool the patient rapidly:
- Immerse the patient in cold water up to his or her neck (preferred method).
- Douse the patient with ice water-soaked towels over the entire body, frequently rotating the cold, wet towels, spraying with

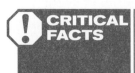 **CRITICAL FACTS**

The most serious of heat-related illnesses is heat stroke. Heat stroke is a life-threatening condition that occurs when the body has become overheated and is no longer able to cool itself down.

In cases of heat stroke, call for more advanced medical personnel immediately. Your next priority is to begin rapid cooling methods, such as cold water immersion. The quicker you can get the body temperature down, the better the outcome.

Hypothermia is the state of the body being colder than the usual core temperature. It is caused by either excessive loss of body heat and/or the body's inability to produce heat.

cold water, fanning the patient or covering the patient with ice towels or bags of ice placed over the body.

- If you are not able to measure and monitor the patient's core temperature, apply rapid cooling methods for 20 minutes or until the patient's LOC improves.

Low blood pressure and rapid pulse are signs of shock, so take steps to prevent or minimize shock. Refer to **Chapter 18** for more information on care for shock. A person in heat stroke may experience respiratory or cardiac arrest. Be prepared to give ventilations or perform CPR, if needed.

COLD-RELATED EMERGENCIES

Hypothermia (Generalized Cold Exposure)

Hypothermia is the state of the body being colder than the usual core temperature. It is caused by either excessive loss of body heat and/or the body's inability to produce heat.

Hypothermia can come on gradually or it can develop very quickly. In hypothermia, body temperature drops below 95° F (35° C).

As the body cools, an abnormal heart rhythm (ventricular fibrillation, or V-fib) may develop. If this happens, the heart will eventually stop and the patient will die if not cared for.

Contributing Factors

As with heat-related illnesses, anyone can develop hypothermia, but predisposing factors put some people at a higher risk (**Fig. 16-5**). These factors include—

- A cold environment. Even if the ambient temperature is not extremely low, hypothermia can occur if a person is not adequately protected from the cold.
- A wet environment. The presence of moisture (e.g., perspiration, rain, snow or water) will increase the speed at which body heat is lost.
- Wind. Wind makes the environment a lot colder than the ambient temperature indicates. The higher the wind chill effect, the lower the temperature actually is.

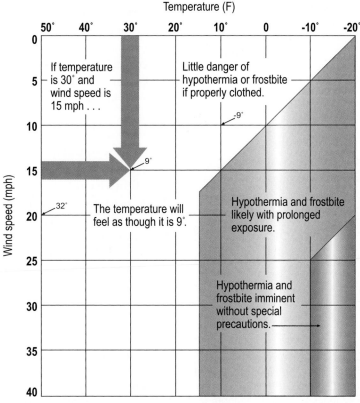

Fig. 16-5: Wind speed is a main factor that could contribute to cold-related emergencies or a decrease in body temperature.

- Age. The very young and the very old may have difficulty keeping warm in cool or cold conditions. Infants may not yet be able to shiver effectively. The elderly may not have enough body mass to retain body heat. Both age groups may be unable to help themselves stay warm by removing themselves from the cold environment or by protecting themselves with warmer clothing. In addition, many elderly people have impaired circulation.
- Medical conditions. People with certain medical conditions, such as generalized infection, hypoglycemia, shock and head injury, may be at higher risk of developing hypothermia.
- Alcohol, drugs and poisoning. Alcohol and certain types of drugs or poisons can reduce a patient's ability to feel the cold, or can cloud judgment and impede rational thought, preventing the patient from taking proper precautions to stay warm.
- Clothing inappropriate for the weather.

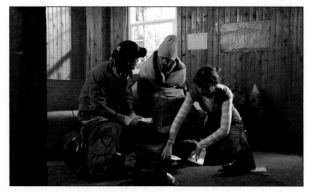

Fig. 16-6: When providing care for a patient with hypothermia, your priority is to move the patient into a warmer environment.

Signs and Symptoms of Hypothermia

The signs and symptoms of hypothermia include—
- Shivering (may be absent in later stages of hypothermia).
- Numbness.
- Glassy stare.
- Apathy or decreasing LOC.
- Weakness.
- Impaired judgment.

In cases of severe hypothermia, the patient may be unconscious. Breathing may have slowed or stopped. The body may feel stiff as the muscles become rigid.

Providing Care for Hypothermia

Your priority is to move the patient into a warmer environment, if possible. Be careful to move the patient gently, as any sudden movements can cause a heart arrhythmia and possibly cardiac arrest. Then—
- Perform a primary assessment, including a pulse check for up to 30 to 45 seconds.
- Call for more advanced medical personnel.
- Remove any wet clothing and dry off the patient.
- Passively rewarm the patient by wrapping all exposed body surfaces with anything at hand, such as warm blankets, clothing or newspapers. Be sure to also cover the head, since a significant amount of body heat is lost through the head (**Fig. 16-6**).
- If you are far from definitive health care, you may begin active rewarming. Place the patient near a heat source and apply heat pads, hot water bottles or chemical hot packs lightly wrapped in a towel or fabric to the wrists, ankles, armpits, groin and back of the neck to warm the blood in major blood vessels. Active rewarming should not delay definitive care.
- Do not immerse the patient in warm water.
- Do not rub or massage the extremities.
- Give warm, not hot, liquids that do not contain alcohol or caffeine if the patient is alert and able to swallow.
- Provide emergency oxygen, if it is available.

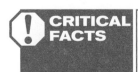

CRITICAL FACTS For hypothermia, your first priority is to move the patient to a warmer environment. Other critical care steps include removing wet clothing, drying the patient, passively rewarming the patient with dry clothes or blankets, giving the patient warm liquids, administering emergency oxygen if available and monitoring the patient's condition.

- Monitor the patient's condition. Capillary refill is affected by cold environments, so refill may be slow and therefore may not be an ideal method for assessing circulation. For more on capillary refill, see **Chapters 7 and 8**.
- Continue to warm the patient.
- Be prepared to perform CPR or use an *automated external defibrillator* (AED), if necessary.

Frostbite (Localized Cold Exposure)

Frostbite is the freezing of body tissues, usually the nose, ears, fingers or toes (**Fig. 16-7**). In both superficial and deep frostbite, the situation is serious and could result in loss of the body part. In fact, frostbite of the fingers and toes can cause enough damage to warrant amputation of hands and feet, and even arms and legs.

In early (or superficial) frostbite, only the first layers of skin are frozen. In late (or deep) frostbite, the skin and underlying tissues are frozen.

Signs and Symptoms of Frostbite

Signs and symptoms of frostbite include—
- Lack of feeling in the affected area.
- Swelling.
- Skin that appears waxy, is cold to the touch or is discolored (flushed, white, yellow or blue).

In more serious cases, blisters may form and the affected part may turn black and show signs of deep tissue damage.

Providing Care for Frostbite

As with hypothermia, the priority is to get the patient out of the cold. Once the patient is removed from the cold, you should also do the following:

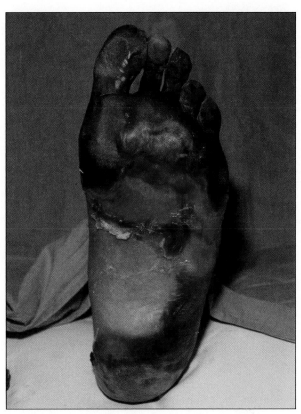

Fig. 16-7: Frostbitten skin features waxy skin that is cold to the touch and flushed or appears white, yellow or bluish in color. *Courtesy of Nigel Vardy and Nottingham University Hospitals NHS Trust.*

- Handle the area gently. Rough handling can damage the body part. *Never* rub the affected area, as this can cause skin damage.
- If there is a chance the body part may refreeze or if you are close to a medical facility, do *not* attempt to rewarm the frostbitten area.
- For minor frostbite, rapidly rewarm the affected part using skin-to-skin contact such as with a warm hand.
- For a more serious injury, rewarm the body part by gently soaking it in water not warmer than about 105°F. If you do not have a thermometer, test the water temperature yourself. If the temperature is uncomfortable to your touch, it is

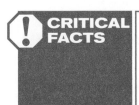

CRITICAL FACTS

Frostbite is the freezing of body tissues, usually the nose, ears, fingers or toes. Frostbite can cause serious damage, including loss of the body part or the need for amputation.

Your priority in caring for a frostbite patient is getting him or her out of the cold. Handle the frostbitten area carefully. Rewarm in warm water, but *only* if there is no risk of the body part refreezing and you are *not* close to a medical facility. Loosely bandage the area. If fingers and toes are frostbitten, place dry, sterile gauze between them. Avoid breaking blisters and take precautions to prevent hypothermia.

too warm. Keep the frostbitten part in the water until normal color returns and it feels warm (for 20 to 30 minutes) (**Fig. 16-8, A–B**).

- Loosely bandage the area with dry, sterile dressings.
- If the fingers or toes are frostbitten, place dry, sterile gauze between them to keep them separated. If the damage is to the feet, DO NOT allow the patient to walk.
- *Avoid* breaking any blisters.
- Take precautions to prevent hypothermia.
- Monitor the person and care for shock.
- Do not give any ibuprofen or other *nonsteroidal anti-inflammatory drugs* (NSAIDs) when caring for frostbite.

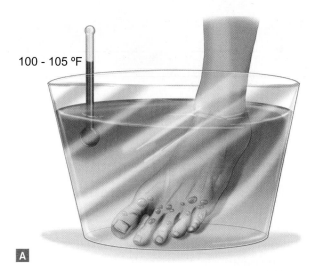

100 - 105 °F

A

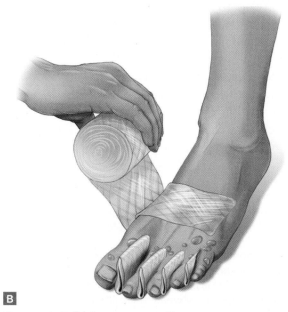

B

Fig. 16-8, A–B: **(A)** Gently warm the affected area by soaking it in warm, not hot, water. **(B)** If the patient's fingers or toes are frostbitten, place dry, sterile gauze between them to keep them separated.

PREVENTING HEAT-RELATED ILLNESSES AND COLD-RELATED EMERGENCIES

Generally, illnesses caused by overexposure to extreme temperatures are preventable. The easiest way to prevent illness caused by temperature extremes is to avoid being outside during the parts of the day when temperatures are most extreme. For instance, if working outdoors in hot weather, it is safer if the work can be done in the early morning and evening hours when the sun is not as strong. In cold weather, outside work is safer during the warmer part of the day.

Appropriate clothing for the weather and activity level adds protection against illness. It is best to wear light-colored clothing in the heat, which helps reflect the sun's rays. In the cold, the best clothing is made of tightly woven fibers, such as wool, to trap warm air against the body. Head coverings should be worn in both heat and cold. A hat or cap protects the head from the sun's rays in the summer and prevents heat from escaping in the winter. Also, other areas of the body, such as the fingers, toes, ears and nose, should be protected from cold exposure by wearing protective coverings.

Take additional precautions, such as changing activity level and taking frequent breaks. For instance, in very hot conditions, it is best to exercise only for brief periods, then rest in a cool, shaded area. Frequent breaks allow the body to readjust to normal body temperature, enabling it to better withstand brief periods of exposure to temperature extremes. Avoid heavy exercise during the hottest or coldest part of the day. Extremes of temperature promote fatigue, which hampers the body's ability to adjust to changes in the environment.

Whether in the heat or cold, it is important to drink enough fluids. Drinking at least six 8-ounce glasses of fluids daily is the most important way to prevent heat-related illness and cold-related emergency. It is best to drink fluids when taking a break. Drink cool fluids in the summer and warm fluids in the winter. Cool and warm fluids help the body maintain a normal temperature. If cool or warm drinks are not available, drink plenty of water. Avoid beverages containing caffeine or alcohol, which hinder the body's temperature-regulating mechanism.

BITES AND STINGS
Insects

In the United States, roughly ½ to 5 percent of the population is severely allergic to stings from bees, wasps, hornets and yellow jackets. For highly allergic patients, even one sting can result in anaphylaxis, a severe allergic reaction in which air passages may swell and restrict breathing. Such highly allergic reactions account for the nearly 50 reported deaths from insect bites and stings each year. However, more people die from lightning strikes than from insect bites and stings.

Providing Care for an Insect Sting

To care for an insect sting, follow standard precautions and examine the sting site to see if the stinger is in the skin. Remove it, if it is still present. Scrape the stinger away from the skin with the edge of a tongue depressor or plastic card, such as a credit card (**Fig. 16-9**). With a bee sting, the venom sac may still be attached to the stinger and can continue to release venom for up to several minutes afterward. If you use tweezers, grasp the base of the stinger, *not* the venom sac. Grasping the venom sac could squeeze it and release more venom.

Cleanse the site and cover with a dressing. Wrapped ice or a cold pack may be applied to the area to reduce pain and swelling. Ask if the patient has any history of allergies to insect bites or stings and observe for signs of an allergic reaction, even if there is no known history. An allergic reaction can range from a minor

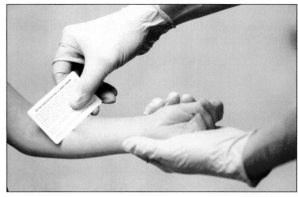

Fig. 16-9: Remove an insect stinger by scraping it away from the skin with the edge of a rigid item, such as a plastic card.

localized skin rash to anaphylaxis. Look for signs of anaphylaxis, including—

- Difficulty breathing, wheezing or shortness of breath.
- Tight feeling in the chest and throat.
- Swelling of the face, neck or tongue.
- Weakness, dizziness or confusion.
- Rash or hives.
- Low blood pressure.
- Shock.

If anaphylaxis occurs, provide emergency care *immediately*, including assisting with the patient's prescribed epinephrine auto-injector, if local protocols allow. (For more information on assisting with an epinephrine auto-injector, see the Enrichment section at the end of this chapter.) Administer emergency oxygen, if available. Call for more advanced medical personnel.

Ticks

Ticks can contract, carry and transmit serious diseases to humans. These include Rocky

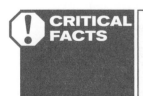
CRITICAL FACTS

In the United States, up to 5 percent of the population is severely allergic to insect stings. Such allergic reactions account for nearly 50 reported deaths each year.

If anaphylaxis occurs, provide emergency care immediately, including assisting with the patient's epinephrine auto-injector if local protocols allow. Administer emergency oxygen, if available, and call for more advanced medical personnel.

Mountain spotted fever, Babesia infection, Ehrlichiosis and Lyme disease (**Fig. 16-10, A–B**).

Providing Care for Tick Bites

If a tick is still embedded in the skin, it must be removed. With a gloved hand, grasp the tick with fine-tipped, pointed, nonetched, *nonrasped* (smooth inside surface) tweezers as close to the skin as possible. Pull slowly, steadily and firmly (**Fig. 16-11**).

- Do not try to burn the tick off.
- Do not apply petroleum jelly or nail polish to the tick.

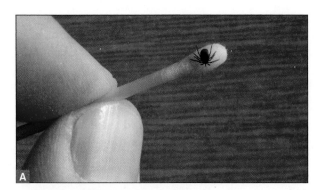

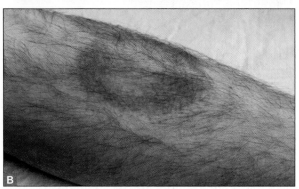

Fig. 16-10, A–B: **(A)** A deer tick can be as small as the head of a pin, *iStockphoto.com/Martin Pietak*; **(B)** A person with Lyme disease may develop a rash, *iStockphoto.com/Heike Kampe.*

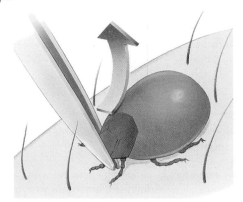

Fig. 16-11: Remove a tick that is still embedded in the skin by pulling slowly, steadily and firmly on the tick with a pair of fine-tipped, pointed, nonetched, nonrasped tweezers.

Table 16-1:

Infections From Ticks

INFECTIOUS DISEASES	SIGNS AND SYMPTOMS
Rocky Mountain Spotted Fever	Fever, nausea, vomiting, muscle pain, lack of appetite, severe headache, rash, abdominal pain, joint pain and diarrhea
Babesia Infection	Non-specific flu-like symptoms, such as fever, chills, sweats, headache, body aches, loss of appetite, nausea or fatigue, and anemia which can lead to jaundice and dark urine
Ehrlichiosis	Fever, headache, fatigue, muscle aches, nausea, vomiting, diarrhea, cough, joint pains, confusion and occasional rash
Lyme Disease	Fever, headache, fatigue and a characteristic skin rash (e.g., "bull's-eye")

Place the tick in a jar containing rubbing alcohol to kill it. Clean the bite area with soap and water, and apply antiseptic or antibiotic ointment if protocols allow and the patient has no known allergies or sensitivities to the medication. Advise the patient to seek medical advice, because of the risk of contracting a tickborne disease. If the tick cannot be removed, the patient should seek more advanced medical care.

Spiders and Scorpions

Few spiders in the United States have venom that causes serious illness or death. However, the bites of black widow and brown recluse spiders can, in rare instances, be fatal (**Fig. 16-12, A–E**). The venom of recluse spiders (known as brown recluse, fiddle back or violin) is necrotizing (tissue destroying), while the venom of widows (black, red and brown) contains neurotoxin and affects neuromuscular function. Symptoms will vary depending on the amount of venom injected and

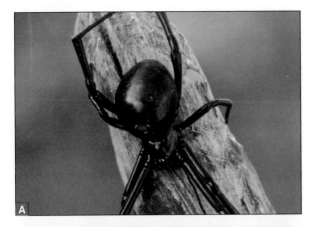

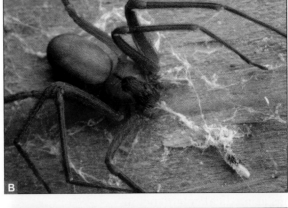

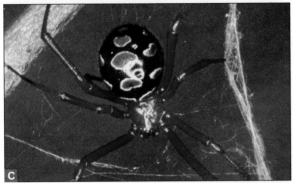

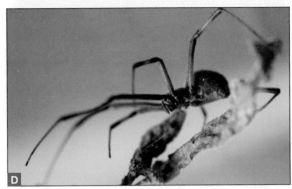

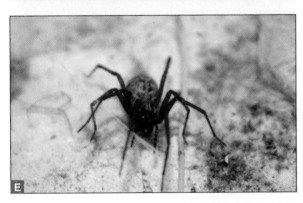

Fig. 16-12, A–E: **(A)** Black widow spider, *iStockphoto.com/ Mark Kostich;* **(B)** Brown recluse spider, *Shutterstock.com/ Miles Boyer;* **(C)** Red widow spider, courtesy of *James Castner, Entomology and Nematology Department, University of Florida;* **(D)** Brown widow spider, *iStockphoto.com/Denis Ananiadis; and* **(E)** Hobo spider, *iStockphoto.com/Rick Jones.*

the patient's sensitivity to the venom. Most spider bites resolve on their own with no adverse effects or scarring. Signs and symptoms of venomous spider bites can mimic other conditions. The only sure way of knowing a person has been bitten by a spider is to have witnessed it.

Bites usually occur on the hands and arms of people reaching into places where spiders are residing. The bite of the black widow spider and its relatives is the more painful and often the more deadly, especially in very young and elderly patients. The bite usually causes an immediate sharp pinprick pain, followed by a dull pain in the area of the bite. Sometimes, however, no pain is felt initially. Other signs and symptoms may include muscular rigidity in the shoulders, chest, back and abdomen; restlessness; anxiety;

dizziness, headache and profuse sweating; weakness; and drooping or swelling of the eyelids.

A brown recluse spider bite may produce little or no pain initially, but localized pain develops an hour or more later. The brown recluse is also called the "fiddle back" or "violin" spider because of the distinctive violin-shaped pattern on the back of its front body section. A blood-filled blister forms under the surface of the skin, sometimes in a target or bull's-eye pattern. Over time, the blister increases in size and eventually ruptures, leading to tissue *necrosis* (destruction) and a black scab.

Another potentially dangerous spider is the northwestern brown, or hobo, spider. It can produce an open, slow-healing wound similar to that of the brown recluse.

An **antivenin** to counteract the poisonous effects of the venom is available for black widow bites. Antivenin is used mostly for children and the elderly, and is rarely necessary when bites occur in healthy adults.

Scorpions live in dry regions, such as the southwestern United States and Mexico (**Fig. 16-13**). Like spiders, only a few species of scorpions have a potentially fatal sting. However, because it is difficult to distinguish highly poisonous scorpions from non-poisonous scorpions, treat *all* scorpion stings as medical emergencies.

General signs and symptoms of spider bites and scorpion stings may include—

- A mark indicating a possible bite or sting.
- Severe pain in the sting or bite area.
- A blister, lesion or swelling at the entry site.
- Nausea and vomiting.
- Stiff or painful joints.
- Chills or fever.
- Difficulty breathing or swallowing or signs of anaphylaxis.
- Sweating or salivating profusely.
- Irregular heart rhythms.
- Muscle aches or severe abdominal or back pain.
- Dizziness or fainting.
- Chest pain.
- Elevated blood pressure and heart rate.
- Infection of the bite.

Providing Care for Spider Bites and Scorpion Stings

If a patient has been bitten by a spider or stung by a scorpion, wash the wound thoroughly and bandage it. Additionally, consider applying a topical antibiotic ointment to the bite to prevent infection, if protocols allow and the patient has no known allergies or sensitivities to the medication. Apply an ice or a cold pack to the site to reduce

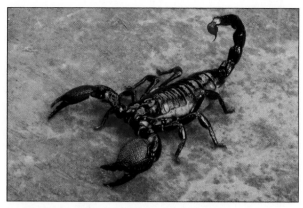

Fig. 16-13: Scorpion. *iStockphoto.com/John Bell.*

swelling and pain. The patient should seek medical attention or, if severe symptoms are present, should be transported to a medical facility, keeping the bitten area elevated and as still as possible.

Venomous Snakes

There are an estimated 7000 to 8000 people reported bitten by venomous snakes annually in the United States. However, fewer than five die. Most deaths occur because the patient goes into anaphylaxis, is in poor health or because too much time passes before receiving medical care. **Figure 16-14, A–D** shows the four kinds of venomous snakes found in the United States. Rattlesnakes account for *most* snakebites and *nearly all* deaths from snakebites.

Signs and symptoms of a venomous snakebite include—

- One or two distinct puncture wounds, which may or may not bleed. The exception is the coral snake, whose teeth leave a semicircular mark.
- Severe pain and burning at the wound site immediately after or within 4 hours of the incident.
- Swelling and discoloration at the wound site immediately after or within 4 hours of the incident.

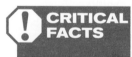

CRITICAL FACTS

If a patient has been bitten by a spider or stung by a scorpion, wash and bandage the wound. Consider applying a topical antibiotic if no known allergies or sensitivities to the medication exist and local protocols allow. Apply an ice or cold pack to reduce swelling and pain.

The patient should seek medical attention. Severe symptoms require immediate transportation to a medical facility. While seeking more advanced medical attention, keep the bitten area elevated and as still as possible.

To care for a venomous snakebite, wash the wound and apply an elastic roller bandage after washing the wound to slow the spread of venom.

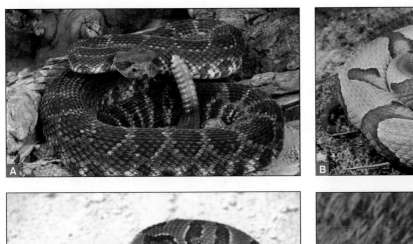

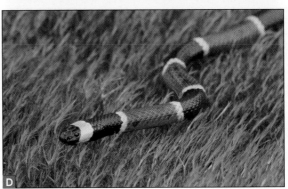

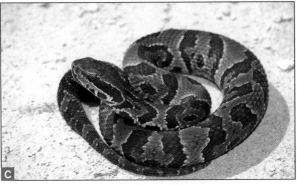

Fig. 16-14, A–D: **(A)** Rattlesnake, *Shutterstock.com/Audrey Snider-Bell;* **(B)** Copperhead, *iStockphoto.com/Jake Holmes;* **(C)** Cottonmouth, *Shutterstock.com/Leighton Photography & Imaging;* **(D)** Coral snake, *iStockphoto.com/Mark Kostich.*

Providing Care for Snakebites

To provide care for a bite from a venomous snake—
- Wash the wound.
- Apply an elastic roller bandage to slow the spread of venom through the lymphatic system by following these steps:
  - Check for feeling, warmth and color of the limb and note changes in skin color and temperature.
  - Place the end of the bandage against the skin and use overlapping turns.
  - The wrap should cover a long body section, such as an arm or a calf, beginning at the point farthest from the heart. For a joint, such as the knee or ankle, use figure-eight turns to support the joint.
  - Check above and below the injury for feeling, warmth and color, especially fingers and toes, after you have applied an

elastic roller bandage. By checking before and after bandaging, you may be able to tell if any tingling or numbness is from the elastic bandage or the injury.
- Check the snugness of the bandaging—a finger should easily, but not loosely, pass under the bandage.
- Keep the injured area still and *lower* than the heart. Transport the patient via stretcher or carry the patient. The patient should walk *only* if absolutely necessary.

For *any* snakebite—
- **Do not** apply ice.
- **Do not** cut the wound.
- **Do not** apply suction.
- **Do not** apply a tourniquet.
- **Do not** administer electric shock, such as from a car battery.

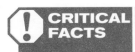 **CRITICAL FACTS** For any snakebite, **never** apply ice, cut the wound, apply suction, apply a tourniquet or administer an electric shock.

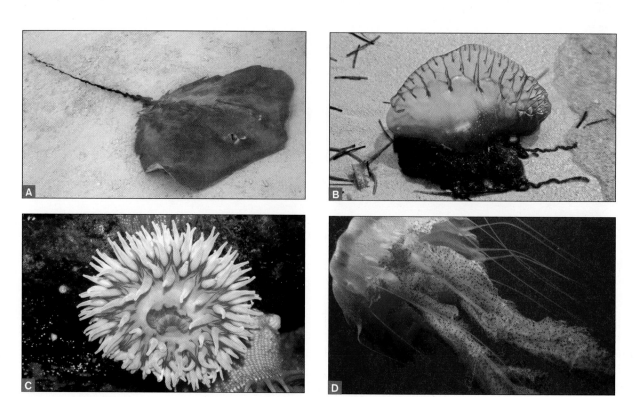

Fig. 16-15, A–D: (A) Stingray, *iStockphoto.com/Dia Karanouh*; (B) Bluebottle jellyfish/Portuguese man-of-war, *iStockphoto.com/ Mark Kostich*; (C) Sea anemone, *iStockphoto.com/Omers*; (D) Jellyfish, *Shutterstock.com/Johan1900*

Aquatic Life

The stings of some forms of aquatic life are not only painful, but they can make you sick, and in some parts of the world, can kill you **(Fig. 16-15, A–D)**. The side effects of a sting from an aquatic creature can include allergic reactions that can cause breathing and heart problems, as well as paralysis and death. If the sting occurs in water, move the patient to dry land as soon as possible. Emergency care is necessary if the patient was stung by a deadly jellyfish, does not know what caused the sting, has a history of allergic reactions to aquatic life stings, is stung on the face or neck, or starts to have difficulty breathing.

Providing Care for Jellyfish Stings

Basic care steps for jellyfish stings are to remove the patient from the water, prevent further envenomation by deactivating or removing (stingers) nematocysts, then control pain. There are some differences in specific care based on the region and the species of jellyfish. EMRs should know the types of jellyfish that are in their area. Contact local marine experts to learn about the types of jellyfish in the region, specific treatment recommendations and photographs to aid in identification.

For most types of jellyfish in most waters in the United States, flush the injured part in vinegar as soon as possible for at least 30 seconds to offset the toxin. A baking soda slurry may also be used if vinegar is not available. For bluebottle jellyfish, also known as the Portuguese man-of-war, which are found in tropical waters, flush with ocean water instead of vinegar. Vinegar triggers further envenomation. Do not rub the wound or apply fresh water, ammonia or rubbing alcohol, because these substances may increase pain.

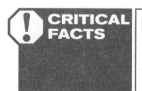

CRITICAL FACTS

The stings of some forms of aquatic life are not only painful, but they can make you sick, and in some parts of the world, can kill you. The side effects of a sting from an aquatic creature can include allergic reactions that can cause breathing and heart problems, as well as paralysis and death.

For most types of jellyfish in most waters in the United States, flush the injured part in vinegar as soon as possible followed by hot-water immersion.

Carefully remove any stingers/tentacles with gloved hands or a towel. When stingers are removed or deactivated, use hot-water immersion (as hot as can be tolerated or about 113°F) for at least 20 minutes or until pain is relieved. If hot water is not available, dry hot packs or, as a second choice, dry cold packs may also be helpful in decreasing pain. Do not apply a pressure immobilization bandage.

If the sting is from a stingray, sea urchin or spiny fish, flush the wound with tap or ocean water. Immobilize the injured part, usually the foot, and soak the affected area in nonscalding hot water (as hot as the patient can stand) for about 30 minutes or until the pain subsides. Toxins from these animals are heat-sensitive and dramatic relief of local pain often occurs from application of hot water.

Carefully clean the wound with soap and water and apply a bandage. It is possible the patient may require a **tetanus** vaccine or booster, so ask when the last immunization or booster was given. *Tetanus*, also called *lockjaw*, is a bacterial disease that enters the body through a break in the skin and attacks the *central nervous system* (CNS). According to the *Centers for Disease Control and Prevention* (CDC), tetanus is fatal in about 10 percent of cases and higher among older people. It is a deadly but preventable disease through vaccination. Stings and wounds to the face, head and neck are the most likely to be fatal because of the proximity of these areas to the brain.

Domestic and Wild Animals

The bite of a domestic or wild animal carries the risk of infection, as well as soft tissue injury.

Dog bites are the most common of all bites from domestic or wild animals.

Providing Care for Animal Bites

A patient who is bitten should be removed from the situation if possible, but only without endangering yourself or others. Do *not* restrain or capture the animal. Your concerns should be for your own safety and caring for the patient. Clean minor wounds with large amounts of saline or clean water and control any bleeding. The patient should be transported or advised to see a health care provider for more advanced medical care. If the wound is bleeding heavily, control the bleeding and transport the patient for further medical care.

Tetanus and **rabies** immunizations may be necessary, so it is vital that bites from any wild or unknown domestic animals be reported to the local health department or other agency according to local protocols. Follow local protocols regarding contacting animal control to capture the animal. Try to obtain and provide a description of the animal and the area in which the animal was last seen.

Humans

Human bites are quite common and differ from other bites because they may be more contaminated, tend to occur in higher-risk areas of the body (especially on the hands) and often receive delayed care. Children are often the inflictors and the recipients of human bite wounds.

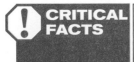

CRITICAL FACTS

For stingray, sea urchin or spiny fish stings, flush the wound with tap or ocean water, immobilize the injured part, and soak it in water as hot as the patient can stand for 30 minutes or until the pain subsides.

___

The bite of a domestic or wild animal carries the risk of infection, as well as soft tissue injury. Dog bites are the most common of all bites from domestic or wild animals.

___

Clean minor wounds from animal bites and control bleeding. Patients should seek more advanced medical care. Heavy bleeding requires immediate control and transportation to a medical facility.

___

Tetanus and rabies immunizations may be necessary. It is vital that wild or unknown domestic animal bites are reported to the local health department or other agency according to local protocols.

___

Human bites are common, tend to be more contaminated than other bites and occur in higher-risk areas, and often receive delayed care. Caring for human bites is the same as for animal bites.

As with animal bites, if the wound is minor, clean it with large amounts of saline or clean water and control any bleeding. Advise the patient to seek follow-up care by a health care provider or medical facility. If the bite is severe, control bleeding and prepare the patient for transport to a medical facility.

WATER-RELATED EMERGENCIES
Drowning Incidents

Drowning is the fifth-most-common cause of death from unintentional injury in the United States among all ages, but rises to second among those from 1–14 years of age. Approximately 4500 Americans die from drowning every year. In addition, an estimated 16,000 drowning incidents result in hospitalization, with many people suffering permanent disability. People drown while in lakes, pools and even bathtubs, especially young children. Children under age 5 and young adults from age 15 to 24 drown more often than others.

Drowning occurs when a person is submerged or immersed in a liquid, usually water, which surrounds the airway and makes air exchange impossible. A drowning is an event in which a victim experiences respiratory impairment due to submersion in water. Drowning may or may not result in death.

Contributing Factors

Drowning cannot just happen on its own. A person must be in a situation that causes the submersion. These situations include—

- Young children left alone or unsupervised around water (e.g., tubs, pools, lakes).
- Use of alcohol and recreational drugs, which may cause people to do things they otherwise would not.
- Traumatic injury, such as diving into a shallow body of water.
- Condition or disability, such as heart disease, seizure disorder or neuromuscular disorder, that may cause sudden weakness or loss of consciousness while in the water.

Shallow Water Blackout

The practice of voluntarily *hyperventilating* (extremely rapid or deep breathing) followed by holding one's breath and then swimming under water or holding one's breath for extended periods of time is dangerous and can be fatal. Some swimmers use this technique to try to swim long distances under water or to try to hold their breath for an extended period while submerged in one place.

People mistakenly think that by taking a series of deep breaths in rapid succession and forcefully exhaling, they can increase the amount of oxygen they breathe, allowing them to hold their breath longer under water. This is not true. Instead, it lowers the carbon dioxide level in the body. The level of carbon dioxide in the blood is what signals a person to breathe.

When a person hyperventilates and then swims under water, the oxygen level in the blood can drop to a point where the swimmer passes out before the carbon dioxide level is high enough to trigger the need to inhale. When the need to inhale finally does trigger instinctively, water rushes into the unconscious person's mouth and nose, causing laryngospasm and allowing the drowning process to begin. Even highly skilled swimmers can die from this practice.

- History of mental illness; for example, depression, suicide attempt, anxiety or panic disorder.

Severity

Whether people die depends on how long they have been submerged and are unable to breathe. It also can depend on the temperature of the water. Children submerged in icy water have been successfully revived after considerable periods of time.

Brain damage or death can occur in as little as 4 to 6 minutes. The sooner the drowning process is stopped by getting the patient's airway out of the water, opening the airway and providing

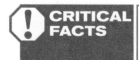

CRITICAL FACTS Contributing factors for submersion incidents include children left alone or unsupervised around or with access to water, use of alcohol and recreational drugs, traumatic injury, sudden illness or mental illness.

resuscitation (ventilations or CPR), the better the chances for survival without permanent brain damage. If the submersion lasts any longer, often the result is death. These times are estimates; brain damage and/or death can occur more quickly.

Signs and Symptoms of Drowning

Signs of a drowning incident include—
- Persistent coughing.
- Shortness of breath or no breathing at all.
- Disorientation or confusion.
- Unconsciousness, although the patient may have regained consciousness.
- Vomiting.
- Respiratory and/or cardiac arrest.

Signs of a fatal drowning incident include—
- Unconsciousness.
- No breathing.
- No pulse.
- Rigor mortis.

Because drowning victims may appear deceased when they are not (imperceptible heart rate and breathing), CPR and emergency efforts are recommended in all cases.

Water Rescues

Before beginning the rescue, consider the patient's condition, the condition of the water and the resources available once you get the patient on dry land. Also consider the rescuers' ability to affect a rescue safely. You should make every effort to assist without entering the water.

Patient's Condition

Ask yourself the following questions:
- Is the patient responsive and able to cooperate with the rescue? If so, the safest method may be a reaching or throwing assist, such as by using a pole or rope.
- What position is the patient in? If the patient is submerged, basic life support will likely be needed right away. Submersion may also make it difficult to find the patient in murky or cloudy water.

- Does the patient seem to be injured? If so, you may have to remove the patient from the water before providing care.
- Is their condition potentially due to head or neck trauma (e.g., a diving incident)? If so, you may need to stabilize the spine while attempting to remove the patient from the water.

Condition of the Water

There are several aspects of the water's condition that will influence how you respond to a water rescue, including—
- Visibility. Are you able to see the patient and visualize any injuries? Are you able to see any hazards under the water?
- Water temperature. You will need to continue resuscitation for a cold-water drowning until the patient is rewarmed at the hospital. Also, consider the type of clothing the patient is wearing. A wetsuit provides much more protection against hypothermia than do street clothes.
- Movement of the water. How fast is the water flowing? Fast-flowing water can be deceivingly strong. If the water is above your knees, do not attempt to wade through without being harnessed. Otherwise, you could be swept away. Also, be aware that a patient's location can change in fast-moving water.
- Depth of the water. Is the depth of the water such that you will be able to stand or will you require additional equipment?
- Additional hazards. In floods or situations where a motor vehicle is submerged, there is the potential for exposure to a hazardous material, such as oil or gas. Hazardous materials may also escape from buildings in a flood.

Resources Available

Determine what other resources are available to assist in a water rescue. Are you the only rescuer? Will there be several other rescuers available once you get the patient on dry land? Are they all able to swim? Are there sufficient *personal flotation devices* (PFDs) for each rescuer?

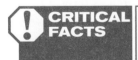

Submersion situations are not always easy to manage. Consider your own safety above all else when working on a water rescue. Water rescues require special training and should only be attempted by properly trained responders.

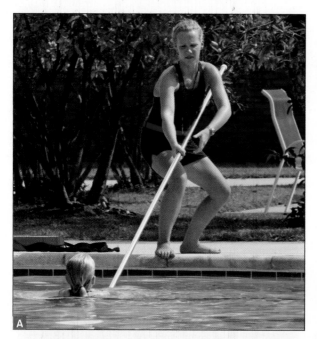

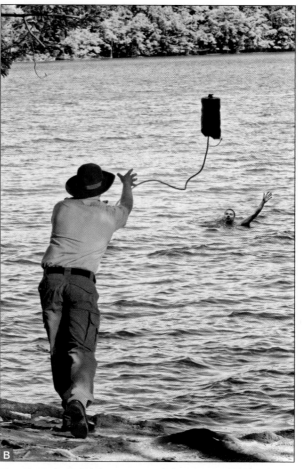

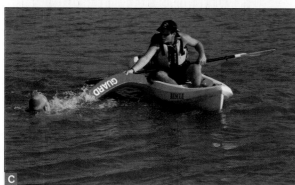

Fig. 16-16, A–C: **(A)** Reach assist; **(B)** Row assist; **(C)** Throw assist. Consider your own safety before following the "reach, throw, row then go" technique to rescue a person from the water. "Go" only if you are trained to do so.

Rescuing the Victim

People who drown are not always in easy-to-manage situations. If the patient is in the water, consider your own safety before all else when attempting a water rescue.

As mentioned earlier, water rescues require special training and should only be attempted by those who are properly trained. To attempt a water rescue, you must be—

- A good swimmer.
- Specially trained in water rescue.
- Wearing a PFD.
- Accompanied by other qualified rescuers.

If you are not trained in water rescue, do not attempt one unless the patient is responsive and close to shore and the emergency has taken place in open, shallow water with a stable bottom.

Before entering the water, be sure you are secure so you will not be pulled in. Any sturdy object that can be grasped will do.

Follow the "reach, throw, row then go" technique (**Fig. 16-16, A–C**). You can reach with an object, such as an oar, a sturdy branch or even a large towel. If the victim is too far for a reaching assist, you can throw out a floating object for the victim to hang on to, such as a life preserver or even an empty picnic cooler. Tie a rope to this object if possible, so you can pull the victim to shore.

If possible, use a boat to get closer (row), but not close enough that the victim can grab the side of the boat and tip it. The "go" part of this technique is only for those who are trained and who can perform deep-water rescue. Further training in water rescue is available in other American Red Cross courses, such as Basic Water Rescue and Lifeguarding.

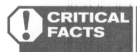 **CRITICAL FACTS** To perform a water rescue, follow the "reach, throw, row then go" technique. "Go" is only for those who are trained to perform deep-water rescue.

Providing Care for Drowning

Remove any victim of a drowning incident from the water as soon as possible. How and when to remove the victim depends on his or her overall condition (e.g., LOC), the victim's size, the potential for spinal injury, how soon help is expected to arrive and whether anyone can help. The priority in providing care in a water emergency is ensuring the patient's face (mouth and nose) is out of the water and appropriate care is given. Ventilations and/or CPR must be initiated immediately on an unresponsive patient who is not breathing and has no pulse. Ventilations may be started in the water; however, chest compressions cannot. If CPR is required, the patient must be removed from the water first. If a spinal injury is suspected, minimize movement to the spine, but priority must be given to airway management. Make sure additional personnel have been summoned.

For the patient who is unresponsive and face-up in shallow water or when a spinal injury is suspected, perform the head-splint technique:

1. Approach the patient's head from behind, or stand behind the patient's head. Lower yourself so the water level is at your neck.
2. Grasp the patient's arms midway between the shoulder and elbow with your thumbs to the inside of each of the patient's arms. Grasp the patient's right arm with your right hand, and the patient's left arm with your left hand. Gently move the patient's arms up alongside the head while you reposition yourself to the patient's side while trapping the patient's head with his or her arms.
3. Squeeze the patient's arms against the head (**Fig. 16-17, A**). This helps keep the head in line with the body. Do not move the patient any more than necessary.
4. Position the patient's head close to the crook of your arm, with the head in line with the body.
5. Check for breathing and a pulse for no more than 10 seconds.
   - If there is breathing, hold the patient steady in the water until additional help arrives. Do not lift the victim.
   - If there is no breathing or pulse, immediately remove the patient from the water and give ventilations or perform CPR as needed.

For the patient who is unresponsive and face-down in shallow water, turn the patient face-up quickly. Use the head-splint technique

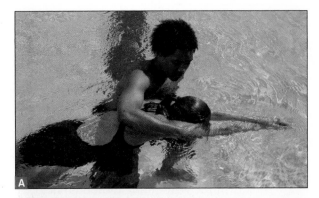

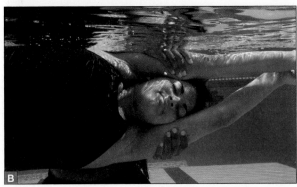

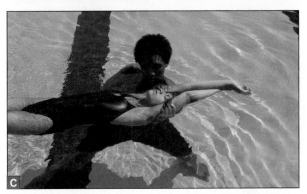

Fig. 16-17, A–C: To care for an unresponsive drowning victim with a suspected head, neck or spinal injury: **(A)** Approach from the side, raise the arms and squeeze the arms against the head to keep it in line with the body, and **(B)** slowly rotate the body. **(C)** When the victim is face-up, keep the head in the crook of your arm and steady until help arrives.

on a face-down victim (if a spinal injury is suspected, take care to minimize movement to the spine):

1. Approach the patient from the side.
2. Move the patient's arms up alongside the head by grasping the patient's arms midway between the shoulder and elbow. Move the patient's right arm with your right hand, and the patient's left arm with your left hand.
3. Squeeze the patient's arms against the head. This helps keep the head in line with the body.
4. Glide the patient forward.
5. Move slowly and rotate the patient toward you until he or she is face-up (**Fig. 16-17, B**). To rotate the patient, push the patient's closer

arm under water while pulling the other arm across the surface toward you. In water with currents, hold the patient's head upstream to keep the body from twisting.

6. Position the patient's head close to the crook of your arm, with the head in line with the body (**Fig. 16-17, C**).

7. Check for breathing and a pulse for no more than 10 seconds.
   - If there is breathing, hold the patient steady in the water until additional help arrives. Do not lift the victim.
   - If there is no breathing or pulse, immediately remove the patient from the water and give ventilations or perform CPR as needed.

Follow local protocols for spinal motion restriction. This may include the application of a *cervical collar* (C-collar) by more advanced medical personnel, as well as backboarding. Before you place the patient on the backboard, make sure there are enough rescuers helping you. Their role is to make sure the patient's face does not become submerged. Once the head and neck are stabilized, slide the board under the patient. Let the board float up until it is against the patient's back. Secure the patient to the backboard.

After the patient is immobilized using the backboard, lift the patient from the water head first. If the patient is wearing a life jacket, do not try to remove it. If needed, place padding under the patient's head to keep the spine aligned.

Many patients who have been submerged vomit because water has entered the stomach or air has been forced into the stomach during ventilations. If the patient vomits, roll him or her to the side to prevent aspiration or choking. This can be done even if the patient is immobilized on a backboard. Simply turn the patient, ensuring the head is securely fastened to the board. To remove vomit from the mouth, use a finger or suction device.

Always take patients who have been involved in a drowning incident to the hospital, even if you think the danger has passed. Complications can develop as long as 72 hours after the incident and may be fatal.

For more information on water rescues, refer to **Chapter 32**.

PUTTING IT ALL TOGETHER

Environmental emergencies include a wide range of situations that often occur during the course of everyday events. As an *emergency medical responder* (EMR), it is important you know how to identify the signs and symptoms of environmental emergencies and be able to provide appropriate care.

Maintaining body temperature is vital for proper cell function. If the body temperature drops below or rises above the acceptable level, the body tries to protect itself but can only do so to a certain extent. If the body cannot protect itself, it begins to shut down. Therefore, it is crucial you be able to identify the various issues that can contribute to heat-related illnesses and cold-related emergencies, including who is at highest risk of falling ill and how to help a patient who is succumbing to such an emergency.

While there are many thousands of species of snakes, spiders and insects, only a few are venomous and pose any danger to humans. Quick action by the EMR can minimize or reduce the effects of a sting or bite that has the potential to cause a serious reaction.

Finally, with all the access to water in this country, be it a bathtub, a bucket full of water, a creek or the ocean, people are constantly exposed to the danger of drowning, particularly young children. As always, it is essential that EMRs ensure their own safety before they try to help others, so you *must* know your limits when it comes to water rescues. You cannot help a drowning person if you become a victim yourself.

Drownings can be caused by other emergencies, such as a spinal injury or a cardiac arrest. An EMR must be prepared for *any* situation when it comes to water rescue.

YOU ARE THE EMERGENCY MEDICAL RESPONDER

Based on your findings, you suspect that the snake was venomous and the patient appears to be reacting to the bite. What initial care can you provide? What else should you do and why?

Enrichment
Assisting with an Epinephrine Auto-Injector

Epinephrine is a form of adrenaline medication used to care for severe allergic reactions. When assisting with an epinephrine auto-injector it is important to keep some precautions in mind.

Determine whether the patient has already taken epinephrine or an antihistamine. If so, only administer a second dose when more advanced medical personnel are not present and if anaphylactic symptoms persist for a few minutes. Check the label to confirm that the prescription of the auto-injector is for the patient. In some areas, responders may be able to carry and use epinephrine auto-injectors on individuals who have not had it prescribed. Check with local protocols before carrying or using an epinephrine auto-injector on individuals who have not had it prescribed. Check the expiration date of the auto-injector. If it has expired, DO NOT USE IT. If the medication is visible, confirm that the liquid is clear and not cloudy. If it is cloudy, DO NOT USE IT. Leave the safety cap on until the auto-injector is ready to use. Carefully avoid accidental injection when assisting a patient by *never* touching the needle end of the device.

An epinephrine auto-injector contains a preloaded dose of 0.3 mg of epinephrine for adults or 0.15 mg of epinephrine for children who weigh between 33 and 66 pounds. The injector has a spring-loaded plunger that, when activated, injects the epinephrine. Forcefully pushing the auto-injector against a large muscle mass, usually the outer thigh, activates the device. *Always* follow medical direction and the manufacturer's instructions for the specific device.

To assist with the administration of an epinephrine auto-injector, follow these general guidelines and local protocols if allowed—

- Size-up the scene and perform a primary assessment.
- Look for a medical *identification* (ID) tag or bracelet.
- If the patient is unconscious, has difficulty breathing, complains of the throat tightening or explains that he or she is subject to severe allergic reactions, call for more advanced medical personnel.
- Provide care for life-threatening conditions.
- Check a conscious patient to determine—
  - The substance (antigen) involved.
  - The route of exposure to the antigen.
  - The effects of the exposure.
- If the patient is conscious and is able to talk, ask—
  - What is your name?
  - What happened?
  - How do you feel?
  - Do you feel any tingling in your hands, feet or lips?
  - Do you feel pain anywhere?
  - Do you have any allergies? Do you have prescribed medications to take in case of an allergic reaction?
  - Do you know what triggered the reaction?
  - How much and how long were you exposed?
  - Do you have any medical conditions or are you taking any medications?
- Check the patient from head to toe. Visually inspect the body.
  - Observe for signs and symptoms of respiratory distress or allergic reactions.
  - Check the patient's head.
    - Assess for swelling of the face or tongue and tightening of the throat.
    - Notice if the patient is drowsy, not alert or exhibiting slurred speech.
  - Check skin appearance. Look at the patient's face and lips. Ask yourself, is the skin—
    - Cold or hot?
    - Unusually wet or dry?
    - Pale, ashen, bluish or flushed?

Continued on next page

Enrichment
Assisting with an Epinephrine Auto-Injector (continued)

- Check the chest.
  - Ask if he or she is experiencing pain during breathing.
  - Notice rate, depth of breaths, wheezes or gasping sounds.
- Care for respiratory distress.
  - Help the patient to rest in a comfortable position, usually sitting.
  - Summon more advanced medical personnel.
  - Calm and reassure the patient.
  - Monitor the patient's condition.
- Document any changes in condition over time.

SKILLsheet

Assisting with an Epinephrine Auto-Injector

NOTE: Always obtain consent, follow standard precautions and wash your hands immediately after providing care. Check the medication to ensure that it is for the patient, that it has not expired and that the liquid is clear and not cloudy.

NOTE: If possible, help the patient self-administer the auto-injector.

To care for a conscious patient if the patient is unable to self-administer the auto-injector, and local protocols allow—

STEP 1
Locate the outside middle of one thigh to use as the injection site.

NOTE: If injecting through clothing, press on the area with a hand to determine that there are no obstructions at the injection site, such as keys, coins, the side seam of trousers, etc.

STEP 2
Grasp the auto-injector firmly in your fist, and pull off the safety cap with your other hand.

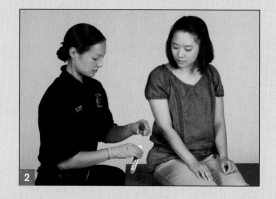

STEP 3

Hold the tip (needle end) near the patient's outer thigh so that the auto-injector is at a 90-degree angle to the thigh.

STEP 4

Quickly and firmly push the tip straight into the outer thigh. You will hear a click.

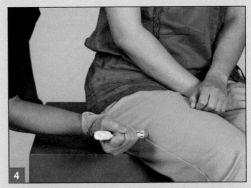

STEP 5

Hold the auto-injector firmly in place for **10** seconds, then remove it from the thigh and massage the injection site with a gloved hand for several seconds.

STEP 6

Perform an ongoing assessment and observe the patient's response to the epinephrine.

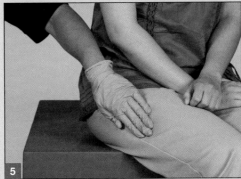

STEP 7

Place the used auto-injector in a proper sharps container and give it to more advanced medical personnel when they arrive.

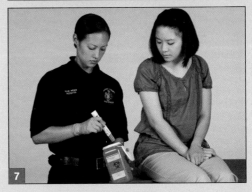

Enrichment
Lightning

On average, *lightning* causes more deaths annually in the United States than any other weather hazard, including blizzards, hurricanes, floods, tornadoes, earthquakes and volcanic eruptions. The *National Weather Service* (NWS) estimates that lightning kills nearly 100 people annually and injures about 300 others.

Lightning occurs when particles of water, ice and air moving inside a storm cloud lose electrons. Eventually, the cloud becomes divided into layers of positive and negative particles. Most electrical currents run between the layers inside the cloud. However, occasionally, the negative charge flashes toward the ground, which has a positive charge. An electrical current travels back and forth between the ground and the cloud many times in the moment you see lightning flash. Anything with demonstrable height (e.g., a tower, tree or person)—can provide a path for electrical current.

Traveling at speeds of up to 300 miles per second, a lightning strike can hurl a person through the air, burn clothes off and cause the heart to stop beating. The most severe lightning strikes carry up to 50 million volts of electricity, enough to light 13,000 homes. Lightning can "flash" over a person's body or, in its more dangerous path, it can travel through blood vessels and nerves to reach the ground.

Besides burns, lightning can also cause neurological damage, fractures and loss of hearing or eyesight. The patient sometimes acts confused and may describe the episode as getting hit on the head or hearing an explosion.

People should use common sense during thunderstorms to prevent being struck by lightning. If a thunderstorm threatens, the NWS advises individuals to—

- Postpone activities promptly and not wait for rain to begin. Thunder and lightning can strike without rain.
- Go quickly inside a completely enclosed building, *not* a carport, open garage or covered patio. If no enclosed building is convenient, a cave is a good option outside, but move as far back as possible from the cave entrance.
- Watch cloud patterns and conditions for signs of an approaching storm.
- Designate safe locations and move or evacuate to a safe location at the first sound of thunder. Every *5 seconds* between the flash of lightning and the sound of thunder *equals 1 mile* of distance.
- Use the *30-30 rule* where visibility is good and there is nothing obstructing your view of the thunderstorm. When you see lightning, count the time until you hear thunder. If that time is 30 seconds or less, the thunderstorm is within 6 miles. Seek shelter immediately. The threat of lightning continues for a much longer period than most people realize. Wait *at least 30 minutes* after the last clap of thunder before leaving shelter.
- If inside during a storm, keep away from windows. Injuries may occur from flying debris or glass if a window breaks.
- Stay away from plumbing, electrical equipment and wiring during a thunderstorm. Water and metal are both excellent conductors of electricity.
- Do *not* use a corded telephone or radio transmitter except for emergencies.

If people are caught in a storm outdoors and cannot find shelter, they should *avoid*—
- Water.
- High ground.
- Open spaces, such as meadows, football fields and golf courses.
- All metal objects, including electric wires, fences, machinery, motors and power tools.
- Unsafe places, such as under canopies, under small picnic shelters or rain shelters, or near trees.

If lightning is striking nearby when people are outside and cannot access shelter, they should—

- Crouch down and limit the amount of the body that is touching the ground **(Fig. 16-18)**. Feet should be placed together. If possible, weight should be placed on only the balls of the feet. Hands can be placed over the ears to minimize possible hearing damage from thunder.
- Avoid proximity to other people. A minimum distance of 15 feet between people should be maintained.

If there is a tornado alert, a previously specified location (as indicated by a disaster plan) should be located as soon as possible. This may be the basement or the lowest interior level of a building.

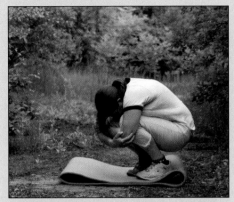

Fig. 16-18: If lightning is striking nearby when people are outside and cannot access shelter, they should crouch down and limit the amount of the body that is touching the ground. *Courtesy of the Canadian Red Cross.*

Enrichment
SCUBA and Free Diving Emergencies

The growing popularity of SCUBA (self-contained underwater breathing apparatus) and **free diving** has increased the number of diving-related accidents that occur each year. Most of these accidents are the result of complications arising from the fact that pressure under water is greater than that on land, with the pressure increasing relative to the depth.

SCUBA

Barotrauma simply means pressure-related (*baro*) injury (*trauma*), and results from the inability to equalize the body's internal pressure with that of the external environment. The most frequent examples of barotrauma occur in air travel and scuba diving. The external pressure exerts a crushing type force on the body parts affected; hence the nickname, "lung squeeze." Barotrauma can affect multiple areas of the body. Signs and symptoms may vary depending on the body part or parts affected. The most common areas affected are the lungs, face and ears, with predominant signs and symptoms including pain in the affected area, disorientation, dizziness, nausea and bleeding from the mouth, nose or ears.

Pulmonary Overinflation Syndrome

Pulmonary Overinflation Syndrome (POIS), or Pulmonary Overpressure Syndrome, occurs because gases under pressure (including air) contract and take up less volume. The air inhaled at depth will expand during ascent as the pressure decreases, and can go beyond the lungs' capacity . If a SCUBA diver holds his or her breath while ascending, the lungs can rupture, hence the common name "burst lung." POIS can also result in **arterial gas embolism**, as the excess volume of air created on ascent can be forced into the bloodstream and travel to the brain. Signs and symptoms may include numbness or tingling of the skin, weakness, paralysis and loss of consciousness.

Under pressure, inert gases from inhaled air—mostly nitrogen—are absorbed into body tissues at higher concentration than normal. The longer time spent at depth, the more this occurs. In addition, at increased depths, more gases are forced into body fluids and tissues due to the increased pressure.

Decompression Sickness

Decompression sickness occurs when a diver ascends too quickly, without sufficient time for gases to exit body tissues and be removed from the body through exhalation. These gases expand as pressure decreases during ascent, creating bubbles in the body. Decompression sickness is often called "the bends" because when these bubbles occur in joints (specifically the elbow, shoulder, knee and/or hip), the joint(s) involved feels better when held bent rather than held straight. Type I decompression sickness signs and symptoms include—
* Rash.
* Dull, deep and/or throbbing pain in the body tissues or joints.
* Itching or burning sensation of the skin or bubbles under the skin (*subcutaneous emphysema*).

Type II signs and symptoms can have delayed onset of up to 36 hours and include the following:
* Pulmonary problems, such as:
  * A burning sensation in the chest upon inhalation
  * Non-productive coughing
  * Respiratory distress
* Hypovolemic shock and neurological symptoms

Nitrogen Narcosis

Another common danger to recreational divers is nitrogen narcosis. This condition occurs at depths over 100 feet when the pressure causes nitrogen to dissolve into brain nerve membranes. This causes a temporary disruption in nerve transmission, resulting in an altered LOC similar to intoxication. It is particularly dangerous because, like any type of intoxication, judgment is impaired and bad judgment under water can lead to the conditions mentioned above or drowning.

FREE DIVING

Free diving is an extreme sport in which divers compete to see how deep they can dive without any underwater breathing apparatus. This is accomplished through excessive breath holding and hyperventilation. It is a dangerous activity because of the risk of loss of consciousness due to lack of oxygen to the brain (*hypoxia*), and subsequent drowning. Some divers utilize buoyancy devices to pull them to the surface if they lose consciousness, but this is not a reliable method of getting to oxygen in time. Other conditions associated with free diving include barotrauma, ear perforation, nitrogen narcosis and drowning.

PROVIDING CARE

All of the conditions mentioned above are life threatening and require immediate medical attention. The diver needs immediate medical attention if he or she loses consciousness, shows paralysis or shows symptoms of stroke within 10 minutes of surfacing.
* If the patient is alert, place him or her in a supine position.
  * If his or her mental state is altered, place the patient in a supine (face-up) position.
  * If a spinal injury is suspected, maintain spinal motion restriction.
* If breathing appears adequate, administer emergency oxygen if available.
* If breathing is inadequate, begin positive pressure ventilation and log the exact time of oxygen delivery.
* If needed, initiate ventilations or CPR and apply the AED.
* Try to obtain the patient's diving log and bring it to the hospital. (Divers keep diving logs to mathematically track how long they have been at a given depth in order to avoid decompression sickness.)
* Transport immediately or call for more advanced medical personnel.
  * Medical control will determine if the patient should be transported directly to a facility with a recompression (hyperbaric) chamber. The *Divers Alert Network* (DAN) at Duke University maintains a list of recompression facilities and can be reached around the clock at 1-919-684-8111 (collect), 1-800-446-2671 (toll-free) or 1-919-684-9111 (Latin America hotline); you can also visit *www.diversalertnetwork.org*

17

Behavioral Emergencies

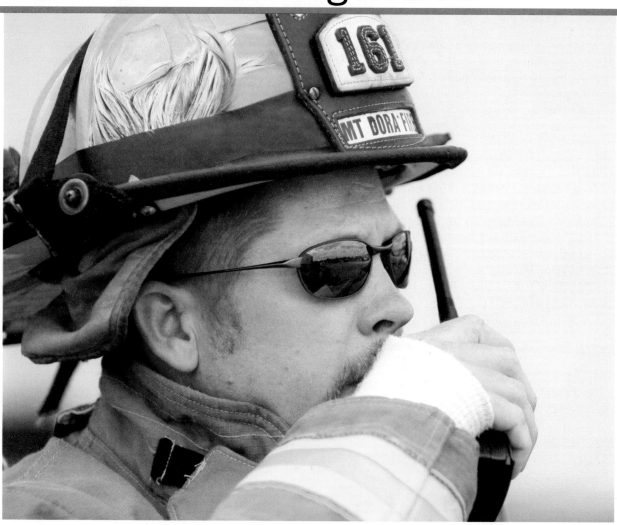

Your fire rescue unit responds to a local mall concerning a man who is threatening violence to anyone who comes near him. When you arrive, police and security guards have the man in protective custody and are trying to calm him down. As you begin interviewing the man and take a history, his mood abruptly swings to one of remorse and sadness. The smell of alcohol on his breath is overpowering. How would you respond to this patient and what are some things you can do to earn his trust?

Key Terms

Anxiety disorder: A condition in which normal anxiety becomes excessive and can prevent people from functioning normally; types include generalized anxiety disorder, obsessive-compulsive disorder, panic disorder, post-traumatic stress disorder, phobias and social-anxiety disorder.

Behavior: How people conduct themselves or respond to their environment.

Behavioral emergency: A situation in which a person exhibits abnormal behavior that is unacceptable or intolerable, for example violence to oneself or others.

Bipolar disorder: A brain disorder that causes abnormal, severe shifts in mood, energy and a person's ability to function; the person swings from the extreme lows of depression to the highs of mania; also called manic-depressive disorder.

Child abuse: Action that results in the physical or psychological harm of a child; can be physical, sexual, verbal and/or emotional.

Child neglect: The most frequently reported type of abuse in which a parent or guardian fails to provide the necessary, age-appropriate care to a child; insufficient medical or emotional attention or respect given to a child.

Clinical depression: A mood disorder in which feelings of sadness, loss, anger or frustration interfere with everyday life for an extended period of time.

Elder abuse: Action that results in the physical or psychological harm of an elderly person; can be physical, sexual, verbal and/or emotional, usually on someone who is disabled or frail.

Elder neglect: A type of abuse in which a caregiver fails to provide the necessary care to an elderly person.

Hallucination: Perception of an object with no reality; occurs when a person is awake and conscious; may be visual, auditory or tactile.

Mania: An aspect of bipolar disorder characterized by elation, hyperexcitability and accelerated thoughts, speech and actions.

Panic: A symptom of an anxiety disorder, characterized by episodes of intense fear and physical symptoms such as chest pain, heart palpitations, shortness of breath and dizziness.

Paranoia: A condition characterized by feelings of persecution and exaggerated notions of perceived threat; may be part of many mental health disorders and is rarely seen in isolation.

Phobia: A type of anxiety disorder characterized by strong, irrational fears of objects or situations that are usually harmless; may trigger an anxiety or panic attack.

Rape: Non-consensual sexual intercourse often performed using force, threat or violence.

Rape-trauma syndrome: The three stages a victim typically goes through following a rape: acute, outward adjustment and resolution; a common response to rape.

Schizophrenia: A chronic mental illness in which the person hears voices or feels that his or her thoughts are being controlled by others; can cause hallucinations, delusions, disordered thinking, movement disorders and social withdrawal.

Self-mutilation: Self-injury; deliberate harm to one's own body used as an unhealthy coping mechanism to deal with overwhelming negative emotions.

Sexual assault: Any form of sexualized contact with another person without consent and performed using force, coercion or threat.

Suicide: An intentional act to end one's own life, usually as a result of feeling there are no other options available to resolve one's problems.

Learning Objectives

After reading this chapter, and completing the class activities, you will have the information needed to—

- Identify behavior that suggests a person may be experiencing a behavioral emergency.
- Describe how to approach and care for a person experiencing a behavioral change or psychological crisis.
- Make appropriate decisions about care when given an example of an emergency in which someone is experiencing a behavioral emergency.
- Identify risk factors for suicide.
- Describe how to assess a person who is contemplating or has already attempted violence toward him- or herself.

INTRODUCTION

Behavior is how people conduct themselves or respond to their environment. A **behavioral emergency** is a situation in which a patient exhibits abnormal behavior that is unacceptable or intolerable. Such is often the case with people who become violent, attempt to take their own lives or believe that other people are out to harm them. A behavioral emergency can pose unique problems that, as an *emergency medical responder* (EMR), you will have to manage.

BEHAVIORAL EMERGENCIES

A behavioral emergency can be present in someone who acts abnormally, or in ways that are unacceptable or dangerous to him- or herself, his or her family or the community at large. People exhibiting abnormal behavior may be violent toward themselves or others. They may appear agitated or speak in a rapid or incoherent manner, or they may be subdued or withdrawn. They may also appear to be intoxicated.

Assessment

Assume that a patient with a behavioral emergency has an altered mental status. Size-up the scene to gather information relevant to safety. Consider the *mechanism of injury* (MOI) or nature of illness. When it is safe to enter the scene, remain cautious as you approach the person (**Fig. 17-1**). Just because the scene may appear safe does not necessarily mean that it is. A person may be carrying a weapon or other object, or have one nearby, that could cause injury. Always be prepared for any potential threat, keep your eyes on the person and never turn your back.

Observe the person's general appearance and behavior as you talk. Determine the person's *level of consciousness* (LOC) and activity level. Is the person

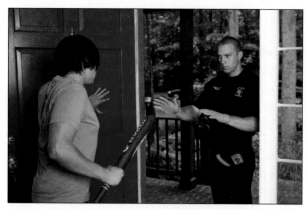

Fig. 17-1: Approach a person having a behavioral emergency with caution.

active or subdued? How does the person speak? Explain what you would like to do, including checking vital signs and providing care for any injuries, such as external bleeding. If family or friends of the patient are available, ask if the patient has a history of aggressive behavior or if there are any underlying medical issues. A seemingly intoxicated person may have an underlying medical condition that is triggering the behavior.

Signs and symptoms commonly seen during a behavioral emergency may present with a rapid onset and include—

- Emotional reactions such as **panic**, anxiety, fear, agitation, depression, withdrawal, confusion and anger.
- Unusual appearance.
- Unusual speech patterns.
- Abnormal or bizarre behavior or thought patterns.
- Loss of contact with reality.
- Aggressive behavior including threats or intent to harm self or others.
- Certain odors on the patient's breath, such as alcohol.
- Pupils that are dilated, constricted or that react unequally.
- Excess salivation.
- Loss of bladder control.
- Visual **hallucinations**.

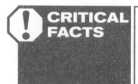

CRITICAL FACTS

A behavioral emergency is a situation in which a patient exhibits abnormal behavior that is unacceptable or intolerable. Such is often the case with people who become violent, attempt to take their own lives or believe that other people are out to harm them.

Signs and symptoms commonly seen during a behavioral emergency may present with a rapid onset and can include emotional reactions, such as fear, panic or anger; unusual appearance or speech; abnormal or aggressive behavior; loss of bladder control and hallucinations.

Behavioral Changes
Causes of Behavioral Emergencies

The primary causes of behavioral emergencies include—

- Injury. Any condition that reduces the amount of oxygen to the brain, such as a head injury, can result in a significant change in behavior. Too little oxygen could make a normally calm person suddenly become anxious or even violent. Cognitive changes associated with head injury can also be factors in behavioral change.
- Physical illness.
- Past history of behavioral emergency.
- Alcohol or drug use or abuse.
- Noncompliance regarding taking prescribed psychiatric medications.
- Adverse effects of prescribed medications.
- Mental illness. Mental illnesses that can alter behavior include depression, **schizophrenia** and **bipolar disorder**. The exact cause of mental illness is not always known, but it is sometimes the result of a chemical abnormality in the brain. The behavior exhibited by a patient with a mental illness can be bizarre and can include excited or depressed behavior.
- Extreme stress. Extreme emotional distress, such as grief at the loss of a loved one, can trigger a change in an individual's behavior. People react differently to stressful situations. The impact of the incident and the way the person copes or fails to cope can lead to an emotional situation that the person cannot handle. People can react with uncontrollable crying, denial, anger or depression.

Other circumstances that can lead to altered behavior include heat or cold exposure, diabetes, low blood sugar, lack of oxygen, shock, head trauma, brain infection, seizure disorders, poisoning or drug overdose, withdrawal from alcohol or drugs, mind-altering substance or substance abuse and problems with the nervous system associated with aging.

Some behavioral emergencies may pose a particular danger to the EMR, to the patient and to others, including when the patient displays agitation, bizarre thinking and behavior, danger to him- or herself or danger to others.

Excited Delirium Syndrome

Excited delirium syndrome poses challenges for police as well as EMS personnel. With excited delirium, the person exhibits some or a combination of the following signs and symptoms:

- Agitation
- Violent or bizarre behavior
- Insensitivity to pain
- Extreme increase in body temperature

Individuals with excited delirium develop high body temperatures. They may also exhibit increased body strength. Unfortunately, this syndrome is life threatening and if immediate advanced medical intervention is not sought out, it usually ends in death. This syndrome is most often associated with incidents involving the police. It can be associated with drug use, particularly cocaine or methamphetamine, but can occur in non-drug users as well.

PSYCHOLOGICAL EMERGENCIES
Anxiety and Panic

While a certain amount of anxiety is a normal reaction to stress, excessive anxiety may be part of an **anxiety disorder**. There are several types of anxiety and panic disorders, all with potential to have dramatic effects on the afflicted person. People having a severe anxiety or panic attack are in real distress and need assistance. A person's anxiety and panic is often based on the feeling that he or she has no control over the situation and a fear of what may happen next. Anxiety attacks can last any length of time, but panic attacks generally last no longer than 30 minutes.

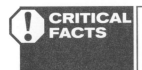

CRITICAL FACTS The primary causes of behavioral emergencies include injury, physical illness, past history of behavioral emergencies, alcohol or drug use/abuse, noncompliance regarding taking prescribed psychiatric medications, adverse effects of prescribed medications, mental illness and extreme stress.

Someone who is experiencing an *anxiety attack* may show any of these signs and symptoms:

- Fatigue
- Headaches
- Muscle tension
- Muscle aches
- Difficulty swallowing
- Trembling or twitching
- Irritability
- Sweating
- Hot flashes

People experiencing a panic attack may have any of the above signs and symptoms, as well as—

- Difficulty breathing.
- Heart palpitations.
- An out-of-control feeling.

Phobias

Phobias are irrational fears of objects or events that are usually harmless. They can cause an anxiety or panic attack. When people have a phobia about a certain situation or event, they may display an exaggerated response of fear, referred to as a *phobic reaction*, when exposed to the situation or event.

A person having a phobic reaction, such as an anxiety or panic attack, may display any of these behaviors:

- Irrational fear
- Unexplained, uncontrolled anxiety
- Desire to flee the situation or avoid the object
- Inability to continue functioning as long as the person is in the situation or the object is present
- Acknowledgement that the fear reaction is out of proportion to the situation or event
- Physical symptoms such as heart palpitations, difficulty breathing and sweating

Clinical Depression

Although **clinical depression** is a chronic illness, people who are clinically depressed can have an emergency that may trigger thoughts of **suicide**. Depression is more than just "the blues." It is a recognized medical illness that may require not only psychological therapy but also medical intervention.

It is important to keep in mind that there are many ways people can exhibit signs and symptoms of depression, including thoughts of impending suicide. For more information about suicide, refer to the section later in this chapter.

Signs and symptoms of clinical depression are numerous. They include but are not limited to—

- Persistent feeling of being useless.
- Loss of interest in regular activities.
- Feeling hopeless or guilty.
- Unexplained sadness.
- Crying spells.
- Irritability and restlessness.
- Insomnia or sleeping too much.
- Lack of appetite or overeating (followed by weight loss or gain).
- Inability to concentrate and make decisions.
- Physical aches and pains with no medical basis.
- Loss of sexual desire.
- Thoughts of suicide.

Bipolar Disorder

Bipolar disorder is a mental illness in which the person swings from the extreme lows of depression to the highs of **mania**. A person with mania exhibits elation, hyperexcitability and accelerated thoughts, speech and actions. Bipolar disorder is sometimes called *manic-depression*. Because of the extreme mood swings, the person can be in danger of self-harm when on either end of the spectrum. When depressed, the person may consider suicide. When manic, self-destructive or risky behaviors could result in severe injury or death.

Someone who is in a depressive episode would exhibit signs and symptoms of depression such as feeling useless or hopeless, alternating between sleeping too much or too little, being unable to go to work and being unable to concentrate. When experiencing the manic phase, the person could show signs and symptoms such as—

- Rapid speech and quickly changing thought patterns.
- Inability to sit still and/or concentrate.
- Inability to finish a task.
- Euphoria.
- Increased physical activity.
- Participating in risky activities.
- Inability to sleep.
- Increased desire to have sex.
- Agitation.
- Aggressive behavior.

Paranoia

Paranoia is a condition characterized by feelings of persecution and exaggerated notions of perceived threat. It may be part of many mental health disorders and, rarely, is seen in isolation. Paranoia is marked by irrational and delusional behavior. Paranoid individuals often believe that someone or several people are "out to get them." Paranoia can be limited to believing that they are being watched or followed, or it can become more fantastical in nature, such as believing there are implants in the brain being monitored by people who want to do the paranoid person harm. Paranoia can also be a side effect of medication or recreational drug use, particularly stimulants.

If a patient is paranoid, it can be difficult for you to provide care because he or she may fear that you are part of the plot or group trying to cause harm.

Patients who are paranoid may display behaviors such as—

- Checking for wiretaps (bugs) in every room.
- Accusing people of following them or listening to their conversations.
- Being suspicious of every person who approaches them.
- Refusing to eat or drink anything that they have not prepared.

Schizophrenia

Schizophrenia is a severe, chronic mental illness in which the person hears voices or feels that his or her thoughts are being controlled by others. These voices or thoughts can instruct the person to do things he or she would otherwise not do, like becoming violent toward a family member or a stranger. For this reason, you must exercise particular caution when attempting to help a patient whom you know or suspect suffers from schizophrenia.

Someone with schizophrenia may display some or all of the following:

- Hallucinations (visual or auditory, but mostly auditory)
- Delusions

- Lack of personal care or hygiene
- Inappropriate emotions for the situation or lack of emotions altogether
- Anger
- Suspicions and paranoid behavior
- Social isolation

VIOLENCE

Behavioral emergencies require extra sensitivity. Every person copes in a different way and every person has a breaking point. People experiencing a behavioral emergency may have no control over what they are feeling at any given moment, and those feelings are real and valid. A behavioral emergency may cause a person to become violent toward self or others. A head injury, low blood sugar in someone with diabetes, a lack of oxygen, and mind-altering substances (such as alcohol, depressants, stimulants or narcotics) can all cause a person to act in a violent manner.

Patients Who Are Violent Toward Themselves

Patients who are violent toward themselves may attempt or threaten suicide. Your primary concern as an EMR is to treat any injuries or medical conditions arising from the violence or suicide attempt and then transport the patient to a facility where he or she can receive medical and psychiatric treatment. If it is necessary to prevent the patient from harming you, him- or herself or others, you may need to use medical restraints to transport the patient.

Suicide

The term suicide refers to an intentional act to end one's own life. People who commit suicide often feel they have no other option for resolving their problems but to end their own lives. Suicide is about four times more likely to end in death for males than for females, although females are much more likely to attempt suicide. People of

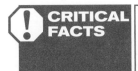

CRITICAL FACTS

People experiencing a behavioral emergency may have no control over what they are feeling at any given moment and can become violent toward themselves or others.

Suicide is about four times more likely to end in death for males than for females, although females are much more likely to attempt suicide. People of any age, race or socio-economic status are at risk of making suicide attempts.

any age, race or socio-economic status are at risk of making suicide attempts.

Those in the 15-to-24 age group are at highest risk of dying by suicide. Suicide is the third-leading cause of death for people in this age group in the United States.

Older people are also at a higher risk than the general population, because depression is common in the geriatric population and it may be misdiagnosed as dementia or confusion. The *National Institutes of Health* (NIH) reported that, in 2004, people aged 65 and over accounted for 16 percent of all suicides, even though they only make up 12 percent of the American population.

Assessing Suicide Risk

Many people who attempt suicide suffer some form of mental or emotional problem or illness, especially depression. Substance misuse or abuse, primarily of alcohol and other drugs, plays a major role in attempted suicides.

In any behavioral emergency, it is important to assess the patient's risk for attempting suicide. Some risk factors include—

- Mental or emotional disorders, especially depression.
- History of substance misuse or abuse.
- Feelings of hopelessness.
- Impulsive or aggressive tendencies.
- Past attempts at suicide.
- Failing or failed relationship with a spouse, family or friend.
- Serious illness or death of a close family member or friend.
- Serious, prolonged or chronic personal illness.
- A long period of failure at work or school or a long period of unemployment.
- Failure to achieve sufficient occupational, educational or financial success.
- Dramatic change in the economy.
- Feelings of isolation.
- Mass suicides (e.g., in a group/cult setting).

- Reluctance to seek help for mental-health problems due to the stigma attached to suicidal thoughts, suicide attempts or general mental health problems.
- Inability to access mental health services.

When assessing a patient for suicide risk, keep the following in mind:

- Take any threat of suicide seriously, and transport the patient for evaluation. Ask if the patient has ever considered suicide.
- Address any injuries or medical conditions related to a suicide attempt.
- Always listen carefully, as the patient may reveal important information indirectly (**Fig. 17-2**).
- Do not dismiss what you may consider to be unimportant feelings.
- Be non-judgmental and remember that people react differently to different problems.
- The patient may tell you that everything is fine but transport the patient anyway, as help may still be needed.
- Make specific plans to help the patient, for example making arrangements for the patient to meet with a particular health care worker or clergy.
- Be careful not to show disgust or fear when caring for the patient. These feelings can be

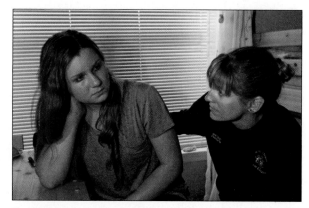

Fig. 17-2: When assessing the suicide risk of a patient, listen carefully for important information that may be communicated indirectly and always take the patient seriously.

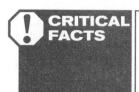
CRITICAL FACTS

Older people are also at a higher risk than the general population, because depression is common in the geriatric population and it may be misdiagnosed as dementia or confusion.

There are many factors to consider when assessing a patient's suicide risk. Risk factors include mental or emotional disorders; history of substance abuse or past suicide attempts; feelings of hopelessness or isolation; impulsiveness or aggressiveness; failed relationships; personal illness; failure at work, school or in financial matters.

revealed through your words and your body language.

- Never deny that the patient attempted suicide. This may give the message that you are unable to accept the patient's feelings.
- Never try to use strong emotions to either shock the person out of attempting suicide or to call the person's bluff and provoke him or her.

To better assess the patient, ask the patient questions to get a better grasp of the situation. These questions include—

- How does he or she feel?
- Is the patient thinking of hurting or killing him- or herself or anyone else?
- Is the patient a threat to him- or herself or others?
- Does the patient have a medical problem?
- Is the patient suffering from a recent trauma?
- Does the patient have any weapons on him- or herself or nearby?
- What interventions are necessary?

Self-Mutilation

Self-mutilation, or self-injury, refers to deliberately harming one's own body, through acts such as burning or cutting. It is not usually meant as an attempt to commit suicide, but is an unhealthy coping mechanism to deal with overwhelming negative emotions such as tension, anger and frustration. The individual experiences momentary calmness and a release of tension but then quickly feels a sense of shame and guilt, in addition to a return of the negative feelings the person was trying to avoid. Self-mutilation may be a component of a mental illness such as depression, an eating disorder or a personality disorder.

Sometimes, a suicidal patient may have a last-minute change of heart and inflict nonlethal wounds (sometimes called *hesitation marks*) to receive help or to punish someone. **Child abuse**

and **rape** survivors may turn to self-mutilation such as nonlethal cutting or burning as a way to cope with the trauma. A patient who has committed self-mutilation will need to be treated for bleeding, shock and other soft-tissue injuries.

Patients Who Are Violent to Others

Patients experiencing a behavioral emergency may become aggressive or violent. The violence may be caused by a medical emergency, a mental health issue, alcohol or drug intoxication, a lack of oxygen or a head injury.

Violent behavior can take many forms, from verbal abuse to punching, kicking, biting and using weapons. While the violence may not be directed toward you, you could easily become an indirect victim caught in the middle. In some cases, these acts may be specifically targeted to people in positions of authority, like you. Attempt to identify exit or escape routes for your safety.

A patient's posture and comments can indicate potential violence. Threatening comments and posture, such as clenching fists or assuming a fighting stance, may indicate the patient's intentions.

Be alert to the following signs:

- Agitation; the patient may pace or move erratically
- Rapid or incoherent speech
- Shouting or making threats
- Clenched fists or a fighting stance
- Using objects as a weapon or throwing objects

Sexual Assault

Sexual assault is defined as any form of sexual contact, against a person's will, often by coercion, force or threat. Victims of rape and sexual assault often know their attackers—a friend, a family member, a relative, a date or a friend of the family. These patients suffer from physical and emotional trauma, and need to be treated with sensitivity.

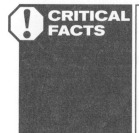

CRITICAL FACTS

Asking the patient questions will help you better assess the situation. These questions can include "How do you feel?"; "Are you thinking of hurting yourself or anyone else?"; "Have you suffered a personal trauma recently?"; or "Do you have a weapon nearby?"

Patients experiencing a behavioral emergency may become aggressive or violent. Violent behavior can take many forms, from verbal abuse to punching, kicking, biting and using weapons. Be alert to signs of violence, such as agitation, rapid or incoherent speech, shouting, making threats, clenched fists or other aggressive stances, throwing objects or using objects as a weapon.

Rape

Rape is defined as non-consensual sexual intercourse often performed using force, threat or violence. It is devastating, and many patients will go into acute emotional distress and shock during and after the attack.

Some common signs and symptoms include—
- Unresponsive, dazed state.
- Nausea, vomiting, gagging or urination.
- Intense pain from assault and penetration.
- Psychological and physical shock and paralysis.
- Possible bleeding or body fluid discharge.
- Torn or removed clothing.

Because of the significant legal issues, it is vital to manage the rape scene appropriately to preserve evidence that will be required for the police investigation. If possible, the patient should be treated by someone of the same gender to avoid further emotional trauma. If present, work with the *sexual assault nurse examiner* (SANE). If possible, transport the victim to a medical facility that has a rape crisis unit and can take the proper specimens as well as comfort the victim.

Tell the patient what you will be doing and why you are doing it. Encourage having the patient treated on a clean white sheet. If the victim must remove clothing or if clothing must be removed from the patient in order to provide care, do so while on the clean white sheet to catch any debris that was left on the patient during the crime. Try to determine the patient's emotional state and complete a patient assessment, checking for trauma around the lower abdomen, thighs, genital and anal areas. Do *not* clean the patient. Prevent the patient from showering, bathing, brushing teeth or urinating, since cleaning can destroy evidence. Police will be responsible for evidence collection. Any evidence you collect while treating the patient for injuries should be isolated and each piece of evidence needs to be bagged individually in a paper bag to prevent cross-contamination. Plastic bags do not allow for air movement and cause the DNA to deteriorate due to moisture buildup. Follow local protocols, and give the evidence to the police as soon as possible.

Most victims of rape experience symptoms of **rape-trauma syndrome** following a rape.

There are three stages:
- Acute. This occurs immediately after the rape, a time when the patient needs critical support. Whether or not a patient suffered physical injuries, a rape victim has experienced significant emotional trauma. This phase lasts anywhere from a few days to a few weeks.
- Outward adjustment. This phase may last weeks or months after the attack. The victim resumes what appears to be his or her "normal" life, but is experiencing turmoil internally, including depression, rage and flashbacks.
- Resolution. Moving on from a rape may take months or years, and may involve professional counseling to assist the patient in dealing with the lasting emotional trauma.

Pediatric Considerations

Child Abuse and Neglect

You may encounter a situation involving an injured child in which you have reason to suspect child abuse. Child abuse is the physical, verbal, psychological or sexual assault of a child resulting in injury and/or emotional trauma. Typically, the child's injuries cannot be logically explained, or a parent or guardian gives an inconsistent or suspicious account of how the injuries occurred.

The signs and symptoms of child abuse include–
- Situations in which the description of the injury does not fit the cause.
- Patterns of injury that include cigarette burns, whip marks and hand prints.
- Obvious or suspected fractures in a child less than 2 years of age.
- Unexplained fractures.
- Injuries in various stages of healing, especially bruises and burns.
- Unexplained lacerations or abrasions, especially around the mouth, lips and eyes.
- Injuries to the genitals; pain when the child sits down.
- More injuries than are common for a child of the same age.
- Repeated calls to the same address.

Child neglect is a type of abuse in which the parent or guardian fails to provide the necessary, age-appropriate care to a child.

Signs and symptoms include–
- Lack of adult supervision.
- A child who appears to be malnourished.

- An unsafe living environment.
- Untreated chronic illness; for example, an asthmatic child with no medications.

When providing care for a child who may have been abused, your first priority is to care for the child's injuries or illness. An abused child may be frightened, hysterical or withdrawn. The child may be unwilling to talk about the incident in an attempt to protect the abuser. If you suspect abuse, explain your concerns to responding police officers or other *emergency medical services* (EMS) personnel, if possible.

If you think you have reasonable cause to believe that abuse has occurred, you must report your suspicions to the proper authorities. Familiarize yourself with the mandatory reporting laws in your state or jurisdiction. Depending on your role and state, you may be considered a mandatory reporter and be required to report suspected incidents of abuse or neglect.

Do not be afraid to report suspected abuse because of fear of getting involved or of being sued. In most states, when you make a report in good faith, you may be immune from civil or criminal liability or penalty, even if you made a mistake. In this instance, "good faith" means you honestly believe that abuse has occurred or the potential for abuse exists and a prudent and reasonable person in the same position would also believe this. You do not need to identify yourself when you report child abuse, although your report will have more credibility if you do.

Refer to **Chapter 25** for more information.

Geriatric Considerations

Elder Abuse and Neglect

As with child abuse, the elderly are also susceptible to abuse from the willful infliction of injury by physical or sexual assault, emotional mistreatment, and neglect. **Elder abuse** is a growing problem in the United States as the population ages. EMRs may encounter a situation that involves the possible abuse of an elderly person.

The signs and symptoms of elder abuse include—
- Any unexplained injury or an injury that has an unlikely explanation.
- Burns, bruises, reddened areas that do not go away.
- Abrasions on arms, legs or torso.
- Unexplained hair loss.

- Injuries in various stages of healing (especially bruises and burns).
- Scratches, cuts or bite marks.
- Cuts and scratches around the breasts, buttocks, genitals; vaginal or rectal bleeding.
- Withdrawn, sad or fearful demeanor and failure to make eye contact.
- Upset or fearful behavior when the abuser enters the same room.

Elder neglect is a type of abuse in which a caregiver fails to provide the necessary care for an elderly person.

The signs and symptoms of elder abuse include—
- An unkempt appearance.
- Improper clothing for the weather conditions.
- Lack of availability of food, water or utilities.
- An unsafe living environment.
- Dehydration.
- Untreated or chronic medical conditions.
- Confusion or disorientation.
- Withdrawn, sad or fearful demeanor and failure to make eye contact.
- Upset or fearful behavior when the abuser enters the same room.

If you think you have reasonable cause to believe that elder abuse has occurred, report your suspicions to the proper authorities **(Fig. 17-3)**. Familiarize yourself with the mandatory reporting laws in your state or jurisdiction. Depending on your role and state, you may be considered a mandatory reporter and be required to report suspected incidents of elder abuse or neglect.

Refer to **Chapter 26** for more information.

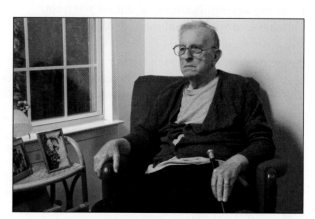

Fig. 17-3: Elder neglect is a type of abuse in which a caregiver fails to provide the necessary care for an elderly person.

PROVIDING CARE FOR BEHAVIORAL EMERGENCIES

Scene Size-Up and Personal Safety

When responding to a possible behavioral emergency, assess the scene to identify any possible sources of harm to yourself, the patient or any bystanders. Do *not* approach the scene unless you feel confident that it is safe to do so. Be wary of sudden behavior changes in the patient, which are the most common cause of injuries to responders.

Be sure to identify and locate the patient before you enter the scene. A disturbed individual may try to jump you from behind or otherwise take you by surprise. Attempt to identify exit or escape routes for your safety and make sure you remain between the patient and an exit, so you can leave the scene if it is necessary for your own safety. As soon as possible, clear the scene of any objects that can be used to injure the patient or others. Do *not* enter the scene if the patient has any kind of weapon. Keep in mind there may be more than one patient (as in a suicide pact).

Assessing the scene can also provide you with hints about what has happened to cause or contribute to the crisis. Are there empty beer, liquor or pill bottles lying around? Do you see drug paraphernalia or signs of injury, such as blood stains?

As with other behavioral emergencies, your first job upon arriving at a scene of a potential suicide is to ensure your own safety. Selected methods of suicide, such as carbon monoxide in fumes from a running vehicle engine in an enclosed area or emissions from a gas stove, can create a dangerous environment for rescuers. In addition, the suicidal individual may further endanger you by attacking or attempting to attack you to prevent your interference.

Some patients may be experiencing hallucinations or delusions. Do *not* play along with these or lie to the patient and say that you believe they are real.

Do *not* think that you can manage a situation involving an emotional crisis by yourself. A suicidal person or a rape victim needs professional counseling. Summon more advanced personnel. This could include law enforcement, EMS personnel or local mental health or rape crisis center personnel. While waiting for others to arrive, continue to talk with the patient.

Establishing Rapport

Once you have entered the scene, you will need to establish rapport with the patient before getting too close. To do this, speak directly to the patient and maintain eye contact. Acknowledge that the patient appears upset and state that you are there to help. Tell the patient who you are and exactly what you want to do to help. Use a calm, reassuring voice, and keep your distance until the patient has indicated it is acceptable to approach. Use slow, deliberate movements. Do not touch the patient without permission. Touch can be very disturbing to some patients, particularly for those who are recent victims of an attack.

Once you have established a rapport with the patient, you can begin to communicate to find out what happened and determine what interventions are needed. Speak directly to the patient and be supportive and empathetic, never threatening, judgmental or confrontational. Show you are listening by repeating and rephrasing the patient's answers to your questions, nodding or stating phrases such as "go on" or "I understand." Make sure that no one interrupts, except in the case of medical necessity.

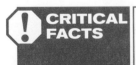

CRITICAL FACTS

When responding to a possible behavioral emergency, assess the scene to identify any possible sources of harm to yourself, the patient or any bystanders.

Do not think that you can manage a situation involving an emotional crisis by yourself. Summon more advanced personnel and continue to talk to the patient while waiting for help to arrive.

Once you have entered the scene, you will need to establish rapport with the patient before getting too close. Once you have established a rapport with the patient, you can begin to communicate to find out what happened and determine what interventions are needed.

Patient Assessment

Observe the patient and look for signs of disorientation or life-threatening conditions, such as a serious injury or difficulty breathing. Also, continue to observe the patient for signs of potential violence, such as a threatening posture or the possession of a weapon. Look for signs of fear, anxiety, confusion, anger, mania, depression, withdrawal or loss of contact with reality. Also look for sudden behavioral changes, such as quiet withdrawal followed by sudden, explosive anger.

Once you get the patient talking, try to find out what happened. Determine the level of orientation and responsiveness and try to find out what the chief complaint is. If the patient allows, take a set of baseline vital signs. Also try to obtain a SAMPLE history. If the patient is unconscious, perform a rapid head-to-toe assessment and try to obtain a SAMPLE history from family, friends or other bystanders.

Calming the Patient

In addition to maintaining a calm voice and slow, deliberate movements, several techniques can be used to help calm a patient. If the patient is disoriented, explain who you are, where you are and what is happening. Reassure the patient that the disorientation is temporary. Do not stand too close to the patient. If the patient's friends or family members are around, ask the patient if it is okay to enlist others to help in calming the patient. Encourage the patient to tell you what the problem is and explain that you are there to listen. Never leave the patient alone, and stay alert to any changes in the patient's emotional state.

Restraining the Patient

When patients are so agitated or violent that they cannot be approached safely and may pose a danger to themselves or others, you may need to assist EMS personnel with the use of restraints. If this occurs, follow their instructions exactly. Try to stay clear of the patient's arms and legs. Do not use restraints unless instructed to do so by more advanced medical or law enforcement personnel.

When using restraints, the goal is to use the minimum force needed. Thus, the amount of force used will depend on factors such as the patient's strength and level of agitation. Soft leather or cloth straps are considered humane restraints, while metal cuffs are not.

Legal Considerations

Restraining a person without justification can give rise to a claim of assault and battery. You may be required to obtain police authorization before you can use patient restraints. Be aware of the laws regarding the use of patient restraints in your jurisdiction. Wait for someone who is authorized to use restraints if you are not legally allowed to do so. Seek medical direction and approval before applying restraints. Be aware of and follow local protocols involving the use of patient restraints.

Be sure a restrained patient can breathe. The patient should be placed in a face-up position, and breathing should be monitored regularly. A struggling patient who appears to calm down may actually be suffering from breathing difficulties or may have lost consciousness.

For legal reasons, it is important to document everything you do while participating in the use of restraints.

PUTTING IT ALL TOGETHER

Behavioral emergencies pose special challenges for EMRs. Patients experiencing behavioral emergencies may act in unexpected ways, and may pose a danger to themselves or others by reacting in a violent or aggressive manner. Behavioral emergencies can be triggered by injury, physical or mental illness, extreme stress or the use of alcohol or other drugs.

When responding to a patient with a behavioral emergency, begin by assessing the scene to identify any possible sources of harm to you, the patient or any bystanders. Do *not* enter the scene unless you feel confident that it is safe to do so. Be wary of sudden behavioral changes in the patient, which is a common cause of injury to responders.

Consider the need for law enforcement personnel. If a patient appears to be a threat to him- or herself or others, or the patient appears to be a victim of sexual assault, rape or child abuse, summon law enforcement support immediately.

When dealing with a rape or sexual assault patient, remember that emotional trauma will be present, even when physical injuries are absent. Acute emotional shock is a normal reaction. Be careful not to disturb any evidence found at the scene.

Cases of child abuse or neglect need to be carefully documented. You must follow local protocols around mandatory reporting if you suspect the injuries are due to abuse or neglect.

Assess both the patient's physical and mental status by asking specific questions in a calm and reassuring manner. Evaluate the patient's mental status by observing appearance, demeanor, level of activity and speech. Ask bystanders if the patient has underlying medical conditions, or a history of mental issues or violent actions. Do *not* leave the patient alone. Good communication skills, respect and empathy can defuse potentially explosive situations.

Restraining a patient should be a last resort, done in consultation with law enforcement and advanced medical direction. Use only as much force as is necessary to restrain the patient, and *always* follow local protocols. Ensure that you clearly document all the circumstances if medical restraints are required, including the names and contact information for any third-party observers, law enforcement personnel and medical personnel.

YOU ARE THE EMERGENCY MEDICAL RESPONDER

As you continue to calmly interview the patient, you gradually earn his trust and soon learn that he has had trouble sleeping and hasn't eaten much in the past 2 weeks. He says he got out of drug rehab 3 months ago. He has not been taking his prescribed medication for about a month and recently lost two very close relatives. The patient says he "sort of went off the wagon." What other steps must you consider in providing proper care for this patient? What additional resources should you consider?

UNIT

6

TRAUMA EMERGENCIES

18

Shock

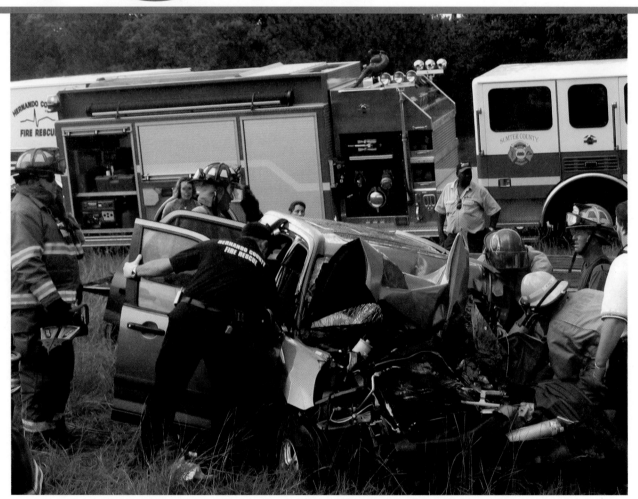

))) YOU ARE THE EMERGENCY MEDICAL RESPONDER

Your ambulance unit is the first to arrive on an isolated road where an 18-year-old male driver lost control of a motor vehicle and collided with a tree. In the crash, the driver's legs were broken and he is pinned in the wreckage. You find the driver conscious, restless and in obvious pain. After a couple of minutes, the patient's condition has changed. He begins to look ill. You notice he responds only to loud verbal stimuli, is breathing fast and looks pale. His skin is cold and moist and his pulse is rapid and weak. What would you do to help the patient?

Key Terms

Cardiogenic shock: The result of the heart being unable to supply adequate blood circulation to the vital organs, resulting in an inadequate supply of nutrients; caused by trauma or disease.

Dilation: The process of enlargement, stretching or expansion; used to describe blood vessels.

Distributive shock: A type of shock caused by inadequate distribution of blood, either in the blood vessels or throughout the body, leading to inadequate volumes of blood returning to the heart.

Hypoperfusion: A life-threatening condition in which the circulatory system fails to adequately circulate oxygenated blood to all parts of the body; also referred to as *shock*.

Hypovolemic shock: A type of shock caused by an abnormal decrease in blood volume.

Neurogenic/vasogenic shock: A type of distributive shock caused by trauma to the spinal cord or brain, where the blood vessel walls abnormally constrict and dilate, preventing relay of messages and causing blood to pool at the lowest point of the body.

Obstructive shock: A type of shock caused by any obstruction to blood flow, usually within the blood vessels, such as a pulmonary embolism.

Respiratory shock: A type of shock caused by the failure of the lungs to transfer sufficient oxygen into the bloodstream; occurs with respiratory distress or arrest.

Septic shock: A type of distributive shock that occurs when an infection has spread to the point that bacteria are releasing toxins into the bloodstream, causing blood pressure to drop when the tissues become damaged from the circulating toxins.

Shock: A life-threatening condition that occurs when the circulatory system fails to provide adequate oxygenated blood to all parts of the body; also referred to as *hypoperfusion*.

Learning Objectives

After reading this chapter, and completing the class activities, you will have the information needed to—

- List conditions that can result in shock.
- List the signs and symptoms of shock.
- Describe how to provide care to minimize shock.
- Make appropriate decisions about care when given an example of an emergency in which shock is likely to occur.

INTRODUCTION

Injuries and medical emergencies can become life threatening as a result of **shock**. When the body experiences injury or sudden illness, it responds in a number of ways. Survival depends on the body's ability to adapt to the physical stresses of injury or illness. When the body's measures to adapt fail, the injured or ill person can progress into a life-threatening condition called *shock*. Shock complicates the effects of injury or sudden illness. In this chapter, you will learn to recognize the signs and symptoms of shock and how to provide care to minimize it.

WHAT IS SHOCK?

Shock, or **hypoperfusion**, is a progressive condition in which the circulatory system fails to adequately circulate oxygenated blood to all parts of the body. When vital organs, such as the brain, heart and lungs, do not receive sufficient oxygenated blood, the body begins a series of responses to protect those organs. The amount of blood circulating to the less important tissues of the arms, legs and skin is reduced so that more can go to the vital organs. This reduction in blood circulation to the skin causes a person in shock to appear pale or *ashen* (grayish) and feel cool. While, in the short term, this can protect the body's most crucial organs, if the situation is not treated quickly shock can lead to death.

When the body is healthy, three conditions are necessary to maintain adequate blood flow—

- The heart must be working well.
- The blood vessels must be intact and able to adjust blood flow.
- An adequate amount of blood must be circulating in the body.

Injury or sudden illness can interrupt normal body functions. In cases of minor injury or illness, this interruption is brief, because the body is able to compensate quickly. With more severe injuries or illnesses, however, the body is unable to adjust. When the body is unable to meet its demands for oxygen because the blood fails to circulate adequately, shock occurs.

WHY SHOCK OCCURS

Shock results from inadequate delivery of oxygenated blood to the body's tissues. There are several possible reasons for shock to occur. It can be the result of—

- Severe bleeding or loss of fluid from the body.
- Failure of the heart to pump enough oxygenated blood.
- Abnormal **dilation** of the vessels.
- Impaired blood flow to the organs and cells.

The Heart

The condition and functioning of the heart can have a significant impact on the likelihood of shock. If the heart rate is too slow, the rate of new oxygenated blood cells reaching each part of the body will not be enough to keep up with demand. If the heart beats too rapidly (ventricular tachycardia [V-tach]) or if the heartbeat becomes erratic (ventricular fibrillation [V-fib]), the oxygenated blood is not sent throughout the body as it should be. Damage to the heart can lead to weak and ineffective contractions; this can be related to disease (e.g., diabetes or cardiovascular disease), poisoning or respiratory distress.

Blood Vessels

If blood vessels are not able to adequately constrict or become abnormally dilated, even though the blood volume is adequate and the heart is beating well, the vessels are not filled completely with blood. Since oxygen is absorbed into the body through the walls of the blood vessels, this condition leads to less oxygen being available to the body. Abnormal dilation of the blood vessels can be caused by neck fractures with spinal cord injury, or by infection or anaphylaxis.

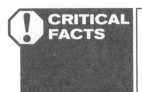

CRITICAL FACTS

Shock, or hypoperfusion, is a progressive condition in which the circulatory system fails to adequately circulate oxygenated blood to all parts of the body.

There are several possible reasons for shock to occur. It can be the result of severe bleeding or loss of fluid, failure of the heart to pump enough oxygenated blood, abnormal dilation of the vessels and impaired blood flow to the organs and cells.

Blood

Insufficient blood volume can lead to shock. Also, if the levels of some components of the blood, such as plasma or fluids, become too low, blood flow will be impaired and shock can result. These conditions can occur due to bleeding, severe vomiting, diarrhea and burns.

Chest and Airway

Shock can also occur following any injury to the chest, obstruction of the airway or any other respiratory problem that decreases the amount of oxygen in the lungs. This means insufficient oxygen enters the bloodstream.

TYPES OF SHOCK

There are four major types of shock: *hypovolemic, obstructive, distributive* and *cardiogenic*. All cause a drop in blood pressure and have the same outcome if not treated quickly.

Hypovolemic

Hypovolemic shock is due to a severe lack of blood and fluid within the body. *Hemorrhagic shock* is the most common type of hypovolemic shock. It results from blood loss, either through external or internal bleeding, which causes a decrease in total blood volume.

Obstructive

Obstructive shock is caused by some type of obstruction to blood flow, usually within the blood vessels, such as a pulmonary embolism, tension pneumothorax or cardiac tamponade.

Distributive

Distributive shock refers to any type of shock caused by inadequate distribution of blood either in the blood vessels or throughout the body, leading to inadequate volumes of blood returning to the heart. It includes the following—

- **Neurogenic/vasogenic shock** is caused by spinal cord or brain trauma. The blood vessel walls normally constrict and dilate to circulate the blood throughout the circulatory system. In neurogenic shock, the messages are not relayed and the blood pools at the lowest point of the body.
- **Anaphylaxis** (also referred to as anaphylactic shock) occurs as the result of exposure to an allergen. It is a whole-body reaction that causes dilation of the blood vessels and constriction (closing) of the airways, which in turn causes blood to pool and trouble breathing. The airways may close completely from inflammation. For more information on anaphylaxis, refer to **Chapter 16**.
- **Septic shock** occurs when an infection has spread to the point that bacteria are releasing toxins into the bloodstream. The blood pressure drops when the tissues become damaged from the circulating toxins.

Cardiogenic

Cardiogenic shock is the result of the heart being unable to supply adequate blood circulation to the vital organs, resulting in an inadequate supply of oxygen and nutrients. Disease, trauma or injury to the heart causes this type of shock.

Other Types of Shock

Other types of shock include hypoglycemic, metabolic, psychogenic and **respiratory shock**. Hypoglycemic shock is a reaction to extremely low blood glucose levels. Metabolic shock is the result of a loss of body fluid, which can be due to severe diarrhea, vomiting or a heat-related illness. Psychogenic shock is due to factors such as emotional stress that cause blood to pool in the body in areas away from the brain, which can result in fainting (syncope). Respiratory shock is the failure of the lungs to transfer sufficient oxygen into the bloodstream and occurs with respiratory distress or arrest.

SIGNS AND SYMPTOMS OF SHOCK

Because this is a progressive condition, the signs and symptoms you see will depend on what stage of shock the person is in, and this will change over

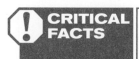
CRITICAL FACTS

There are four major types of shock: hypovolemic, obstructive, distributive and cardiogenic. All cause a drop in blood pressure and have the same outcome if not treated quickly.

Other types of shock include hypoglycemic, metabolic, psychogenic and respiratory shock.

Early Stages of Shock

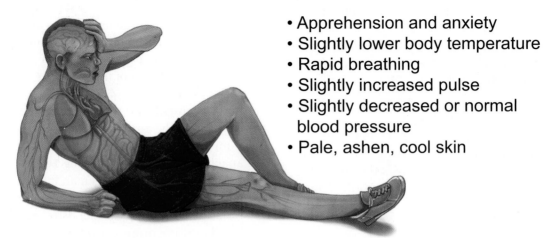

- Apprehension and anxiety
- Slightly lower body temperature
- Rapid breathing
- Slightly increased pulse
- Slightly decreased or normal blood pressure
- Pale, ashen, cool skin

Later Stages of Shock

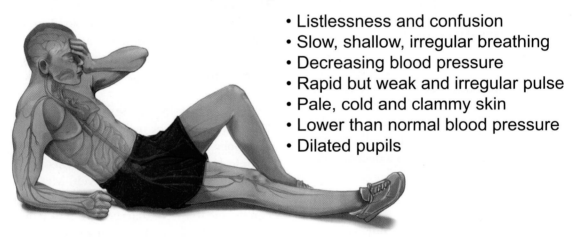

- Listlessness and confusion
- Slow, shallow, irregular breathing
- Decreasing blood pressure
- Rapid but weak and irregular pulse
- Pale, cold and clammy skin
- Lower than normal blood pressure
- Dilated pupils

Fig. 18-1: Shock is a progressive condition, so the stage the person is in determines what signs and symptoms you see.

time (**Fig. 18-1**). At first, the signs and symptoms may seem minor, but responding to them promptly will increase the patient's chance of survival.

Early Signs and Symptoms

You may observe that—
- The patient expresses feelings of apprehension and anxiety.
- The patient's body temperature is slightly lower than normal.
- The patient is breathing quickly.
- The patient's pulse is slightly increased.
- The patient's blood pressure is normal or slightly decreased.
- The patient's skin is pale or ashen, (grayish) and cool.

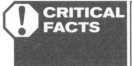
CRITICAL FACTS
Early signs and symptoms may include feelings of apprehension and anxiety; slightly low body temperature; rapid breathing; slight increase in pulse rate; normal or slightly decreased blood pressure and pale, ashen and cool skin.

Later Signs and Symptoms

You may observe that—

- The patient is listless and confused, and may have difficulty speaking.
- The patient's breathing has slowed down and is shallow and irregular.
- The patient's blood pressure is decreasing; diastolic blood pressure may reach zero.
- The patient's pulse is rapid, but the pulse is weak and irregular.
- The patient's skin is pale, cold and clammy, and the body temperature is much lower than normal.
- The patient's pupils are dilated and slow to respond to light.

Pediatric Considerations

Early signs of shock may be absent in young children or infants, because their bodies can compensate for some of the factors that cause shock by maintaining blood pressure at normal levels. If the conditions continue, however, the situation can suddenly deteriorate into severe shock. Because a child is smaller than an adult, blood volume is less and losing what seems like a small amount of blood can be serious, making children more susceptible to shock. Do *not* wait for signs and symptoms of shock to develop when treating a young child or infant, but treat promptly based on your assessment of the injuries or trauma.

PROVIDING CARE

Once you have assessed the patient and determined that there are signs and symptoms of shock present, quick response is essential—

- Be sure the patient's airway is open and clear. Perform a primary assessment. Administer emergency oxygen, if available, and provide appropriate ventilatory support (**Fig. 18-2, A**).
- Take steps to control any bleeding if present and prevent further blood loss.
- Since you may not be sure of the patient's condition, leave him or her lying flat.
- If you see any suspected broken bones or dislocated or damaged joints, immobilize them to prevent movement. Broken bones or dislocated or damaged joints can cause more bleeding and damage.
- Cover the patient with a blanket to prevent loss of body heat (**Fig. 18-2, B**). It is important not to overheat the patient—your goal should be to maintain a normal body temperature. If the patient is lying on cold ground and if it is possible to do so without causing harm, you may want to put a blanket under the patient as well.
- Talk to the patient in a calm and reassuring manner to reduce the harmful effects of emotional stress. If you can help the patient rest in a comfortable position and reduce

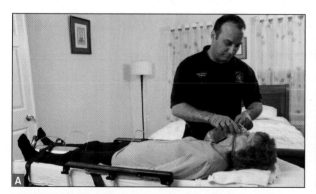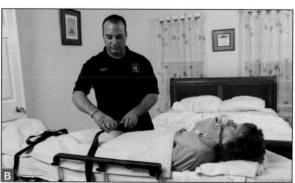

Fig. 18-2: **(A)** If it is available, administer emergency oxygen to a patient who is showing signs and symptoms of shock. **(B)** Cover a patient in shock with a blanket to prevent loss of body heat in order to maintain a normal body temperature.

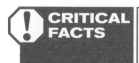 **CRITICAL FACTS** Later signs and symptoms of shock can include listlessness; confusion; difficulty speaking; irregular breathing; decreased blood pressure (diastolic blood pressure may reach zero); rapid yet weak or irregular pulse; pale, cold and clammy skin with a low body temperature and dilated pupils.

the pain, this will also be beneficial; pain intensifies the body's reactions and can accelerate the progression of shock.

- Do not give any food or drinks, even if the patient asks for them. The patient is likely to be thirsty due to the fluid loss. However, depending on the condition, surgery may be needed and it is better for the patient's stomach to be empty if that is the case. More advanced emergency medical personnel will be able to provide fluid replacement intravenously.
- Treat any specific injuries or conditions, and have the patient transported to a hospital as soon as possible.

PUTTING IT ALL TOGETHER

Any condition or trauma situation where the body's ability to get oxygenated blood to the vital organs is compromised can lead to shock. Left untreated, shock is a progressive condition that can be fatal.

Shock can be caused by loss of blood or body fluids, when the heart is not pumping blood effectively, by over-dilation of the blood vessels or by damage to the chest or airways. If any of these conditions are present, it is important to watch the patient for signs and symptoms of shock. These include decreasing blood pressure; increasing heart rate; increasing respiratory rate; pale or ashen, cool, clammy skin; pupils that are dilated and slow to respond; and anxiety and apprehension at first, turning into confusion and listlessness as shock progresses.

To treat shock, first ensure the patient has an open and clear airway and is breathing. Administer emergency oxygen or artificial ventilation as appropriate. Control bleeding, if present, and, keep the patient laying flat. Splint any broken bones or joints and keep the patient warm by covering the patient with a blanket. Reassure and comfort the patient; try to keep the patient comfortable and reduce any pain. Do *not* give food or drink. Treat any specific injuries, call for more advanced medical personnel and transport the patient to a hospital as soon as possible.

YOU ARE THE EMERGENCY MEDICAL RESPONDER

After extrication teams arrive, they finally free the driver from the vehicle and he is removed from the car. You notice that the patient looks worse. He now responds only to painful physical stimuli. His breathing has become very irregular. You know that the hospital is 20 minutes away. How would you respond? What should you do to provide care until the patient arrives at the hospital?

19

Bleeding and Trauma

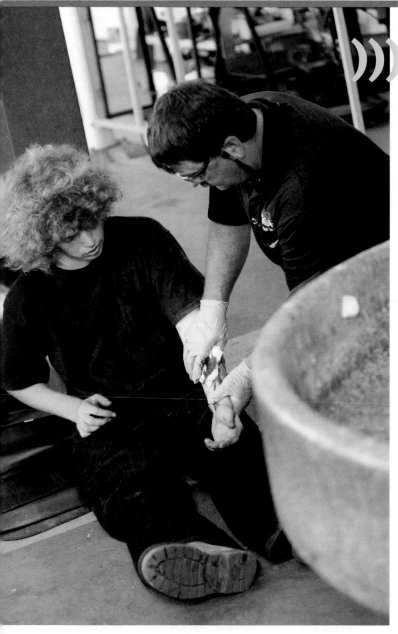

))))

YOU ARE THE EMERGENCY MEDICAL RESPONDER

As a member of your company's *medical emergency response team* (MERT), you are called to assist a worker whose arm has been lacerated by a part that came loose from a lathe. The man's arm is bleeding severely. You arrive to find a co-worker attempting to stop the bleeding. How would you respond?

Key Terms

Adult respiratory distress syndrome (ARDS): A lung condition in which trauma to the lungs leads to inflammation, accumulation of fluid in the alveolar air sacs, low blood oxygen and respiratory distress.

Arteries: Large blood vessels that carry oxygen-rich blood from the heart to all parts of the body, except for the pulmonary arteries, which carry oxygen-poor blood from the heart to the lungs.

Bandage: Material used to wrap or cover a part of the body; commonly used to hold a dressing or splint in place.

Bandage compress: A thick gauze dressing attached to a gauze bandage.

Bleeding: The loss of blood from arteries, veins or capillaries.

Blood volume: The total amount of blood circulating within the body.

Capillaries: Tiny blood vessels linking arteries and veins that transfer oxygen and other nutrients from the blood to all body cells and remove waste products.

Clotting: The process by which blood thickens at a wound site to seal an opening in a blood vessel and stop bleeding.

Contusion: An injury to the soft tissues that results in blood vessel damage (usually to capillaries) and leakage of blood into the surrounding tissues; caused when blood vessels are damaged or broken as the result of a blow to the skin, resulting in swelling and a reddish-purple discoloration on the skin; commonly referred to as a bruise.

Direct pressure: Pressure applied on a wound to control bleeding.

Dressing: A pad placed directly over a wound to absorb blood and other body fluids and to prevent infection.

Elastic bandage: A bandage designed to keep continuous pressure on a body part; also called an *elastic wrap*.

External bleeding: Bleeding on the outside of the body; often, visible bleeding.

Golden Hour: A term sometimes used to describe the first hour after a life-threatening traumatic injury; providing early interventions and advanced medical care during this time frame can result in the best chance of survival.

Head-on collision: A collision in which a vehicle hits an object, such as a tree or other vehicle, straight on.

Hemorrhage: The loss of a large amount of blood in a short time or when there is continuous bleeding.

Hemostatic agent: A method of external hemorrhage control that uses a substance that absorbs or adsorbs moisture from blood and speeds the process of coagulation and clot formation to achieve *hemostasis* (control of bleeding).

Internal bleeding: Bleeding inside the body.

Occlusive dressing: A special type of dressing that does not allow air or fluid to pass through.

Perfusion: The circulation of blood through the body or through a particular body part for the purpose of exchanging oxygen and nutrients with carbon dioxide and other wastes.

Pressure bandage: A bandage applied snugly to create pressure on a wound, to aid in controlling bleeding.

Pressure points: Sites on the body where pressure can be applied to major arteries to slow the flow of blood to a body part.

Roller bandage: A bandage made of gauze or gauze-like material that is wrapped around a body part, over a dressing, using overlapping turns until the dressing is covered.

Rollover: A collision in which the vehicle rolls over.

Rotational impact: A collision in which the impact occurs off center and causes the vehicle to rotate until it either loses speed or strikes another object.

Side-impact collision: A collision in which the impact is at the side of the vehicle; also known as a *broadside* or *t-bone collision*.

Tourniquet: A tight, wide band placed around an arm or a leg to constrict blood vessels in order to stop blood flow to a wound.

Trauma dressing: A dressing used to cover very large wounds and multiple wounds in one body area; also called a *universal dressing*.

Trauma system: A system of definitive care facilities offering services within a region or community in various areas of medical expertise in order to care for injured individuals.

Triangular bandage: A triangle-shaped bandage that can be rolled or folded to hold a dressing or splint in place; can also be used as a sling to support an injured shoulder, arm or hand.

Veins: Blood vessels that carry oxygen-poor blood from all parts of the body to the heart, except for the pulmonary veins, which carry oxygen-rich blood to the heart from the lungs.

Learning Objectives

After reading this chapter, and completing the class activities, you will have the information needed to—

- Describe the components of a trauma system.
- Differentiate among arterial, venous and capillary bleeding.
- Describe how to care for external bleeding.
- List appropriate standard precautions to follow when controlling external bleeding.
- Explain the functions of dressing and bandaging.
- List the signs of internal bleeding.
- Describe how to care for a patient who exhibits the signs and symptoms of internal bleeding.
- Make appropriate decisions about care when given an example of an emergency in which a patient is bleeding.

Skill Objectives

After reading this chapter, and completing the class activities, you should be able to—

- Demonstrate how to control external bleeding with direct pressure, dressings and bandages, including caring for shock.
- Demonstrate how to control severe, uncontrollable external bleeding using a manufactured tourniquet (*Enrichment skill*).

INTRODUCTION

Bleeding is the loss of blood from **arteries**, **veins** or **capillaries**. Bleeding is either internal or external. **External bleeding** is usually obvious because it is typically visible. **Internal bleeding** is often difficult to recognize. Uncontrolled bleeding, whether internal or external, is a life-threatening emergency. A large amount of bleeding occurring in a short time is called a **hemorrhage**.

If left untreated, severe bleeding can result in shock and, eventually, death. Check for and control severe bleeding during the primary assessment after you check for breathing and a pulse. You may not identify internal bleeding until you perform a more detailed check during the physical exam and history.

INCIDENCE/SIGNIFICANCE OF TRAUMA

The **Golden Hour** is that time period when a severely injured patient requiring surgery has the best chance of survival if the surgery is performed within an hour's timeframe. The danger of dying from shock or bleeding during this period is most likely.

Trauma is a physical injury, wound or shock caused by an agent, force or mechanism. The trauma patient requires rapid assessment and care of the conditions found. This is often done by a multidisciplinary team, supported by the appropriate health care professionals, to minimize or eliminate the risk of death or permanent disability. A **trauma system** must determine the necessary level of care for the injury.

TRAUMA SYSTEM

A trauma system is a system of definitive care facilities offering services within a region or community in various areas of medical expertise in order to care for injured individuals. These systems consist of many different components that provide medical services for injury prevention, prehospital care, acute care facilities and post-hospital care. The value of a trauma system is that it provides a seamless transition for patients to move between each phase of care, leading to improved patient outcomes.

There are four levels of medical treatment facilities:

- *Level I:* This facility must have the capability to deal with all levels and types of patient injury on a 24-hour basis. These facilities are leading medical care facilities, often university-based teaching hospitals, and must have an adequate depth of resources and personnel to deal with all levels of patient care.

- *Level II:* This facility is expected to be able to provide definitive care to patients, despite the type of injury the patient may have suffered. However, this facility may have to send a patient with more severe injuries to a Level I facility in some cases. A Level II facility may be the most prominent health care facility in a given region or community.

- *Level III:* These facilities are found in smaller communities that do not have access to larger Level I or Level II medical centers. They can provide prompt assessment, resuscitation and emergency operations and arrange for transport to a Level I or II facility as required. They are generally *not* required in major urban or suburban centers within the trauma system.

- *Level IV:* These facilities are often rural clinics in remote areas and can generally only offer patient care until arrangement for transportation can be made. These facilities may not even have a physician on site. Treatment protocols for resuscitation, transfer protocols, data reporting and participation in system performance improvement are essential at a Level IV facility.

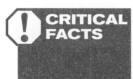

CRITICAL FACTS

Bleeding is the loss of blood from arteries, veins or capillaries. Bleeding is either internal or external. External bleeding is usually obvious because it is typically visible. Internal bleeding is often difficult to recognize.

A trauma system is a system of definitive care facilities offering services within a region or community in various areas of medical expertise in order to care for injured individuals. These systems consist of many different components that provide medical services for injury prevention, prehospital care, acute care facilities and post-hospital care. The value of a trauma system is that it provides a seamless transition for patients to move between each phase of care, leading to improved patient outcomes.

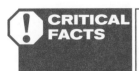

CRITICAL FACTS

The most serious bleeding is arterial bleeding, followed by venous bleeding.

Hemorrhaging occurs when a large amount of blood is lost in a short period of time or when there is continuous bleeding.

In selecting the appropriate level facility, transport considerations must also be taken into account. State guidelines dictate the maximum transport time depending on the acuity of the patient; for example, whether the patient has a compromised airway. Pediatric trauma patients are often transported to the nearest children's hospital, even if it is further away than other hospitals.

MULTI-SYSTEM TRAUMA

Patients who are subjected to significant forces are at an increased risk for injuries to multiple organs within the body at the same time. A multi-system trauma is one involving more than one body system. For example, a patient who was in a major accident may have broken bones (skeletal system), but may also be experiencing difficulty breathing (respiratory system). Multi-system trauma patients are also at a greater risk of developing shock (see **Chapter 18**). Suspect multi-system trauma in any patient subjected to significant external forces.

PERFUSION

Perfusion is the circulatory system's method of delivering oxygen and nutrients while eliminating carbon dioxide and other wastes. The entire body requires perfusion, but different parts of the body require different amounts. Some organs are especially sensitive to changes in the efficiency of perfusion. For example, a major organ such as the heart, when denied constant perfusion, cannot function properly. Both the brain and spinal cord can only last about 4 to 6 minutes without constant perfusion before irreversible damage is done. Kidneys can last up to 45 minutes without perfusion. The skeletal system can withstand a lack of perfusion for as long as 2 hours before damage becomes permanent.

BLEEDING
General Considerations

To reduce the risk of disease transmission when controlling bleeding, *always* follow standard precautions, including—

- Avoiding contact with the patient's blood, directly or indirectly, by using barriers such as disposable gloves and protective eyewear.
- Avoiding eating, drinking and touching your mouth, nose or eyes while providing care or before washing your hands.
- Always washing your hands thoroughly before (if practical) and after providing care, even if you wore gloves or used other barriers.

The severity of blood loss can be estimated based on the signs and symptoms with which the patient presents, as well as your general impression of the amount of blood loss. It is important to control bleeding. Uncontrolled bleeding, or significant blood loss, will lead to shock and possibly death. Do *not* wait for shock to develop before providing care to someone who is injured or suddenly ill.

Types of Bleeding

Bleeding is the loss of blood from arteries, veins or capillaries and can result in either internal or external bleeding. The most serious of these is arterial bleeding, followed by venous bleeding. Hemorrhaging occurs when a large amount of blood is lost in a short period of time or when there is continuous bleeding.

Arterial Bleeding

Arterial bleeding is the most urgent type of bleeding (**Fig. 19-1, A**). Arterial blood is oxygenated and is being pumped from the heart to supply the body with nutrients. Arterial bleeding is most often caused by blunt trauma but can also occur when internal organs are damaged.

Arterial blood—
- Is bright red.
- Spurts from the wound as it is being pushed by the heart's pumping action.
- Will not clot or stop easily because of the pumping pressure.
- Decreases in pressure as the patient's blood pressure drops, due to decreased **blood volume**.

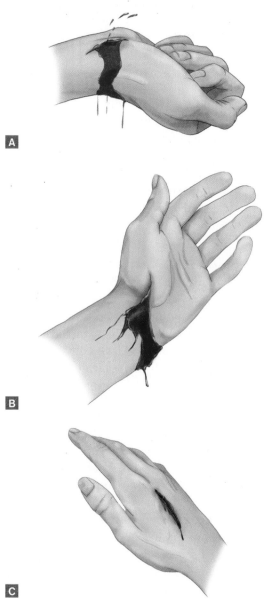

A

B

C

Fig. 19-1, A–C: **(A)** Arterial bleeding is the most serious type of bleeding, followed by **(B)** venous bleeding. **(C)** Capillary bleeding is not usually a concern in healthy people.

Venous Bleeding

Venous bleeding is usually the result of an outside force causing trauma or an internal force breaking through a vein, such as a broken bone or organ damage (**Fig. 19-1, B**). The blood is returning to the heart so it does not have the pumping action to move it forward. Bleeding from a vein can be severe.

Venous blood—
- Is darker red than arterial blood.
- Flows steadily, but the flow can still be quick and severe.
- May be easier to stop because it does not have the pressure from the pumping heart.

Capillary Bleeding

Capillary bleeding is not usually a concern in healthy people (**Fig. 19-1, C**). It is usually slow because the vessels are small and the blood is under low pressure.

Capillary blood—
- Is darker red than arterial blood.
- Oozes from the capillaries.
- Usually clots spontaneously.

DRESSINGS AND BANDAGES

All open wounds need some type of covering to help control bleeding, absorb drainage and prevent contamination and infections. These coverings are commonly referred to as **dressings** and **bandages**. There are many different types of both.

Dressings

Dressings are pads placed directly on the wound to absorb blood and other fluids and to prevent infection. To minimize the chance of infection, dressings should be sterile. Most dressings are porous, allowing air to circulate to the wound to help promote healing. Standard dressings include varying sizes of cotton gauze (sterile and nonsterile), commonly ranging from 2- to 4-inch squares (i.e., 2-inch x 2-inch pads). Much larger dressings called universal dressings or **trauma dressings** are used to cover very large wounds and multiple wounds in one body area (**Fig. 19-2**). Some dressings have nonstick surfaces to prevent the dressing from sticking to the wound.

A special type of dressing, called an **occlusive dressing**, does not allow air to pass through. Plastic wrap and petroleum jelly-soaked gauze are examples of this type

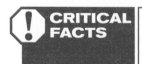

CRITICAL FACTS

All open wounds need some type of covering to help control bleeding, absorb drainage and prevent contamination and infections. These coverings are commonly referred to as dressings and bandages. There are many different types of both.

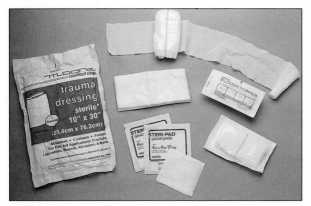

Fig. 19-2: Dressings are placed directly on the wound to absorb blood and prevent infection.

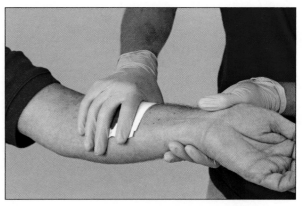

Fig. 19-4: To care for external bleeding, place pressure directly on the wound with your gloved fingers or hand over a dressing.

of dressing (**Fig. 19-3**). Occlusive dressings are used for sucking chest wounds and open abdominal wounds. For more information on the use of an occlusive dressing, refer to **Chapter 21**.

Application of Dressings

For most dressings, place pressure directly on the wound with a sterile gauze pad. Place your fingers or hand over the gauze pad and apply firm, **direct pressure (Fig. 19-4)**. If you do not have gauze available, apply pressure with your own gloved hand or have the injured person apply pressure with the hand.

Bandages

A bandage is any material used to wrap or cover any part of the body. Bandages are used to hold dressings in place, to apply pressure to control bleeding, to help protect a wound from dirt and infection and to provide support to an injured limb or body part. Many different types of

bandages are available commercially (**Fig. 19-5**). A bandage applied snugly to create pressure on a wound or injury is called a **pressure bandage**.

A common type of bandage is a commercial adhesive compress. Available in assorted sizes, an adhesive compress consists of a small pad of nonstick gauze (the dressing) on a strip of adhesive tape (the bandage) applied directly to small injuries. Also available is the **bandage compress**, a thick gauze dressing attached to a gauze bandage. This bandage can be tied in place. Because it is designed to help control severe bleeding, the bandage compress usually comes in a sterile package.

A **roller bandage** is usually made of gauze or gauze-like material. Some gauze bandages are made of a self-adhering material that easily conforms to different body parts. Roller bandages are available in assorted widths from 1/2 to 12 inches and lengths from 5 to 10 yards. A roller bandage is generally wrapped around the body part, over a dressing, using overlapping turns until the dressing is completely covered. It

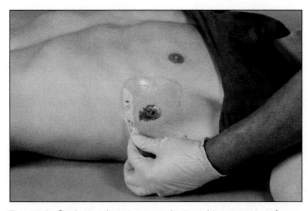

Fig. 19-3: Occlusive dressings are designed to prevent air from passing through.

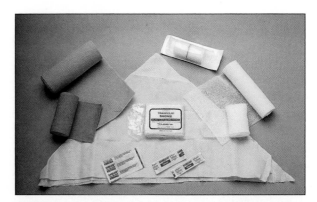

Fig. 19-5: Bandages are used to hold dressings in place, apply pressure, protect a wound from infection and provide support to an injured limb or body part.

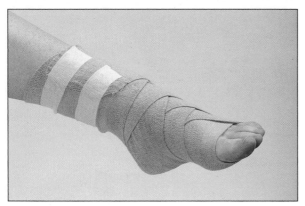

Fig. 19-6: An elastic roller bandage is designed to keep continuous pressure on a body part.

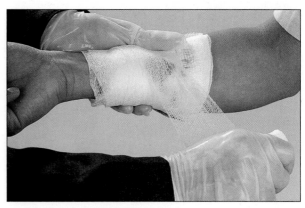

Fig. 19-8: A pressure bandage can be applied to maintain direct pressure.

can be tied or taped in place. A folded strip of roller bandage may also be used as a dressing or compress. In **Chapter 22**, you will learn to use roller bandages to hold splints in place.

A special type of roller bandage is an **elastic bandage**, sometimes called an *elastic wrap*. Elastic bandages are designed to keep continuous pressure on a body part (**Fig. 19-6**). When properly applied, they can effectively control swelling or support an injured limb. Elastic bandages are available in assorted widths from 2 to 6 inches. They are very effective in managing injuries to muscles, bones and joints. Elastic bandages are frequently used in athletic environments and should be applied only by those who are trained and proficient in their use.

Another commonly used bandage is the **triangular bandage**. When it is folded, it can hold a dressing or splint in place on most parts of the body. Used as a sling, the triangular bandage can support an injured shoulder, arm or hand (**Fig. 19-7**).

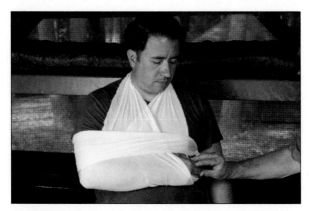

Fig. 19-7: Used as a sling, the triangular bandage can support an injured shoulder, arm or hand.

Application of Bandages

A pressure bandage will hold gauze pads in place while maintaining direct pressure (**Fig. 19-8**). If blood soaks through, add additional dressings and bandages and reapply direct pressure. Do not remove any blood-soaked dressings or bandages.

To apply a roller bandage, follow these general guidelines:

- Secure the end of the bandage in place. Wrap the bandage around the body part until the dressing is completely covered and the bandage extends several inches beyond the dressing. Tie or tape the bandage in place (**Fig. 19-9, A–C**).
- Do not cover fingers or toes, if possible. By keeping these parts uncovered, you will be able to tell if the bandage is too tight (**Fig. 19-9, D**). If fingers or toes become cold, numb or begin to turn pale, ashen or blue, the bandage is too tight and should be loosened slightly.
- If blood soaks through the bandage, apply additional dressings and another bandage and reapply direct pressure. Do not remove the blood-soaked ones.

Elastic bandages can easily restrict blood flow if not applied properly. Restricted blood flow is not only painful but also can cause tissue damage if not corrected. **Figure 19-10, A–D** shows the proper way to apply an elastic bandage.

EXTERNAL BLEEDING

External bleeding is usually easy to control. Follow standard precautions when providing care. Wash your hands before *and* after providing

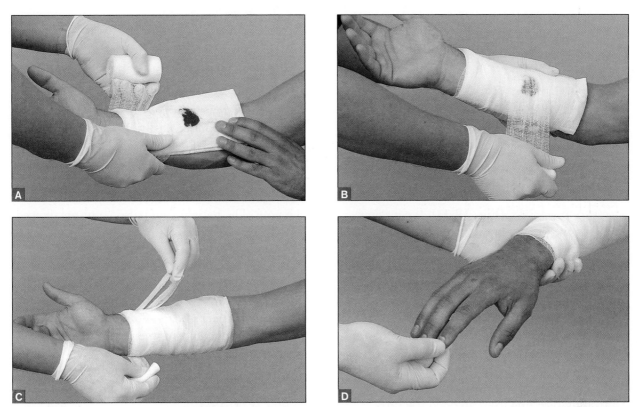

Fig. 19-9, A–D: To apply a roller bandage: **(A)** Start by securing the bandage in place. **(B)** Use overlapping turns to cover the dressing completely. **(C)** Tie or tape the bandage in place. **(D)** Check the fingers for feeling, warmth and color.

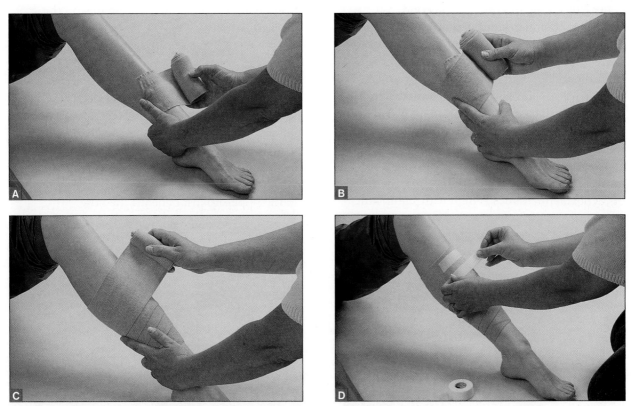

Fig. 19-10, A–D: To apply an elastic bandage: **(A)** Start the elastic bandage at the point farthest from the heart. **(B)** Anchor the bandage. **(C)** Wrap the bandage using overlapping turns. **(D)** Tape the end of the bandage in place.

care, and wear gloves. You may use alcohol-based hand sanitizers if there is no visible matter present and soap and water are not available.

Providing Care

When treating a bleeding patient, apply a sterile, gauze dressing or trauma pad over the wound and then apply direct pressure to the wound with your gloved hand. If necessary, use your gloved hand to begin applying direct pressure to the wound while someone else obtains the necessary material(s) (**Fig. 19-11**). If conscious and able, the patient may use his or her hand to apply pressure while you obtain the necessary equipment or perform other, more urgent duties.

For serious bleeding, apply strong, direct pressure to the wound to counter the pressure from the beating heart. Use fingertip pressure (using the flat part of fingers) first to control bleeding. If the wound is large and fingertip pressure does not work, use hand pressure with gauze dressings to stop the bleeding. If you are controlling bleeding from an open fracture, do *not* apply direct pressure over the bones but instead pack sterile gauze around the area to control bleeding and prevent infection.

If the dressing becomes saturated with blood while you are applying pressure, *do not remove it*. Instead, place additional dressings over the soaked bandage and reapply direct pressure. Then cover the dressings with a bandage to hold them in place. Keep the patient warm and position the patient flat on his or her back. Care for other conditions, including shock.

Part of your care for serious bleeding is to always assess and care for shock, since the risk of (hypovolemic) shock is high with significant blood loss (see **Chapter 18** for more information on shock). Do not give food or drink if shock is suspected.

Nosebleeds

Nosebleeds are usually self-contained and can most often be stopped easily. They can be caused by trauma or develop from a medical reason, such as dryness or high blood pressure. In your assessment of the patient, you can expect to find pain or tenderness in the area and bleeding from the nose. The patient could also vomit swallowed blood. For an unconscious patient, a nosebleed can potentially block the airway.

To care for a nosebleed—
- Ensure the conscious patient is sitting in an upright position.
- Tilt the patient's head and upper body forward slightly, if possible, to prevent swallowing or choking on the blood.
- Pinch the patient's nostrils together firmly for about 5 to 10 minutes to slow down the blood flow (**Fig. 19-12**).
- Tell the patient not to sniffle or blow his or her nose.
- Do not pack the patient's nose to stop the bleeding.

As with bleeding from external wounds, monitor the patient for signs of shock if the bleeding does not stop. If you suspect a fractured skull, do *not* try to stop a nosebleed as this might increase pressure on the brain. Instead, cover the nostrils loosely with sterile gauze. Other methods of controlling bleeding include applying an ice pack to the bridge of the nose or putting pressure on the upper lip just beneath the nose.

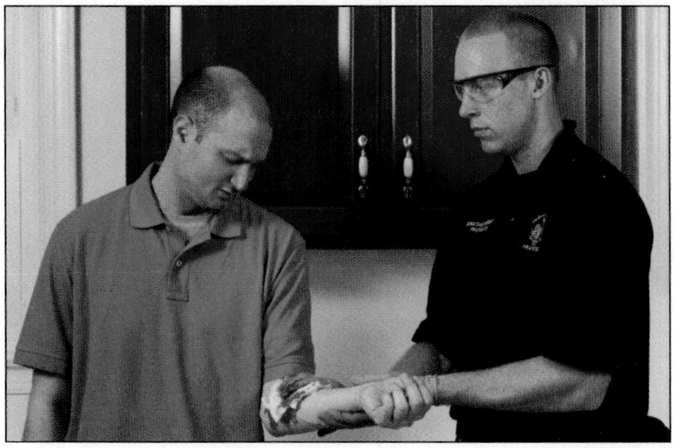

Fig. 19-11: When treating a bleeding patient, apply a dressing or trauma pad and use a gloved hand to apply direct pressure to the wound.

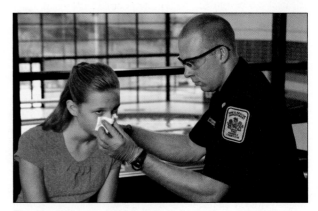

Fig. 19-12: To care for a nosebleed, firmly pinch or have the patient pinch the nostrils together for about 5 to 10 minutes.

Other Methods of Bleeding Control

If the bleeding is not controlled by direct pressure alone, other methods of controlling bleeding may be considered and should be followed according to local protocols.

Tourniquets

A **tourniquet** is a tight band placed around an arm or leg to constrict blood vessels, to stop blood flow to a wound. Because of the potential for adverse effects, a tourniquet should *only be used as a last resort* in cases of delayed-care or delayed EMS response situations when direct pressure does not stop the bleeding or you are not able to apply direct pressure. Application of a tourniquet is considered an *emergency medical technician* (EMT) level or higher skill in most jurisdictions and requires proper training. There are several types of manufactured tourniquets available, and these are preferred over makeshift devices. For a manufactured tourniquet, always follow the manufacturer's instructions and medical control.

In general, apply the tourniquet around the wounded extremity, just above the wound, and route the tag end of the strap through the buckle. Pull the strap tightly and secure the tourniquet in place. Twist the rod (windlass) to tighten the tourniquet, until the bright red bleeding stops, then secure the rod in place (**Fig. 19-13, A–B**). The tourniquet should *not* be removed in the prehospital setting once it is applied. Note and record the time that the tourniquet was applied and give this information to more advanced medical personnel.

Blood pressure cuffs are sometimes used to slow the flow of blood in an upper extremity as a tourniquet. Another technique is to use a bandage 4-inches wide and six- to eight-layers deep. Always follow local protocols when the use of a tourniquet is considered.

Hemostatic Agents

Hemostatic agents generally use substances that remove moisture from blood and speed up the process of clot formation. Chemical composition varies depending on the product, but ingredients include—
- Mineral zeolite.
- Micropourous polysaccharide hemosphere.

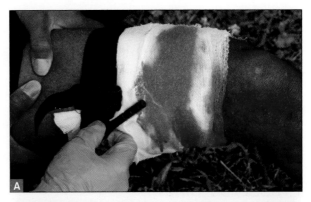

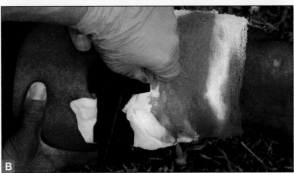

Fig. 19-13, A–B: To apply a tourniquet: **(A)** Secure the tourniquet in place around the injured body part. **(B)** Tighten it by twisting the rod and securing it into place. Note and record the time the tourniquet was applied.

- Microporous hydrogel-forming polyacrylamide.
- Poly-N-acetylglucosamine.

Hemostatic agents are available in a variety of forms, including treated sponge or gauze pads and powder or granular forms. The powder or granular forms are poured directly on the bleeding vessel. Some hemostatic agents are used in conjunction with direct pressure.

Over-the-counter versions of hemostatic bandages are available. There are also hemostatic agents intended for professional rescuers that are available. Local protocols and procedures for the use of hemostatic agents may vary. *Always* follow local protocols for use in the prehospital setting.

Hemostatic agents are not for routine use. Do not use hemostatic agents in place of direct pressure or a tourniquet. Use hemostatic agents only if direct pressure or use of a tourniquet fails or is not possible.

Elevation

Elevation uses gravity to slow the flow of blood to an area of the body and may encourage **clotting**. Elevation should be used only if the patient does not have a painful, swollen deformity or possible fracture. Elevate the injured area above the level of the heart while maintaining direct pressure.

Immobilization

Immobilize the limb to restrict movement while maintaining direct pressure. This will restrict blood flow. Encourage the patient to be still.

Pressure Points

If other methods do not control severe bleeding, consider taking other measures. In an effort to further slow bleeding, you can compress the artery supplying the area against an underlying bone at specific sites on the body called **pressure points**. Remember to maintain direct pressure while using pressure points. The main pressure points used to control bleeding in the arms and legs are over the brachial (inside the elbow) and femoral (in the groin) arteries.

Once you have controlled the bleeding, cover the area with a sterile bandage (or pressure bandage) and fasten firmly and securely with tape. Monitor and provide care for shock. If bleeding resumes or blood seeps through the bandages, apply additional gauze and reapply direct pressure.

Splints

In an open wound to an extremity where the bone or joint is also injured, the bone ends or fragments can be displaced and cause damage to soft tissues and blood vessels, causing further bleeding. Using a splint to immobilize the extremity can help prevent this problem. If the wound is over an open fracture (on the bones), do *not* apply direct pressure but instead pack sterile gauze around the area to control bleeding and prevent infection.

Internal Bleeding
Causes

Internal bleeding is the escape of blood from arteries, veins or capillaries into spaces in the body. Internal bleeding can be caused by a variety of injuries or conditions, including blunt force trauma. For example, the impact of the chest or head against the steering wheel during a motor-vehicle collision can cause internal bleeding. It can also be caused by a fracture, which may cause bones to pierce internal organs. Because this type of damage may not be visible, it may lead to extensive concealed bleeding. It may also cause unexplained shock.

Internal bleeding can also occur along with external bleeding. For example, if a patient is bleeding from a knife wound, the blade may have penetrated an organ, which then begins bleeding inside the body.

The patient may experience injuries to extremities, causing pain, swelling or deformity. This may lead to serious internal blood loss from long bone fractures. Internal bleeding is not always easy to recognize unless the patient is losing blood from the ears, mouth, vagina, rectum or possibly from the nose.

As with external bleeding, arterial bleeding is the most serious. The strength of the heartbeat will cause the blood to flow from the blood vessels into the interior of the body quickly and with great force.

Signs and Symptoms of Internal Bleeding

Some signs and symptoms of internal bleeding include—

- Discoloration of the skin around the area (bruising) on the neck, chest, abdomen or side.
- Nausea, vomiting or coughing up blood.
- Discolored, painful, tender, swollen or firm tissue (e.g., the abdomen).
- Tenderness and guarding (protecting the area).

Signs and symptoms of shock may be present, including—

- Anxiety or restlessness.
- Rapid, weak pulse.
- Rapid breathing.
- Skin that feels cool or moist or that looks pale, ashen or bluish.

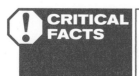 **CRITICAL FACTS** Some signs and symptoms of internal bleeding include bruising on the neck, chest, abdomen or side; nausea, vomiting or coughing up blood; patient guarding the area; rapid pulse or breathing; skin that is cool or moist or looks pale, ashen or bluish; excessive thirst; declining LOC and drop in blood pressure.

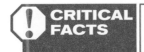
- Excessive thirst.
- Declining *level of consciousness* (LOC).
- Drop in blood pressure.

Providing Care

If a patient is bleeding internally—
- Call for more advanced medical personnel if serious internal bleeding is suspected.
- Ensure the patient remains as still as possible, to reduce the heart's blood output.
- Care for shock.

When internal bleeding is from the capillary blood vessels, the result is bruising around the wound area and is not serious. To reduce discomfort for the patient, you can apply ice or a cold pack, ensuring that the ice does *not* come in direct contact with the patient's skin.

PUTTING IT ALL TOGETHER

One of the most important things you can do in any emergency is to recognize and control severe bleeding. External bleeding is easily recognized and should be cared for immediately. Check and care for severe bleeding during the primary assessment. Severe external bleeding is life threatening. Although internal bleeding is less obvious, it also can be life threatening. Recognize when a serious injury has occurred and suspect internal bleeding. You may not identify internal bleeding until you perform the physical exam and patient history. When you identify or suspect severe bleeding, quickly transport or arrange for transport of the patient to a hospital. Continue to provide care until more advanced medical personnel take over.

Do *not* wait for shock to develop before providing care to someone who is injured or suddenly ill, especially if there is blood loss or if the normal function of the heart is interrupted. Care for life-threatening conditions, such as severe external bleeding, before caring for lesser injuries. Remember that managing shock effectively begins with recognizing a situation in which shock may develop, and providing appropriate care. Summon more advanced medical personnel *immediately* if you notice signs and symptoms of shock. Shock can often be reversed by advanced medical care, but *only* if the patient is reached in time.

YOU ARE THE EMERGENCY MEDICAL RESPONDER

You have called for more advanced medical personnel. Blood is spurting with each beat of the patient's heart. The bandage is soaked with blood and your partner notices that the patient is turning pale and his LOC is changing. How would you respond? What other concerns do you have and what additional steps should you take until EMS personnel arrive?

SKILLsheet

Controlling External Bleeding

REMEMBER: Always follow standard precautions and summon more advanced medical personnel if necessary.

STEP 1

Cover the wound with a dressing, such as a sterile gauze pad.

STEP 2

Apply direct pressure firmly against the wound until bleeding stops.

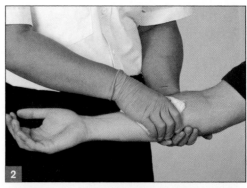

STEP 3

Cover the dressing with a roller bandage and secure directly over the wound.

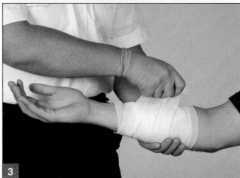

STEP 4

Check for circulation beyond the injury (check for pulse, skin temperature and feeling).

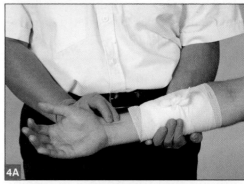

If the bleeding does *not* stop–
- Apply additional dressings and bandages on top of the first ones and continue to apply direct pressure.
- Take steps to minimize shock.
- Summon more advanced medical personnel.
- Follow local protocols when considering other methods of bleeding control.

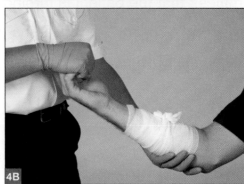

Enrichment
Mechanisms of Injury—The Kinematics of Trauma

VEHICLE COLLISIONS

Motor-vehicle collisions are one of the most frequent scenes to which an *emergency medical responder* (EMR) may be called. Collisions are categorized as head-on impact, rear impact, **side impact, rotational impact** and **rollover**. Each collision category shows a predictable pattern of injury, which is influenced by the type of restraint the occupant was using at the time of the collision.

A **head-on collision** is one in which a vehicle hits an object, such as a tree or a stopped vehicle, straight on. When the car makes impact in a head-on collision, the bodies of the occupants will continue to move. Injuries common to head-on collisions include face, head, neck, chest and abdominal injuries. This is also true for rear-impact collisions.

In **side-impact collisions**, also known as broadside or t-bone collisions, the person on the impact side of the accident sustains more injuries than do occupants on the opposite side. Due to the impact sustained during a side-impact collision, the body moves one way and the head the other. This makes head and neck injuries more common. Chest and pelvic injuries are also possible in this situation.

Rotational impact occurs off center, when the car strikes an object and rotates around it until the car either loses speed or strikes another object. Injuries similar to head-on and side-impact collisions can be expected in these cases.

Rollovers see the occupants of the car changing positions as the car does **(Fig. 19-14)**. In these cases, predicting injury is impossible, as every object in the car becomes potentially lethal. If occupants are not wearing seat belts, it is more likely that they may be thrown from the car. Common injuries in rollovers include soft tissue injuries, multiple broken bones and crushing injuries.

When someone is struck by or falls against a blunt object—one with no sharp edges or points—the resulting injuries are often closed wounds. This means that, although the soft tissues of skin, muscle, nerves and blood vessels may be damaged, the skin is not broken and there is no visible bleeding. The patient may look unharmed, but there may be serious, even fatal, injury to the internal organs and significant internal bleeding.

Proper use of restraints in a vehicle will help to lessen the likelihood of injury for the occupants. However, injuries can still be sustained. Restraints vary based on the type of vehicle and some can be more effective than others in preventing injury.

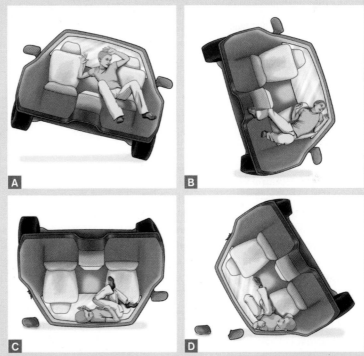

Fig. 19-14, A–D: In a rollover, unrestrained occupants of the car change positions as the car does

- Lap Belt
  - Prevents occupants from being thrown from a car.
  - Does not prevent head, neck and chest injuries.
  - Can cause internal injuries if not worn properly.
  - Can cause injury to the diaphragm.

Continued on next page

Enrichment
Mechanisms of Injury—The Kinematics of Trauma (continued)

- Lap and Shoulder Belts
  - Prevent occupants from striking the steering wheel and dashboard.
  - Severe impact can cause damage to the clavicle.
  - Do not prevent head and neck injury.
- Air Bag
  - Located in the steering wheel, dashboard and/or side curtains.
  - Must have high impact to deploy.
  - Occupants must be wearing seat belts for full effect.
  - Can cause burns, **contusions** (bruises) and other, more serious injuries.

Pediatric Considerations

Because an airbag could seriously injure or even kill a child, or even an adult of short stature, these individuals are safest in the rear seat. A child or an infant in a rear-facing seat is close to the dashboard and could easily be struck by the airbag with sufficient force to cause serious harm or even death. Older children who have outgrown child seats are also at risk from a deploying air bag, if not properly restrained.

Infants should *always* be transported in car seats. However, as with seat belts and air bags, car seats vary based on type and some can be more effective than others in preventing injury.
- Infant car seats facing backward help prevent head and neck injuries.
- The greatest danger is to the infant's neck.
- Seats vary, based on the age and size of the occupant.

In motorcycle accidents, there are four potential scenarios: head-on, angular, ejection and laying the bike down **(Fig. 19-15)**. The purpose of laying the bike down is to minimize impact in the case of an impending crash. The rider may turn the motorcycle sideways and drag a leg along the ground to lose speed in order to get off the bike. This can result in severe burns and abrasions, but lessens the likelihood of internal injuries.

Head-on impacts will usually result in the driver impacting the handle bars at the same speed the bike is traveling. Multiple injuries can result.

Angular impact can result in severe amputations, as the rider strikes an object at an angle. Ejection from the bike causes the rider to fly over the handle bars, which can result in severe head, spinal and face injury, especially if the rider is not wearing a helmet.

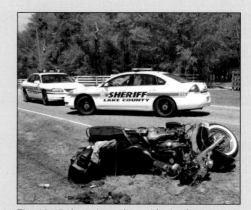

Fig. 19-15: In motorcycle accidents, there are four potential scenarios: head-on, angular, ejection or laying the bike down (shown). *Courtesy of Captain Phil Kleinberg, EMT-P, Lake-Sumter EMS.*

All-terrain vehicle (ATV) crashes commonly result in head, neck and extremity injuries similar to those seen in motorcycle collisions. These vehicles are prone to crashes and rollovers.

FALLS

A significant number of trauma-related injuries each year are caused by falls, particularly in the elderly. The severity of the injury depends on—
- The distance of the fall.
- Any interruptions during the fall.
- Which body parts impact first.
- The surface on which the patient lands.
- The patient's physical condition *before* the fall took place.

There are two types of falls. *Feet-first falls* cause energy to travel up the skeleton as the patient lands **(Fig. 19-16)**. When a patient's knees are bent on landing, injury will be less severe. Spine, hip socket, femur, heel and ankle are the most common sites for injury from these falls. If hands are outstretched to help "break" a fall, then wrists will be also be impacted. Broken shoulders and clavicles are also common.

Head-first falls begin with the arms and extend to the shoulders on impact. Therefore, spine and head injuries are common. Chest, lower back and pelvis injuries often occur as the body is falling and the torso and legs are thrown forward or backward.

Falls on the side of the head (as in skiing accidents) often do not show signs and symptoms until 1 to 2 hours after the injury. Be sure to tell this to patients, so that they are aware of it. Strongly encourage patients to get checked out by a health care provider before symptoms occur.

Fig. 19-16: In a jump or fall from a height, the impact can be transmitted up the legs, causing injures to the thigh, pelvis, head, neck or back.

PENETRATING INJURIES

When an object is pushed through the surface and soft tissue of the body, a *penetrating injury* occurs. There are *low-velocity* and *medium-high velocity* penetrating injuries. Low-velocity injuries occur most commonly with the use of hand-powered weapons such as knives or arrows. The severity of the injury can be determined by the location of the injury and the length of the weapon. The strength and force capacity of the attacker is also a determining factor.

Medium-high velocity injuries are caused by guns. Tissue damage can be much more widespread in a patient with a gunshot wound than may be indicated by the surface wound. Little external bleeding can still be a result of a devastating internal injury.

BLAST INJURIES

Explosions can produce unique patterns of injury, often inflicting multiple life-threatening injuries on several patients simultaneously. Blast injuries are divided into four categories: primary, secondary, tertiary and miscellaneous.

Primary blast injury is caused by the direct effect of blast overpressure on a patient's tissue, resulting in injury to air-filled structures such as the lungs, ears and gastrointestinal tract. A primary blast injury damages organs and tissue solely by the shock of the blast wave.

Secondary blast injury is caused when a patient is struck by flying objects and is responsible for the majority of casualties in many explosions. Injuries most commonly include penetrating thoracic trauma, including lacerations of the heart and major blood vessels, which is a common cause of death by secondary blast injuries.

Tertiary blast injuries are caused by individuals flying through the air and striking other objects, generally from high-energy explosions. The patient is usually very close to the explosion source when injured this way.

Miscellaneous blast-related injuries, sometimes termed quaternary blast injuries, encompass all other injuries a patient may experience caused by explosions, including burns, crush injuries and inhalation of toxic fumes or substances. It is probable that wheezing associated with a blast injury is from one of the following:
* Pulmonary contusion
* Inhalation of toxic gases or dusts
* Pulmonary edema from myocardial contusion
* **Adult respiratory distress syndrome (ARDS)**

If possible, try to determine—
* What material caused the explosion.
* The patient's location relative to the center of the explosion.
* If there is evidence of radiation and/or chemicals.

Enrichment
Tourniquets

A tourniquet can be used on an arm or a leg if blood loss is *uncontrolled* by direct pressure, or direct pressure is not possible. For example, a tourniquet may be appropriate if you cannot reach the wound because of entrapment, there are multiple injuries or the size of the wound prohibits application of direct pressure. Tourniquets are rarely necessary, but if one is needed to control bleeding, manufactured tourniquets are safer, more effective and preferred over makeshift devices. If used, the tourniquet should be applied and kept it in place continuously until more advanced medical personnel take over or the person reaches a medical facility.

In general, apply the tourniquet around the wounded extremity, just above the wound, and route the tag end of the strap through the buckle. Pull the strap tightly and secure the tourniquet in place. Twist the rod (windlass) to tighten the tourniquet, until the bright red bleeding stops, then secure the rod in place. The tourniquet should *not* be removed in the prehospital setting once it is applied. Note and record the time that the tourniquet was applied and give this information to more advanced medical personnel.

SKILLsheet

Using a Manufactured Tourniquet

NOTE: Always follow standard precautions and summon more advanced medical personnel. Always follow the manufacturer's instructions and medical control when applying a tourniquet.

STEP 1

Position the tourniquet around the limb, approximately 2 inches (approximately two finger widths) above the wound but not over a joint.

STEP 2

Route the tag end of the strap through the buckle, if necessary.

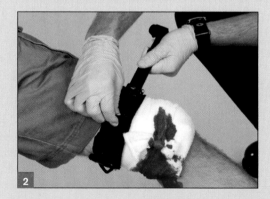

STEP 3

Pull the strap tightly and secure it in place.

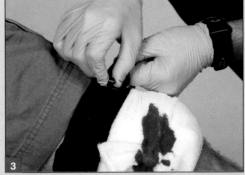

STEP 4

Tighten the tourniquet by twisting the rod until the flow of bleeding stops and secure the rod in place.

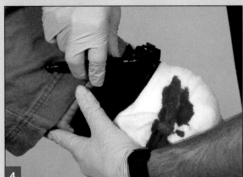

STEP 5

Note and record the time that you applied the tourniquet and give this information to more advanced medical personnel. *Do not* cover the tourniquet with clothing.

20 Soft Tissue Injuries

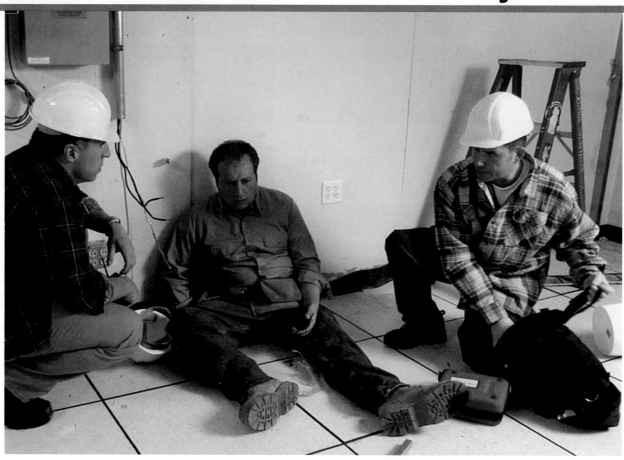

))) YOU ARE THE EMERGENCY MEDICAL RESPONDER

You are on the *medical emergency response team* (MERT) responding to a call at a power plant that at least one worker has suffered an electrical shock from a live junction box. Plant workers thought that a colleague had turned off the power, but when the injured worker reached inside and touched a wire, he received a shock and an electrical burn. The injured worker has lost consciousness. A second worker at the scene moved away from his co-worker and called for help. When you arrive, the co-worker who placed the call relates what happened. How should you respond? What are your immediate concerns?

Key Terms

Abrasion: The most common type of open wound; characterized by skin that has been rubbed or scraped away.

Amputation: The complete removal or severing of an external body part.

Avulsion: An injury in which a portion of the skin, and sometimes other soft tissue, is partially or completely torn away.

Burn: An injury to the skin or other body tissues caused by heat, chemicals, electricity or radiation.

Chemical burn: A burn caused by strong, caustic chemicals damaging the skin.

Closed wound: A wound in which soft tissue damage occurs beneath the skin and the skin is not broken.

Compartment syndrome: Condition in which there is swelling and an increase in pressure within a limited space that presses on and compromises blood vessels, nerves and tendons that run through that limited space; usually involves the leg, forearm, arm, thigh, shoulder or buttock.

Critical burn: Any burn that is potentially life threatening, disabling or disfiguring; a burn requiring advanced medical care.

Crush injury: An injury to a body part, often an extremity, caused by a high degree of pressure; may result in serious damage to underlying tissues and cause bleeding, bruising, fracture, laceration and compartment syndrome.

Dermis: The deeper layer of the skin; contains the nerves, sweat glands, oil glands and blood vessels.

Electrical burn: A burn caused by contact with an electrical source, which allows an electrical current to pass through the body.

Epidermis: The outer layer of the skin; provides a barrier to bacteria and other organisms that can cause infection.

Full-thickness burn: A burn injury involving all layers of skin and underlying tissues; skin may be brown or charred, and underlying tissues may appear white; also referred to as a *third-degree burn.*

Hypodermis: A deeper layer of skin, located below the epidermis and dermis, that contains fat, blood vessels and connective tissues.

Laceration: A cut, usually from a sharp object, that can have either jagged or smooth edges.

Open wound: A wound resulting in a break in the skin's surface.

Partial-thickness burn: A burn injury involving the epidermis and dermis, characterized by red, wet skin and blisters; also referred to as a *second-degree burn.*

Puncture/penetration: A type of wound that results when the skin is pierced with a pointed object.

Radiation burn: A burn caused by exposure to radiation, either nuclear (e.g., radiation therapy) or solar (e.g., radiation from the sun).

Rule of Nines: A method for estimating the extent of a burn; divides the body into 11 surface areas, each of which comprises approximately 9 percent of the body, plus the genitals, which are approximately 1 percent.

Soft tissues: Body structures that include the layers of skin, fat and muscles.

Superficial burn: A burn injury involving only the top layer of skin, characterized by red, dry skin; also referred to as a *first-degree burn.*

Wound: An injury to the soft tissues.

Learning Objectives

After reading this chapter, and completing the class activities, you will have the information needed to—

- List the types of soft tissue injuries.
- Describe the emergency medical care for a patient with a soft tissue injury.
- Describe the emergency medical care for a patient with an injury from an embedded object.
- Describe the emergency medical care for a patient with an open wound.
- Describe the emergency medical care for a patient with an amputation.

- List the signs and symptoms of closed wounds.
- List the causes of a burn injury.
- List conditions under which you would summon more advanced medical personnel for a burn injury.
- Describe the emergency medical care for burns.
- Describe the kinds of injuries that might occur from a thermal, electrical, chemical and radiation burn.
- Describe how to care for thermal, chemical, electrical and radiation burns.

INTRODUCTION

An infant falls and bruises an arm while learning to walk; a child needs stitches in the chin after tumbling from the "monkey bars" on the playground; a teenager gets a sunburn during a weekend at the beach; and an adult cuts a hand while working in a woodshop. What do these injuries have in common? They are all **soft tissue** injuries.

In the course of growing up and in our daily lives, soft tissue injuries occur often and in many different ways. Fortunately, most soft tissue injuries are minor, requiring little attention. Often, only an *adhesive bandage* or ice and rest are needed. Some injuries, however, are more severe and require immediate medical attention.

Burns are a special kind of soft tissue injury. Like other types of soft tissue injury, burns can damage the top layer of skin or the skin and the layers of fat, muscle and bone beneath. In this chapter, you will learn how to recognize and care for soft tissue injuries.

SKIN AND SOFT TISSUE INJURIES

Soft Tissues

The soft tissues include the layers of skin, fat and muscle that protect the underlying body structures (**Fig. 20-1**).

In **Chapter 4**, you learned that the skin is the largest single organ in the body and that, without it, the human body could not function. The skin provides a protective barrier for the body; it helps regulate the body's temperature and it receives information about the environment through the nerves that run through it.

The outer layer of skin, the **epidermis**, provides a barrier to bacteria and other organisms that can cause infection. The deeper layer, the **dermis**, contains the important structures of the nerves, the sweat and oil glands and the blood vessels. The **hypodermis**—located beneath the epidermis and dermis—contains fat, blood vessels

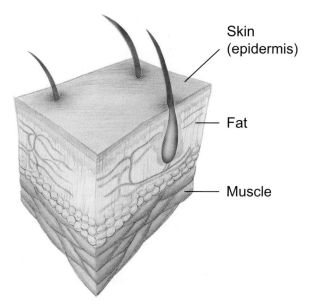

Fig. 20-1: Layers of skin, fat and muscle protect underlying structures of the body.

and connective tissues. Because the skin is well supplied with blood vessels and nerves, most soft tissue injuries are likely to bleed and be painful.

Beneath the skin layers lies a layer of fat. This layer helps insulate the body, to help maintain body temperature. The fat layer also stores energy. The amount of fat varies in different parts of the body and in each person.

The muscles lie beneath the fat layer and comprise the largest segment of the body's soft tissues. Most soft tissue injuries involve the outer layers of tissue. However, violent forces, such as those that cause deep burns or cause objects to penetrate the skin, can injure *all* the soft tissue layers. Muscle injuries are discussed more thoroughly in **Chapter 22**, along with other musculoskeletal injuries.

Types of Soft Tissue Injuries

An injury to the soft tissues is called a **wound**. Soft tissue injuries are typically classified as either **closed wounds** or **open wounds**. A wound is considered closed when the soft tissue damage occurs beneath the surface of the skin, leaving the outer layer intact; this often results in internal

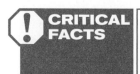

CRITICAL FACTS

The skin is the largest organ in the body. The outer layer, called the epidermis, provides a barrier to bacteria and other organisms that can cause infection.

An injury to the soft tissues is called a wound. Soft tissue injuries are typically classified as either closed wounds or open wounds.

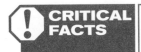

CRITICAL FACTS   Burns are a soft tissue injury that has three classifications: superficial, partial thickness and full thickness.

bleeding. A wound is considered open when there is a break in the skin's outer layer; this usually results in external bleeding.

Burns are a special kind of soft tissue injury. A burn injury occurs when intense heat, certain chemicals, electricity or radiation contact the skin or other body tissues. Burns are classified as superficial, partial thickness or full thickness.

CLOSED WOUNDS

Closed wounds occur beneath the surface of the skin. The simplest closed wound is a *bruise*, also called a *contusion* (**Fig. 20-2**). Bruises result when the body is subjected to blunt force, such as when you bump your leg on a table or chair. Such a blow usually results in damage to soft tissue layers and blood vessels beneath the skin, causing internal bleeding.

A much more serious closed wound can be caused by a violent force hitting the body. This type of force can injure larger blood vessels and deeper layers of muscle tissue, causing heavy bleeding beneath the skin, which causes a localized tissue mass that can be discolored by the internal bleeding. These injuries are referred to as *hematomas*.

Signs and Symptoms of Closed Wounds

When blood and other fluids seep into the surrounding tissues, the area discolors (turns black and blue) and swells. The amount of discoloration and swelling varies depending on the severity of the injury. At first, the area may only appear red. Over time, more blood may leak into the area, making the area appear dark red or purple. Violent forces can cause more severe soft tissue injuries involving larger blood vessels, the deeper layers of muscle tissue and even organs deep within the body. These injuries can result in profuse internal bleeding. With deeper injuries, you may or may not see bruising immediately.

Providing Care for Closed Wounds

Many closed wounds, such as bruises, do *not* require special medical care. To care for a closed wound, be sure to keep the injured area still. Applying cold can be effective early on in helping control both pain and swelling (**Fig. 20-3**). Use an ice pack and apply it to the injured area for about 20 minutes. Place a damp or wet thin barrier such as a cloth between the ice pack and bare skin to prevent tissue damage. Remove the ice for 20 minutes before applying it again. If 20 minutes cannot be tolerated, apply ice for periods of 10 minutes. If an ice pack is not available, you can fill a plastic bag with ice (crushed or cubed) and water or wrap ice with a damp cloth. Elevating the injured part may help reduce swelling. However, *do not* elevate the injured part if this causes more pain.

Do *not* assume that all closed wounds are minor injuries. Take the time to find out whether more serious injuries could be present. With the cases that follow, the patient may be bleeding internally and need emergency

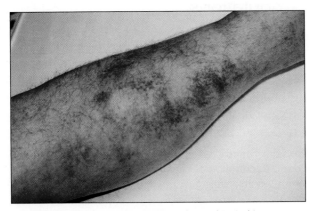

Fig. 20-2: Bruises result when the body is subjected to blunt force. *Courtesy of Ted Crites.*

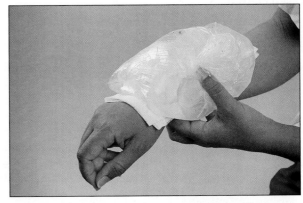

Fig. 20-3: Applying cold to a closed wound can be effective in helping control pain and swelling.

medical care. Call for more advanced medical care if—

- The patient complains of severe pain or cannot move a body part without pain.
- The force that caused the injury seems great enough to cause serious damage.
- An injured extremity is blue or extremely pale.
- The patient is extremely thirsty after being hit in the abdominal area.
- The patient shows signs and symptoms of shock.

With all closed wounds, help the patient rest in the most comfortable position, keep the patient from getting chilled or overheated (care for shock), and reassure and comfort the patient. If a patient has an injured lower extremity, ensure that the patient does *not* bear weight on the extremity until advised to do so by a medical professional.

OPEN WOUNDS

Open wounds are injuries that break the skin. These breaks can be as minor as a scrape of the surface layers or as severe as the loss of a body part. The amount of bleeding depends on the severity of the injury. Any break in the skin provides an entry point for disease-producing microorganisms, or *pathogens*.

There are six main types of open wounds, including—

- **Abrasions.**
- **Amputations.**
- **Avulsions.**
- Crush injuries.
- Punctures/penetrations.
- **Lacerations.**

Types of Open Wounds
Abrasions

An *abrasion* is the most common type of open wound. It is characterized by skin that has been rubbed or scraped away, such as when someone falls and scrapes the hands or knees **(Fig. 20-4)**. An abrasion is sometimes called a "*rug burn*," "*road rash*" or "*strawberry*." Because the scraping

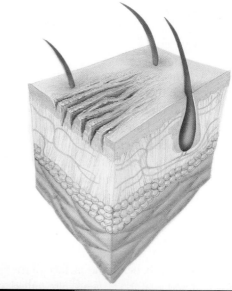

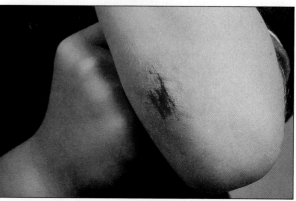

Fig. 20-4: An abrasion is characterized by skin that has been rubbed or scraped away.

of the outer skin layers exposes sensitive nerve endings, an abrasion is usually painful. Bleeding is easily controlled and not severe, since only the capillaries are affected. Because of the way the injury occurs, dirt and other matter can easily become embedded in the skin, making it especially important to clean the wound.

Amputations

In some severe injuries, the force is so violent that a body part, such as a finger, may be severed. A complete severing of a part (usually involving a bone or limb) is called an *amputation* **(Fig. 20-5)**. Although damage to the tissue is severe, bleeding may not be as profuse as you might expect. The

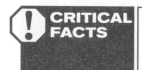

Open wounds are injuries that break the skin. These breaks can be as minor as a scrape of the surface layers or as severe as a deep penetration or even body part loss. The six types of open wounds are abrasions, amputations, avulsions, crush injuries, punctures/penetrations and lacerations.

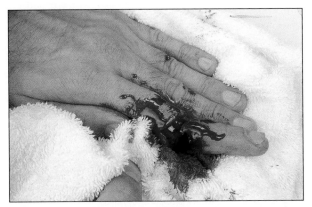

Fig. 20-5: An amputation is a complete severing of a part of the body.

blood vessels usually constrict and *retract* (pull in) at the point of injury, slowing bleeding and making it relatively easy to control with direct pressure. In the past, a completely severed body part could not be successfully reattached. With today's technology, reattachment is often successful, making it important to carefully

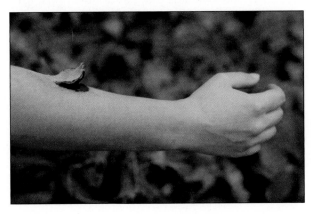

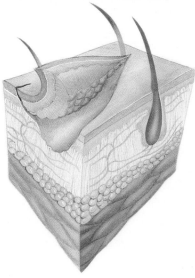

Fig. 20-6: In an avulsion, part of the skin and other soft tissue is torn away. *Courtesy of the Canadian Red Cross.*

handle and send the severed part to the hospital with the patient.

Avulsions

An avulsion is an injury in which a portion of the skin and sometimes other soft tissue is partially or completely torn away (**Fig. 20-6**). A partially avulsed piece of skin may remain attached but hang like a flap. Bleeding can be heavy because avulsions often involve deeper soft tissue layers.

Crush Injuries

A **crush injury** is the result of a body part, usually an extremity, being subjected to a high degree of pressure, in most cases after being compressed between two heavy objects (**Fig. 20-7**). This type of injury may result in serious damage to underlying tissues and cause bleeding, bruising, fracture, laceration and **compartment syndrome**. In a severe crush injury to the torso, internal organs may rupture. Crush injuries can be open or closed.

Crush syndrome is common in people who are trapped in collapsed structures due to, for example, an earthquake or act of terrorism. The injury does not happen at the time that the tissue is crushed, but once the crushed muscle is released from compression and the tissue is re-perfused with blood. At that point, multiple adverse processes occur, as the products of muscle breakdown are released into the blood. The patient may suffer major shock and renal failure, and death may occur.

Punctures/Penetrations

A **puncture/penetration** wound results when the skin is pierced with a pointed object,

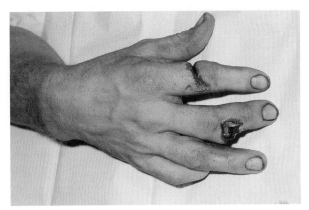

Fig. 20-7: Crush injuries occur when a body part is subjected to a high degree of pressure.

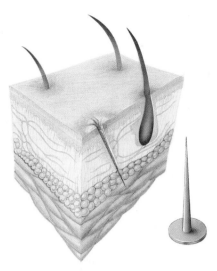

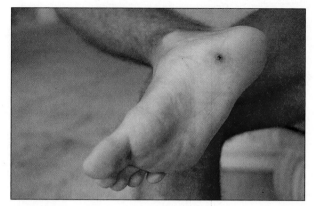

Fig. 20-8: A puncture wound results when skin is pierced by a pointed object.

such as a nail, piece of glass, splinter or knife **(Fig. 20-8).** A bullet wound is also considered a puncture wound. Because the skin usually closes around the penetrating object, external bleeding is generally not severe. However, internal bleeding may be quite severe if the penetrating object damages major blood vessels or internal organs. An object that remains in the open wound is called an *embedded object.* An object may also pass completely through a body part, creating two open wounds—one at the *entry point* and one at the *exit point.*

Although puncture wounds generally do *not* bleed profusely, they are potentially more dangerous than wounds that bleed more, because they are more likely to become infected. Objects penetrating the soft tissues carry microorganisms that cause infections. Of particular danger is the microorganism that causes tetanus, a severe infection.

Lacerations

A laceration is a cut, usually from a sharp object. The cut may have jagged or smooth edges **(Fig. 20-9).** Lacerations are commonly caused by sharp-edged objects, such as knives, scissors or broken glass. A laceration can also result when a blunt force splits the skin. Such splits occur

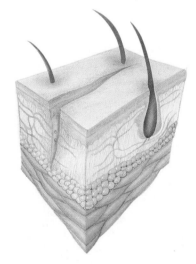

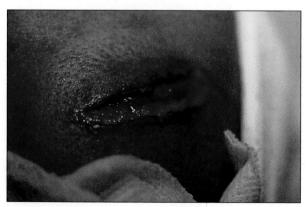

Fig. 20-9: A laceration is a cut in the skin. It may have either jagged or smooth edges.

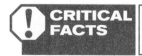 **CRITICAL FACTS** With any open wound, always follow standard precautions to avoid contact with blood and other body fluids.

in areas where bone lies directly under the skin's surface, such as the jaw. Deep lacerations can also affect the underlying layers of fat and muscle, damaging both nerves and blood vessels. Lacerations usually bleed freely and, depending on the structures involved, can bleed profusely. Because the nerves may also be injured, lacerations are not always immediately painful.

Providing Care for Open Wounds

With any open wound, always follow standard precautions to avoid contact with blood and other body fluids.

Major Open Wounds

A major open wound involves serious tissue damage and may bleed severely. As you learned in **Chapter 19,** the main priority of care for a major open wound is to control bleeding *immediately* with direct pressure using sterile dressings and *pressure bandages* and care for shock.

Minor Open Wounds

A minor open wound, such as an abrasion or small cut, is one in which damage is only superficial and bleeding is minimal. To care for a minor wound, follow these general guidelines—

- Control any bleeding.
  - Place a sterile dressing over the wound.
  - Apply direct pressure until bleeding stops.
- Clean the wound with soap (if available) and water.
- If possible, irrigate the wound with clean, warm running water for about 5 minutes to remove any dirt and debris. Use saline or any source of clean water if clean running water is not available.
- If bleeding continues, use a new sterile dressing and apply more pressure.
- After bleeding stops, remove the dressing and apply antibiotic ointment, if one is available, the patient has no known allergies or sensitivities to the medication and local protocols allow you to do so.
- Cover the wound with a sterile dressing and a bandage (or with an adhesive bandage).

Impaled Objects

An impaled object is one that has been embedded into an open wound (**Fig. 20-10**). There are two situations in which it is appropriate to remove an

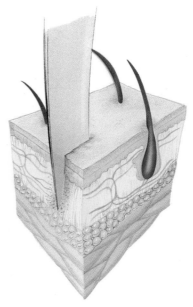

Fig. 20-10: An impaled object is one that has been embedded into the body.

impaled object. The first is if the impalement is through the cheek, with uncontrolled bleeding and interference with airway management. The second is if the object impales the chest and interferes with CPR. When providing emergency care for an impaled object, securing the object is highly important so that it cannot move and cause further damage.

Carefully secure the object manually, remove any clothing from the area if possible and control bleeding by applying direct pressure with sterile dressings to the edges of the wound. Avoid placing pressure on or moving the object. Once bleeding has stopped, apply a bulky dressing around the object, pack dressings around it and secure everything in place (**Fig. 20-11**).

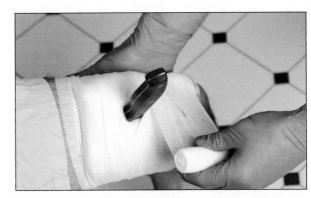

Fig. 20-11: To care for an impaled object: Use bulky dressings to support the embedded object. Use bandages over the dressing to control bleeding.

Amputations

First, provide emergency care. Control external bleeding. While it is important to care for the severed body part, it is vital to care for the patient first. Ask another responder to search for and provide care for the body part while you tend to the patient.

If the amputation is incomplete (i.e., an avulsion), *never* remove the body part. Care for it as you would any soft tissue injury, stabilizing the part.

If the body part is completely severed, find it, wrap it in sterile gauze, moistened in sterile saline if available. Then place it in a plastic bag, seal the bag, label it with the patient's name and the time and date it was placed in the bag. Keep the bag cool by placing it in a larger bag or container of an ice and water slurry, *not* on ice alone and *not* on dry ice (**Fig. 20-12**). Transfer the bag to the *emergency medical services* (EMS) personnel transporting the patient to the hospital.

BURNS

Burns are another type of soft tissue injury, caused primarily by heat. They can also occur when the body is exposed to certain chemicals, electricity or radiation.

When burns occur, they first affect the top layer of skin, called the *epidermis*. If the burn progresses, the *dermis*, or the second layer, can also be affected. Deep burns can damage underlying tissues. Burns that break the skin can cause infection, fluid loss and loss of temperature control. They can also damage the respiratory system and eyes.

The severity of a burn depends on the —
- Temperature of the source of the burn.
- Length of exposure to the source.
- Location of the burn.
- Size of the burn.
- Patient's age and medical condition.

In general, patients under 5 years of age and over age 60 have thinner skin and often burn more severely. People with chronic medical problems also tend to have more severe burns, especially if they are not well nourished, have heart or kidney problems or are exposed to the

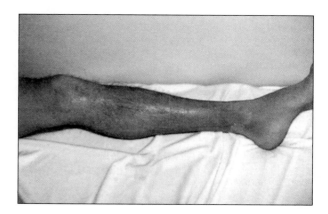

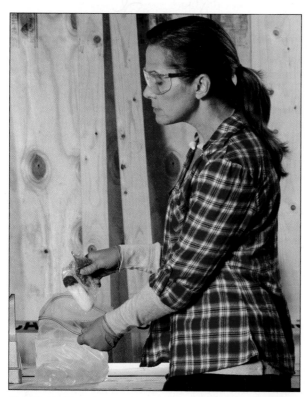

Fig. 20-12: Wrap a severed body part in sterile gauze, seal it in a plastic bag and put the bag in an ice and water slurry.

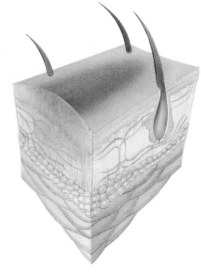

Fig. 20-13: A superficial burn involves only the top layer of skin. *Image courtesy of Alan Dimick, M.D., Professor of Surgery, Former Director of UAB Burn Center.*

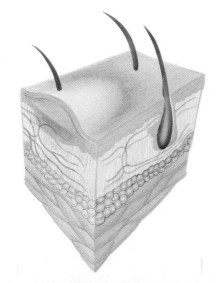

sunburns are superficial burns. Superficial burns generally heal in 5 to 6 days without permanent scarring.

Partial-Thickness Burns

A **partial-thickness burn** involves both the epidermis and the dermis (**Fig. 20-14**). These injuries are also red and have blisters that may open and weep clear fluid, making the skin appear wet. The burned skin may look *mottled* (blotchy). These burns are usually painful, and the area often swells. The body loses fluid and the burn is susceptible to infection. Although the burn usually heals in 3 or 4 weeks, extensive partial-thickness burns can be serious, requiring more advanced medical care. Scarring may occur from partial-thickness burns.

Full-Thickness Burns

A **full-thickness burn** destroys both layers of skin, as well as any or all of the underlying structures: fat, muscles, bones and nerves (**Fig. 20-15**). These burns may look brown or *charred* (black), with the tissues underneath sometimes appearing white. They can be either extremely painful or relatively painless if the

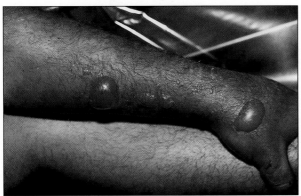

Fig. 20-14: A partial-thickness burn involves the epidermis and the dermis. *Image courtesy of Alan Dimick, M.D., Professor of Surgery, Former Director of UAB Burn Center.*

burn source for a prolonged period because they are unable to escape.

Classifying Burns

Burns are classified in several ways, including their depth, their extent, whether or not there is respiratory involvement, the body part burned and the cause of the burn.

Depth of Burn

One of the main ways burns are classified is by their depth. The deeper the burn, the more severe it is. Generally, three depth classifications are used: superficial (first degree), partial thickness (second degree) and full thickness (third degree).

Superficial Burns

A **superficial burn** involves only the top layer of skin, the epidermis (**Fig. 20-13**). The skin is red and dry, and the burn is usually painful. The area may swell. Most

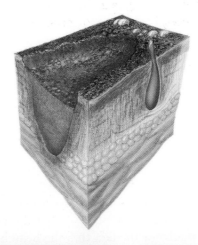

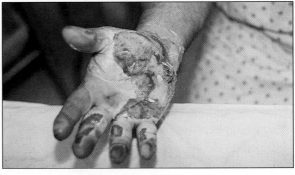

Fig. 20-15: A full-thickness burn destroys both layers of the skin in addition to any or all of the underlying structures, including fat, muscles, bones and nerves. *Image courtesy of Alan Dimick, M.D., Professor of Surgery, Former Director of UAB Burn Center.*

burn destroys nerve endings in the skin. Full-thickness burns are often surrounded by painful partial-thickness burns.

Full-thickness burns can be life threatening. Because the burns are open, the body loses fluid, and shock is likely to occur. These burns also make the body highly prone to infection. Scarring occurs and may be severe. Many burn sites eventually require skin grafts.

Extent of Burn

The extent of a burn is another important aspect of the severity of the burn. It is commonly described using the **Rule of Nines**. This method is used in the field to quickly determine if patients need to go to a specialty burn center for treatment. It approximates the percentage of burned surface area of the patient. In an adult, the body surface is divided into the following 11 sections, each comprising approximately 9 percent of the body's skin coverage (**Fig. 20-16**):

- Head
- Right arm
- Left arm
- Chest
- Abdomen
- Upper back
- Lower back
- Right thigh
- Left thigh
- Right leg (below the knee)
- Left leg (below the knee)

These body parts equal 99 percent, leaving the genitals to make up the last one percent. The Rule of Nines is applied by adding up all the areas of the body that have partial- or full-thickness burns. Partial areas are approximated.

With pediatric patients, considerations must be made for the fact that the head is a proportionally larger contributor to body surface area and the upper legs contribute less. The pediatric Lund-Browder diagram reflects this difference (**Fig. 20-17**).

The patient's palm can be used to estimate the size of a patchy burn. Assume that the patient's palm represents approximately 1 percent of a body's total surface area.

If you do not remember the Rule of Nines, simply communicate to more advanced medical personnel or the specialty burn center how the burn occurred, the body parts involved and

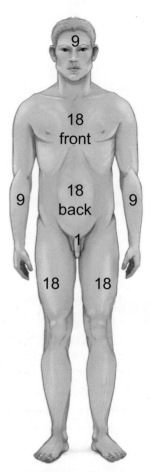

Fig. 20-16: The rule of nines is used to estimate what percentage of the body is affected by burns.

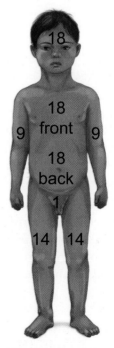

Fig. 20-17: The Lund-Browder diagram is used to assess the severity of burns in pediatric patients.

the approximate type of burn. For example, "The patient was injured when an overheated car radiator exploded. The patient has partial-thickness burns on the face, neck, chest and arms."

Respiratory Involvement

The respiratory system may also be damaged when a patient is burned. If you note soot or burns around the mouth, nose or the rest of the face, this may be a sign that air passages or lungs have been burned (**Fig. 20-18**). Respiratory damage may include airway closure due to swelling of the face and throat. Consider a hoarse voice a sign of respiratory involvement.

There may also be swelling of the larynx due to inhalation of superheated air, which may also cause fluid accumulation in the lungs. With more severe inhalation of smoke and toxic gases, there may be respiratory arrest or compromise, or poisoning. Burns around the chest can reduce the patient's ability to expand the chest. This can cause trouble breathing.

Circumferential burns are also of concern. Circumferential burns refer to burns that circle an entire body part. Circulatory compromise in that extremity can be the result of a circumferential burn to an extremity. A circumferential burn to the chest is of critical concern because of expansion and contraction during respiration.

Body Part Burned

The particular part of the body burned also determines the seriousness of the burn. Burns to certain parts of the body are more critical than to others. In particular, burns to the head, face, eyes and ears may be associated with respiratory problems and may be disfiguring. Burns to the hands and feet are serious because of the potential impact on the patient's function. Burns to the genitals or groin area are considered critical because of the potential loss of function and because these areas are susceptible to infection. Burns in any area where there is a significant joint (e.g., hips and shoulders) are serious because of potential loss of joint function.

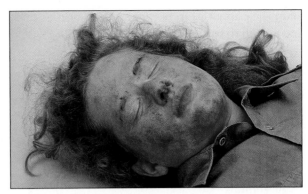

Fig. 20-18: Soot burns around the mouth, nose or the rest of the face may indicate air passages or lungs have been burned.

Cause of Burn

It is also important to take into account the source of the burn. *Thermal burns* include those caused by an open flame; contact with a hot object, steam or gas; or scalding by hot liquid. Burns can also be caused by chemicals, electricity and radiation.

Expect that burns caused by flames or hot grease will require medical attention, especially if the patient is under 5 or over 60 years of age. Hot grease is slow to cool and difficult to remove from the skin. Burns that involve hot liquid or flames contacting clothing will also be serious, since the clothing prolongs the heat contact with the skin.

Some synthetic fabrics melt and stick to the body. The melted fabrics may take longer to cool than the soft tissues. Although these burns may appear minor at first, they can continue to worsen for a short time.

Severity of the Burn

It is important to be able to identify a **critical burn**. A critical burn requires the immediate attention of more advanced medical personnel. Critical burns are potentially life threatening, disfiguring and/or disabling.

Knowing whether you should summon more advanced medical personnel for a burn injury can sometimes be difficult. It is not always easy or possible to assess the severity of a burn immediately after injury. Even superficial burns to large areas of the body or to certain body parts can be critical. You cannot judge severity by the

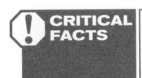
CRITICAL FACTS Consult with medical control for a decision on when to transport the patient involved in a burn incident. Advanced medical personnel must assist in the care of serious burn injuries, such as those causing difficulty breathing, burns covering more than one body part or to delicate body parts, any serious burns to a child or elderly patient, and any burns from chemicals, explosions or electricity.

pain the patient feels, because nerve endings may have been destroyed.

Consult with medical control for a decision on when to transport the patient. Call for more advanced medical personnel immediately for assistance in caring for the following:

- Burns causing breathing difficulty
- Signs of burns around the mouth and nose
- Burns covering more than one body part
- Burns to the head, face, neck, hands, feet or genitals
- Any partial-thickness or full-thickness burn to a child or an elderly person
- Burns resulting from chemicals, explosions or electricity

Patients should be referred to a burn unit if they have—

- Partial- or full-thickness burns that cover more than 10 percent of the body surface, for those patients under the age of about 5 or over about 60.
- Partial- or full-thickness burns that cover more than 2 percent of the body surface, for those in other age groups.
- Partial- or full-thickness burns that involve the face, hands, feet, genitalia, perineum or major joints.
- Full-thickness burns that cover more than 5 percent of the body surface, in patients of any age.
- **Electrical burns**, including injury caused by lightning.
- **Chemical burns**.
- Inhalation injury.
- Circumferential burns.
- A burn injury and a pre-existing medical condition that could make their care more complicated or lengthy, or that could affect mortality (e.g., diabetes).
- Both burns and other injuries (e.g., fractures or blast injury) where the burn injury poses the greatest risk of morbidity or mortality.
- A burn injury (in a child) and the hospital lacks qualified personnel or equipment. In this case, the child with burns should be transferred to a burn center with the required personnel and equipment needed to look after a child with burns.

- A burn injury (in a child) where there are special circumstances (e.g., suspected child abuse or substance abuse) and where social/emotional and/or long-term rehabilitative support will be needed.

Thermal Burns
Signs and Symptoms of Thermal Burns

The signs and symptoms of thermal burns depend upon the extent of the burn. The signs and symptoms, based on the degree of the burns, are as follows:

- Superficial burns. Painful, red area that turns white when touched; no blisters; moist-appearing skin
- Partial-thickness burns. There are two kinds of signs and symptoms—superficial and deep:
  - Superficial signs and symptoms: Painful, red area that turns white to touch; mottling, blisters, moist skin; hair is still present
  - Deep signs and symptoms: May or may not be painful (nerve endings may be destroyed); may be moist or dry (sweat glands may be destroyed); may or may not turn white when area is touched; hair is usually gone
- Full-thickness burns. Painless, no sensation to touch, pearly white or charred, dry and may appear leathery

Providing Care for Thermal Burns

As you approach the patient, decide if the scene is safe. Look for fire, smoke, downed electrical wires and warning signs for chemicals or radiation. If the scene is *not* safe and you have not been trained to manage it, summon specially trained personnel.

If the scene *is* safe, approach the patient cautiously. If the source of the burn is still in contact with the patient, take steps to remove and extinguish it. Doing so may require you to smother the flames or extinguish them with water or to remove smoldering clothing. For example, if the burn is caused by hot tar or plastic, cool the area with water but do *not* attempt to remove the tar or plastic.

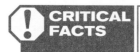 **CRITICAL FACTS** To care for a thermal burn, remove the patient from the source, cool and cover the burned area and take steps to minimize shock.

Perform a primary assessment. Pay close attention to the patient's airway. Note soot or burns around the mouth, nose and the rest of the face, which may be a sign that air passages or lungs have been burned. If you suspect a burned airway or burned lungs, continually monitor breathing and call for advanced medical personnel immediately. Air passages may swell, impairing or stopping breathing. Administer emergency oxygen if it is available.

As you do a physical exam, look for additional signs of burn injuries. Also look for other injuries, especially if there was an explosion or electrical shock.

If thermal burns are present, once you have removed the patient from the source, follow these three basic care steps:

1. Cool the burned area.
2. Cover the burned area.
3. Minimize shock.

Cool the Burned Area

Even after the source of the burn has been removed, soft tissue will continue to burn, causing more damage. Therefore, it is essential to cool any burned areas *immediately* with large amounts of cold tap water at least until pain is relieved (**Fig. 20-19, A**). Do *not* use ice or ice water. Ice or ice water can cause critical body heat loss and may make the burn deeper. Flush the area using whatever resources are available (e.g., a tub, shower or garden hose). You can apply soaked towels, sheets or other wet cloths to a burned face or other area that cannot be immersed. Be sure to keep these compresses cold by frequently resoaking with cold tap water; otherwise, they will not absorb the heat from the skin's surface.

Allow adequate time for the burned area to cool. If pain continues or if the edges of the burned area are still warm to the touch when the cooling source is removed, continue cooling. When the burn is cool, remove any remaining clothing from the area by carefully removing or cutting material away. Do *not* try to remove any clothing that is stuck to skin. Remove any jewelry only if doing so will not further injure the patient, as swelling may occur.

In some jurisdictions, you may be provided more specific directions for when and how to cool burns. Follow your local protocols.

Cover the Burned Area

Burns often expose sensitive nerve endings. Cover the burned area to keep out air and help reduce pain (**Fig. 20-19, B–C**). Use dry, sterile dressings, and loosely bandage them in place. The bandage should *not* put pressure on the burn surface. If the burn covers a large area of the body, cover it with clean, dry sheets or other clean cloth.

Covering the burn helps prevent infection. Do not put ointments, butter, oil or other commercial or home remedies on any burn that will receive medical attention. These products seal in heat and do not relieve pain. Other home remedies can contaminate open skin areas, causing infection. Do not break blisters. Intact skin helps prevent infection.

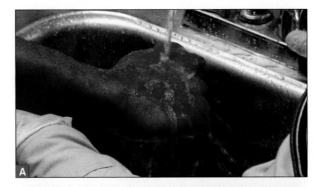
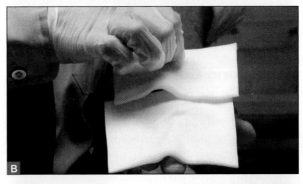
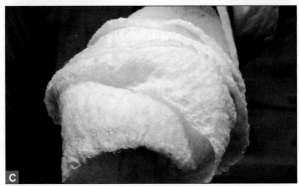

Fig. 20-19, A–C: To stop the burning of soft tissue: **(A)** Cool burned areas with large amounts of cold water. **(B–C)** Cover and wrap it with sterile dressings when fully cooled.

For small superficial burns or small burns with open blisters that are not sufficiently severe or extensive enough to require medical attention, care for the burned area as an open wound. Wash the area with soap and water. Cover the burn with a dressing and bandage. Apply antibiotic ointment if your protocols permit you to do so, one is available and the patient has no known sensitivities or allergies to the medication. Tell the patient to watch for signs of infection.

Minimize Shock

Full-thickness burns and large partial-thickness burns can cause shock as a result of pain and loss of body fluids. Lay the patient down unless the patient is having trouble breathing. Administer emergency oxygen if it is available and it is safe to do so.

Risk of Hypothermia

Patients who have sustained a burn have an impaired ability to regulate the body's temperature. Therefore, there is a tendency to chill. Keep the patient warm to prevent hypothermia. Help the patient maintain normal body temperature by protecting the patient from drafts. Remember that cooling burns over a large area of the body also risks inducing hypothermia in the burned patient. Be cautious and aware of this risk when cooling a burn that covers a large area.

Pediatric Considerations

Providing Care for Burns

Children have a larger body surface area relative to their weight than do adults. Body surface area is a major factor in determining how much water is lost through evaporation in burn patients. Therefore, children with burns lose more water through evaporation than do adult patients. This means that children usually tend to have greater fluid needs during resuscitation. Evaporative water loss leads to greater heat loss, so children or infants with burns are prone to hypothermia. Keep the room temperature high.

When dealing with pediatric burn patients, be aware of the possibility that the burns are the result of child abuse. Inflicted burns often leave characteristic patterns of injury that cannot be concealed. A detailed history, including previous trauma, presence of recent illnesses and immunization records, will help determine if your suspicions are correct.

Chemical Burns

Chemical burns are common in industrial settings, but also occur in the home. Cleaning solutions, household bleach, oven or drain cleaners, toilet bowl cleaner, paint strippers and lawn or garden chemicals are common sources of caustic chemicals that can eat away or destroy tissue. Caustic chemicals cause chemical burns.

Typically, burn injuries result from chemicals that are strong acids or alkalis. These substances can quickly injure the skin. As with heat burns, the stronger the chemical and the longer the contact, the more severe the burn. The chemical will continue to burn as long as it is on the skin. You must remove the chemical from the skin as quickly as possible, and then call for more advanced medical personnel immediately. If you suspect a chemical burn, also check to see whether the eyes are burned.

Signs and Symptoms of Chemical Burns

Signs and symptoms of chemical burns include—
- Pain.
- Burning.
- Numbness.
- Change in *level of consciousness* (LOC).
- Respiratory distress.
- Oral discomfort or swelling.
- Eye discomfort.
- Change in vision.

Providing Care for Chemical Burns

Always brush dry or powdered chemicals off with a gloved hand or a cloth, if possible. If not, flush them off with water. In some cases, a continuous flow of water will remove a dry substance before the water can activate it. Continue flushing until more advanced medical personnel arrive or for at least 20 minutes. If the substance is a liquid, flush the burn continuously with large amounts of *cool*, running water until more advanced medical personnel arrive or for at least 20 minutes (**Fig. 20-20**). Have the patient remove contaminated clothing and jewelry, if possible. Take steps to minimize shock.

Chemical burns to the eyes can be exceptionally traumatic. Ensure more advanced medical personnel have been called. If an eye is burned by a chemical, flush the affected eye until more advanced medical personnel arrive or for at

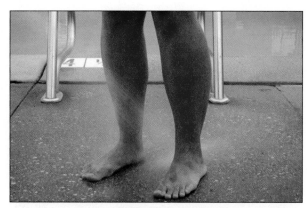

Fig. 20-20: Flush a chemical burn with large amounts of cool, running water.

least 20 minutes. Flush the affected eye from the nose outward and downward to prevent washing the chemical into the unaffected eye.

Electrical Burns

The human body is a good conductor of electricity. When someone comes into contact with an electrical source, such as a power line, a malfunctioning household appliance or lightning, electricity is conducted through the body. Body parts resist electrical current; some body parts, such as the bones, resist the electrical current more strongly than others. This resistance produces heat, which can cause electrical burns along the flow of the current (**Fig. 20-21**).

Signs and Symptoms of Electrical Burns

The severity of an electrical burn depends on the type and amount of contact, the current's path through the body and how long the contact lasted. Electrical burns are often deep; although these wounds may look superficial, the tissues

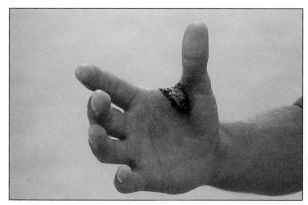

Fig. 20-21: Although electrical burns may look superficial, they are often deep, following the current's path through the body, and may severely damage underlying tissues.

beneath may be severely damaged. Some electrical burns will be marked by entry and exit wounds indicating where the current has passed through the body.

The signs and symptoms of electrical injury include—
- Unconsciousness.
- Dazed, confused behavior.
- Obvious burns on the skin's surface.
- Trouble breathing or no breathing.
- Burns both where the current entered and where it exited the body, often on the hand or foot.

Providing Care for Electrical Burns

Scene safety is of utmost importance. Once it is determined that the electrical current is secured and no longer passing through the patient, perform a primary assessment and care for any immediate life-threatening conditions. During the physical exam, look for two burn sites (entry and exit wounds). Cool any electrical burns with cold tap water as you would a thermal burn, until pain is relieved; then cover any burn injuries with a dry, sterile dressing, and provide care to minimize shock. Look for painful, swollen and deformed extremities, because the resistance to the electrical current can cause severe muscle contractions, which may produce musculoskeletal injuries.

With someone who has been struck by lightning, look for and provide care for life-threatening conditions such as respiratory or cardiac arrest. The patient may also have fractures, including spinal fracture, so do not move the patient unless evacuation is required due to the scene becoming unsafe. Caring for any immediate life-threatening conditions takes priority over caring for burns.

Exposure to high- or even low-voltage electric current can cause dangerous cardiac arrhythmias in addition to electrical burns. Be prepared to perform CPR and use an AED. Anyone who suffers an electrical shock needs an advanced medical assessment to determine the extent of injury.

Radiation Burns

Radiation burns may occur from exposure to nuclear radiation, X-rays or as a side effect of radiation therapy. It can also be caused by tanning beds, or as the result of solar radiation from the sun. Solar burns are similar to heat burns, often resulting in superficial and sometimes partial-thickness burns. Usually they are mild, but they can be painful (**Fig. 20-22**). They may blister, involving more than one layer of skin. Care for sunburn as you would any other burn. Cool the burn and protect the burned area from further damage by keeping it away from the source of the burn.

People are rarely exposed to other types of radiation unless working in special settings, such as certain medical, industrial or research sites. If you work in such settings, you will be informed and will be required to take precautions to prevent overexposure.

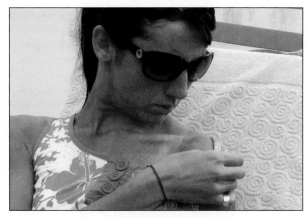

Fig. 20-22: Radiation burns, such as sunburns, are usually mild but they can be painful and blister when involving more than one layer of skin.

PUTTING IT ALL TOGETHER

Caring for wounds involves controlling bleeding and minimizing the risk of infection. Your primary concern with minor wounds is to clean the wound to prevent infection. For major wounds, control the bleeding quickly and summon more advanced medical personnel. *Always* use a barrier such as disposable gloves, dressings or a clean folded cloth, to avoid contact with blood. Dressings and bandages, when correctly applied, help control bleeding, reduce pain and minimize the risk of infection. Apply pressure to help stop bleeding.

Burns damage the layers of the skin and sometimes the internal structures, which can be life threatening. Heat, chemicals, electricity and radiation all cause burns. When caring for someone who has sustained a burn, *always* ensure the scene is safe. Approach the patient and check for life-threatening conditions and for non-life-threatening conditions, if necessary.

Once the patient has been removed from the burn source, follow the steps of burn care:
- Cool the burned area with water to minimize additional tissue destruction.
- Protect the burned area by covering it with sterile dressings, clean sheets or other cloth.
- To minimize shock, keep the patient from getting chilled or overheated.
- Summon more advanced medical personnel for any critical burn.

In addition, *always* check for inhalation injury if the person has a heat or chemical burn involving the face. With electrical burns, check carefully for other problems, such as difficulty breathing, cardiac problems and painful, swollen, deformed areas.

Remember to take care with pediatric patients, especially infants, as they are prone to hypothermia. With electrical burns, check carefully for additional conditions, such as difficulty breathing, cardiac arrest and fractures.

))) YOU ARE THE EMERGENCY MEDICAL RESPONDER

The safety officer quickly verifies that power has been shut off and it is safe to approach the scene. You perform a primary assessment. The patient regains consciousness and complains of pain in his hand and elbow. Your partner has called for more advanced medical personnel. What types of injuries or conditions should you suspect and what emergency care should be provided? Is calling for EMS personnel appropriate? Why or why not?

21

Injuries to the Chest, Abdomen and Genitalia

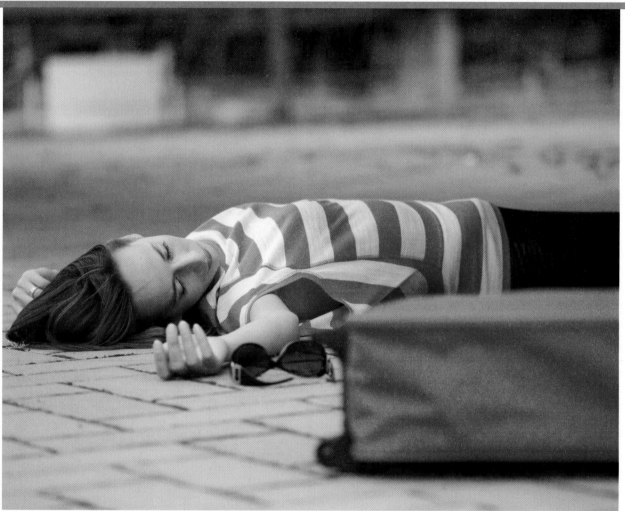

))) **YOU ARE THE EMERGENCY MEDICAL RESPONDER**

Your police unit responds to a call in a part of town plagued by violence. When you arrive, you find the scene is empty except for a young woman lying on the sidewalk. After sizing up the scene and approaching the young woman, you notice that she has been shot and is bleeding profusely. How would you respond?

Key Terms

Chest tube: A tube surgically inserted into the chest to drain blood, fluid or air, and to allow the lungs to expand.

Evisceration: A severe injury that causes the abdominal organs to protrude through the wound.

Flail chest: A serious injury in which multiple rib fractures result in a loose section of ribs that does not move normally with the rest of the chest during breathing and often moves in the *opposite* direction.

Hemopneumothorax: An accumulation of blood and air between the lungs and chest wall.

Hemothorax: An accumulation of blood between the lungs and chest wall; caused by bleeding that may be from the chest wall, lung tissue or major blood vessels in the thorax.

Hypotension: Abnormally low blood pressure.

Impaled object: An object that remains embedded in an open wound; also referred to as an *embedded object*.

Intercostal: Located between the ribs.

Parenchyma: Tissue that is involved in the functioning of a structure or organ as opposed to its supporting structures.

Percussion: A technique of tapping on the surface of the body and listening to the resulting sounds, to learn about the condition of the area beneath.

Peritoneum: The membrane that lines the abdominal cavity and covers most of the abdominal organs.

Pleural space: The space between the lungs and chest wall.

Pneumothorax: Collapse of a lung due to pressure on it caused by air in the chest cavity.

Subconjunctival hemorrhage: Broken blood vessels in the eyes.

Subcutaneous emphysema: A rare condition in which air gets into tissues under the skin that covers the chest wall or neck; may occur as a result of wounds to those areas.

Sucking chest wound: A chest wound in which an object, such as a knife or bullet, penetrates the chest wall and lung, allowing air to pass freely in and out of the chest cavity; breathing causes a sucking sound, hence the term.

Tension pneumothorax: A life-threatening injury in which the lung is completely collapsed and air is trapped in the pleural space.

Thoracic: Relating to the *thorax*, or chest cavity.

Traumatic asphyxia: Severe lack of oxygen due to trauma, usually caused by a thoracic injury.

Learning Objectives

After reading this chapter, and completing the class activities, you will have the information needed to—

- Describe general care steps for injuries to the chest, abdomen and pelvis.
- List the different types of chest injuries.
- List the signs and symptoms of chest injuries.
- Describe how to care for a sucking chest wound.
- Describe how to care for an impaled or embedded object in the chest.
- List different types of abdominal injuries.
- List the signs and symptoms of abdominal injuries.
- Explain assessment techniques for abdominal injuries.
- Describe how to care for closed and open abdominal injuries.
- List the signs and symptoms of genital injuries.
- Describe how to care for genital injuries.

INTRODUCTION

Many injuries to the chest and abdomen involve only soft tissues. Often these injuries, like those that occur elsewhere on the body, are only minor cuts, scrapes, burns and bruises. Occasionally, a violent force or mechanism, known as *trauma*, results in more severe injuries. These include fractures and injuries to organs, which can cause severe bleeding or impair breathing. Occupants who are not wearing seat belts during motor-vehicle collisions often suffer fractures and lacerations. Falls, athletic injuries and many other forms of trauma may also cause such injuries. Injuries to the pelvis may be minor soft tissue injuries or serious injuries to bone and internal structures.

Because the chest, abdomen and pelvis contain many organs important to life, injury to these areas can be fatal if left untreated. You may recall from the previous chapter that a force capable of causing severe injury in these areas may also cause injury to the spine.

General care for these injuries includes—
- Calling for more advanced medical personnel.
- Limiting movement.
- Monitoring breathing and other vital signs.
- Controlling bleeding.
- Minimizing shock.

ANATOMY OF THE CHEST, ABDOMEN AND GENITALIA

The chest cavity, also called the ***thoracic*** *cavity*, is the second-largest body cavity and contains the heart and lungs (**Fig. 21-1**). The ribs, sternum and upper portion of the spine (*thoracic vertebrae*) frame the wall of the thoracic cavity, also referred to as the *thoracic cage*. The *diaphragm*, a large muscular partition, separates the thoracic cavity from the abdominal cavity.

Below the diaphragm is the abdominal cavity. The abdominal cavity contains the major organs of several of the body's systems:

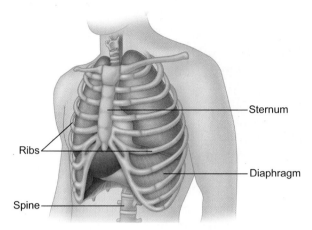

Fig. 21-1: The thoracic cavity

the digestive system, urinary system and endocrine system (**Fig. 21-2**). The abdominal cavity is lined with a thick membrane called the **peritoneum**, which supports the organs, including the stomach, gallbladder, urinary bladder, intestines, liver, spleen, pancreas and kidneys. It also contains important vascular structures such as the *abdominal aorta* and *inferior vena cavae*.

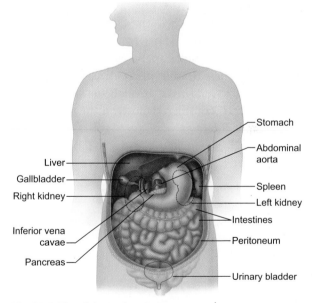

Fig. 21-2: The abdominal cavity

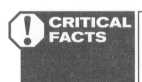

Because the chest, abdomen and pelvis contain many organs important to life, injury to these areas can be fatal if left untreated. General care for these injuries includes calling for advanced medical personnel, limiting movement in the patient, monitoring breathing and other vital signs, controlling bleeding and taking steps to minimize shock.

Genitalia are part of the reproductive systems of women and men. The male genitalia include the testicles, a duct system and the penis. The female genitalia include the ovaries, fallopian tubes, uterus and vagina (**Fig. 21-3**).

CHEST INJURIES

Chest injuries are the second-leading cause of trauma deaths each year in the United States. About 35 percent of deaths from motor-vehicle collisions involve chest injuries. Crushing forces, direct blows and falls can also lead to such injuries (**Fig. 21-4, A–C**).

Chest wounds can be either *open* or *closed*. Open chest wounds occur when an object, such as a knife or bullet, penetrates the chest wall. Open chest wounds also can be caused by fractured ribs that break through the skin. A chest wound is considered closed if the skin is not broken. Closed chest wounds are generally caused by a blunt object.

Types of Chest Injuries

Certain types of chest injuries may be life threatening, and others merely cause discomfort. You will likely be able to recognize severe injuries. It is important to summon more advanced medical personnel in those situations.

Blunt Trauma

Blunt trauma is injury caused by the force of an object that impacts with, but does not penetrate, the body. Signs and symptoms include severe shortness of breath, chest pain and rapid, possibly irregular pulse. The possibility of blunt trauma should be considered in patients who sustain a blow to the abdomen or chest and show signs of respiratory distress.

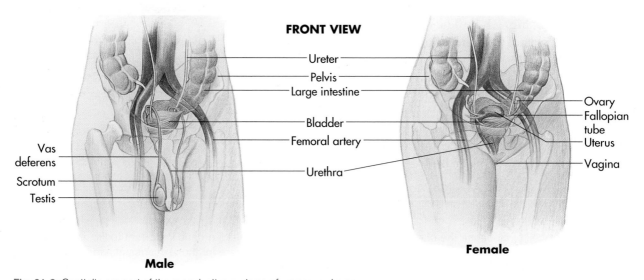

FRONT VIEW

Ureter
Pelvis
Large intestine
Bladder
Femoral artery
Urethra

Vas deferens
Scrotum
Testis

Ovary
Fallopian tube
Uterus
Vagina

Male

Female

Fig. 21-3: Genitalia are part of the reproductive systems of women and men.

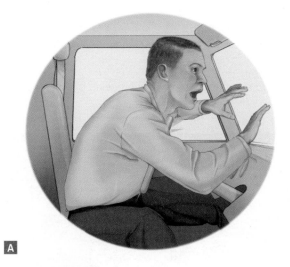

A

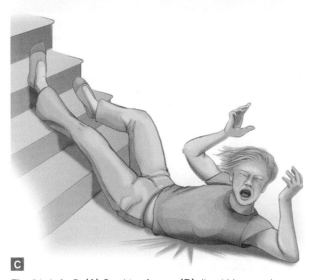

B

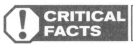

C

Fig. 21-4, A–C: **(A)** Crushing forces, **(B)** direct blows and **(C)** falls can lead to chest injuries, which are the second-leading cause of trauma deaths in the U.S. each year.

Often, associated injuries will occur with blunt trauma, including major trauma to the spleen or liver. Therefore, it is not unusual for patients with these injuries to go into hypovolemic shock, a type of shock in which there is multiple organ failure due to major fluid loss—usually blood.

Traumatic Asphyxia

Traumatic asphyxia, or severe lack of oxygen due to trauma, can result from chest injury. These injuries often are caused by a strong crushing mechanism or by situations in which patients have been pinned under a very heavy object.

Signs and symptoms of traumatic asphyxia include—

- Shock.
- Distended neck veins.
- Bluish discoloration of the head, tongue, lips, neck and shoulders (*cyanosis*).
- Broken blood vessels in the eyes (**subconjunctival hemorrhage**).
- Black eyes.
- Pinpoint-sized red dots (*petechiae*) on the head and neck.
- Rounded, "moon-like" facial appearance.
- Bleeding from the nose or ear.
- Coughing up or vomiting blood.
- Loss of consciousness, seizures or blindness.

Traumatic asphyxia is a very serious emergency that requires immediate intervention. If it is suspected, call for more advanced *emergency medical services* (EMS) personnel immediately. Assess the patient for associated chest and abdominal injuries. Elevate the patient's head to approximately 30° to decrease pressure to the head. Establish and maintain adequate airway and breathing and administer emergency oxygen, if needed.

Broken Ribs

Rib fractures are usually caused by a forceful blow to the chest. Although painful, a simple rib

CRITICAL FACTS | Rib fractures are usually caused by a forceful blow to the chest.

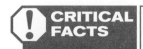

CRITICAL FACTS

A flail chest injury is a serious, life-threatening rib fracture. It results from a severe blow or crushing injury in which multiple ribs fracture in multiple places, causing loose sections of ribs that move abnormally in the chest.

Pneumothorax is the collapse of a lung due to air in the chest cavity pressing on the lung and preventing it from expanding.

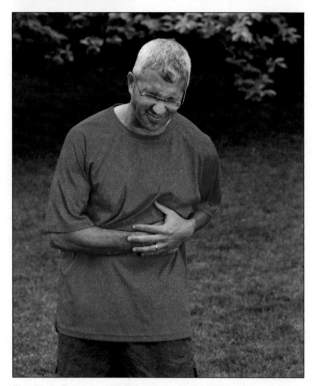

Fig. 21-5: Patients with rib injuries usually attempt to ease the pain by creating an anatomical splint with their hand or arm and leaning toward the side of the injury.

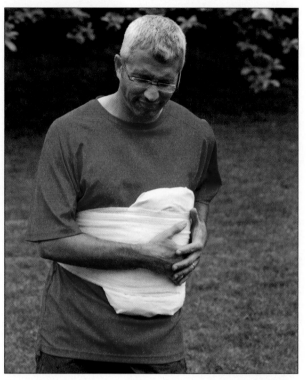

Fig. 21-6: Give a patient with fractured ribs or a flail chest a pillow or rolled blanket to hold against the injury/immobilize the injured area. Continue to monitor breathing.

fracture is rarely life threatening. The patient will usually attempt to ease the pain by leaning toward the side of the fracture and pressing a hand or arm over the injured area, thereby creating an *anatomical splint* (**Fig. 21-5**). When ribs are broken, suspect the possibility of internal injuries.

The first priority with broken ribs is adequate breathing. A patient with a fractured rib often has shallow breathing because normal or deep breathing is painful. Give the patient a blanket or pillow to hold against the fractured ribs (**Fig. 21-6**). Use a sling and binder to hold the patient's arm against the injured side of the chest. Monitor breathing.

Possible complications of broken ribs include—
- Collapse of a lung due to air in the chest cavity pressing on the lung (**pneumothorax**).
- Accumulation of blood between the lungs and chest wall (**hemothorax**).
- Air in the tissues under the skin (**subcutaneous emphysema**).

- Bruising or piercing of the lung and injuries to the spleen or liver.
- Lacerated blood vessels between the ribs.

Flail Chest

In situations involving severe blows or crushing injuries, multiple ribs can fracture in multiple places. These fractures can produce a loose section of ribs that does not move normally with the rest of the chest during breathing. Usually, the loose section will move in the opposite direction from the rest of the chest. This injury is called a **flail chest**, which is considered a serious rib fracture and can be life threatening (**Fig. 21-7**). When a flail chest involves the breastbone, the breastbone is separated from the rest of the ribs.

In flail chest, the lung tissues may be bruised, leading to inadequate oxygenation of the heart. There is also a risk of the ribs puncturing a lung. If you suspect a fractured rib or ribs, have the patient rest in a position that will make breathing easier.

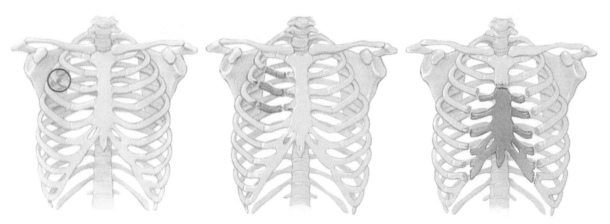

Fig. 21-7: Severe blows or crushing injuries can cause flail chest, in which multiple ribs fracture in multiple places, creating a loose section of ribs.

Binding the patient's arm to the chest on the injured side will help support the injured area and make breathing more comfortable. You can use an object such as a pillow or rolled blanket to help support and immobilize the injured area. Serious fractures often cause severe bleeding and trouble breathing, and shock is likely to develop. Administer emergency oxygen if it is available, and continue to monitor the patient's vital signs.

Pneumothorax

Pneumothorax is the collapse of a lung due to air in the chest cavity pressing on the lung and preventing it from expanding (**Fig. 21-8, A**). Pneumothorax can occur in two ways. In blunt chest trauma, it may result when a fractured rib penetrates the lung, causing air to leak. It can also occur when air enters the chest cavity because of a **sucking chest wound**.

Pneumothorax reduces lung pressure and leads to respiratory distress.

Patients may report pain while breathing, and pain at the site of the rib fractures. Decreased breath sounds will be present upon examination, and many patients with traumatic pneumothorax also have some element of severe bleeding (hemorrhage), causing a **hemopneumothorax**. Patients with pneumothorax will require a **chest tube** in order to fully re-expand the lung.

Hemothorax

Hemothorax is an accumulation of blood between the lungs and chest wall (**pleural space**), which creates pressure on the heart and lungs and prevents the lungs from expanding, resulting in the same symptoms as those which occur in pneumothorax (**Fig. 21-8, B**). The bleeding that leads to hemothorax may

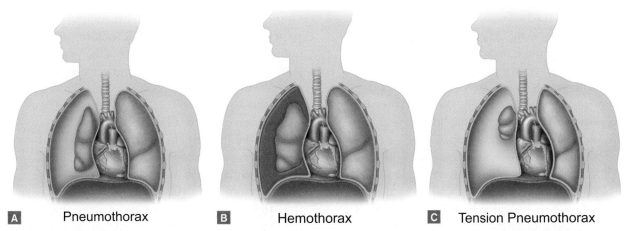

A Pneumothorax   **B** Hemothorax   **C** Tension Pneumothorax

Fig. 21-8, A–C: In the term hemothorax, "hemo" refers to blood. In pneumothorax and tension pneumothorax, "pneumo" refers to air.

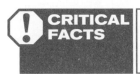

CRITICAL FACTS

Hemothorax is an accumulation of blood between the lungs and chest wall (pleural space), which creates pressure on the heart and lungs and prevents the lungs from expanding.

be from the chest wall, the lung's functional tissue (**parenchyma**), or major blood vessels in the thorax. It may occur following blunt or penetrating injury to the chest, and often occurs together with pneumothorax.

Again, patients will complain of pain and shortness of breath, and the condition may cause shock. During patient assessment, if trained to do so, you likely will note a decrease in breath sounds and dullness when tapping and listening to breath sounds (**percussion**) over the affected area. A massive hemothorax will also cause abnormal or unstable blood pressure.

A chest tube is required with a patient who has a hemothorax, and close monitoring of the initial and cumulative hourly chest tube drainage will help determine if there is a need for surgery.

Tension Pneumothorax

Tension pneumothorax is a serious, life-threatening injury in which there is complete collapse of the lung. Air enters the space around the lungs and remains trapped there (**Fig. 21-8, C**). It is caused by the same traumas as those that produce a simple pneumothorax. Tension pneumothorax causes air to continue leaking from an underlying injury to the functional lung tissue (*pulmonary parenchymal injury*), which increases pressure within the affected side of the chest cavity.

Patients are typically in respiratory distress with reduced breath sounds or a complete absence of breath sounds, and that side of the chest produces abnormal breath sounds during percussion. Because the trachea is shifted away from the side of the injury and the space between the lungs, contents are shifted away from the affected side, and decreased return of blood to the heart results. The patient will show signs of unstable blood pressure, such as abnormally low blood pressure (*hypotension*), which can quickly develop into complete cardiovascular collapse.

Extreme pressure in the chest cavity prevents blood from returning to the heart and the blood is no longer pumped out. Death can occur quickly. Immediate care provided by advanced medical professionals for this life-threatening condition includes decompression of the affected lung by inserting a large-bore needle through the second **intercostal** space, along an imaginary line that passes through the midpoint of the clavicle (*midclavicular line*). A chest tube is then inserted.

Signs and Symptoms of Chest Injuries

You should know the signs and symptoms of serious chest injury. These may occur with both open and closed wounds. They include—

- Shortness of breath and difficulty breathing.
- Pain during breathing.
- Pain at the site of the injury that increases with deep breathing or movement.
- Obvious deformity, such as that caused by a fracture.
- Flushed, pale, ashen or bluish discoloration of the skin.
- Coughing up blood.
- Distended (*protruding*) neck veins.
- Drop in blood pressure.

Providing Care
Providing Care for a Sucking Chest Wound

Puncture wounds to the chest range from minor to life threatening. A forceful puncture may penetrate the rib cage and allow air to enter the chest through the wound. This prevents the lungs from functioning normally (**Fig. 21-9**).

Puncture wounds cause varying degrees of internal or external bleeding. If the injury penetrates the rib cage, air can pass freely in and out of the chest cavity and the patient cannot breathe normally. With each breath the patient takes, you may hear a sucking sound coming from the wound. This is the primary sign of a penetrating chest injury, called a *sucking chest wound*.

Without proper care, the patient's condition will worsen quickly. The affected lung or lungs will fail to function, and breathing will become more difficult. Your main concern is the breathing problem. To care for a sucking chest wound, cover the wound with an occlusive dressing, one that does not allow air to pass through it (**Fig. 21-10, A–B**). Tape the dressing in place on all sides except for one side that

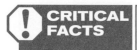 **CRITICAL FACTS** Tension pneumothorax is a serious, life-threatening injury in which there is complete collapse of the lung. Air enters the space around the lungs and remains trapped there.

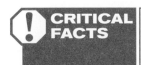
Signs and symptoms of serious chest injury are similar in both open and closed wounds. They include trouble breathing, including shortness or breath and pain when breathing (especially deep breathing); pain at the site of the injury; obvious deformity; pale or bluish skin; coughing up blood; protruding neck veins and a drop in blood pressure.

Puncture wounds to the chest range from minor to life threatening. A forceful puncture may penetrate the rib cage and allow air to enter the chest through the wound. This prevents the lungs from functioning normally.

Occlusive dressings are used to care for a sucking chest wound. When applied properly, this dressing will prevent air from entering the wound during inhalation but allow it to escape during exhalation.

should remain loose. (For more information on occlusive dressings, see **Chapter 19**.) Taping the dressing this way keeps air from entering the wound during inhalation but allows it to escape during exhalation. If none of these materials is available, a folded cloth or, as a last resort, your gloved hand, may be used. Administer emergency oxygen if it is available, and take steps to minimize shock. If no spinal injury is suspected, have the patient sit or lie in a comfortable position.

Providing Care for Impaled Objects in the Chest

An **impaled object** or *embedded object* is one that remains in an open wound. In the case of an impaled object in the chest, it is extremely

important *not* to remove the object, unless it interferes with chest compressions. Instead, the object must be stabilized to keep it from moving. This can be accomplished by using a bulky dressing or gauze around the object. This will also assist in controlling bleeding.

Emergency care for an impaled object includes the following steps—

- Stabilize the object to prevent further damage.
- Remove clothing to expose the wound.
- Control bleeding by applying direct pressure to the edges of the wound (but avoid placing direct pressure on the object).

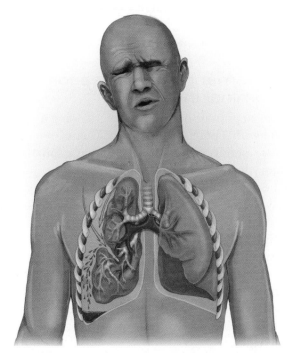

Fig. 21-9: If a puncture wound penetrates the rib cage, air can pass freely in and out of the chest cavity and the patient cannot breathe normally.

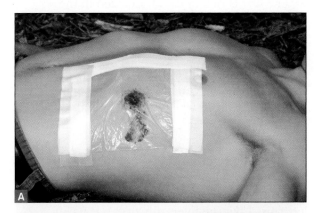

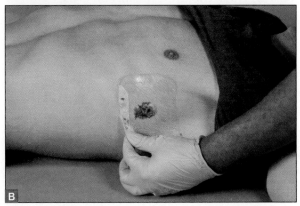

Fig. 21-10, A–B: **(A)** A makeshift occlusive dressing; **(B)** A commercially manufactured occlusive dressing

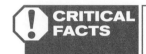
- Use a sterile bulky dressing to help hold the object in place. Carefully pack the dressing around the object.
- Secure the sterile bulky dressing in place with gauze, a cravat or tape.

ABDOMINAL INJURIES

The *abdomen* is the area immediately below the chest and above the pelvis. It is easily injured because it is not surrounded by bones, although it is protected at the back by the spine and ribs. The upper abdomen is only partially protected in front by the lower ribs. The muscles of the back and abdomen also help protect the internal organs, many of which are vital. Certain organs are easily injured or tend to bleed profusely when injured, such as the liver, spleen and stomach.

The *liver* is rich in blood. Located in the upper right quadrant of the abdomen, the lower ribs somewhat protect this organ. However, it is delicate and can be torn by blows from blunt objects or penetrated by a fractured rib. The resulting bleeding can be severe and quickly be fatal. The liver, when injured, can also leak bile into the abdomen, which can cause severe infection.

The *spleen* is located in the upper left quadrant of the abdomen, behind the stomach, and is protected somewhat by the lower left ribs. Like the liver, this organ is easily damaged. The spleen may rupture when a blunt object strikes the abdomen forcefully. Since the spleen stores blood, a spleen injury can cause a severe loss of blood in a short time and can be life threatening.

The *stomach* is one of the main digestive organs. The upper part of the stomach changes shape depending on its contents, the stage of digestion and the size and strength of the stomach muscles. Many blood vessels and nerves line the stomach. It can bleed severely when

injured, and food contents may empty into the abdomen and possibly cause infection.

Acute Abdomen

Abdominal pain is common and often not serious. However, acute and severe abdominal pain, referred to as acute abdomen, is usually a symptom of intra-abdominal disease such as appendicitis or peritonitis.

Signs and Symptoms of an Abdominal Injury

The signs and symptoms of serious abdominal injury include—
- Severe abdominal pain.
- Bruising.
- External bleeding.
- Nausea and vomiting (sometimes vomit containing blood).
- Pale or ashen, cool, moist skin.
- Weakness.
- Thirst.
- Pain, tenderness or a tight, swollen feeling in the abdomen.
- Organs possibly protruding from the abdomen.

Assessment Techniques for Abdominal Injury

Several steps must be taken when assessing a patient with a potential abdominal injury—
- First, establish spinal stabilization if a spinal injury is suspected.
- Check the patient's position. Knees flexed toward the chest are a good indication the patient has suffered an abdominal injury **(Fig. 21-11)**.
- Inspect the abdomen for contusions, lacerations, abrasions and punctures.
- Look for signs of potential internal bleeding, including a distended abdomen as well as discoloration and bruising around the navel and sides.

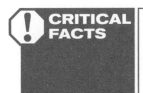
- Inspect the patient for internal organs protruding from an open abdominal wound (abdominal **evisceration** or disembowelment).
- Palpate the abdomen from the furthest point away from the pain, noting tenderness or masses.
- If the patient has a decreased mental status, it is important to note grimacing or signs of pain as you palpate. Keep in mind that the patient may be contracting stomach muscles to avoid pain, or the contractions may be the result of muscle spasms.
- Assess both the upper and lower extremities for injury and a pulse, as abdominal aortic injury may cause the pulses of the lower extremities to be weaker than the upper. If no foot pulses are found, check the pulses at the back of the knee or thigh. These should be equal to or stronger than the radial pulse, even in the case of shock.
- Assess motor and sensory function.
- Log roll the patient and inspect for signs of trauma.
- Assess baseline vital signs, especially for indications of blood loss and shock.

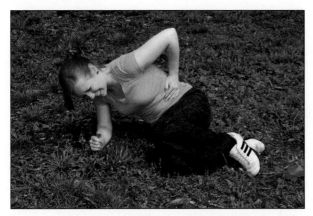

Fig. 21-11: Patients who have suffered abdominal injuries often guard the injury by flexing their knees toward their chests.

Symptoms such as low blood pressure, rapid heartbeat or pale, cool, moist skin are all indications of shock.

- Ensure that the airway is open and the patient is able to breathe adequately. If inspection of the airway shows signs of bloody vomitus, suctioning may be required. If the patient is not breathing adequately, begin positive pressure ventilation with emergency oxygen.

Providing Care for Abdominal Injury

Like a chest injury, an injury to the abdomen is either open or closed. Even with a closed wound, the rupture of an organ can cause serious internal bleeding that can quickly result in shock. Injuries to the abdomen can be extremely painful. Serious reactions can occur if organs leak blood or other contents into the abdominal cavity.

To care for a closed abdominal injury—

- Carefully position the patient on the back.
- Avoid applying direct pressure.
- Bend the patient's knees slightly. Doing so allows the muscles of the abdomen to relax. Place rolled-up blankets or pillows under the patient's knees. If moving the patient's legs causes pain, or you suspect spinal injury, leave the legs straight.
- Administer emergency oxygen, if available.
- Take steps to minimize shock.
- Summon more advanced medical personnel.

Providing Care for Eviscerations

A severe open injury may result in evisceration, a situation in which abdominal organs protrude

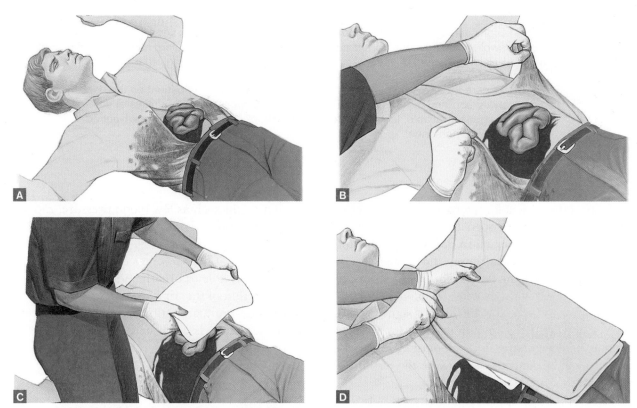

Fig. 21-12, A–D: **(A)** Severe injuries to the abdominal cavity can result in protruding organs. **(B)** Carefully remove clothing from around the wound. **(C)** Apply a large, moist, sterile dressing over the wound and cover it with plastic wrap. **(D)** Place a folded towel over the dressing to maintain warmth.

through the wound (**Fig. 21-12, A**). To care for an open wound in the abdomen, follow these steps (**Fig. 21-12, B–D**)—

- Summon more advanced medical personnel.
- Carefully position the patient on the back.
- Avoid applying direct pressure.
- Avoid pushing the organs back in.
- Remove clothing from around the wound.
- Apply moist (warm tap water can be used), sterile or clean dressings loosely over the wound.
- Cover the dressings loosely with plastic wrap, if available.
- Cover the dressings lightly with a folded towel to maintain warmth.
- Keep the patient from getting chilled or overheated.
- Administer emergency oxygen, if available.

Providing Care for Impaled Objects in the Abdomen

If the patient has been impaled by an object in the abdomen, it is important not to remove the object. Instead, dress the wound around the object to control the bleeding. Stabilize the object with bulky dressings to prevent movement.

Gastrointestinal Bleeding

There are multiple causes of gastrointestinal bleeding, and these tend to be classified as either upper or lower, depending on the location of the problem within the gastrointestinal tract. Bleeding in the upper gastrointestinal tract originates in the esophagus, stomach or duodenum (first part of the intestine) and may include such problems

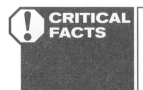

CRITICAL FACTS

A severe open injury may result in evisceration, a situation in which abdominal organs protrude through the wound. To care for an evisceration: summon more advanced medical personnel; position the patient on the back; remove clothing from around the wound; apply moist, sterile or clean dressings loosely over the wound; cover the dressings loosely with plastic wrap, if available, then cover lightly with a folded towel; keep the patient from getting chilled or overheated; and administer emergency oxygen, if available.

as peptic ulcers, gastritis, stomach cancer or ingestion of caustic poisons. Bleeding in the lower gastrointestinal tract originates in the small intestine, large intestine, rectum or anus, and includes diverticular disease, polyps, hemorrhoids and anal fissures, as well as cancer and inflammatory bowel disease.

A patient with gastrointestinal bleeding may experience vomiting of blood, bloody bowel movements or black, tarry stools. Symptoms that may accompany the bleeding include fatigue, weakness, abdominal pain, pale appearance and shortness of breath.

Serious gastrointestinal bleeding can have a significant impact on vital signs—for example, causing blood pressure to drop sharply and heart rate to increase. Summon more advanced medical personnel, as the patient may require a blood transfusion or surgery.

GENITAL INJURIES

Assessing and treating a patient with a genital injury requires a calm and professional approach, as it can be embarrassing not only for the patient, but also for you. Using a sensitive approach to the patient's situation, such as clearing onlookers from the scene, supplying a drape for privacy and reassuring the patient, will help the process be less embarrassing. If possible, someone of the same gender should treat the patient.

Injuries to the penis usually occur as a result of an accident or assault. They can be either closed wounds, such as a bruise, or open wounds, such as an avulsion or laceration. Regardless, genital injuries are extremely painful.

The female organs, like those of the male, can cause extreme pain when injured. However, these types of injuries are rare, as the female genitals are smaller and much more protected. Straddle injury and sexual assault are the most common situations in which the female genitals can be injured, as well as childbirth. Injuries

can cause severe bleeding and pain due to the large amount of blood vessels in this area. Despite excessive bleeding, these injuries are rarely life threatening.

Signs and Symptoms of Genital Injuries

Signs and symptoms of genital injury are similar as those for an abdominal injury. They include—

- Severe pain.
- Bruising.
- External bleeding.
- Nausea.
- Vomiting (sometimes containing blood).
- Weakness.
- Thirst.
- Pain, tenderness or a tight feeling in the area.
- Protruding organs.
- Rigid abdominal muscles.
- Other signs of shock.

Providing Care for Genital Injuries

Care for a closed wound to the male genitals as you would for any closed wound. Wrap the penis in a soft, sterile dressing moistened with saline solution and apply a cold compress to reduce pain and swelling. As with any injury, *never* remove an impaled object. Stabilize the object and bandage it in place for transport.

If the injury is an open wound, apply a sterile dressing and direct pressure with your gloved hand or the patient's hand, or use a protective barrier to avoid contact. In the case where the penis is partially or completely amputated, apply a sterile pressure dressing to help stop bleeding, which may be significant. Aggressive direct pressure may also be needed if bleeding is excessive. As with an avulsion, if the penis is found, follow the procedure for preserving and transporting parts. If any parts are avulsed or completely amputated, wrap them in sterile gauze, moistened in sterile saline if available. Then place them in a plastic bag, labeled with

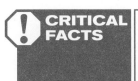

CRITICAL FACTS

Signs and symptoms of genital injury are the same as those for an abdominal injury.

To care for injuries to the male genital region, remember never to remove an impaled object. Closed wounds to this area should be treated as any other closed wound injury. For open wounds, apply sterile dressing and direct pressure, either with your gloved hand or allow the patient to do it.

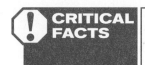

CRITICAL FACTS

To provide care for injury to the female genitals, control bleeding with pressure using compresses moistened with saline. Use a diaper-like dressing for the wound and stabilize any impaled objects with a bandage. Use ice packs over the dressing to reduce swelling and ease pain.

the patient's name and the time and date they were placed in the bag. Keep the bag cool by placing it in a larger bag or container of ice and water slurry, *not* on ice alone and *not* on dry ice. Transfer the bag to the EMS personnel transporting the patient to the hospital.

It is also possible for injuries to affect the scrotum and testicles. A blow to this area can rupture the scrotum and can cause pooling of blood, which is extremely painful. A ruptured testicle requires surgery. Apply an ice pack to the area to reduce swelling and pain and, if the scrotal skin has become avulsed, try to find it. Wrap the skin in sterile dressing and transport with the patient. The scrotum should be dressed with gauze sterilized and moistened with saline. Apply pressure to control bleeding.

To provide care for injury to the female genitals, control bleeding with pressure using compresses moistened with saline. Use a diaper-like dressing for the wound and stabilize any impaled objects with a bandage. Use ice packs over the dressing to reduce swelling and ease pain. *Never* place anything in the vagina, including dressing. Treat the patient for shock as required.

Remember your training regarding a crime scene if you suspect a patient has been a victim of sexual assault. Take care to provide the patient with privacy by clearing the area of onlookers and draping a sheet or blanket over the patient. Do *not* touch the genitals; discreetly ask if the patient has suffered any other injuries, such as to the head. If bleeding is life threatening, this will take priority over maintaining the integrity of the crime scene. Do *not* allow the patient to bathe or douche and discourage the patient from washing the hair or cleaning under the fingernails. Unless injuries are life threatening, do *not* clean or touch any wounds. Handle the patient's clothing as little as possible, bagging them separately from any other items. If there is blood on the items, do *not* use plastic bags and be sure to follow local protocols.

PUTTING IT ALL TOGETHER

Injuries to the chest, abdomen or genitalia can be serious. They can damage soft tissues, bones and internal organs. Although many injuries are immediately obvious, some may be detected only as the patient's condition worsens over time. Watch for signs and symptoms of serious injuries that require immediate medical attention.

Care for any life-threatening condition and then give any additional care needed for specific injuries. *Always* call for more advanced medical personnel as soon as possible. Have the patient remain as still as possible. For open wounds to the chest, abdomen or genitalia, control bleeding. If you suspect a fracture, immobilize the injured part. Use occlusive dressings for sucking chest wounds and for open abdominal wounds when these materials are available. Your actions can make the difference in the patient's chances of survival.

 YOU ARE THE EMERGENCY MEDICAL RESPONDER

As you begin your assessment, you notice that the young woman has multiple gunshot wounds to her chest and abdomen. How should you care for this patient?

22 Injuries to Muscles, Bones and Joints

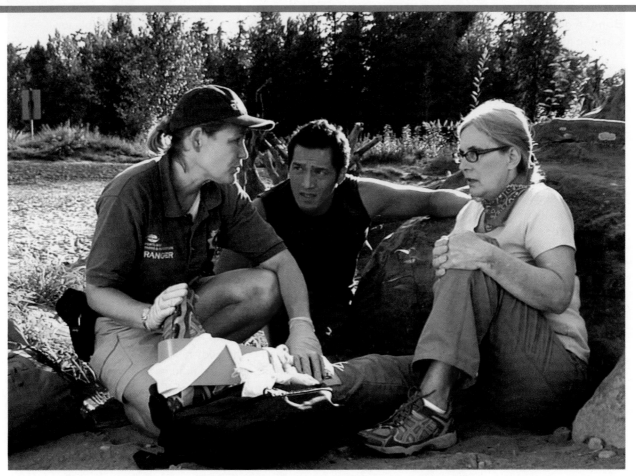

))) YOU ARE THE EMERGENCY MEDICAL RESPONDER

You are patrolling the state park where you are the emergency medical responder (EMR) on duty. You come across two hikers walking on the trail; one appears to be assisted by the other. As you approach, you notice that the hiker that is being assisted is not putting any weight on the right leg. How would you respond?

Key Terms

Air splint: A hollow, inflatable splint for immobilizing a part of the body.

Anatomic splint: A splint formed by supporting an injured part of the body with an uninjured, neighboring body part; for example, splinting one finger against another; also called a *self-splint*.

Angulation: An angular deformity in a fractured bone.

Binder: A cloth wrapped around a patient to securely hold the arm against the patient's chest to add stability; also called a *swathe*.

Bone: A dense, hard tissue that forms the skeleton.

Cardiac muscle: A specialized type of muscle found in the heart.

Circumferential splint: A type of splint that surrounds or encircles an injured body part.

Closed fracture: A type of fracture in which the skin over the broken bone is intact.

Cravat: A folded triangular bandage used to hold splints in place.

Crepitus: A grating or popping sound under the skin that can be due to a number of causes, including two pieces of bone rubbing against each other.

Direct force: A force that causes injury at the point of impact.

Dislocation: The displacement of a bone from its normal position at a joint.

Extremity: A limb of the body; *upper extremity* is the arm; *lower extremity* is the leg.

Fracture: A break or disruption in bone tissue.

Immobilize: To use a splint or other method to keep an injured body part from moving.

Indirect force: A force that transmits energy through the body, causing injury at a distance from the point of impact.

Joint: A structure where two or more bones are joined.

Ligament: A fibrous band that holds bones together at a joint.

Muscle: A tissue that contracts and relaxes to create movement.

Open fracture: A type of fracture in which there is an open wound in the skin over the fracture.

Rigid splint: A splint made of rigid material such as wood, aluminum or plastic.

Self-splint: A splint formed by supporting one part of the body with another; also called an *anatomic splint*.

Smooth muscles: Muscles responsible for contraction of hollow organs such as blood vessels or the gastrointestinal tract.

Soft splint: A splint made of soft material such as towels, pillows, slings, swathes and cravats.

Splint: A device used to immobilize body parts.

Sprain: The partial or complete tearing or stretching of ligaments and other soft tissue structures at a joint.

Strain: The excessive stretching and tearing of muscles or tendons; a pulled or torn muscle.

Swathe: A cloth wrapped around a patient to securely hold the arm against the patient's chest, to add stability; also called a *binder*.

Tendon: A fibrous band that attaches muscle to bone.

Traction splint: A splint with a mechanical device that applies traction to realign the bones.

Twisting force: A force that causes injury when one part of the body remains still while the rest of the body is twisted or turns away from it.

Vacuum splint: A splint that can be molded to the shape of the injured area by extracting air from the splint.

Voluntary muscles: Muscles that attach to bones; also called *skeletal muscles*.

Learning Objectives

After reading this chapter, and completing the class activities, you will have the information needed to—

- List the three mechanisms of muscle, bone and joint injuries.
- Describe different types of musculoskeletal injuries.
- Describe how to assess for muscle, bone and joint injuries.
- List the signs and symptoms of muscle, bone and joint injuries.

- Describe general care for muscle, bone and joint injuries.
- List general guidelines for splinting.
- List the purposes of immobilizing an injury.
- Describe typical agricultural and industrial injuries *(Enrichment)*.
- List safety factors associated with agricultural and industrial injuries *(Enrichment)*.

Skill Objectives

After reading this chapter, and completing the class activities, you should be able to—

- Demonstrate how to immobilize muscle, bone and joint injuries.

INTRODUCTION

Although musculoskeletal injuries are almost always painful, they are rarely life threatening. However, when not recognized and taken care of properly, they can have serious consequences and even result in permanent disability or death. Broken **bones**, dislocated **joints**, strained **muscles** and similar injuries are common, and most people will experience one or more of these during their lifetime. Injuries to muscles, bones and joints range from simple, minor problems such as a **sprained** finger, to serious situations such as a **fractured** pelvis.

In this chapter, you will learn how to recognize and care for muscle, bone and joint injuries. Developing a better understanding of the structure and function of the body's framework will help you assess musculoskeletal injuries and give appropriate care.

MUSCULOSKELETAL SYSTEM

The musculoskeletal system is a combination of two body systems—the muscular and skeletal systems. It consists of the bones, muscles, **tendons** and **ligaments**. The skeletal system creates a structural framework for the body and is comprised of approximately 206 bones of varying shapes and sizes. There are six sections that comprise the skeleton: the skull, spine, thorax, pelvis, upper extremities and lower extremities.

FRONT VIEW

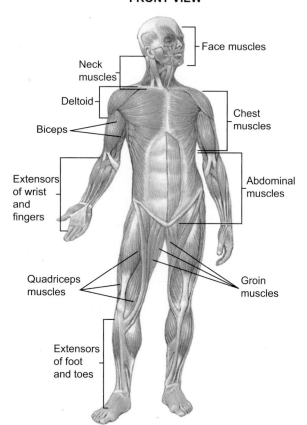

BACK VIEW

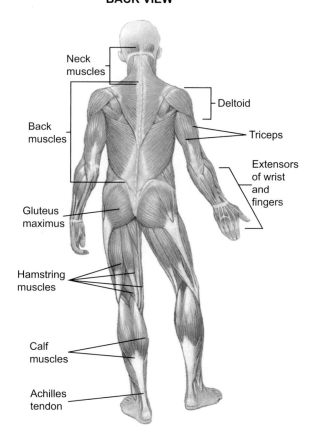

Fig. 22-1: The major muscles of the body

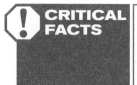 **CRITICAL FACTS**

The musculoskeletal system is a combination of two body systems–the muscular and skeletal systems. It consists of the bones, muscles, tendons and ligaments.

There are three types of muscles: the voluntary muscles, smooth muscles of the walls of organs, and cardiac muscles of the heart.

Muscles, bones and joints are injured when force is applied to them. The three basic *mechanisms of injury* (MOIs) are direct force, indirect force and twisting force.

There are three types of muscles: the **voluntary muscles**, **smooth muscles** of the walls of organs, and **cardiac muscles** of the heart. Voluntary muscles, also called skeletal muscles, are the major muscles that make up the body and enable movement (**Fig. 22-1**).

Ligaments and tendons join structures of the musculoskeletal system together. Ligaments hold the bones at a joint together and tendons connect muscle to bone. All joints have a normal range of movement—an area in which they can move freely without too much stress or strain. When joints are forced beyond this range, ligaments can stretch and tear. Muscles and tendons can also become stretched or torn when placed under a lot of stress or worked too hard.

INJURIES TO MUSCLES, BONES AND JOINTS

Causes of Injury

Muscles, bones and joints are injured when force is applied to them. Knowing the specific mechanism, or cause, of injury can give you important clues about which parts of the body may be injured, what other hidden injuries may exist along with the more obvious ones, and how serious the injuries may be.

There are three basic *mechanisms of injury* (MOIs):

- **Direct force** causes injury at the point of impact (**Fig. 22-2, A**). For example, the patient may have been hit by a loose pitch during a baseball game, fracturing the bone in the ankle.
- **Indirect force** transmits energy through the body and causes injury at some distance from the original point of impact (**Fig. 22-2, B**). For example, the patient might have a fall from a galloping horse, and stretch out the arms while landing so that the hands hit the ground first. The collarbone is broken when the force is transmitted up the arm to the shoulder.
- **Twisting force**, or rotating force, causes injury when one part of the body remains still while the rest of the body is twisted or turned away from it (**Fig. 22-2, C**). For example, a patient may be skiing and fall to the side, causing a leg to twist while still in a ski boot that is pointing downhill.

Types of Injuries

The four basic types of injuries to muscles, bones and joints are fractures, **dislocations**, **strains** and sprains.

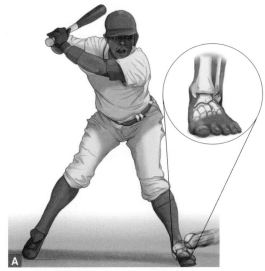
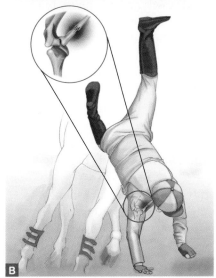
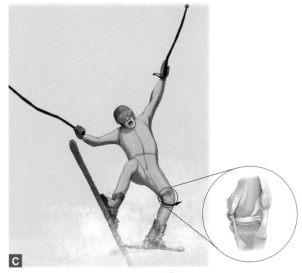

Fig. 22-2, A–C: The three basic MOIs are **(A)** direct force, **(B)** indirect force and **(C)** twisting force.

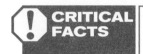

> **CRITICAL FACTS**
>
> The four basic types of injuries to muscles, bones and joints are fractures, dislocations, strains and sprains.

Fractures

A fracture is a break or damage to a bone. Fractures can involve bones that are broken all the way through, chipped or cracked (**Fig. 22-3**). A fall, a blow or sometimes even a twisting movement can cause a fracture. Some fractures are obvious, but others may not be easy to detect without an X-ray. While most isolated fractures are not considered critical or life threatening, if the femur or pelvis is fractured, the patient is at serious risk of excessive blood loss, shock and death. These two bones contain many blood vessels and any injury tends to cause heavy bleeding. Fracture to the spine can also result in damage to the spinal cord.

There are two kinds of fractures—

- **Closed fractures:** The skin over the broken bone is intact (**Fig. 22-4, A**).
- **Open fractures:** There is an open wound in the skin over the fracture. In some cases, the broken bone actually protrudes from the skin or is visible through the wound (**Fig. 22-4, B**).

While closed fractures are more common, open fractures are more dangerous because

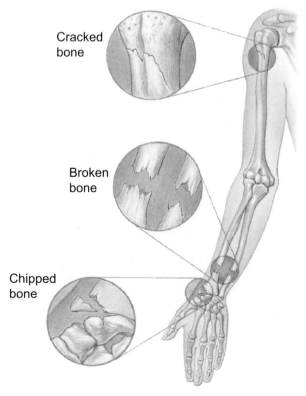

Fig. 22-3: Fractures include chipped or cracked bones and bones broken all the way through.

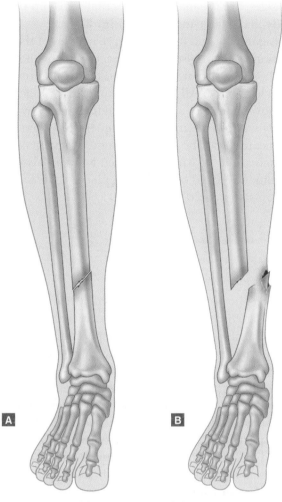

Fig. 22-4, A–B: **(A)** Closed fracture; **(B)** Open fracture

they carry a risk of infection and severe bleeding. In general, fractures are life threatening only if they involve breaks in large bones such as the femur, sever an artery or affect breathing. Since you cannot always tell if a person has a fracture, you should consider the MOI. A fall from a height or a motor-vehicle crash could signal a possible fracture. When in doubt, suspect a fracture and provide care accordingly.

Dislocations

Dislocations are usually more obvious than fractures. A dislocation is the displacement of a bone at a joint away from its normal position (**Fig. 22-5**). The bones in the human body are linked together at joints. When the bones that normally meet at a particular joint have been

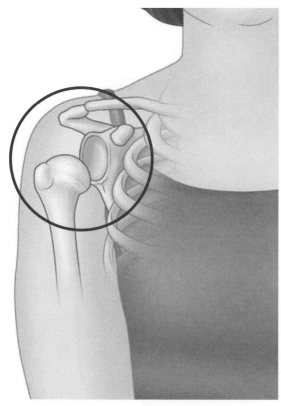

Fig. 22-5: A dislocation is the movement of a bone at a joint away from its normal position.

displaced or separated from each other, and the ligaments or tendons have been stretched, displaced or torn, this is called a dislocation.

Some joints, such as the shoulder and fingers, dislocate more easily because they are relatively exposed and not as well protected by ligaments. Other joints, such as the elbow, are less likely to become dislocated, but are just as serious as any joint dislocation. In general, dislocation requires a severe force. However, if a joint has become dislocated once and the ligaments holding the bones in place were damaged, subsequent dislocations are then more likely to occur. In some cases, dislocation can become chronic so that relatively minor movements can cause joint instability.

A force strong enough to cause an initial dislocation can also cause a fractured bone, bleeding and damaged nerves, so it is important to check for those injuries as well. A dislocation can be extremely painful.

Sprains

A sprain is the partial or complete tearing or stretching of ligaments and other tissues at a joint (**Fig. 22-6, A**). If the bones that meet at a joint are forced beyond their usual range of movement, the ligaments can be stretched or torn even though the bones are not actually

dislocated. The greater the number of ligaments torn, the more severe is the injury. Severe sprains, caused by a great deal of force being applied, can also involve fractured or dislocated bones. Milder sprains are caused when the only injury is stretched ligaments.

Patients generally find that the pain of these mild sprains is quickly resolved and they return to their normal activities. However, this often leads to reinjury of the joint that was sprained. Proper care should always be given once ligaments have been stretched or torn, even if the injury is mild. Otherwise, the joint may become less stable and the partially healed, less-stable joint will be much more susceptible to reinjury. The joints most easily injured are at the ankle, knee, wrist and fingers.

Strains

A strain is the excessive stretching and tearing of muscles or tendons, sometimes called a "pulled muscle" or a tear (**Fig. 22-6, B**). Tendons are

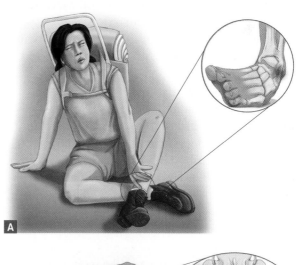

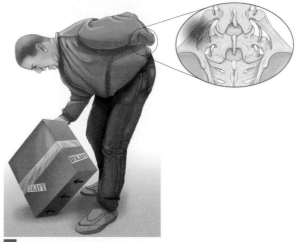

Fig. 22-6, A–B: **(A)** A sprain is the partial or complete tearing or stretching of ligaments and other tissues at a joint. **(B)** A strain is the excessive stretching and tearing of muscles or tendons.

stronger than muscles and more resistant to injury, so damage more often happen in muscles or at the attachment between the muscle and tendon. Strains can result from overexertion, such as lifting something too heavy, or from working a muscle for too long. They can also result from sudden or uncoordinated movements. Strains most often involve the muscles in the neck, back, thigh or calf.

Like sprains, strains are often neglected and this may lead to re-injury. The muscles need time and rest to repair the damage. Repeated strains of the neck and back are common causes of workers being absent from work.

Assessing Signs and Symptoms of Injuries to Muscles, Bones and Joints

Injuries to the musculoskeletal system are identified during the physical examination. Because these injuries often appear to be similar, it may be difficult for you to determine exactly what type of injury has occurred. As you complete the physical examination, think about how the body normally looks and feels. Check for deformity; compare the injured side to the uninjured side.

Ask how the injury happened. The cause of the trauma may alert you to the possibility that the muscles, bones and joints have been injured. As the patient or bystanders explain how the injury occurred, listen for clues, such as a fall from a height or a serious motor-vehicle accident. Also ask the patient if any areas are painful. Then carefully examine the entire body, starting with the head.

Keep in mind as you assess the patient that if there was sufficient force present to fracture a bone or dislocate a joint, that force may also cause bleeding, internal injuries and shock. Fractures can cause severe pain and there may be so much focus on this that the patient will not mention other problems such as abdominal pain, which may actually indicate more serious injuries.

Some common signs and symptoms associated with musculoskeletal injuries include:
- A snapping sound. If a bone has fractured, the patient may report hearing or feeling the bone snap or break.
- Deformity or **angulation (Fig. 22-7)**. If you suspect injury in one arm or leg but not the other, compare the two arms or two legs to

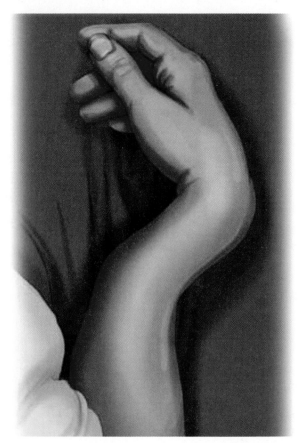

Fig. 22-7: Serious bone or joint injuries may appear deformed.

see if the injured limb is bent at an abnormal angle, or has changed in shape compared to the uninjured one. Other fractured bones may show indentations, and a dislocated joint often shows an indentation where the bones would normally meet.
- Pain and tenderness. The pain of a fractured bone or dislocated joint is often severe.
- **Crepitus**. There may be a grating sound or feeling when attempting to move the fractured bone, caused by the two pieces of bone rubbing against each other.
- Swelling. Swelling may be present and may obscure some indentations.
- Restricted movement. The patient may be unable to move the affected area, due to pain or because of a dislocated joint.
- Visible break. In an open fracture, the broken ends of the bones may be visible.
- Bruising or discoloration. Internal bleeding may cause bruising as blood pools under the skin.
- Loss of circulation or sensation. There may be a loss of circulation or sensation in an **extremity** (the shoulders to the fingers; the hips to the toes).

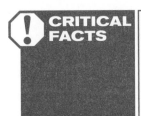

CRITICAL FACTS

Signs and symptoms of musculoskeletal injuries include a snapping sound, deformity/angulation, pain and tenderness, crepitus, swelling, restricted movement, bruising and loss of circulation or sensation.

Call for more advanced medical personnel if you suspect a fracture to an area other than a digit; if the injury involves severe bleeding or impairs walking or breathing, involves the head, neck or spine; or you see or suspect multiple injuries.

It is often impossible to determine whether a patient has experienced a fracture, dislocation, sprain or strain at the initial examination. X-rays and other tests by a health care provider will determine the precise nature of the injuries. Fortunately, it is not necessary to know whether the swelling of an ankle, for example, is caused by a fracture or a sprain to provide appropriate care.

Providing Care for Injuries to Muscles, Bones and Joints

A gentle, reassuring approach is important in caring for patients with muscle, bone and joint injuries. The patient is likely to be experiencing severe pain and may be frightened. Avoid moving the injured parts of the patient's body as much as possible, as this is likely to increase the pain and may cause further injury. Keep the injured area stable in the position found until more advanced medical personnel take over.

For any muscle, bone or joint injury, follow these general guidelines when providing care—

- Follow standard precautions.
- Ensure that the patient is breathing effectively, and administer emergency oxygen if needed.
- Control bleeding if present.
- If a spinal injury is suspected, stabilize the head, neck and spine and keep the patient flat.
- Avoid any movements or changes in position that cause pain. The patient will usually find the most comfortable position. Keep the injured area immobile in that position.
- Remove any jewelry or restrictive clothing in the affected area so that swelling does not cause more pain or injury.
- Clean and bandage any open wounds before splinting.
- Follow the steps on pages **492–499** to **immobilize** the injured joint or bones with **splints** only if you must transport the patient to definitive medical care *and* you can do so without causing more pain.

- Check for circulation and sensation to the limb. Feel for the patient's distal pulse, skin temperature and ability to move and detect touch in the injured parts, before and after splinting.

Call for more advanced medical personnel if—
- You suspect a fracture to an area other than a finger or toe.
- The injury involves severe bleeding.
- The injury impairs walking or breathing.
- The injury involves the head, neck or spine.
- You see or suspect multiple injuries.

The general care for all musculoskeletal injuries is similar: *rest, immobilize, cold* and *elevate* or "RICE" (**Fig. 22-8**). Another common interpretation of the acronym RICE is known as *rest, ice, compression* and *elevation*.

Rest

Avoid any movements or activities that cause pain. Help the patient find the most comfortable position. If you suspect head, neck or spinal injuries, leave the patient lying flat.

Immobilize

Stabilize the injured area in the position it was found. In most cases, it will *not* be necessary to apply a splint. For example, the ground can

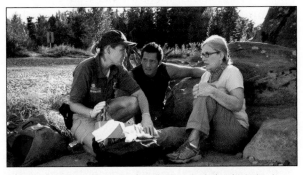

Fig. 22-8: The general care for all musculoskeletal injuries is rest, immobilize, cold and elevate, or RICE, also interpreted as rest, ice, compression and elevation.

provide support to an injured leg, ankle or foot or the patient may cradle an injured elbow or arm in a position of comfort.

Cold

Apply ice or a cold pack for periods of 20 minutes. If 20 minutes cannot be tolerated, apply ice for periods of 10 minutes. If continued icing is needed, remove the pack for 20 minutes, and then replace it.

Cold helps reduce swelling and eases pain and discomfort. Commercial cold packs can be stored in a kit until ready to use, or you can make an ice pack by placing ice (crushed or cubed) with water in a plastic bag and wrapping it with a towel or cloth. Place a thin layer of gauze or cloth between the source of cold and the skin to prevent injury to the skin. Do *not* apply an ice or cold pack directly over an open fracture, because doing so would require you to put pressure on the open fracture site and could cause discomfort to the patient. Instead, place cold packs *around* the site. Do *not* apply heat, as there is no evidence that applying heat helps.

Elevate

Elevating the injured area above the level of the heart helps slow the flow of blood, helping to reduce swelling. Elevation is particularly effective in controlling swelling in extremity injuries. However, *never* attempt to elevate a seriously injured area of a limb unless it has been adequately immobilized.

SPLINTING

When an injury to bones, muscles or joints is suspected, immobilizing the affected body part is an important step in treatment. Preventing the bones, joints and ligaments from moving helps to reduce the risk of further injury, and minimizes the risks of some possible complications such as—
- Broken bone ends injuring blood vessels, nerves or muscles as they move. This can cause loss of sensation in the affected area or increase the bleeding.
- Broken bone ends breaking through the skin.

- Blood vessels being compressed by broken or dislocated bones, thus reducing blood flow.
- Paralysis caused by damage to the spine.

The purposes of immobilizing an injury are to—
- Lessen pain.
- Prevent further damage to soft tissues.
- Reduce the risk of serious bleeding.
- Reduce the possibility of loss of circulation to the injured part.
- Prevent closed extremity injuries from becoming open extremity injuries.

A tool or device used to immobilize an injury is called a *splint*. There are many commercially manufactured types of splints, but if necessary one can be improvised from items available at the scene.

Rules for Splinting

No matter where the splint will be applied, or what the injury is, there are some general rules for splinting—
- Splinting should *only* be performed if you have to move or transport the patient to receive medical care *and* you can do so without causing more pain.
- Assess the patient's distal pulse, skin temperature, ability to move and ability to feel at the body part that is on the other side of the injury from the heart. For example, if the elbow has been injured, check pulse, skin temperature, mobility and sensation at the wrist. If a leg bone is injured, check at the ankle. Continue to assess these three signs every 15 minutes after the splint has been applied. This will let you know if the splint, or swelling under the splint, has impaired circulation to the affected area.
- If a fracture is suspected, immobilize the bones or joints above and below the injury (**Fig. 22-9**). For example, if a bone in the lower leg is broken, you would immobilize the ankle and the knee.
- Cut off or remove any clothing around the injury site. If the patient is wearing a watch or jewelry near the injury, these should also be removed. Swelling may occur beyond the actual injury site. If an elbow is injured, for

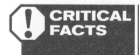 **CRITICAL FACTS**

Immobilizing an injury is important. It lessens pain, prevents further damage to soft tissues, reduces the risk of serious bleeding, reduces the possibility of loss of circulation to the injured part and prevents closed injuries from becoming open injuries.

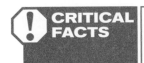Splints can be commercially made or improvised with items you have on hand. There are six different types of splints: soft, rigid, traction, circumferential, vacuum and anatomic (self-splint).

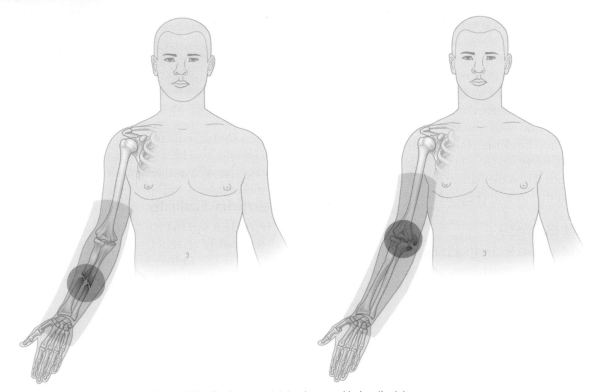

Fig. 22-9: If a fracture is suspected, immobilize the bones or joints above and below the injury.

example, any bracelets, watches or rings on the wrist and hand should be removed.

■ Cover any bleeding or open wounds, including open fractures, with sterile dressings and carefully bandage with minimal pressure.

■ Do *not* try to push protruding bones back below the skin.

■ Do *not* attempt to straighten any angulated fracture; always splint the limb in the position found.

■ Do *not* allow the patient to bear weight on an injured lower extremity.

■ Pad the splints you are using so that they will be more comfortable and conform to the shape of the injured body part.

■ Secure the splint in place with folded triangular bandages, roller bandages or other wide strips of cloth.

■ Elevate the splinted part, if possible.

Types of Splints

Whether commercially made or improvised, there are six general types of splints: soft, rigid,

traction, circumferential, vacuum and anatomic or **self-splint**.

Soft Splints

Soft splints include folded blankets, towels, pillows, slings, **swathes**, and **cravats (Fig. 22-10)**. Many improvised splints are made from soft materials such as bed pillows or blankets, and they can be effective if secured properly. A swathe is a

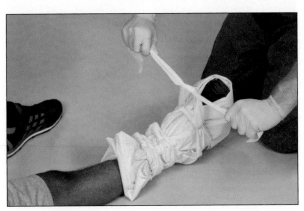

Fig. 22-10: Soft splints use soft, pliable materials, such as folded blankets or towels, to immobilize an injury.

cloth wrapped around a patient to securely hold the arm against the patient's chest, to add stability. Cravats are folded triangular bandages used to hold splints in place.

A sling is a type of soft splint made from a triangular bandage. It can provide stability when the shoulder, elbow or upper arm has been injured. The sling will support the weight of the arm. To immobilize the injury, you should then apply a **binder**—wrapping the cloth around the patient and the arm to hold the arm securely against the side of the patient's chest. With both the sling and binder in place, the arm will not be able to move, the weight of the arm will be supported and the patient's pain should be significantly reduced (**Fig. 22-11**).

Rigid Splints

A **rigid splint** is one that is made of a rigid material such as wood, aluminum, plastic, cardboard or composite materials (**Fig. 22-12**). Some are specially shaped to be used for a particular body part, such as an arm or a finger. Some are designed to be pliable so they can be shaped to the body part. They may come with padding or require padding to be added at the time of use.

If commercial splinting materials are not available, improvised rigid splints can be created from cardboard boxes, rolled-up magazines, an athlete's shin guards, or other items available at the scene. Look for an item that is light but rigid, and strong enough to resist breaking. It should be long enough to prevent movement on either side of the injury, and wide

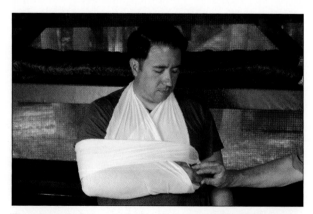

Fig. 22-11: A sling made from a triangular bandage can provide stability to an injury to the shoulder, elbow or upper arm, while a binder wrapping the injured body part to the chest can be used to immobilize.

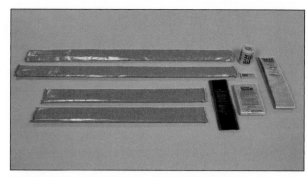

Fig. 22-12: Commercially manufactured rigid splints

enough that it will cover the entire injured area. You should also be able to pad it effectively to protect the skin and any wounds.

Traction Splints

A **traction splint** contains a mechanical device that is attached to the body part above and below the injury and provides a steady counter-pull (**Fig. 22-13**). This is not the same as applying manual traction to realign the bones, and these splints are not intended to reposition fractured bones. Instead, they reduce pain and blood loss by immobilizing bones that might otherwise move in the direction opposite to the splint's pull. Each brand or type of traction splint will have instructions about correct use.

Circumferential Splints

A **circumferential splint** surrounds or encircles the injured body part. One example is a commercial **air splint**, which begins as a soft, pliable splint that can be positioned around the injured area. It is then filled with air and becomes rigid and applies pressure to the injured area. **Air splints** have the potential to interfere with circulation, making it difficult to check the patient's pulse or temperature. They can, however, be helpful in reducing bleeding in cases of serious injury to the pelvis. Air splints should only be used under medical direction.

Vacuum Splints

A **vacuum splint** starts out soft and pliable so that it can be shaped to fit the area that has been injured. Once it is in place, the air can be sucked out, creating a vacuum inside and making the splint rigid and immobilizing.

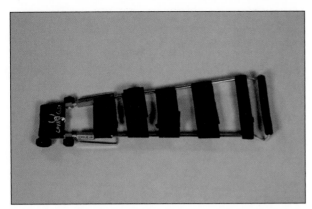

Fig. 22-13: A traction splint

Anatomic or Self-Splints

In many cases, the patient's own body can act as a splint. This is called an ***anatomic splint*** or *self-splint*. For example, if the right leg is broken, the left leg can be used as a splint (**Fig. 22-14**). The legs are fastened together using cravats or roller bandages. Any gaps between the legs are filled with padding.

Splinting Upper Extremities

The upper extremities are the arms and hands. The bones in the upper extremities are the collarbone, shoulder blade, humerus, radius and ulna, as well as the bones in the hand, wrist and fingers. The upper extremities are the most commonly injured parts of the body. Since people who are falling or about to crash instinctively try to protect themselves by throwing out their arms and hands, these areas receive the force of the impact. Often, the result is a fracture, sprain or dislocation.

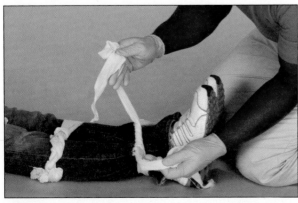

Fig. 22-14: In an anatomic splint, the patient's own body is used to immobilize an injured body part.

Splinting the Collarbone

When the collarbone is broken, the patient's shoulder may look lower than the uninjured side. You may see obvious deformity in the collarbone. It is best splinted with a sling, to reduce the pull from the arm's weight, and a binder to immobilize the arm against the chest.

Splinting the Shoulder

A dislocated shoulder will appear deformed and a hollow may be visible in the upper arm below the shoulder. This injury is extremely painful. There is a risk that nerves and arteries near the shoulder can be damaged by movement, so be cautious as you apply any splints. A sling and binder should be used, with some padding between the arm and the chest to maintain a reasonably comfortable position (**Fig. 22-15**).

Splinting the Upper Arm

The humerus is a strong bone, so if it is broken (most often near the shoulder or partway towards the elbow) check for other injuries, as considerable force probably was involved. This injury can be splinted with a padded rigid splint on the outside of the arm. If the elbow can be comfortably bent, you can then use a sling and binder. If the elbow cannot be bent without causing more pain, or if the rigid splint you are using is longer than the

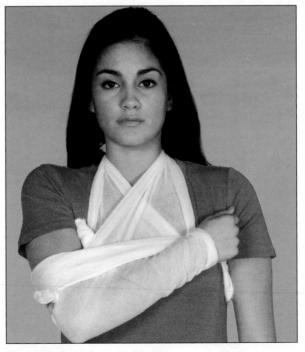

Fig. 22-15: Splint for a shoulder injury

upper arm, keep the arm straight at the patient's side and wrap the bandages or binders around the arm and chest (**Fig. 22-16**).

Splinting the Elbow

Do not attempt to straighten or bend the elbow or change its position. If the elbow is bent, even if it is deformed, splint with a sling and binder (**Fig. 22-17**). You may use a flat pillow or towel wrapped around the injured area and then secured to the chest. If the elbow is straight, use rigid splints along the length of both sides of the arm, from fingertips to underarm.

Splinting the Forearm and Wrist

A rigid splint extending from the elbow to the fingertips should be applied first. Then a sling and binder can be applied to support the arm against the chest (**Fig. 22-18**). If there is no open wound, a circumferential air splint, extending from elbow to past the fingertips, can be applied instead of the rigid splinting.

Splinting the Hands and Fingers

If a single finger has a broken bone, you may be able to create a self-splint or anatomic splint

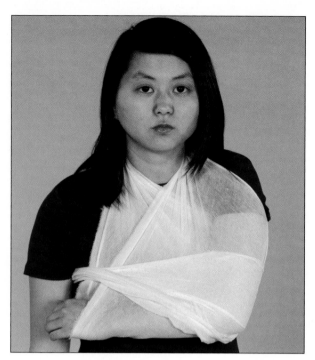

Fig. 22-17: Splint for an elbow injury

by taping the injured finger to the one beside it. A tongue depressor or similar-sized piece of cardboard can also work as a rigid splint, taped to the finger (**Fig. 22-19**).

When several fingers have broken bones or the back of the hand is involved in the injury, you will need to splint the entire hand. To immobilize the hand, place a small ball, or a

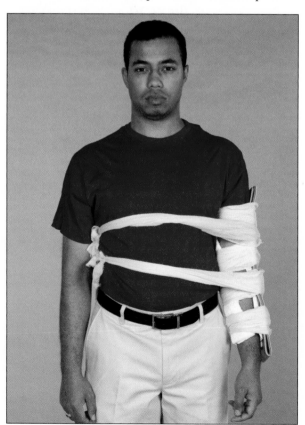

Fig. 22-16: Splint for an upper arm injury

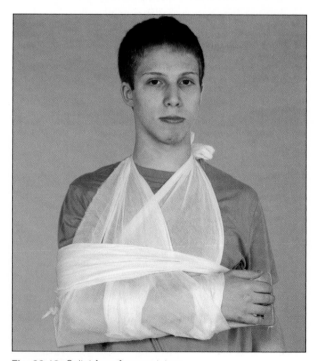

Fig. 22-18: Splint for a forearm injury

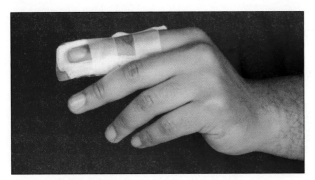

Fig. 22-19: Splint for a finger injury

rolled-up bandage or face cloth, inside the palm of the person's hand, with the fingers curled naturally around it. Then wrap the entire hand and splint the lower arm and wrist with a rigid splint or arm board. A sling can be added to help support the arm.

Splinting Lower Extremities
Splinting the Pelvis

Injuries to the pelvis are potentially life threatening because of the risk of heavy bleeding in this area. Assess the patient for shock and internal blood loss. To immobilize a pelvic fracture, a pelvic wrap can be used, following the manufacturer's instructions and if you are trained to apply one (**Fig. 22-20**). If a pelvic wrap is not available, one can be improvised using a sheet that is repeatedly folded lengthwise to create a thick, eight-inch wide strip. This strip is pushed under the small of the patient's back and pulled through until equal lengths appear on each side of the patient's body. Using the extended ends of the fabric, pull the strip of fabric down so that it is behind the injured pelvis, and cross the ends in front of the pelvis. Twist the ends together

so that the fabric is tightly secured around the pelvis. Tuck the leftover fabric ends under the patient or tie them in a knot.

The patient should then be placed on a long backboard. Use a blanket or pillow for padding between the patient's legs and add padding on both sides of the patient's hips. Then secure the patient to the backboard. Minimize movement of the pelvis and legs.

Splinting the Hip

The hip is the joint where the thigh bone, or femur, fits into the pelvis (**Fig. 22-21**). Like the pelvis, the femur has significant blood vessels, and any injury in this area can cause dangerous bleeding, which can be difficult to detect. Look for swelling in the thigh area. Assess and treat for bleeding and shock before beginning to splint. To immobilize the hip you will need to splint the patient's entire body on a long backboard.

Splinting the Femur

As mentioned previously, injuries to the femur can be very serious because of the risk of bleeding, which may be internal and not noticed. A broken femur causes a great deal of pain and significant swelling; the deformity of the thigh is usually quite noticeable and the muscle often

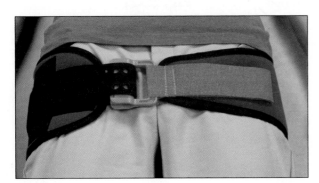

Fig. 22-20: Splint for a pelvis injury

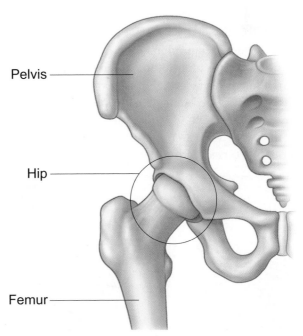

Pelvis

Hip

Femur

Fig. 22-21: The hip joint

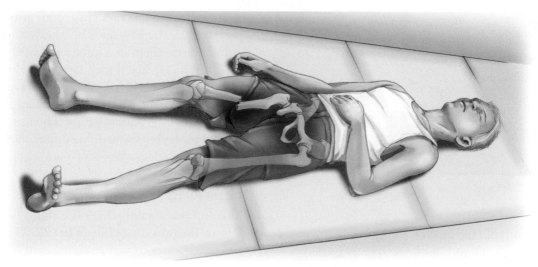

Fig. 22-22: The deformity of the thigh from a broken femur is usually quite noticeable.

contracts (shortens) with this type of break (**Fig. 22-22**). The leg may also be turned inward or outward. Use a traction splint if one is available and you have the training to apply this type of splint correctly.

If a traction splint cannot be applied, you can use two long rigid splints instead, with padding to fill any gaps between the splint and the patient's body (**Fig. 22-23**). One splint or board must start at the patient's groin area and extend past the bottom of the patient's foot, on the inside of the affected leg. The other should go from the patient's armpit to below the bottom of the patient's foot. Wrap the boards tightly, using cravats at the chest, hips, knees and ankles to immobilize the body.

Splinting the Knee

Knees may be injured in either a bent or straight position. Do *not* attempt to change the position of the knee. If it is straight, use two padded rigid splints, one on the outside and one on the inside of the leg. The inside splint should start at the groin and extend past the bottom of the foot. The outside splint should start at the hip

and also extend past the foot. Use cravats to keep the splints in place. If the knee is bent, use a pillow or folded blanket under the knee to maintain the bent position. Then use short, padded rigid splints running along either side of the knee to immobilize the upper and lower leg in relationship to the knee.

Splinting the Tibia and Fibula (Lower Leg Bones)

The tibia (shinbone) and fibula are the two bones that extend from the knee to the ankle. The tibia is covered by only a thin layer of skin, so open fractures of this bone are common. The fibula is not a weight-bearing bone and fractures of this bone may not be as easily detected. Injuries to either bone are splinted in the same way, using a circumferential air splint, extending from above the knee to below the foot. Or you can use two padded rigid splints, one on the inside running from the groin to below the foot, and the other on the outside running from the hip to below the foot (**Fig. 22-24**).

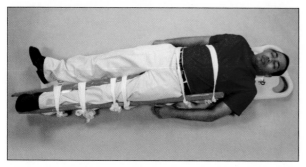

Fig. 22-23: Splint for a femur injury

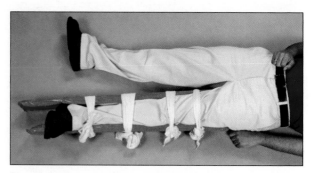

Fig. 22-24: Splint for a tibia or fibula injury

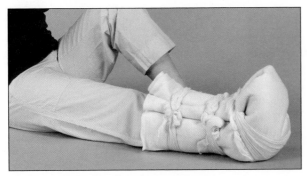
Fig. 22-25: Splint for an ankle or a foot injury

Splinting the Ankle and Foot

Injuries to the foot or ankle are often caused by heavy objects falling on the foot, or when a falling person lands on the feet. Twisting forces during a fall or while running can also cause an ankle injury. Whether the injury is a break or a sprain, *both* should be splinted in the same way, by immobilizing the entire foot and ankle (**Fig. 22-25**). A circumferential air splint is a good choice, but a pillow or thick blanket wrapped around the foot and ankle and secured in place will also work.

PUTTING IT ALL TOGETHER

Injuries to bones, muscles and joints are generally caused by significant force, so careful assessment should be done to identify or rule out other injuries. Injuries can include fractures to bones; dislocations of joints; and strains and sprains involving muscles, ligaments and tendons. It is not always easy to identify the type of injury present.

Injuries to the pelvis or femur are potentially critical because of the major blood vessels running through these parts of the body. Assess the patient for bleeding and shock.

Ensure that the patient is breathing effectively and provide emergency oxygen if needed. Assess for bleeding and take steps to control bleeding if necessary. If a spinal injury is suspected, stabilize the spine and keep the patient flat. Avoid any movements or changes in position that cause pain. Help the patient find the most comfortable position. Remove any jewelry or restrictive clothing in the affected area.

Clean and bandage any open wounds before splinting. Follow guidelines to immobilize the injured joint or bones with splints. Check the patient's pulse and ability to move and detect touch in the injured parts before and after splinting. Apply ice or a cold pack to reduce swelling and ease pain and discomfort. If there is no spinal injury, and the limb has been securely immobilized, elevate it so that it is above the level of the patient's heart.

In most cases, splinting the injured area will help prevent further damage, reduce bleeding and reduce pain. A variety of commercial splints are available for this purpose; many splints can be improvised if commercial products are not available. After splinting, check every 15 minutes to see that the patient's pulse, ability to move, skin temperature, color and ability to detect touch in the part of the body past the injured area are still stable.

))) YOU ARE THE EMERGENCY MEDICAL RESPONDER

After approaching the hikers, you find out that they were attempting to jump from rock to rock when one landed in an awkward position and could no longer put weight on the right leg without much pain. You are close to the entrance to the park but must move the injured hiker off the trail in order for emergency medical services (EMS) personnel to arrive and take over care. How should you respond? What actions should you take?

SKILLsheet

Applying a Rigid Splint

To apply a rigid splint—

STEP 1
Follow standard precautions and obtain consent.

STEP 2
Support the injured body part *above and below* the site of the injury.

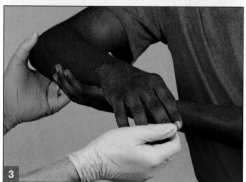

STEP 3
Check for circulation and sensation beyond the injured area.

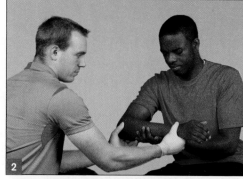

STEP 4
Place an appropriately sized rigid splint (e.g., padded board) under the injured body part.

NOTE: Place padding, such as a roller gauze, under the palm of the hand to keep it in a normal position.

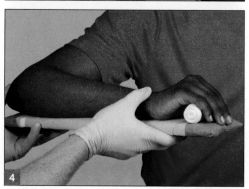

STEP 5

Tie several folded triangular bandages *above and below* the injured body part.

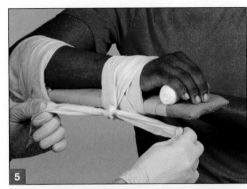

STEP 6

Recheck for circulation and sensation beyond the injured area.

NOTE: If a rigid splint is used on an injured forearm, immobilize the wrist and elbow. Bind the arm to the chest using folded triangular bandages or apply a sling. If splinting an injured joint, immobilize the bones on either side of the joint.

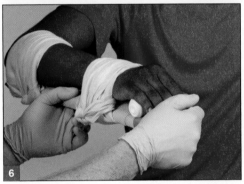

SKILLsheet

Applying a Sling and Binder

To apply a sling and a binder–

STEP 1
Follow standard precautions and obtain consent.

STEP 2
Support the injured body part *above and below* the site of the injury.

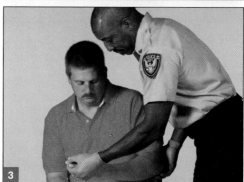

STEP 3
Check for circulation and sensation beyond the injured area.

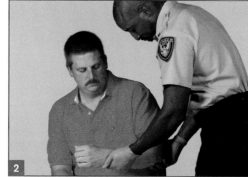

STEP 4
Place a triangular bandage under the injured arm and over the uninjured shoulder to form a sling.

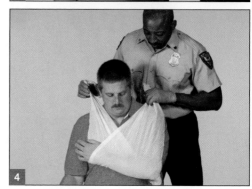

STEP 5

Tie the ends of the sling at the side of the neck.

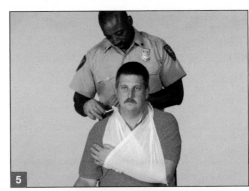

STEP 6

Bind the injured body part to the chest with a folded triangular bandage.

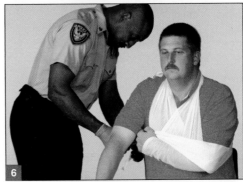

STEP 7

Recheck for circulation and sensation beyond the injured area.

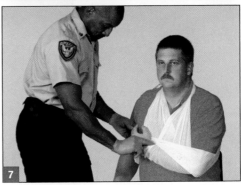

SKILLsheet

Applying an Anatomic Splint

To apply an anatomic splint–

STEP 1
Follow standard precautions and obtain consent.

STEP 2
Support the injured body part *above and below* the site of the injury.

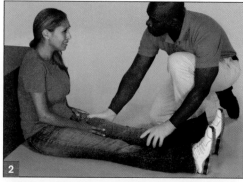

STEP 3
Check for circulation and sensation beyond the injured area.

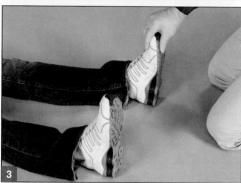

STEP 4
Place several folded triangular bandages *above and below* the injured body part.

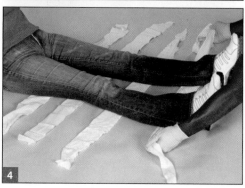

STEP 5

Place the uninjured body part next to the injured body part.

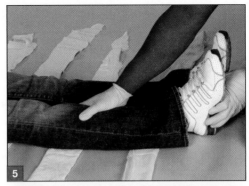

STEP 6

Tie triangular bandages securely.

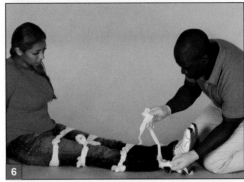

STEP 7

Recheck for circulation and sensation beyond the injured area.

NOTE: If you are not able to fully check circulation because a sock or shoe is in place, check for sensation.

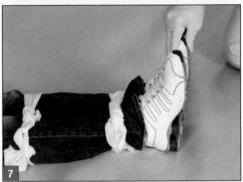

SKILLsheet

Applying a Soft Splint

To apply a soft splint—

STEP 1
Follow standard precautions and obtain consent.

STEP 2
Support the injured body part *above and below* the site of the injury.

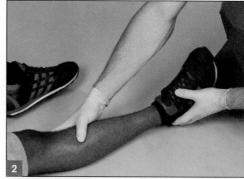

STEP 3
Check for circulation and sensation beyond the injured area.

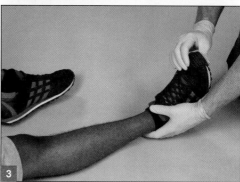

STEP 4
Place several folded triangular bandages *above and below* the injured body part.

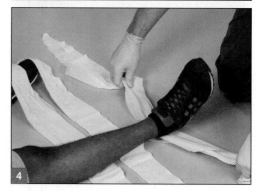

STEP 5

Gently wrap a soft object (e.g., a folded blanket or pillow) around the injured body part.

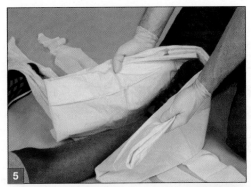

STEP 6

Tie triangular bandages securely with knots.

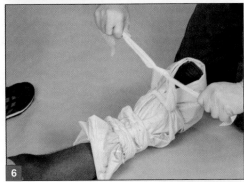

STEP 7

Recheck for circulation and sensation beyond the injured area.

NOTE: If you are not able to fully check circulation because a sock or shoe is in place, check for sensation.

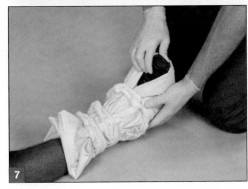

Enrichment
Agricultural and Industrial Emergencies

Because of the heavy equipment involved, some of the most serious accidental injuries occur on agricultural and industrial sites. You can expect to see crush injuries, avulsions, amputations and other major open and closed soft tissue and musculoskeletal injuries.

SCENE SIZE-UP AND SAFETY

As always, size-up the scene of an agricultural or industrial emergency before entering. *Never* enter a scene if there is any risk to your safety. Look out for toxic chemicals, fires or fire hazards, unstable or running machinery and unsecured livestock. If necessary, call specialized personnel, such as the fire department or a *hazardous materials* (HAZMAT) removal team, to stabilize the scene before entering **(Fig. 22-26)**.

Be sure to observe *lockout/tagout procedures*. Lockout/tagout refers to a set of procedures and practices that safeguard against the unexpected startup of machinery and equipment, or the possible release of hazardous energy when machinery is being maintained. The individual using the machinery turns off and disconnects it from its energy source before performing maintenance, and an authorized employee either locks or tags the energy-isolating device to prevent accidental release of energy.

Machinery that is on and/or that might be leaking fuel or hydraulic fluid should *not* be approached. An agricultural storage area should *not* be entered alone.

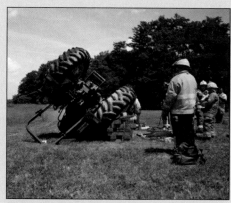

Fig. 22-26: Emergencies occurring on industrial sites often involve heavy, powerful, mechanized equipment, and injuries are often compounded by exposure to gases, fumes and chemicals. *Courtesy of David Denniston, Director, National FARMEDIC Training Program*

Working in confined spaces is another safety concern. A confined space is one with restricted openings for entry and exit; poor ventilation with possible air contaminants; and physical hazards related to engulfment (being surrounded and overwhelmed by a substance such as soil or grain) or collapse. Such scenes might include pits, tunnels, storage tanks, sewers, ventilation and exhaust ducts, underground utility vaults and pipelines.

A rescuer who is required to enter a confined space should follow these guidelines:

* An emergency rescue involving entry into a confined space must *never* be attempted without training in safe confined space entry and rescue procedures.
* Assume a confined space is hazardous.
* A person qualified to do so must ensure that structures are safe from collapse prior to anyone entering the confined space.
* An attendant must be present immediately outside the space to provide help to the rescuer inside, and there must be a plan for emergency rescue.
* There must be a safe method of communication between the rescuer inside the space and the attendant.
* Appropriate PPE must be worn by the rescuer entering. Exact equipment is determined by the specific hazards encountered in the confined space (e.g., eye/face and head and foot protection, respiratory protection, safety belts, lifelines and harnesses).
* Once a confined space has been identified, warning signs should be posted and, when possible, the entry physically blocked.
* The conditions must be tested prior to entry and continuously monitored during entry. Testing must be performed by someone who is properly trained and has the appropriate equipment; one's senses should *never* be trusted to determine if the air in a confined space is safe. Many toxic gases and vapors cannot be seen or smelled. This is also not a reliable way to determine if sufficient oxygen is present.
* Adequate air conditions *must* be maintained in the confined space, through proper ventilation.
* If safe atmospheric conditions cannot be maintained, the absolute necessity of entering should be evaluated. If it is necessary to enter, an appropriate respirator must be worn, and this equipment must be evaluated by someone with the proper training to do so.

- Properly trained workers must control utilities prior to entry into confined spaces, including, for example, electrical services, gas, propane, water, sanitary systems, communications, and any secondary service systems.
- If an unsafe condition develops, the space should be exited *immediately*.

AGRICULTURAL EMERGENCIES

On an agricultural site, the combination of long hours, powerful mechanized equipment that may or may not be properly maintained and remote locations can be deadly. Expect severe trauma, patients left unfound for hours and a high incidence of spinal injury.

Typical Injuries

On an agricultural site, injuries most often involve the hands and arms, which can get caught in machinery. The most common injuries include—
- Abrasions.
- Amputations.
- Animal bites.
- Avulsions.
- Burns.
- Concussions.
- Contusions.
- Eye injuries.
- Fractures.
- Lacerations.
- Punctures.
- Sprains.
- Strains.

Working with the Equipment

Injuries associated with different types of machinery each involve a different approach. It is important to have a basic understanding of how each piece of equipment works and how it can cause harm in order to avoid injuries to yourself or further injury to the patient.

Before trying to extricate a patient from agricultural equipment, the equipment must be stabilized and shut down. If necessary, call a specialized crew to do this.

As a general principle, agricultural equipment can be stabilized by blocking or chocking the wheels, putting on the parking brake or tying the equipment to another vehicle. The equipment should be shut down by entering the cab to access the main controls. The engine should be slowed down with the throttle and then the machine switched off using the ignition key. Some diesel-powered machines are shut down via an air shut-off lever rather than an ignition key.

The engine can also be shut off by shutting the fuel line. This is done using the shut-off valve at the bottom of the fuel tank or using vice-grip pliers. If a diesel engine cannot be shut down and the patient is in a life-threatening situation, a 20-pound CO_2 fire extinguisher can be emptied into the air intake. This will shut down the engine but will also cause considerable damage.

Never touch a control on a piece of agricultural machinery unless you are sure you know what it does.

Tractors

Be aware that tractors can be fueled by diesel, gasoline or propane, and that fuel leaks, fires and explosions are a real possibility. Tractors often cause injuries by rolling over onto the rider. Do *not* approach the site until the tractor has been stabilized.

A patient trapped by a tractor can be freed by digging a trench underneath the patient's body or by cutting off a piece of the machine, such as the steering wheel. In some cases, however, the tractor may need to be lifted off the patient by a specialized team.

Continued on next page

Enrichment
Agricultural and Industrial Emergencies (continued)

Combines

Some common trouble spots on a combine include the auger, which is the rotating part of the screw conveyor; the heads, with their oscillating cutting bars; the reels, steel tines that can impale someone; and the snapping rollers, which can cause crush injuries **(Fig. 22-27)**.

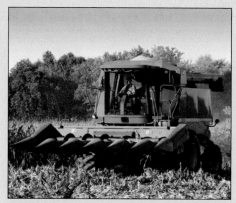

Fig. 22-27: Combine parts such as the auger, heads, reels and snapping rollers can cause serious injuries. *Courtesy of Michelle Lala Clark.*

The reverse feature should *never* be used in an attempt to extricate a patient from a combine. The safest approach is to keep the machinery from moving, so pry bars and other tools should be used to jam the moving parts into place before beginning extrication. The hydraulic system must be locked. Usually a bar near the hydraulic cylinder will lock the header. If possible, the combine header should be divided from the drive mechanism. An acetylene torch can be used to cut pieces of the combine to free a patient, but the combine and surrounding soil should first be washed down and the inside of the combine flushed, to reduce the risk of fire.

If a patient is trapped in the auger, the auger may need to be first cut free, and it should be transported with the patient. First, a large pipe wrench should be wedged on the shaft to prevent it from reversing, and then the auger drive disconnected. No attempt should be made to extricate a patient in the field if the auger has caused an avulsion.

On older equipment, rescue tools can be used to spread snapping rollers, but this approach will *not* work on newer equipment.

Hay Balers

To free a patient caught in a hay baler, the tines may need to be disassembled by unscrewing the bolts holding it together. The drive belts that drive the cross auger or raise the auger may need to be disassembled with rescue tools. To prevent reverse motion, a pipe wrench can be used to hold on to the input shaft as the auger is cut free. To release a patient from the smooth rollers, the mounting bolts at each end should be removed, to remove the bearings.

An acetylene torch should *never* be used to take apart a hay baler, as the combustible dust inside the baler may ignite.

Other Areas

In addition to the fields, agricultural emergencies may occur in silos, manure storage devices and places where livestock are held. Each of these areas carries its own hazards.

Silos

The major hazard in a silo is the gas formed during fermentation of stored crops, which, when inhaled, can kill within minutes **(Fig. 22-28)**. Keep in mind that "silo gas" can leak out to the surrounding area. Signs of this gas include a bleach-like smell, the presence of dead birds and insects, a yellowish or reddish vapor and sick livestock nearby. A *self-contained breathing apparatus* (SCBA) must be worn to rescue a patient in the presence of silo gas. Administer emergency oxygen to the patient if it is available, and transport as soon as possible.

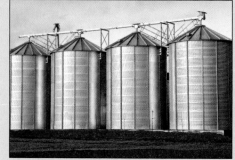

Fig. 22-28: The gas formed during fermentation of crops stored in a silo can kill within minutes when inhaled. © *Shutterstock.com/Jorg Hackemann.*

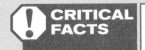
Manure Storage

Manure is often flushed from livestock facilities into a holding pond or a closed structure. The hazards include toxic fumes and risk of drowning. To rescue a patient in a manure storage area, you must wear an SCBA and lifeline. Treat an immersed patient as you would a victim of drowning. If the patient is breathing, connect the patient to an SCBA. Also administer emergency oxygen if it is available. Before transporting the patient, remove any contaminated clothing and flush the patient's body with water. Do *not* bring any contaminated materials into the transport vehicle. Anyone and everything that came into contact with manure will require decontamination.

Livestock

Never enter an area with unsecured livestock. Treat injuries inflicted by livestock as you would any similar injury but be sure to flush animal feces from any wound.

Chemicals Used in Farming

Many types of chemicals, particularly pesticides and fertilizers, are used in farming. Use protective clothing before entering a scene that may contain pesticides or other chemicals. If necessary, call a HAZMAT removal team. If you know what pesticide was involved in a particular emergency, check the label for instructions and precautions, and take the label with you to the hospital. Before transporting a patient, remove all clothing and flush the patient's body with water.

INDUSTRIAL EMERGENCIES

The hazards of industrial emergencies often mimic those of agricultural emergencies and include exposure to gases, fumes or other chemicals and to unstable machinery. The specific hazards depend on the site.

Scene Size-Up and Safety

Once again, it is important to size-up the scene and not enter it until it has been secured. Keep in mind that even small industrial sites, such as newspaper printers and garages, may present significant hazards. These may include dangerous equipment and machinery, hazardous materials, a risk of explosion or fire, and confined spaces.

When responding to the scene of an industrial emergency, determine whether there are hazardous materials present at the scene before entering. Communicate with staff about potential hazards, especially if you are unfamiliar with the operations. Determine if more than one patient is ill or has been injured and if so, how many. Also determine the type of environment in which the emergency occurred; was it on the main level, in an elevated location or in a confined space?

Once you have performed the scene size-up, communicate with safety or management personnel at the site, prior to entering the scene. Call for any specialized teams that may be needed, for example, to manage hazardous materials. Find out if the site has an emergency plan and whether or not that plan has already been activated. Also initiate the incident command system. Always ensure your safety and that of others in the area before entering the scene.

Safety Equipment and Guidelines

Before attempting a rescue in an industrial site, locate and speak to the industrial safety or management personnel. They can guide you through the emergency protocols that should be in place at every industrial site.

Equipment

Hazardous equipment that you may find at industrial sites includes all types of dangerous chemicals and machinery. Chemicals can cause toxic inhalations or absorptions, as well as burns. Be sure to use proper protective gear any time you approach a scene that is suspected of being contaminated with toxic chemicals.

Continued on next page

Enrichment
Agricultural and Industrial Emergencies (continued)

Dangerous types of machinery include presses, hoists, conveyors and crushing devices. As with agricultural emergencies, never approach any equipment that has not been stabilized and shut down. Enlist the help of the safety or management personnel to properly stabilize and shut down machinery.

Dangerous Locations

Dangerous locations on industrial sites include trenches and confined spaces, especially if there are toxic chemicals that can collect there, and elevated locations. A confined space should *not* be entered until the need for an SCBA has been determined and the possible risk of collapse has been evaluated by a person trained to do so. Sick or injured people in elevated (above ground) locations may require rescue by specialized high-angle rescue teams.

Chemicals

A wide range of industrial chemicals is used across various industries, and may be found in a gas, aerosol, liquid or solid state. These chemicals can be hazardous either because of the chemicals they contain (e.g., carcinogens, reproductive hazards, corrosives or agents that affect the lungs or blood) or because of their physical properties (e.g., flammable, combustible, explosive or reactive). Large quantities of these chemicals are present throughout the United States and may pose a risk because of exposure through either routine use or through acts of terrorism. If these hazardous chemicals are released, they could have extremely serious effects on exposed individuals.

In any of their states (gas, aerosol, liquid or solid), these toxic industrial chemicals could enter the body by being inhaled, absorbed through the skin or ingested. The time it takes for these substances to have an effect depends mainly on the route they use to enter the body. Generally, poisoning occurs more quickly if the chemical enters the body through the lungs. *Material Safety Data Sheets* (MSDS) or chemical information cards will provide information on the effects of each chemical on humans, and the symptoms of exposure.

If you or someone you are helping is exposed to a toxic industrial chemical, get yourself and the patient away from the area as quickly as you can. Avoid passing through the contaminated area, if possible.

Employers should have an effective plan in place to assist employees in reaching shelter safely. They may be required to "shelter-in-place" if they cannot get out of a building or if the nearest place with clean air is indoors. Health and safety plans should take into account the possible impact of a release of toxic industrial chemicals. Plans should include guidelines such as monitoring, detection, awareness training, PPE, decontamination and medical surveillance of acutely exposed workers.

Rescuers may have available to them a wide variety of direct reading instruments, as well as procedures for analytical sampling and analysis, to detect toxic industrial chemicals.

During or after a toxic chemical release, and if the duration of the chemical release or airborne concentration of chemicals is unknown, *Occupational Safety and Health Administration* (OSHA) PPE Level B protection should be considered a minimum. Level B requires the highest level of respiratory protection but a lower level of skin protection. Required equipment would include an SCBA, hooded chemical-resistant clothing, special gloves, boots with covers and a hard hat.

23

Injuries to the Head, Neck and Spine

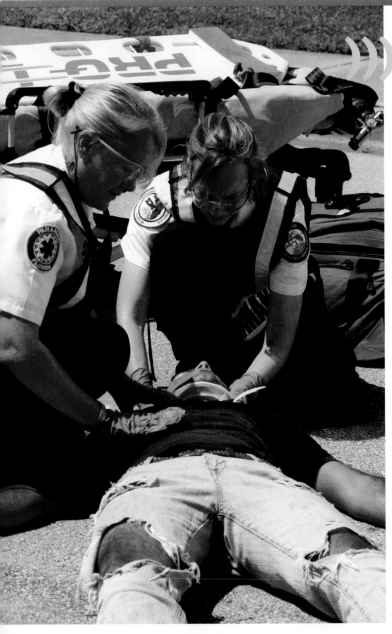

))) YOU ARE THE EMERGENCY MEDICAL RESPONDER

You are the *emergency medical responder* (EMR) with an ambulance crew responding at the scene of a motorcycle accident. As you round a curve and approach the scene, you begin your size-up and see that the motorcycle driver is lying on the road, not moving, and two bystanders appear to be rendering assistance. The motorcycle is a considerable distance from where the driver is located. The motorcyclist is wearing a helmet. As you begin your primary assessment, how should you adjust your methods? What types of injuries should you suspect?

Key Terms

Cerebrospinal fluid: A clear fluid that flows within the ventricles of the brain and around the brain and spinal cord.

Cervical collar: A commercially produced rigid device that is positioned around the neck to limit movement of the head and neck; also called a *C-collar*.

Concussion: A temporary loss of brain function caused by a blow to the head.

In-line stabilization: A technique used to minimize movement and align the patient's head and neck with the spine.

Manual stabilization: A technique used to achieve spinal motion restriction by manually supporting the patient's head and neck in the position found *without* the use of any equipment.

Spinal column: The series of vertebrae extending from the base of the skull to the tip of the tailbone (coccyx); also referred to as the *spine*.

Spinal cord: A cylindrical structure extending from the base of the skull to the lower back, consisting mainly of nerve cells and protected by the spinal column.

Spinal motion restriction: A collective term that includes all methods and techniques used to limit the movement of the spinal column of a patient with a suspected spinal injury.

Learning Objectives

After reading this chapter, and completing the class activities, you will have the information needed to—

- Relate the mechanism of injury to potential injuries of the head, neck and spine.
- List signs and symptoms of head, neck and spinal injuries.
- Describe general care for head, neck and spinal injuries.
- Describe care for specific head injuries.
- Describe the method of determining if a responsive patient may have a spinal injury.

- Explain the importance of minimizing the movement of a victim with a possible head, neck or spinal injury.
- Discuss various ways of preventing head, neck and spinal injuries.
- Explain the methods for removing helmets and other equipment (*Enrichment*).
- Discuss the proper use of *cervical collars* (C-collars) and backboarding (*Enrichment*).

Skill Objectives

After reading this chapter, and completing the class activities, you should be able to—

- Perform the proper care for specific head injuries.
- Demonstrate manual stabilization of the head, neck and spine.

- Demonstrate how to immobilize a head, neck or spinal injury (*Enrichment skill*).

INTRODUCTION

Although injuries to the head, neck and spine account for only a small percentage of all injuries, they cause more than half of the fatalities. Each year, nearly 2 million Americans suffer a head, neck or spinal injury serious enough to require medical care. Most of those injured are males between the ages of 15 and 30. Motor-vehicle collisions account for about half of all head, neck and spinal injuries. Other causes include falls, sports-related mishaps, accidents related to recreational activities and violent acts such as assault (**Fig. 23-1**).

Besides those who die each year in the United States from head, neck and spinal injury, nearly 80,000 people become permanently disabled. These survivors have a wide range of physical and mental impairments including paralysis, speech and memory problems and behavioral disorders.

Fortunately, prompt, appropriate care can help minimize the damage from most head, neck and spinal injuries. In this chapter, you will learn how to recognize when a head, neck or spinal injury may be serious. You will also learn how to provide appropriate care to minimize these injuries.

ANATOMY OF THE HEAD, THE NECK AND THE SPINE

The head contains special sense organs (e.g., eyes, nose and ears), the brain, mouth and related structures. The head is formed by the skull and the face. The four flat bones of the skull are fused together to form a hollow shell. This hollow shell, the *cranial cavity*, contains the brain. The face is

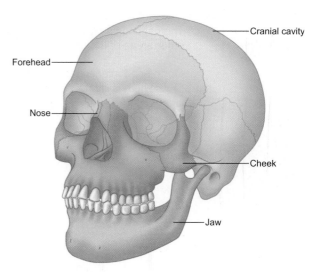

Fig. 23-2: The head

on the front of the skull. The bones of the face include the bones of the cheek, forehead, nose and jaw (**Fig. 23-2**).

The neck contains the esophagus, larynx and part of the trachea. It also contains major blood vessels, muscles and tendons and the cervical bones of the spine.

The back is made up of soft tissue, bones, cartilage, nerves, muscles, tendons and ligaments. It supports the skull, shoulder bones, ribs and pelvis and protects the **spinal cord** and other vital organs.

INJURIES TO THE HEAD
Head Injuries

The head is easily injured because it lacks the padding of muscle and fat that are found in other areas of the body. The most common

Causes of Head, Neck and Spinal Injuries

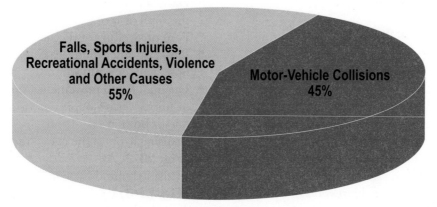

Fig. 23-1: Motor-vehicle collisions account for about half of all head, neck and spinal injuries.

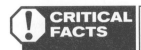
cause of death in patients with head injuries is a lack of oxygen to the brain. Also, swelling of the brain tissues or bleeding within the brain can cause increased pressure inside the skull that, in turn, can cause damage to the brain. A brain injury may lead to altered consciousness with airway and breathing problems. The two types of head injury are open and closed.

Open Head Injuries

Open head injuries involve a break in the skull or occur when an object penetrates the skull. There is direct damage to the skull and brain damage may be involved. Head injuries bleed profusely and a patient may lose blood quickly. With open head injuries, it is important that you—

- Control bleeding promptly with dressings, direct pressure and a pressure bandage, while restricting spinal movement.
- Do *not* apply direct pressure over where there is an obvious skull fracture or depression.
- Do *not* remove any penetrating object; instead stabilize it with thick dressings.

Closed Head Injuries

Closed head injuries occur when the brain is struck against the skull but the skull remains intact. They can also occur from impact with a blunt object. This type of injury may be more challenging to detect as there may *not* be any visible damage to the skull although, in some cases, swelling or a depression is evident. In addition to the general signs of head injury, there may be a softness or depression on the

skull and blood or **cerebrospinal fluid** may be leaking from the nose or ears. If you suspect a closed head injury, do *not* control bleeding using direct pressure, as this could cause further injury by pushing bone fragments into the brain. Because of the rigid nature of the skull, if swelling or bleeding in the brain occurs, brain damage may occur depending on the nature and force of the injury.

Skull Fractures

You should suspect a skull fracture any time there has been significant trauma to the head, even if the patient has suffered a closed head injury. Skull fractures may be accompanied by brain damage, caused by bleeding or swelling within the brain, which is a life-threatening condition. If the patient is showing any of the signs of head injury, a skull fracture may be present and brain injury is possible. A patient with a skull injury should be seen by a more advanced medical professional immediately.

The signs and symptoms of a skull fracture with brain injury include—

- Damage to the skull, including deformity to the skull or face.
- Pain or swelling at the site of injury.
- Blood or other fluids leaking from the mouth, nose, ears or scalp wound.
- Unequal facial movements; drooping, unequal or unresponsive pupils; or vision problems in one or both eyes.
- Bruising around the eyes ("raccoon eyes") **(Fig. 23-3, A)**.
- Bruising behind the ear ("Battle's sign") **(Fig. 23-3, B)**.

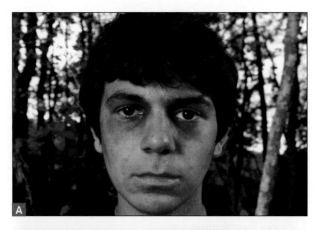

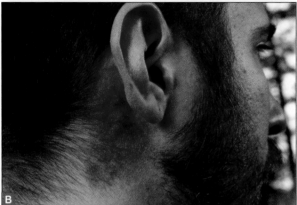

Fig. 23-3, A–B: **(A)** Bruising around the eyes or **(B)** behind the ear indicates a skull fracture with a possible brain injury.

Concussion

A **concussion** is a temporary loss of brain function caused by a blow to the head. It is considered a brain injury, although there may be no detectable damage to the brain. A person who suffers a concussion may *not* always lose consciousness. Concussions are classified from mild to severe, depending on how long it takes the patient to become responsive. However, no matter how mild it may seem, every suspected concussion should be treated seriously.

The effects of a concussion can appear immediately or very soon after the blow to the head occurs. Symptoms can last for days or even longer. Other symptoms may not appear for hours or even days, including mood and cognitive disturbances, sensitivity to light and noise and sleep disturbances. The signs and symptoms of a concussion include—

- Confusion, which may last from moments to several minutes.
- Headache.

- Repeated questioning about what happened.
- Temporary memory loss, especially for periods immediately before and after the injury.
- Brief loss of consciousness.
- Nausea and vomiting.
- Speech problems (patient is unable to answer questions or obey simple commands).
- Blurred vision or light sensitivity.

The mortality rate from a concussion is almost zero and patients usually recover quickly. However, a patient with a suspected concussion should be seen by a medical professional promptly to ensure that the injury is not more serious. The risk of permanent brain damage caused by repeated concussions is significant. An athlete should *not* be allowed to return to play until advised it is okay to do so by a health care provider.

Penetrating Wounds

If an object such as a bullet, knife or nail passes through the skull and lodges in the brain, it is considered a penetrating wound. Penetrating wounds can cause long-term damage.

Do *not* try to remove an object that is impaled in the skull. Stabilize the object and the wound site with bulky dressings, and then dress the surrounding area with sterile gauze. If you suspect an object has penetrated the skull, but it is not visible, cover the area lightly with sterile dressings. *Never* apply firm, direct pressure to a head injury that shows bone fragments, exposed brain tissue or where a depression is visible. Do *not* stop the flow of blood or cerebrospinal fluid draining from the ears or nose. Apply loose gauze dressings. Keep the patient still and minimize movement of the head and neck.

Scalp Injuries

Scalp bleeding can be minor or severe. A scalp injury may bleed more than expected due to the large number of blood vessels in the scalp. The bleeding is usually easily controlled with direct pressure. Because the skull may be injured, be careful to press gently at first. If you feel a depression, a spongy area or bone fragments, do *not* put direct pressure on the wound. Attempt to control bleeding with pressure on the area *around*

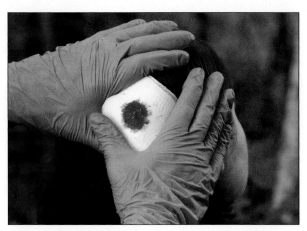
Fig. 23-4: Control bleeding from a scalp injury by applying pressure around the wound. Avoid direct pressure.

the wound (**Fig. 23-4**). Examine the injured area carefully because the patient's hair may hide part of the wound. If you are unsure of the extent of the scalp injury, summon more advanced medical personnel who will be better able to evaluate the injury. Severe bleeding from the scalp can cause shock in young children and infants.

Once bleeding is controlled, apply several dressings and hold them in place with a gloved hand. Secure the dressings with a roller bandage. Use a pressure bandage if necessary.

Signs and Symptoms of Head and Brain Injury

Some of the typical signs and symptoms of head and brain injury include the following:
- Damage to the skull, including deformity to the skull or face
- Pain or swelling at the site of the injury
- Irregular breathing
- A sudden, debilitating headache
- Nausea or vomiting
- Incontinence (involuntary urination or defecation)
- High blood pressure and slowed pulse
- Paralysis or droopiness, often on one side of the body; rigidity of limbs
- Loss of balance

- Asymmetrical facial movements
- Confusion, unresponsiveness or other type of altered mental state
- Facial bruising, including "raccoon eyes" (visible bruising around the eyes)
- External bleeding of the head
- Unusual bumps or depressions on the head
- Blood or other fluids draining from the ears, mouth or nose
- Bruising behind the ears ("Battle's sign")
- Unequal pupil size and unresponsive pupils; disturbance of vision in one eye or both
- Speech problems
- Seizures

Providing Care

Your first step should be to summon more advanced medical care. Making sure to follow standard precautions to prevent disease transmission, provide the following care while waiting for more advanced medical personnel to arrive:
- Establish **manual stabilization** of the head and neck (**Fig. 23-5, A–C**), perform a primary assessment and maintain manual stabilization while at the scene.
- Maintain an open airway. Monitor the airway, suction if needed and administer emergency oxygen, if available.
- Control any bleeding and apply dressings to any open wounds.
- Do *not* apply direct pressure if there are any signs of an obvious skull fracture.
- If there is leaking of cerebrospinal fluid from the ears or a wound in the scalp, cover the area loosely with a sterile gauze dressing.
- Do *not* attempt to remove any penetrating object; instead stabilize it with a bulky dressing.
- Maintain manual stabilization until other *emergency medical services* (EMS) responders relieve you and immobilize the patient on a backboard. If you are trained to do so and protocols allow, apply a **cervical collar** (also called a *C-collar*). (For more information on backboards, refer to **Chapter 5**.)

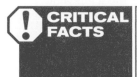
CRITICAL FACTS

There are numerous signs and symptoms of head or brain injury, including irregular breathing, high blood pressure and slowed pulse, loss of balance, external bleeding of the head, bruising behind the ears and seizures—among others.

To provide care for a head injury, maintain an open airway and manual stabilization until other *emergency medical services* (EMS) responders relieve you and immobilize the patient on a backboard.

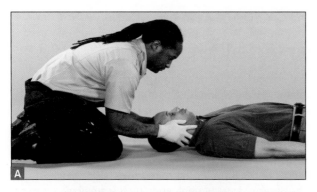

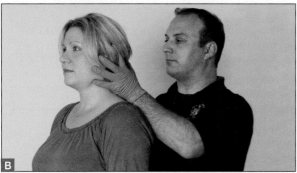

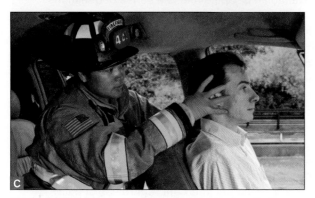

Fig. 23-5, A–C: After summoning more advanced medical care, care for a suspected head and neck injury by establishing manual stabilization, keeping the head in the position found.

- Monitor the patient's vital signs and mental status closely, and watch for any changes in the patient's status.
- Try to calm and reassure the patient. Encourage the patient to engage in conversation with you; it may prevent loss of consciousness.

Nosebleed

Nose injuries often result from a blow by a blunt object. A broken nose may be deformed and will swell. Nosebleeds can also be caused by dryness and high blood pressure. Nosebleeds can

be painful or the nose may be tender, there can be bleeding only from the nose or the patient could vomit swallowed blood. If the patient is unresponsive, the airway can become blocked by blood. Care for soft tissue injuries to the nose as you would other soft tissue injuries. Apply cold packs to reduce swelling and take special care to maintain an open airway. You can usually control bleeding by having the patient sit with the head slightly forward while pinching the nostrils together for about 10 minutes (**Fig. 23-6**). Alternatively, you can apply an ice pack to the bridge of the nose, or put pressure on the upper lip just beneath the nose if there is no trauma to the mouth, teeth or upper jaw. Ice should *not* be applied directly to the skin, as it can damage the skin tissue. Place a cloth between the ice and the skin.

Advanced medical care is needed if the bleeding does not stop, recurs or the patient has a history of high blood pressure. Tell the patient *not* to sniffle or blow his or her nose. If the patient loses consciousness, place the patient on the side to allow the blood to drain away from the airway.

Children may have objects in the nose. Do *not* attempt removal, as special lighting and instruments are required. Reassure the child and parent and call for more advanced medical personnel.

Eye Injuries

Injuries to the eye can involve the eyeball, the bone and the soft tissue surrounding the eye. Blunt objects, like a fist or a baseball, may injure

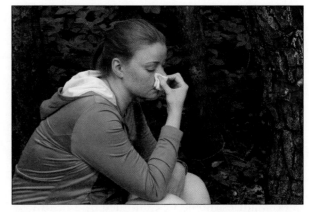

Fig. 23-6: Control a nosebleed by having the patient sit with the head slightly forward, pinching the nostrils together.

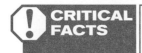 **CRITICAL FACTS** | Nose injuries often result from a blow by a blunt object. A broken nose may be deformed and will swell. Nosebleeds can also be caused by dryness and high blood pressure.

Clearing the Cervical Spine

There are two techniques that can be used to clear a cervical spine. The National Emergency X-Radiography Utilization Study (NEXUS) Low-Risk Criteria and the Canadian Cervical Spine (C-Spine) rule. According to the NEXUS Low-Risk Criteria, in order to clear a cervical spinal injured patient, C-spine radiography is indicated for trauma patients unless they exhibit all of the following criteria:

- No posterior midline C-spine tenderness (Do *not* clear the patient if there is tenderness upon palpation of the C-spine.)
- No evidence of intoxication (Do *not* clear the patient if the patient or a bystander noted they had been drinking or if you find evidence of intoxication during the secondary assessment, such as the smell of alcohol on the patient's breath.)
- Normal level of alertness (Do *not* clear the patient if during the secondary assessment, you note that the patient is not fully alert.)
- No focal neurological deficit (A focal neurologic deficit is a problem in nerve, spinal cord or brain function that affects a specific location, such as the left face. It also refers to any problem with a specific nervous system function, such as memory.)
- No painful distracting injuries (Painful distracting injuries can include, but are not limited to, a long bone fracture, a large laceration or critical burns.)

The Canadian C-Spine rule is used for alert (Glasgow Coma Scale [GCS] score of 15) and stable trauma patients where C-spine injury is a concern. The Canadian C-Spine rule is a series of questions that indicate whether you can clear the spine.

- Are there any high-risk factors which mandate spinal motion restriction? These include being over 65 years of age, a dangerous *mechanism of injury* (MOI) (axial load to head, for example from diving; motor-vehicle collision at a high speed, rollover or ejection; injury sustained while riding motorized recreational vehicles; or bicycle collision), and numbness or tingling in the extremities. If the answer is yes, continue spinal motion restriction. If the answer is no, continue with the questions.
- Are there any low-risk factors which allow safe assessment of range of motion? These include a simple rear-end motor-vehicle collision (excludes being pushed into oncoming traffic, being hit by a bus or large truck, a rollover or being hit by a high speed vehicle), a sitting position, being ambulatory at any time, a delayed onset of neck pain, and absence of midline C-spine tenderness. If the answer is no, continue spinal motion restriction. If the answer is yes, continue with the questions.
- Is the patient voluntarily able to actively rotate the neck 45° to the left and right regardless of pain? If the patient is unable, continue spinal motion restriction. If the patient is able, it is acceptable to clear the spine.

the eye and surrounding area or a smaller object may penetrate the eyeball. Care for open and closed wounds around the eye as you would for any other soft tissue injury.

Injuries to the eyeball itself require different care. Injuries that penetrate the eyeball or cause the eye to be removed from its socket are very serious and can cause blindness. *Never* put direct pressure on the eyeball. Remember that *all* eye injuries should be examined by a health care provider. It is *not* necessary to cover both the injured and the uninjured eyes, because sympathetic or involuntary eye movement occurs even when both eyes are covered and not exposed to outside stimuli. Covering both eyes can also cause fear and increase anxiety, especially in children, and pose a safety risk to the patient.

Assessment

To assess what type of care the patient will need, first determine when the injury occurred, whether one or both eyes were injured and when the patient first noticed the symptoms. Then, using a small penlight, follow these guidelines:

- Check the eye sockets and eyelids for bruising, lacerations, swelling or deformity.
- Check the whites of the eyes for foreign objects, discoloration or discharge.
- Check that the eyes can move in all directions, and that the pupils react equally to light.

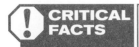
Do *not* attempt to remove an object that is impaled in the eye. Keep the patient in a supine position and enlist someone to help stabilize the patient's head.

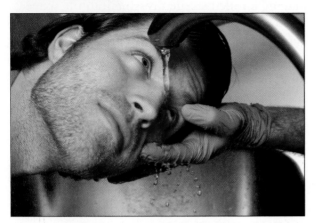

Fig. 23-7: Gently flush an eye with a foreign object or one that has undergone chemical exposure with water.

Ensure that there is no pain when the eyes move.
- Check that the pupils are equal in size.
- Check that there are no lacerations or foreign objects in the eyeballs.

Foreign Bodies

Foreign bodies that get in the eye, such as dirt or slivers of wood or metal, are irritating, painful and can cause significant damage to the cornea. It is important to tell the patient *not* to rub the eyes. *Never* touch the eye and always follow standard precautions when caring for the patient.

If you determine there is a foreign body in the eye, try to remove it by telling the patient to blink several times. If the object is visible on the lower eyelid, pull the eyelid down and try to remove the object with the corner of a sterile gauze pad. Be careful *not* to touch the eyeball.

Next, gently flush the eye with irrigation/saline solution or water (**Fig. 23-7**). After irrigating, if the object is visible on the upper eyelid, gently roll the upper eyelid back over a cotton swab and attempt to remove the object with the corner of a sterile gauze pad, being careful *not* to touch the eyeball. If the object remains, the patient should receive advanced medical care. Cover the injured eye with an eye pad/shield.

Chemical Exposure to the Eye

If chemicals have been in contact with the patient's eyes, irrigate the affected eye or eyes with clean water for at least 20 minutes. If only one eye is affected, make sure you do *not* let the water run into the unaffected eye. Continue care while transporting the patient, if you can.

Impaled Objects

Do *not* attempt to remove an object that is impaled in the eye. Keep the patient in a face-up position and enlist someone to help stabilize the patient's head. Stabilize the object by encircling the eye with a gauze dressing or soft sterile cloth, being careful *not* to apply any pressure to the area. Position bulky dressings around the impaled object, such as roller gauze, and then cover it with a shield such as a paper cup (**Fig. 23-8, A–B**). *Do not* use Styrofoam®-type

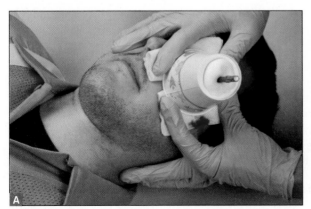

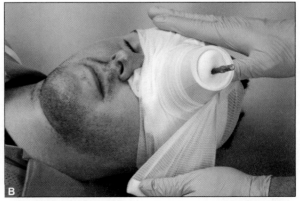

Fig. 23-8, A–B: To care for an impaled object in the eye, do not attempt to remove an impaled object from the eye. Instead, **(A)** stabilize the object with a shield such as a paper cup and **(B)** bandage the cup in place.

materials, as small particles can break off and get into the eye.

The shield should *not* touch the object. Bandage the shield and dressing in place with a self-adhering bandage and roller bandage covering the patient's injured eye, to keep the object stable and minimize movement. Comfort and reassure the patient. Do *not* leave the patient unattended.

Oral Injuries

Patients with facial injuries may have injuries to the teeth or jaws. Situations that fracture or dislocate the jaw can also cause head, neck or spinal injuries. Maintaining an open and clear airway and restricting spinal motion should be priorities.

The signs and symptoms of oral injuries include—

- Teeth that do not meet or are uneven, loose or missing.
- A patient who is unable to open or close the mouth.
- Saliva mixed with blood.
- Pain in areas around the ears.
- Difficulty or pain when speaking.

If the patient is bleeding from the mouth, and a head, neck or spinal injury is *not* suspected, place the patient in a seated position with the head tilted slightly forward or on the side to allow any blood to drain from the mouth.

If the injury has penetrated the lip, place a rolled dressing between the lip and the gum and another dressing on the outer surface of the lip. If the tongue is bleeding, apply a dressing and direct pressure. Cold compresses may alleviate pain and swelling.

If the injury has knocked out a tooth, try to find it. Handle the tooth by the crown, rinse it gently under running water and place it in a glass of milk. If milk is not available, place the tooth in clean water or moistened sterile gauze. If the patient is conscious and able to cooperate, rinse out the mouth with cold tap water if available. Control the bleeding by placing a rolled sterile dressing into the space left by the missing tooth. Have the patient gently bite down to maintain pressure. Do *not* try to reimplant the tooth yourself. Do *not* allow the tooth to dry out. Contact a dentist or bring the tooth and the patient to an emergency care center as soon as possible.

Leave intact dentures in position to support the mouth structure. Remove broken dentures and send them with the patient to assist the oral surgeon with jaw alignment.

INJURIES TO THE NECK AND SPINE

Injuries to the neck or spine can damage both bone and soft tissue, including the spinal cord. It is difficult to determine the extent of damage in neck or spinal injuries. Since generally only X-rays, *computerized tomography* (CT or CAT) scans or *magnetic resonance imaging* (MRI) scans can show the severity of these injuries, you should always care for them as if they are serious.

Mechanism of Injury

Consider the possibility of a serious neck or spinal injury in a number of situations. These may include—

- Any injury caused by entry into shallow water.
- Injury as a result of a fall greater than a standing height.
- An injury involving a diving board, water slide or entering water from a significant height, such as an embankment, cliff or tower.
- Any injury, such as from a car or other vehicle collision, involving severe blunt force to the person's head or trunk.
- A motor-vehicle, motorized cycle or bicycle collision involving a pedestrian or driver or

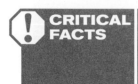
CRITICAL FACTS

Injuries to the neck or spine can damage both bone and soft tissue, including the spinal cord. It is difficult to determine the extent of damage in neck or spinal injuries. Always care for these types of injuries as if they are serious.

You should suspect possible serious neck or spinal injury in many situations, including but not limited to diving board accidents, motor-vehicle accidents where a person has been thrown from the vehicle and situations where hard hats or helmet have been broken.

passengers not wearing safety belts or one that results in a broken windshield or a deformed steering wheel.
- Injury as the result of a hanging.
- Any unresponsive trauma patient.
- Injury involving a penetrating trauma to the head, neck or torso.
- Any person thrown from a motor vehicle.
- Any injury in which a patient's industrial hard hat or helmet is broken, including a motorcycle, bicycle, football or other sports helmet.
- A person who has other painful injuries, especially of the head and neck.
- A person complaining of neck or back pain or tenderness, tingling in the extremities or weakness.
- An injured person who appears to be frail or over 65 years of age.
- A person who is not fully alert or appears to be intoxicated.
- Someone with an obvious head or neck injury.
- Has sensory deficit or muscle weakness involving the torso or upper extremities.
- Children less than 3 years of age with evidence of head or neck trauma.

Lacerations of the Neck

The carotid artery and jugular vein are both located in the neck, and injuries to one or both will produce serious, possibly fatal bleeding (**Fig. 23-9**). An open wound in the neck may result in an air embolism, which is caused by air being sucked into the wound. A fractured larynx or collapsed trachea is also a common neck injury. If the laceration is caused by an object impaled in the neck, do *not* attempt to remove it.

Signs and Symptoms of Neck and Spinal Injuries

The signs and symptoms of neck injuries may include—
- Obvious lacerations, swelling or bruising.
- Objects impaled in the neck.
- Profuse external bleeding.
- Impaired breathing as a result of the injury.
- Difficulty speaking or complete loss of voice.
- A crackling sound when the patient is speaking or breathing, due to air escaping from an injured trachea or larynx.
- Obstructed airway caused by swelling of the throat.

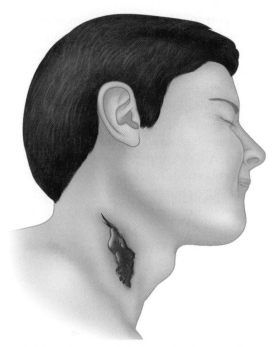

Fig. 23-9: Injuries to the carotid artery or jugular vein will produce serious, possibly fatal, bleeding.

The signs and symptoms of spinal injuries may include—
- Pain or pressure in the back, independent of movement or palpation.
- Tenderness in the area of the injury.
- Pain associated with moving.
- Numbness, weakness, tingling, or loss of feeling or movement in the extremities.
- Partial or complete loss of movement or feeling below the suspected level of injury.
- Difficulty breathing or shallow breathing.
- Loss of bladder and/or bowel control.

If the patient can walk, move and has feeling in the arms and legs, it does *not* necessarily rule out the possibility of injury to the bones of the spine or to the spinal cord.

Providing Care

If you suspect a patient has a neck or spinal injury, restrict spinal motion and control any bleeding. Do *not* move the patient or ask the patient to move to try to find a pain response. It is essential when treating neck injuries to maintain an open airway. If the patient is wearing a helmet, do *not* remove it unless you have been trained to do so, or unless it is necessary to access and assess the patient's airway. Because movement of an injured neck or spine can irreversibly damage the spinal cord, keep the patient still. To restrict spinal motion, use manual stabilization. Perform a primary assessment on the scene while maintaining manual stabilization. Assess the patient's pulse, movement and feeling in the extremities.

Approach patients from the front so they can see you without turning their heads, and tell patients to respond verbally to your questions. Ask the responsive patient the following questions, while maintaining manual stabilization, to further assess the situation:

- Does your neck or back hurt?
- What happened?
- Where does it hurt?
- Can you move your hands and feet?
- Can you feel where I am touching?

For an unresponsive patient, maintain an open airway using the jaw-thrust (without head extension) maneuver and assist ventilation if needed. You *should not* attempt to align the head and neck with the body unless you cannot maintain an open airway, you need to remove a helmet or you need to assist with the application of a C-collar.

Administer emergency oxygen if it is available. While obtaining further information, manually stabilize the head and neck in the position in which it was found. Obtain any further information from others at the scene to determine MOI and the patient's mental status before your arrival.

Keeping the head, neck and spine from moving (spinal motion restriction) helps prevent further damage to the **spinal column**. If a second rescuer is available, that person can provide care for any other conditions while you keep the head and neck stable.

Assist more advanced medical personnel upon arrival by maintaining manual stabilization. More advanced medical personnel will then apply a cervical collar to further immobilize the head and neck. If you must move the patient, secure the patient to a backboard prior to moving.

Helmet Removal

When you encounter a patient who has sustained injuries while wearing a helmet, you must assess whether it is necessary to remove the helmet. As always, assess breathing and pulse and determine your course of action.

Since properly fitted helmets fit snugly to the head, it is difficult to remove one without moving the patient's head and neck. Removing a helmet requires a minimum of two rescuers. When providing care to a patient with a helmet, you should only remove it if it is impeding your care, you are unable to access and assess the airway or if the patient is in cardiac arrest. Otherwise, do *not* try to remove it. If the patient is breathing and the airway is clear, maintain manual stabilization with the helmet in place.

Some helmets are closed in front with face protectors. If the protector cannot be lifted out of the way, it is preferable that it be cut it off rather than the helmet removed.

Situations that may require removing the helmet include those in which—

- You cannot access or assess the patient's airway and breathing.
- The airway is impeded and cannot be opened with the helmet on.
- The patient is in cardiac arrest.
- You cannot immobilize the spine.

If a helmet is loose, this does *not* necessarily mean you must remove it. Try to stabilize the helmet by adding padding between the helmet and the patient's head.

Preventing Head, Neck and Spinal Injuries

While some injuries are unavoidable, many others are preventable by being aware of potential dangers in the environment and taking appropriate safety measures. To prevent head, neck and spinal injuries, take the following steps:

- Know your risk. Be aware of your surroundings and wear appropriate safety equipment and protective devices such as padding, footwear, helmets and eye protection.
- Do not dive into a body of water if you are unsure of the depth.
- Wear your seatbelt in a motor vehicle. Insist that passengers wear seatbelts and *always* transport children in approved child safety seats in the back of the vehicle, according to state and local regulations.
- To prevent falls, safety-proof your home and workplace. Ensure that hallways and stairways are well lit and stairways have handrails.

- Always use a stepstool or a stepladder to reach objects out of reach. Do *not* attempt to pull heavy objects that are out of reach over your head.
- Use good lifting techniques when lifting and carrying heavy objects.
- Use nonslip treads or carpet on stairways, and secure any area rugs with double-sided tape.
- Use nonslip mats in the bathtub, or install handrails.
- Know your risk for osteoporosis, a bone disease responsible for many spine, hip, wrist and other fractures. Make sure you have enough calcium in your diet, and engage in weight-bearing exercises like walking or weight training to increase bone density and stimulate new bone formation.

PUTTING IT ALL TOGETHER

In this chapter, you learned how to recognize and care for serious head, neck and spinal injuries. To decide whether an injury is serious, you must consider its cause. Often the cause is the best indicator of whether an injury to the head, neck or spine should be considered serious. You must also carefully assess the signs and symptoms. If you have any doubts about the seriousness of an injury, summon more advanced medical personnel.

Like injuries elsewhere on the body, injuries to the head, neck and spine often involve both soft tissues and bones. Control bleeding as necessary, usually with direct pressure on the wound. With scalp injuries, however, be careful *not* to apply pressure to a possible skull fracture. With eye injuries, remember *not* to apply pressure on the eyeball.

If you suspect that the patient may have a serious head, neck or spinal injury, minimize movement of the injured area when providing care. Minimizing movement is best accomplished by manual stabilization. Administer emergency oxygen if it is available. Apply a cervical collar and secure the patient to a backboard if you must move the patient, you are trained to do so and local protocols allow.

Many injuries are preventable if simple safety precautions are followed. Know your risks and mitigate your danger of injury.

YOU ARE THE EMERGENCY MEDICAL RESPONDER

As you assess the patient, you find that you cannot determine the status of the airway or breathing because of the patient's helmet. What injuries should you suspect? What can you do to access and assess the airway?

SKILLsheet

Manual Stabilization

NOTE: Call for more advanced medical personnel for a head, neck or spinal injury, while minimizing movement of the head, neck and spine.

STEP 1

Minimize movement by placing your hands on *both* sides of the patient's head.

STEP 2

Support the head in the position found.

NOTE: Do *not* align the head and neck with the spine if the head is sharply turned to one side, there is pain on movement or if you feel any resistance when attempting to align the head and neck with the spine. Instead, gently maintain the head and neck in the position found.

STEP 3

Maintain an open airway. Control any external bleeding and keep the patient from getting chilled or overheated.

NOTE: Gently position the patient's head in line with the body if you cannot maintain an open airway, you need to remove a helmet or you need to apply a C-collar.

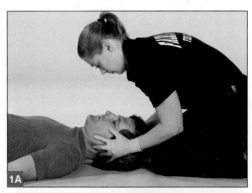

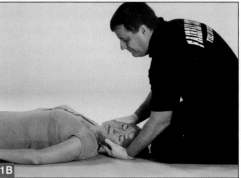

SKILLsheet

Controlling Bleeding from an Open Head Wound

NOTE: Always follow standard precautions and summon more advanced medical personnel if necessary.

STEP 1

Apply direct pressure.
- ◆ Place a sterile dressing or clean cloth over the wound and press gently against the wound with your hand.
- ◆ Do *not* put direct pressure on the wound if you feel a depression, spongy area or bone fragments.
- ◆ Press gently on the area *around* the wound.

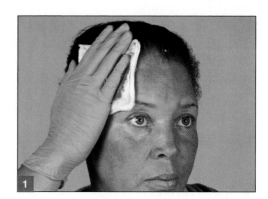

STEP 2

Elevate the body part.
- ◆ Elevate the head and shoulders *unless* you suspect an injury to the spine.

STEP 3

Apply a pressure bandage.
- ◆ Using a roller bandage, cover the dressing completely, using overlapping turns.
- ◆ Tie or tape the bandage in place.
- ◆ If blood soaks through the bandage, place additional dressings and bandages over the wound.

STEP 4

If bleeding stops–
- ◆ Determine if further care is needed.

STEP 5

If bleeding does *not* stop–
- ◆ Summon more advanced medical personnel.

SKILLsheet

Bandaging an Eye with an Injury from an Impaled Object

NOTE: Do not attempt to remove an object that is impaled in the eye. Keep the patient in a face-up position and enlist someone to help stabilize the patient's head.

STEP 1

Stabilize the object by encircling the eye with a gauze dressing or soft sterile cloth.

◆ Do *not* apply any pressure to the area.

STEP 2

Position bulky dressings around the impaled object, such as roller gauze, and then cover it with a shield such as a paper cup.

◆ The shield should *not* touch the object.

NOTE: Do not use Styrofoam®-type materials, as small particles can break off and get into the eye.

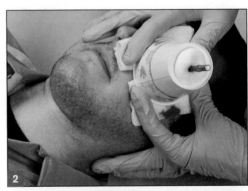

STEP 3

Bandage the shield and dressing in place with a self-adhering bandage and roller bandage covering the patient's injured eye to keep the object stable and minimize movement.

STEP 4

Comfort and reassure the patient.

NOTE: Do *not* leave the patient unattended.

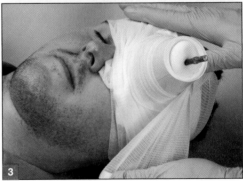

SKILLsheet

Caring for Foreign Bodies in the Eye

NOTE: Tell the patient *not* to rub the eyes. *Never* touch the eye and always follow standard precautions when caring for the patient.

STEP 1

Remove the foreign object from the eye.
- ◆ Tell the patient to blink several times.
- ◆ If the object is visible on the lower eyelid, pull the eyelid down and try to remove the object with the corner of a sterile gauze pad.

NOTE: Be careful *not* to touch the eyeball.

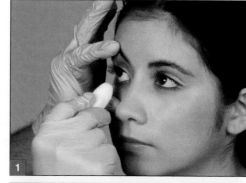

STEP 2

Gently flush the eye with irrigation/saline solution or water.

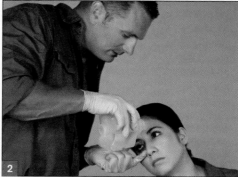

STEP 3

If the object is visible on the upper eyelid, gently roll the upper eyelid back over a cotton swab and attempt to remove the object with the corner of a sterile gauze pad, being careful *not* to touch the eyeball.

NOTE: If the object remains, the patient should receive advanced medical care. Cover the injured eye with an eye pad/shield.

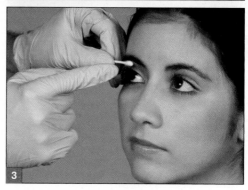

Enrichment
Removing Helmets and Other Equipment

If you determine that it is necessary to remove a helmet from a patient to provide care, you must do so correctly to avoid causing further harm to the patient.

Helmets fall into multiple categories including sports helmets and motorcycle helmets. Sports helmets usually have an opening in front, which allows for easier access to the airway. You can usually remove the face mask on a football helmet by unsnapping the plastic clips that hold the face mask to the helmet, or by cutting the plastic clips. It is more difficult to access the airway with a motorcycle helmet in place, as they usually cover the full face and the airway.

The steps for a *non-athletic* helmet removal require two rescuers and are as follows:

1. If the patient is wearing glasses, remove them first before attempting helmet removal.
2. The first rescuer applies stabilization by holding both sides of the helmet, with fingers on the patient's lower jaw **(Fig. 23-10, A)**. This will prevent the helmet from moving around if the strap is loose.
3. The second rescuer loosens the strap at the D-rings while the first rescuer maintains stabilization **(Fig. 23-10, B)**.
4. The second rescuer then places one hand on the patient's mandible at an angle, with the thumb on one side, and the long and index fingers on the other. With the other hand, the second rescuer holds the back of the patient's head (occipital region).
5. The first rescuer then removes the helmet halfway, making sure to clear the ears, while the second rescuer readjusts hand position under the patient's head. The first rescuer then removes the helmet the rest of the way, making sure to tilt backward to avoid hitting the nose **(Fig. 23-10, C)**.
6. The second rescuer maintains manual stabilization throughout, from below, preventing head tilt. After the helmet has been removed, the first rescuer replaces the hands over the ears, taking over responsibility for stabilization **(Fig. 23-10, D)**.
7. The first rescuer maintains manual stabilization from above until a cervical collar can be applied and complete immobilization is achieved with a backboard **(Fig. 23-10, E)**.

For an *emergency medical responder* (EMR), the removal of athletic equipment, such as football helmets, is usually more challenging than the removal of a motorcycle helmet. Unlike a motorcycle helmet, removal of a football or hockey helmet alone without removal of the athlete's shoulder pads increases the risk of cervical movement and further spinal injury. If an athlete is suspected of having a spinal injury, the helmet should *only* be removed when–

- The face mask cannot be removed after a reasonable period of time to gain access to the airway.
- The design of the helmet and chin strap, even in the absence of the face mask, does not allow for a controlled airway or adequate ventilation.
- The design of the helmet and chin straps do not hold the head securely in place (immobilization of the helmet does not also immobilize the head).
- The helmet prevents immobilization of the patient for transport in an appropriate position.

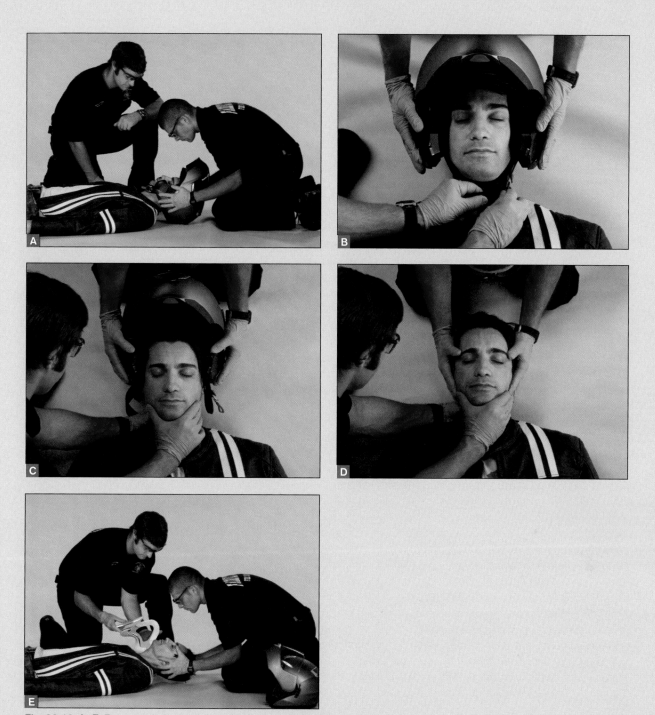

Fig. 23-10, A–E: Remove a helmet only if it is impeding care or blocking access to the airway or if the patient is in cardiac arrest.

Continued on next page

Enrichment
Removing Helmets and Other Equipment (continued)

The face mask *should* be removed after an athlete is suspected of having a spinal injury, even if the patient is still conscious. A face mask is held in place using four loop-straps, two on the top and one on either side. Each of these loop-straps must be removed by one EMR while a second responder minimizes neck movement and maintains the neck in a neutral position **(Fig. 23-11, A)**. The loop-straps can be removed using a variety of tools such as a screwdriver, pruner shear and several other commercial devices designed specifically for this task **(Fig. 23-11, B)**. However, this is a skilled task, requiring practice. The two side loop-straps are removed first, followed by the two top loop-straps **(Fig. 23-11, C)**. *Never* use items such as razor blades, scalpels or *emergency medical technician* (EMT) or trauma shears to remove the loop-straps, as these items increase the risk of injury to the athlete and the EMR and may delay removal of the face mask.

To remove a helmet and shoulder pads, one EMR must provide manual stabilization while a second EMR cuts away the chin strap, shoulder pad straps and jersey. This is followed by removal of the internal cheek pads (using a tongue depressor) and deflating the helmet's air bladder system, if necessary (using a syringe or air pump), while another trained rescuer stabilizes the chin and back of the neck. Two to four other trained rescuers are placed at strategic locations along the body to support the shoulders, upper torso and other locations based on the size of the athlete. The athlete is lifted and the helmet is slid off the head by rotating the helmet in an anterior direction. Do *not* attempt to spread the helmet by the ear holes, as this will only tighten the helmet on the head causing further spinal movement and possible injury. Once the helmet is off, the shoulder pads are immediately removed by spreading apart the front panels and pulling them around the head. Remove any clothing or equipment under the shoulder pads. Lower the athlete back to the ground.

Removal of protective equipment such as a football helmet and shoulder pads is a skilled technique, requiring hours of practice. It often requires a minimum of five rescuers trained in this skill. If this type of situation is encountered during an athletic event, look to the certified athletic trainer to assist in removal of the face mask, helmet and shoulder pads, as the necessary tools will be included in athletic emergency kits. Prior planning and interdisciplinary practice among the EMR, certified athletic trainer and emergency department personnel is recommended prior to the beginning of the athletic season, particularly for football.

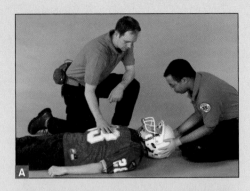
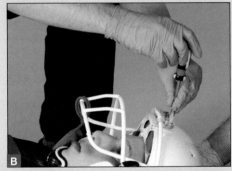
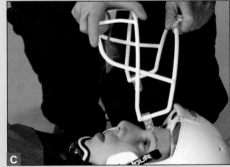

Fig. 23-11, A–C: To remove a face mask:
(A) One EMR should minimize neck movement, maintaining a neutral position for the neck.
(B) A second EMR removes the loop-straps.
(C) Once the loop-straps are removed, the face mask can be removed.

Enrichment
Cervical Collars and Backboarding

A cervical collar (also called a *C-collar*) is a rigid device positioned around the neck to limit movement of the head and neck **(Fig. 23-12)**. Once you have **in-line stabilization**, a rigid C-collar should be applied if local protocols and medical direction permit. This collar helps minimize movement of the head and neck and keeps the head in-line with the body. Applying a C-collar requires two rescuers. While one rescuer maintains in-line stabilization, another carefully applies an appropriately sized C-collar. An appropriately sized collar is one that fits securely, with the patient's chin resting in the proper position and the head maintained in-line with the body **(Fig. 23-13)**. Some C-collars come with specific manufacturer's instructions for proper sizing. Do *not* apply a C-collar in a circumstance in which you would not want to align the head with the body.

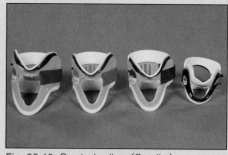

Fig. 23-12: Cervical collars (C-collar)

Once a C-collar has been applied and in-line stabilization maintained, the patient's entire body should be immobilized. This can be done using the following equipment:

- A backboard
- Head immobilizer
- Straps

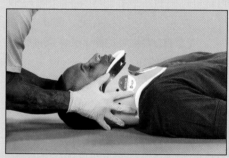

Fig. 23-13: A C-collar should fit securely, with the patient's chin resting in proper position.

If you do not have a backboard available, support the patient in the position in which the patient was found until more advanced medical personnel arrive. Once a C-collar is in place, the patient is positioned on a backboard. This is done by "log-rolling" the patient onto the board. This technique keeps the head in-line with the body. It requires a minimum of two rescuers: one to support the head and maintain in-line stabilization and another to position the backboard and roll the patient's body. However, it is highly preferable to have at least *three* rescuers available to perform this technique. One rescuer can provide in-line stabilization and the others can log-roll the patient and position the backboard.

Once the patient is on the board, use several straps to secure the patient's body to the backboard. There are several ways to apply the straps used to secure the patient onto the board. A common way is to secure the chest by crisscrossing the straps. Regardless of which method is used, the straps should be snug but not so tight as to restrict movement of the chest during breathing. With the remaining straps, secure the patient's hips, thighs and legs. Secure the hands in front of the body.

Once the patient's body is secured to the backboard, secure the patient's head. If the patient's head does not appear to be resting in-line with the body, you may need to place a small amount of padding, such as a small folded towel, to support the head. Normally, approximately 1 inch of padding is all that is needed to keep the head in-line with the body and at the same time provide comfort for the patient. Next, use a commercially made head-immobilization device. Many of these devices use Velcro® straps to secure the head. You should follow the manufacturer's directions when using these devices.

SKILLsheet

Immobilizing a Head, Neck or Spinal Injury

NOTE: Call for more advanced medical personnel for a head, neck or spinal injury, while minimizing movement of the head, neck and spine.

STEP 1

Apply in-line stabilization.
- Place your hands on *both* sides of the patient's head.
- Gently position the head in-line with the body, if necessary.
- Support the head in that position.

NOTE: Do *not* align the head and neck with the spine if the head is sharply turned to one side, there is pain on movement or if you feel any resistance when attempting to align the head and neck with the spine. Instead, gently maintain the head and neck in the position found.

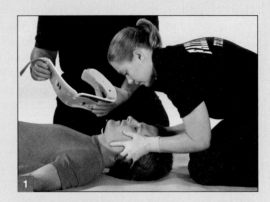

STEP 2

Apply a cervical collar (C-collar).
- One rescuer maintains in-line stabilization.
- Second rescuer applies appropriately sized C-collar (correct size as determined by manufacturer's instructions).

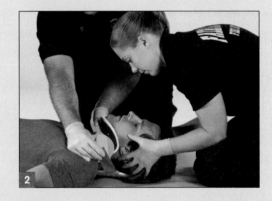

STEP 3

Log-roll the patient onto a backboard.
- One rescuer maintains in-line stabilization of the head.
- Additional rescuers support patient's shoulders, hips and legs.
- Roll the patient in unison, keeping the patient's head and spine in alignment until the patient is resting on his or her side.

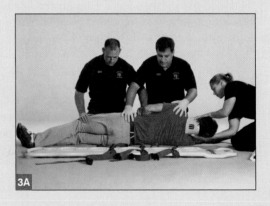

- Position the backboard.
- Log-roll the patient onto the backboard.

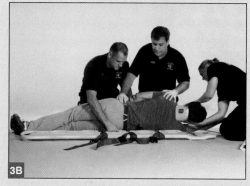

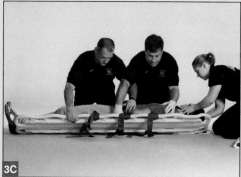

STEP 4

Secure the patient's body.
- Secure the patient's chest.
- Secure the patient's arms, hips, thighs and legs with the remaining straps.
- If necessary, secure the patient's hands in front of the body.

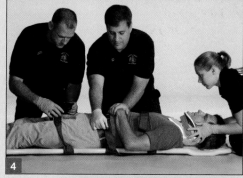

STEP 5

Secure the patient's head.
- Place padding beneath the head if it is not resting in-line with the body.
- If a commercial head immobilizer is not available, place a folded or rolled blanket around the head and neck.
- Secure the forehead.

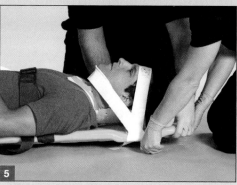

UNIT

7

SPECIAL POPULATIONS

24 Childbirth

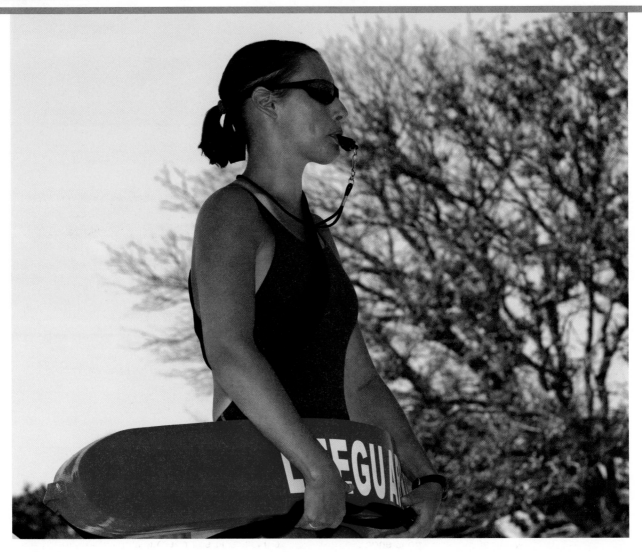

))) **YOU ARE THE EMERGENCY MEDICAL RESPONDER**

You are the lifeguard at a local pool and are working as the *emergency medical responder* (EMR) at that facility for the day. A young woman runs over to you and tells you that she thinks her older sister is in labor. How should you respond?

Key Terms

Abruptio placentae: Placental abruption; a life-threatening emergency that occurs when the placenta detaches from the uterus.

Amniotic fluid: The fluid in the amniotic sac; bathes and protects the fetus.

Amniotic sac: "Bag of waters"; sac that encloses the fetus during pregnancy and bursts during the birthing process.

APGAR score: A mnemonic that describes five measures used to assess the newborn: Appearance, Pulse, Grimace, Activity and Respiration.

Birth canal: The passageway from the uterus to the outside of the body through which a baby passes during birth.

Bloody show: Thick discharge from the vagina that occurs during labor as the *mucous plug* (mucus with pink or light red streaks) is expelled; often signifies the onset of labor.

Braxton Hicks contractions: False labor; irregular contractions of the uterus that do not intensify or become more frequent as genuine labor contractions do.

Breech birth: The delivery of a baby's feet or buttocks first.

Bulb syringe: Small nasal syringe to remove secretions from the newborn's mouth and nose.

Cervix: The lower, narrow part of the *uterus* (womb) that forms a canal that opens into the vagina, which leads to the outside of the body; upper part of the birth canal.

Cesarean section: C-section; delivery of a baby through an incision in the mother's belly and uterus.

Contraction: During labor, the rhythmic tightening and relaxing of muscles of the uterus.

Crowning: The phase during labor when the baby's head is visible at the opening of the vagina.

Dilation: The process of enlargement or stretching; during delivery, refers to the opening of the cervix to allow the baby to be born.

Dropping: "Engagement" or "lightening"; when the baby drops into a lower position and is engaged in the mother's pelvis; usually takes place a few weeks before labor begins.

Eclampsia: A complication during pregnancy in which the patient has convulsions or seizures associated with high blood pressure.

Ectopic pregnancy: A pregnancy outside of the uterus; most often occurs in the fallopian tubes.

Embryo: The term used to describe the early stage of development in the uterus, from fertilization to the beginning of the third month.

Fetal monitoring: A variety of tests used to measure fetal stress, either internally or externally.

Fetus: The term used to describe the stage of development in the uterus after the embryo stage, beginning at the start of the third month.

Hemorrhagic shock: Shock due to excessive blood loss.

Implantation: The attachment of the fertilized egg to the lining of the uterus, 6 or 7 days after conception.

Labor: The birth process, beginning with the contraction of the uterus and dilation of the cervix and ending with the stabilization and recovery of the mother.

Meconium aspiration: Aspiration of the first bowel movement of the newborn; can be a sign of fetal stress and can lead to meconium aspiration syndrome.

Miscarriage: A spontaneous end to pregnancy before the 20th week; usually because of birth defects in the fetus or placenta; also called a *spontaneous abortion.*

Mucous plug: A collection of mucus that blocks the opening into the cervix and is expelled, usually toward the end of the pregnancy, when the cervix begins to dilate.

Multiple birth: Two or more births in the same pregnancy.

Obstetric pack: A first aid kit containing items especially helpful in emergency delivery and initial care after birth; items can include personal protective equipment, towels, clamps, ties, sterile scissors and bulb syringes.

Placenta: An organ attached to the uterus and unborn baby through which nutrients are delivered; expelled after the baby is delivered.

Placenta previa: Placental implantation that occurs lower on the uterine wall, touching or covering the cervix; can be dangerous if it is still covering part of the cervix at the time of delivery.

Preeclampsia: A type of toxemia that occurs during pregnancy; a condition characterized by high blood pressure and excess protein in the urine after the 20th week of pregnancy.

Premature birth: Birth that occurs before the end of the 37th week of pregnancy.

Prolapsed cord: A complication of childbirth in which a loop of the umbilical cord protrudes through the vagina before delivery of the baby.

Stabilization: The final stage of labor in which the mother begins to recover and stabilize after giving birth.

Stillbirth: Fetal death; death of a fetus after 20 weeks gestation or of a fetus weighing more than 350 grams.

Toxemia: An abnormal condition associated with the presence of toxic substances in the blood.

Trimester: A three-month period; there are three trimesters in a normal pregnancy.

Umbilical cord: A flexible structure that attaches the placenta to the fetus, allowing for the passage of blood, nutrients and waste.

Uterus: A pear-shaped organ in a woman's pelvis in which an embryo forms and develops into a baby; also called the *womb*.

Vagina: Tract leading from the uterus to the outside of the body; often referred to during labor as the *birth canal*.

Learning Objectives

After reading this chapter, and completing the class activities, you will have the information needed to—

- Describe each trimester of pregnancy.
- Describe the four stages of labor.
- Describe how to help the mother with labor and normal delivery.
- Describe how to assess a newborn.
- Describe how to control bleeding after birth.

- Describe how to care for the newborn and mother.
- List complications during pregnancy.
- Describe complications during delivery.
- Describe additional complications during pregnancy and delivery *(Enrichment)*.

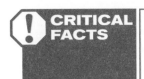

The duration of a full-term pregnancy spans a 9-month period, or 38 weeks from the time in which the embryo becomes implanted into the woman's uterus. The due date is usually calculated as 40 weeks from the woman's last menstrual period. Pregnancy is broken down into 3 trimesters, each lasting approximately 3 months.

INTRODUCTION

Someday, you may be faced with a situation requiring you to assist with childbirth. If you have never seen or experienced childbirth, your expectations probably consist of what others have told you.

Terms such as exhausting, stressful, exciting, fulfilling, painful and scary are sometimes used to describe a planned childbirth, one that occurs in the hospital or at home under the supervision of a health care provider. If you find yourself assisting with the delivery of a baby, however, it is probably not happening in a planned situation. Therefore, your feelings, as well as those of the expectant mother, may be intensified by fear of the unexpected or the possibility that something might go wrong.

Take comfort in knowing that things rarely go wrong. Childbirth is a natural process. Thousands of children all over the world are born each day, without complications, in areas where no medical assistance is available during childbirth.

By following a few simple steps, you can effectively assist in the birth process. This chapter will help you better understand the birthing process, how to assist with the delivery of a baby, how to provide care for both the mother and newborn, how to recognize complications and what complications could require more advanced care.

ANATOMY AND PHYSIOLOGY OF PREGNANCY

The developing **fetus** is contained in the **uterus** and surrounded by **amniotic fluid**. The uterus is made up of a special arrangement of smooth muscle and blood vessels that allow it to enlarge significantly during pregnancy and to forcibly contract during **labor** and delivery. The ability of the uterus to produce strong **contractions** helps pass the baby from the uterus into the **birth canal**. Strong contractions also help the

uterus constrict blood vessels, thus preventing hemorrhage, and help the uterus return to its previous size.

The **cervix** (or neck of the uterus) is the lower, narrow part of the uterus that forms a canal that opens into the **vagina**, which contains a **mucous plug** up to the time of labor. The mucous plug seals the uterine opening and prevents any contamination. Once labor begins and the cervix begins to dilate (widen), the mucous plug is expelled. The fetus is pushed through the cervix and vagina.

The **placenta**, or "organ of pregnancy," begins to develop inside the uterus after the egg attaches itself to the uterine wall. It is rich in blood vessels and its purpose is to deliver oxygen and nourishment to the fetus from the mother, and remove carbon dioxide and waste products.

NORMAL PREGNANCY

The duration of a full-term pregnancy spans a 9-month period, or 38 weeks from the time in which the **embryo** becomes implanted into the woman's uterus. The due date is usually calculated as 40 weeks from the woman's last menstrual period (**Fig. 24-1**). Pregnancy is broken down into 3 **trimesters**, each lasting approximately 3 months.

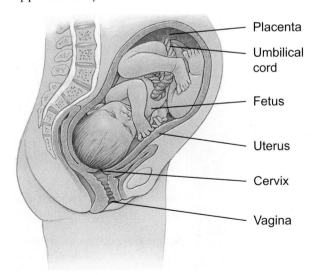

Placenta

Umbilical cord

Fetus

Uterus

Cervix

Vagina

Fig. 24-1: Mother and fetus at 40 weeks

First Trimester

Implantation and rapid development of the embryo occur during the first trimester of pregnancy. Usually implantation takes place with no noticeable symptoms, although slight bleeding may occur in some women. The gradual appearance of morning sickness is common during the first trimester. Morning sickness occurs in 70 percent of pregnant women and usually disappears by the second trimester. Also, the first trimester is generally the time in which a **miscarriage**, also called a *spontaneous abortion*, might occur.

As the embryo grows, its organs and body parts develop. After about 8 weeks, the embryo is called a fetus. To continue developing properly, the fetus must receive nutrients, which it receives from the mother through the placenta. The placenta is attached to the fetus by a flexible structure called the **umbilical cord**.

Second Trimester

Pregnant women commonly experience a feeling of re-energization during the second trimester. This is also when a woman will begin to "show," putting on more weight with the growth of the fetus. The mother can now detect "quickening," or movement of the fetus. The fetus has begun to produce insulin and is urinating, and the placenta is fully developed. Teeth are visible inside the gums and it is now possible to determine if the fetus is male or female.

Third Trimester

The mother gains the most weight during the third trimester, when the fetus grows most rapidly. An expanding abdomen sometimes causes the mother's navel to become convex. Growth of the baby can cause discomfort for the mother, including weak bladder control and backache. The size and movement of the baby may also cause pain or discomfort when pressure is applied to the woman's ribs and spine. The baby moves into a head-down position in preparation for birth, which is known as **dropping**. Babies born during the third trimester, but prior to full term, have a good chance of surviving, due to ever-advancing technology and improved intensive care practices.

BIRTH AND LABOR PROCESS

Pregnancy culminates in the *birth process*, or labor, during which the baby is delivered. Labor begins with rhythmic contractions of the uterus. As these contractions continue, they dilate the cervix. When the cervix is sufficiently dilated, it allows the baby to travel from the uterus through the birth canal and into the outside world. For first-time mothers, this process normally takes between 12 and 24 hours. Subsequent deliveries usually require less time. The labor process has four distinct stages. The length and intensity of each stage vary.

First Stage: Dilation

In the first stage of labor, the mother's body prepares for the birth. This stage covers the time from the first contraction until the cervix is fully dilated. A contraction is a rhythmic tightening and relaxing of the muscles in the uterus. Like a wave, it begins gently, rises to a peak of intensity and then subsides. A break occurs between contractions, and a contraction usually lasts about 30 to 60 seconds. Contractions cause **dilation**, the process that allows the mother's cervix to expand enough for the baby to pass through during the birth (**Fig. 24-2, A**).

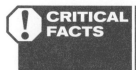

CRITICAL FACTS

Implantation and rapid development of the embryo occur during the first trimester of pregnancy.

Pregnant women commonly experience a feeling of re-energization during the second trimester. This is also when a woman will begin to "show," putting on more weight with the growth of the fetus.

The mother gains the most weight during the third trimester, when the fetus grows most rapidly. An expanding abdomen sometimes causes the mother's navel to become convex.

Pregnancy culminates in the birth process, or labor, during which the baby is delivered. Labor begins with rhythmic contractions of the uterus. The labor process has four distinct stages. The length and intensity of each stage vary.

During this stage of labor, the mucous plug may emerge. The release of the mucous plug, referred to as the **bloody show,** may also have occurred prior to labor. Before or during labor the **amniotic sac** will break, releasing the amniotic fluid. When this happens, people often say the woman's "water has broken." As the time for delivery approaches, the contractions occur closer together, last longer and feel stronger. Normally, when contractions are less than 3 minutes apart, delivery is near. The woman may be in considerable discomfort at this time. This stage is the longest, and may last for 18 hours or more, especially for a first delivery. For a woman who has already gone through labor, this stage may last only a few hours.

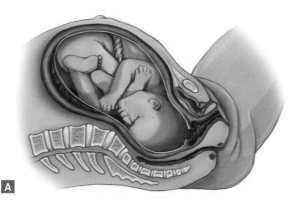

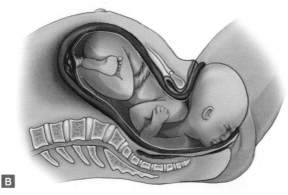

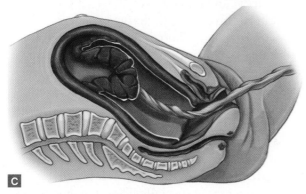

Fig. 24-2, A–C: The stages of labor include **(A)** dilation, **(B)** expulsion and **(C)** placental delivery.

Second Stage: Expulsion

The second stage of labor begins when the cervix is completely dilated and includes the baby's movement through the birth canal and delivery (**Fig. 24-2, B**). During this stage of labor, the mother will experience enormous pressure, similar to the feeling she has to have a bowel movement. This sensation is an indication that it is time for her to push or "bear down," to help ease the baby through the birth canal. Considerable blood may come from the vagina at this time. Contractions are more frequent during this stage, and may last between 45 and 90 seconds each. In a normal delivery, the baby's head becomes visible as it emerges from the vagina. When the top of the head begins to emerge, called **crowning**, birth is imminent and you must be prepared to receive the baby (**Fig. 24-3**).

Third Stage: Placental Delivery

Once the baby's body emerges, the third stage of labor begins. During this stage, the placenta usually separates from the wall of the uterus and exits from the birth canal (**Fig. 24-2, C**). This process normally occurs within 30 minutes of the delivery of the baby.

Fourth Stage: Stabilization

The final stage of labor involves the initial recovery and **stabilization** of the mother after childbirth. Normally, this stage lasts approximately 1 hour. During this time, the uterus contracts to control bleeding, and the mother begins to recover from the physical and emotional stress that occurred during childbirth.

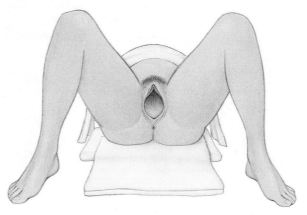

Fig. 24-3: When crowning begins, birth is imminent.

Assessing Labor

If you are called to assist a pregnant woman, you will need to determine whether she actually is in labor. The woman may be experiencing **Braxton Hicks contractions**, or *false labor contractions*. During false labor, the contractions do *not* get closer together, do *not* increase in how long they last and do not feel stronger as time goes on—as they would with true labor. Also, false labor contractions tend to be sporadic; true labor has regular intervals of contractions. But because there is no real, safe way to determine if the labor is false, transporting the woman to a medical facility is a prudent decision.

If the woman is in labor, you should determine how far along she is in the pregnancy, including when the baby is due, and whether she expects any complications. You can determine these factors by asking a few key questions and making some quick observations.

To determine if the birth is imminent, ask the woman her due date. Time the contractions to determine how far apart they are. Take the following steps:

1. Feel the mother's abdomen with a gloved hand for involuntary tightening and relaxing of the uterine muscles (**Fig. 24-4**).
2. Time the length of the movements in seconds from the time the abdomen tightens to the time it relaxes.
3. Time the start of one contraction to the start of the next in minutes.

If the contractions are 5 minutes apart or longer, the woman should be transported to a medical facility if possible. If the contractions are 2 minutes apart, you will not have time to transport the woman because the birth is imminent.

Calm the mother and make her feel confident you are there to keep her and the baby safe. Continue with the following questions:

- Is there a chance of a **multiple birth**? Labor does not usually last as long in a multiple birth situation. Also, if you know it is a multiple birth, you can prepare what you will need to help in the delivery of more than one baby. Additional information on multiple births is presented in the Enrichment section of this chapter.
- Is this a first pregnancy? The first stage of labor normally takes longer with first pregnancies than with subsequent ones.
- Is there a bloody discharge? A pink or light red, thick discharge from the vagina is the mucous plug that falls from the cervix as it begins to dilate, which also signals the onset of labor. This discharge is also referred to as the bloody show.
- Has the amniotic sac ruptured? When this happens, fluid flows from the vagina in a sudden gush or a trickle. Some women think they have lost control of their bladder. The breaking of the sac usually signals the beginning of labor. People often describe the rupture of the sac as "the water breaking."
- Does she have an urge to bear down? If the expectant mother expresses a strong urge to push, labor is far along.
- Is the baby crowning? If the baby's head is visible, the baby is about to be born.

PREPARING FOR DELIVERY

The realization that you are about to assist with childbirth can be as intimidating as it is exciting. Childbirth involves a discharge of watery, sometimes bloody, fluid and other body fluids or substances, such as urine or feces, at stages one and two of labor in addition to what appears to be a rather large loss of blood after stage two. Fluid discharge sometimes creates splashes, and it is important for the *emergency medical responder* (EMR) to follow standard precautions using appropriate *personal protective equipment* (PPE) (see **Chapter 6**). An **obstetric pack** is a first aid kit containing items especially helpful in emergency delivery and can include items such as PPE,

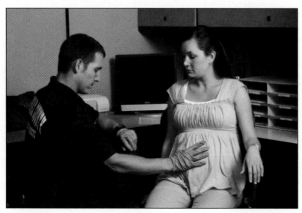

Fig. 24-4: To assess labor, feel the mother's abdomen for tightening and relaxing of the uterine muscles, known as contractions, and time how long they are and how far apart they are.

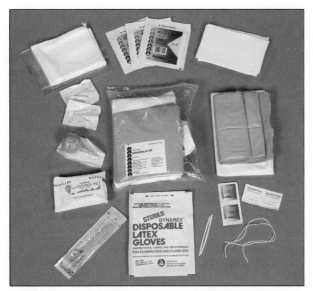

Fig. 24-5: Obstetric pack

towels, clamps, ties, sterile scissors and **bulb syringes** (**Fig. 24-5**). Try not to be alarmed at the loss of blood. It is a normal part of the birth process. Only bleeding that cannot be controlled after the baby is born is a problem. Take a deep breath and try to relax. Remember that you are only assisting in the process; the expectant mother is doing all the work.

Helping the Mother with Labor and Delivery

As part of your primary assessment, check the woman's breathing and pulse. Check for a potentially closed airway. Breathing rate may be increased due to pain, anxiety or blood loss. Heart rate may be increased, peripheral pulses may be weak or absent, skin may be cool and clammy and shock is possible where there has been excessive bleeding. The woman's vital signs may show normal blood pressure; however, blood pressure will decrease in case of shock and increase in the case of **preeclampsia**. Your physical exam will include evaluating the contractions, inspecting for crowning and preparing for delivery.

If the woman is conscious and seems to be experiencing normal symptoms of labor, find out any other pertinent medical history.

Explain to the expectant mother that the baby is about to be born. Be calm and reassuring. A woman having her first child often feels fear and apprehension about the pain and the condition of the baby. Labor pain ranges from discomfort similar to menstrual cramps to intense pressure or pain. Many women experience something in between. Factors that can increase pain and discomfort during the first stage of labor include—
- Irregular breathing.
- Tensing up because of fear.
- Not knowing what to expect.
- Feeling alone and unsupported.

You can help the expectant mother cope with the discomfort and pain of labor. By staying calm, firm and confident and offering encouragement, you can help reduce her fear and apprehension. Reducing fear will aid in reducing her pain and discomfort. Begin by reassuring her that you are there to help. Explain what to expect as labor progresses. Suggest specific physical activities that she can do to relax, such as regulating her breathing. Ask her to breathe slowly and deeply, in through the nose and out through the mouth. Ask her to focus on one object in the room while regulating her breathing.

Breathing slowly and deeply in through the nose and out through the mouth during labor can help the expectant mother in several ways because it:
- Aids muscle relaxation.
- Offers a distraction from the pain of strong contractions as labor progresses.
- Ensures adequate oxygen delivery to both the mother and the baby during labor.

Taking childbirth classes, usually offered at local hospitals, may help you become more competent in techniques to help an expectant mother relax.

Expect delivery to be imminent when you observe the following signs and symptoms:
- Intense contractions are 2 minutes apart or less and last 60 to 90 seconds.

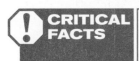

CRITICAL FACTS

If you find yourself helping the mother with labor and delivery, check the woman's breathing and pulse as part of your primary assessment. Check for a potentially closed airway. Breathing rate may be increased due to pain, anxiety or blood loss.

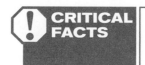
- The woman's abdomen is very tight and hard.
- The mother reports feeling the infant's head moving down the birth canal or has a sensation like an urge to defecate.
- Crowning occurs (the infant's head appears at the opening of the birth canal).
- The mother reports a strong urge to push.

If these signs and symptoms are present, contact medical direction for assistance. The decision will need to be made whether to deliver on-site. If an on-site delivery does not occur within 10 minutes, you will need medical direction's decision to transport.

DELIVERY

Assisting with the delivery is often a simple process. The expectant mother does all the work; your job is to create a clean environment and to help guide the baby from the birth canal, minimizing injury to the mother and baby. Begin by positioning the mother. She should be lying on her back, with her head and upper back raised, *not* lying flat. Her legs should be bent, with the knees drawn up and apart (**Fig. 24-6**). Position the mother in a way that will make her more comfortable.

Establish a clean environment for delivery. Because it is unlikely that you will have sterile supplies, use items such as clean sheets, blankets, towels or clothes. To make the area around the mother as sanitary as possible, place these items over the mother's abdomen and under her buttocks and legs. Keep a clean, warm towel or blanket handy to wrap the newborn. Because you will be coming in contact with the mother's and baby's body fluids, be sure to wear disposable gloves. Wear protective eyewear and a disposable gown, if they are available, to protect yourself from splashing.

Other items that can be helpful include emergency oxygen; a bulb syringe to suction secretions from the infant's mouth and nose; gauze pads or sanitary pads to help absorb secretions and vaginal bleeding and a large plastic bag or towel to hold the placenta after delivery.

Continually check the mother for indications the baby is crowning. You may actually see the head of the baby appear, or the vagina may be bulging. Once crowning takes place, take the following steps to assist with delivery:

- As crowning occurs, place a hand on the top of the baby's head and apply light pressure (**Fig. 24-7**). By doing so, you allow the head to emerge slowly, not forcefully. Gradual emergence will help prevent tearing of the vagina and injury to the baby.
- At this point, the expectant mother should stop pushing. Instruct the mother to concentrate on her breathing techniques. Have her pant. This technique will help her stop pushing and help prevent a forceful birth.
- You may have to puncture the amniotic sac with your fingers if the water has not yet broken.

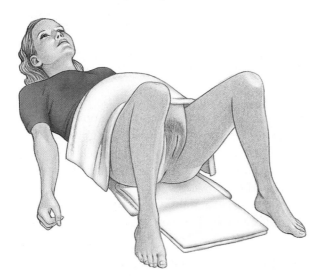

Fig. 24-6: To assist with delivery, begin by positioning the mother on her back, with her head and upper back raised, in a clean environment.

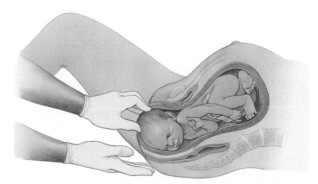

Fig. 24-7: As crowning occurs, apply light pressure to the top of the baby's head to encourage a gradual emergence and prevent a forceful birth.

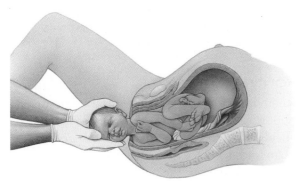

Fig. 24-8: Support the head as it emerges and the baby turns, which allows the shoulders and rest of the body to pass through the birth canal.

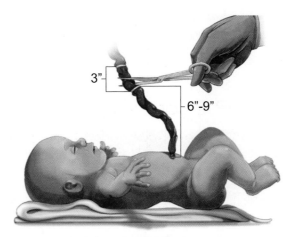

Fig. 24-9: Clamping the umbilical cord

- As the head emerges, the baby will turn to one side, which enables the shoulders and the rest of the body to pass through the birth canal (**Fig. 24-8**).
- Check to see if the umbilical cord is looped around the baby's neck. If it is, gently slip it over the baby's head. If you cannot slip it over the head, slip it over the baby's shoulders as they emerge. The baby can slide through the loop.
- Guide one shoulder out at a time. Do *not* pull the baby.
- As the baby emerges, he or she will be wet and slippery. Use a clean towel to receive/hold the baby.
- Place the baby on its side, between the mother and you. By doing so, you can provide initial care without fear of dropping the newborn.
- If possible, note the time the baby was born.

CARING FOR THE NEWBORN AND MOTHER

An obstetric pack contains items useful for help in caring for the newborn after delivery.

Caring for the Newborn
Cutting the Umbilical Cord

The umbilical cord will stop pulsating not long after the baby is born. When it does, clamp or tie the cord very securely with gauze in two places between the mother and child. The clamp closest to the newborn should be about 6 inches from the baby. There should only be about 3 inches between the two clamps (**Fig. 24-9**). Follow local protocols and medical direction for guidance on cutting the cord.

Assessing the Newborn

The **APGAR** scoring system is the universally accepted method of assessing a newborn at 1 minute and again at 5 minutes after birth. However, if the baby is in distress and needs life-saving care, the APGAR Score is not a priority.

APGAR stands for *Appearance, Pulse, Grimace, Activity and Respiration*. The baby is assigned a number from 0 to 2 for each part of the assessment, for a total possible score of 10.

Tally the five scores for a total score out of 10. Here are the guidelines for interpreting that score:
- 7 to 10 points: Active and vigorous newborn; ready for routine care.
- 4 to 6 points: Moderately depressed; provide stimulation and oxygen.
- 1 to 3 points: Severely depressed; provide extensive care including administering emergency oxygen with bag-valve-mask ventilations and CPR. Also, stimulate the baby to encourage breathing by flicking the soles of the feet or rubbing the back.

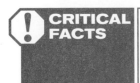

CRITICAL FACTS

The APGAR (Appearance, Pulse, Grimace, Activity and Respiration) scoring system is the universally accepted method of assessing a newborn at 1 minute and again at 5 minutes after birth. However, if the baby is in distress and needs life-saving care, the APGAR Score is not a priority. The baby is assigned a number from 0 to 2 for each part of the assessment, for a total possible score of 10.

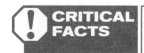
Table 24-1:
APGAR Scoring System

APGAR	SCORE
Appearance	
Cyanotic (blue) skin appearance all over	0
Cyanotic limbs but pink body	1
Pink body all over	2
Pulse (Count the heart rate for 30 seconds. If possible, use a stethoscope. If not, measure the pulse where the umbilical cord meets the abdomen or at the brachial artery.)	
No pulse	0
Pulse rate less than 100 beats per minute	1
Pulse rate more than 100 beats per minute	2
Grimace (reflex irritability) (Gently flick the soles of the newborn's feet, or observe during suctioning.)	
No activity or reflex	0
Some facial grimace	1
Grimace and cough, sneeze or cry	2
Activity (Observe movement/reflexes of the extremities or the degree of flexion of the extremities and the resistance to straightening them.)	
Limp, with no movement of extremities	0
Some flexion, without active movement	1
Actively moving around	2
Respirations (Observe for regular breathing and a vigorous cry. Poor signs include irregular, shallow, gasping or absent respirations.)	
No respiratory effort	0
Slow or irregular breathing effort with weak cry	1
Good respirations and strong cry	2

Routine Care

When handling a newborn, *always* be sure to support the newborn's head. Newborns lose heat quickly; therefore, it is important to keep them warm and dry. Dry the newborn, particularly the head, and wrap the baby in a clean, warm towel or blanket. Place the dried and wrapped newborn on his or her side, with the head slightly lower than the trunk.

It is vital you ensure that you clear the nasal passages and mouth thoroughly. You can do this by using your finger, a gauze pad or a bulb syringe (**Fig. 24-10**). Squeeze a bulb syringe *before* insertion in the mouth and nose. Clear or suction the mouth before the nose. Repeat this until you are sure the airway is clear. If the newborn does not breathe, you must begin giving ventilations.

Most newborns begin crying and breathing spontaneously. If the newborn has not made any sounds, stimulate a cry reflex by flicking your fingers on the soles of the feet.

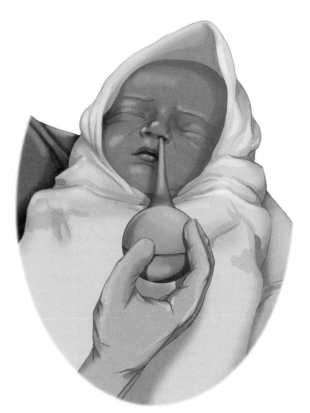

Fig. 24-10: A bulb syringe can be used to clear the newborn's mouth and nasal passages.

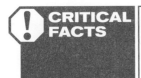
Resuscitation of a newborn begins immediately if respirations fall to less than 30 respirations per minute or the newborn is gasping or not breathing; if pulse is less than 100 beats per minute; or if cyanosis (bluish skin) around the chest and abdomen persists after administering emergency oxygen.

Resuscitation of the Newborn

Resuscitation of a newborn begins immediately if any of these conditions exist:

- Respirations fall to less than 30 respirations per minute or the newborn is gasping or not breathing.
- Pulse is less than 100 beats per minute.
- Cyanosis (bluish skin) around the chest and abdomen persists after administering emergency oxygen.

If the newborn's respirations are low (less than 30 breaths per minute) and/or the pulse rate is below 100 beats per minute, provide positive-pressure ventilations.

If the newborn's respirations are less than 30 breaths per minute or the newborn is unresponsive—

- Flick the bottom of the foot to stimulate a reflex (**Fig. 24-11, A**).
- Rub the lower back, firmly but gently (**Fig. 24-11, B**).
- Clear the airway again, with a bulb syringe.
- Administer high-concentration oxygen (**Fig. 24-12**).

Remember that a newborn's lungs are very small and they need very small puffs of air. You may use a mask only if you have the appropriate size for a newborn. If the newborn's pulse drops to less than 60 beats per minute or does not rise to more than 60 beats per minute during ventilation, begin CPR.

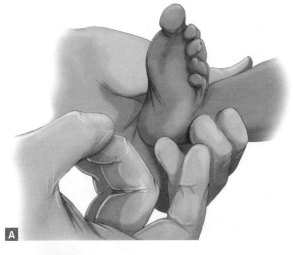

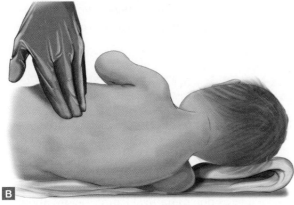

Fig. 24-11, A–B: You may need to stimulate the infant to breathe by (**A**) flicking the bottom of the foot or (**B**) rubbing the lower back.

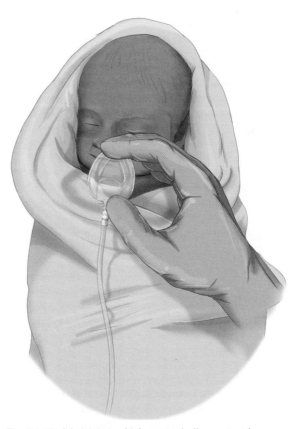

Fig. 24-12: Administering high-concentration oxygen to a newborn

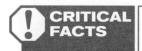

Caring for the Mother
Delivery of the Placenta

Following delivery of the newborn, the placenta will still be in the uterus, attached to the baby by the umbilical cord. Uterine contractions usually expel the placenta within 10 minutes of delivery and almost always within 30 minutes. The mother may experience strong contractions, similar to childbirth, and you may have to tell her to bear down in order for the placenta to be expelled. When the placenta appears, slowly guide it out of the vagina (do *not* pull) and place it in a clean towel or container.

Controlling Bleeding After Birth

Expect some additional vaginal bleeding when the placenta is expelled. Using gauze pads or clean towels, gently clean the mother. Place a sanitary pad or towel over the vagina; do *not* insert anything into the vagina. Instruct the mother to place her legs together.

Feel her abdomen for the uterus, which will feel like a grapefruit-sized mass in the lower sector. Massage the uterus to help expel large blood clots and to help the uterus contract. This should slow the bleeding. Watch for signs of shock from uncontrolled bleeding. If signs and symptoms of shock appear, care for the mother accordingly.

Providing Care

After delivery, be sure to continue caring for the mother, both emotionally and physically. Keep her calm and comfortable and continue to monitor her vitals until more advanced medical care takes over. If available, offer her a drink of water and a cloth to dry her face, as well as a clean blanket if she is cold. Remove any bloody sheets, blankets and other supplies used for delivery from the immediate area.

Caring for the Mother's Emotions with Stillborn/Aborted Fetuses

Stillbirth, or *fetal death,* is the term for the death of a baby prior to delivery but *after* 20 weeks gestation. The term miscarriage usually refers to a pregnancy lost *prior* to 20 weeks gestation. Another means of defining stillbirth is by the weight of the fetus at the time of death; a weight of 350 grams (approximately 12.3 ounces) or more is considered a stillbirth. Whether the loss occurs early in the pregnancy or at 40 weeks of pregnancy or beyond, it can be devastating to the family.

The couple should have time to grieve. The bond parents make with the unborn fetus begins early on in the pregnancy, so it is normal to experience a powerful sense of loss when their baby dies. Sensitivity on the part of the EMR is of utmost importance. It may be helpful to suggest a referral to a counselor or clergy member who has experience dealing with this kind of loss. Some people find it helpful to join a support group of parents who have had a similar experience where they can share their feelings with others who understand what it is like. Encourage them to seek out a bereavement group in their area.

COMPLICATIONS DURING PREGNANCY

Complications during pregnancy are rare.

Spontaneous Abortion

A miscarriage, or spontaneous abortion, is the loss of a fetus due to natural causes before about 20 weeks of pregnancy. About 85 percent of miscarriages occur during the first 12 weeks of

pregnancy. During miscarriage, the woman will experience vaginal spotting, bleeding and discharge, as well as cramping. Miscarriage later in pregnancy is accompanied by severe cramping, resulting in the expulsion of the fetus. The blood lost in these cases often contains mucous or clots.

Ectopic Pregnancy

In a normal pregnancy, the fertilized egg attaches itself to the lining of the uterus. With an **ectopic pregnancy**, the fertilized egg most commonly implants in one of the fallopian tubes, which carry eggs from the ovaries to the uterus. This type of ectopic pregnancy is known as a *tubal pregnancy*. Less commonly, an ectopic pregnancy occurs in the abdomen, ovary or cervix.

The fertilized egg of an ectopic pregnancy cannot survive, and the growing tissue may destroy various maternal structures. Therefore, if left untreated, life-threatening blood loss is possible. Early treatment of an ectopic pregnancy, in the form of termination, is necessary to preserve the chance for healthy pregnancies in the future.

Symptoms of an ectopic pregnancy include—
- Light vaginal bleeding (can be life threatening as it can lead to severe bleeding).
- Lower abdominal pain.
- Cramping on one side of the pelvis.

In the case of the fallopian tube rupturing, symptoms include—
- Sharp, stabbing pain in the pelvis, abdomen or even the shoulder and neck.
- Dizziness.
- Light-headedness.

Preeclampsia (Toxemia) and Eclampsia

Preeclampsia, or **toxemia**, is a common problem during pregnancy and is sometimes referred to as pregnancy-induced hypertension. If left untreated, **eclampsia**, the final and most severe phase of

preeclampsia, occurs. Eclampsia can cause coma and even death of the mother and baby, and can occur before, during or after childbirth.

The only cure for preeclampsia is delivery of the baby and, when it occurs near the end of pregnancy, delivery is advised. Signs and symptoms of preeclampsia include—
- High blood pressure.
- Excess protein in the urine after 20 weeks of pregnancy.
- Severe headaches.
- Changes in vision, such as temporary loss of vision, blurred vision or light sensitivity.
- Upper abdominal pain, usually under the ribs on the right side.
- Nausea or vomiting.
- Dizziness.
- Decreased urine output.
- Sudden weight gain, more than 2 pounds per week.
- Swelling (edema), particularly in the face and hands.
- Seizures, if eclampsia develops.

Vaginal Bleeding in Pregnancy

Vaginal bleeding during the first trimester does *not* typically require treatment. Spotting, or light, irregular discharges of a small amount of blood, may be normal. More bleeding may indicate a problem that needs a health care provider's attention.

When the thick plug of mucous that seals the opening of the cervix is dislodged, a thick or stringy discharge tinged with blood may appear. This "bloody show" is normal when it occurs near the end of pregnancy, and indicates delivery may occur in a week or two.

Since the nature and extent of most complications related to pregnancy can only be determined by a medical professional through examination, you should *not* be concerned with trying to diagnose a particular problem.

Instead, concern yourself with recognizing signs and symptoms that suggest a serious complication; two such symptoms are vaginal bleeding and abdominal pain. Any persistent or profuse vaginal bleeding, or bleeding in which tissue passes through the vagina during pregnancy, is abnormal, as is any abdominal pain.

When bleeding is accompanied by the following symptoms, immediate attention is required:
- Pain
- Cramping
- Fever
- Chills
- Contractions
- Passing tissue from the vagina

An expectant mother exhibiting these signs and symptoms needs to receive more advanced medical care quickly. While waiting for an ambulance or other transport vehicle, take steps to minimize shock. These include—
- Helping the woman into the most comfortable position.
- Controlling bleeding.
- Keeping the woman from getting chilled or overheated.
- Administering emergency oxygen if it is available.

Trauma During Pregnancy

Trauma during pregnancy can be caused by motor-vehicle collisions, falls, assaults or penetrating injuries. When the placenta peels away from the inner wall of the uterus before delivery, it is called **abruptio placentae**. This occurs in 1 to 5 percent of patients with minor trauma and 20 to 50 percent of patients with major trauma. Hemorrhage can occur from disruption of the placenta and spontaneous or traumatic uterine rupture. Pregnant women who have suffered an injury should be evaluated by a health care provider in the emergency room.

If the patient appears to be in shock, remember that the treatment of shock in a pregnant patient differs from the treatment of shock in other adults in two important respects. First, the organ systems change during pregnancy. Second, *two* patients are vulnerable: the mother *and* the fetus. Therefore, obstetric critical care involves simultaneous assessment and management of both the mother and fetus.

The management of **hemorrhagic shock** requires immediate administration of emergency oxygen. **Fetal monitoring** should be performed to detect fetal distress or fetal hypoxia.

Pregnant patients in the third trimester should be placed on their *left* side to avoid compression of the inferior vena cava. If spinal injury is suspected, the spine board should be tilted to the left after the patient is fully secured.

COMPLICATIONS DURING DELIVERY

The vast majority of all births occur without complication, but this is only reassuring if the one you are assisting with is not complicated. For the few births that do have complications, delivery can be stressful and even life threatening for the expectant mother and the baby. All require the help of more advanced medical personnel.

Hemorrhage

The most common complication of childbirth is persistent vaginal bleeding, known as *postpartum hemorrhage*. It is defined as the loss of more than 1 pint of blood following delivery of the placenta. It can occur right after delivery or as late as 1 month later. Hemorrhage can occur when the uterus fails to contract after delivery, as this contraction facilitates the closing of blood vessels that were opened during detachment of the placenta. It can also occur if the uterus was stretched too much during pregnancy or if a piece of placenta remains inside the uterus following delivery. It occurs more commonly following the birth of multiples, a prolonged or abnormal labor or when a woman has been pregnant several times. Women who have bled excessively following labor in the past are at increased risk of reoccurrence.

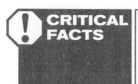
CRITICAL FACTS

The vast majority of all births occur without complication. The few births with complications require the help of more advanced medical personnel.

The most common complication of childbirth is persistent vaginal bleeding, known as postpartum hemorrhage.

In the case of hemorrhage, summon more advanced medical care and take steps to minimize shock. Massaging the lower abdomen and encouraging breastfeeding can also help stimulate the uterus to contract.

Other childbirth complications include a **prolapsed cord**, **breech birth**, limb presentation, multiple births, **premature birth** and **meconium aspiration**.

Prolapsed Umbilical Cord

A prolapsed cord occurs when a loop of the umbilical cord protrudes from the vaginal opening while the baby is still in the birth canal (**Fig. 24-13**). This can threaten the baby's life, because as the baby moves through the birth canal, the cord will be compressed against the unborn child and the birth canal, cutting off blood flow. Without this blood flow, the baby will die within a few minutes from lack of oxygen.

If you notice a prolapsed cord, have the expectant mother assume a knee-chest position as shown in **Figure 24-14**. This will help take the pressure off the cord. Administer emergency oxygen to the mother if it is available. Summon more advanced medical personnel, if they have not already been contacted.

Breech Birth

Most babies are born head-first but, on rare occasions, the baby is delivered feet- or buttocks-first. This condition is commonly called breech

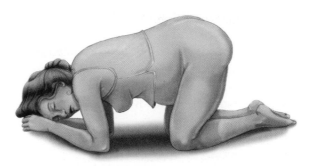

Fig. 24-14: If you notice a prolapsed cord or there is a limb presentation, place the mother in a knee-chest position.

birth. If you encounter a breech delivery, support the baby's body as it exits the birth canal while you are waiting for the head to deliver. Do *not* pull on the baby's body. Pulling will not help to deliver the head.

The weight of the baby's head lodged in the birth canal will reduce or stop blood flow to the baby by compressing the umbilical cord. The baby will also be unable to breathe spontaneously because the face will be pressed against the wall of the birth canal. As a result, if the head has not delivered after 3 minutes, you will need to help create an airway for the baby to breathe.

To help the baby breathe, place the index and middle fingers of your gloved hand into the vagina next to the baby's mouth and nose. Spread your fingers to form a V (**Fig. 24-15**). Though this will not lessen the compression

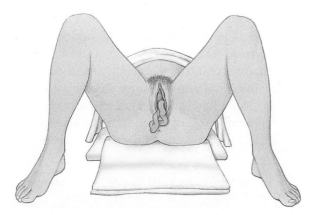

Fig. 24-13: A prolapsed cord can threaten the baby's life.

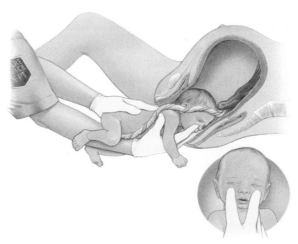

Fig. 24-15: During a breech birth, position your index and middle fingers to allow air to enter the baby's mouth and nose.

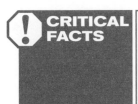
CRITICAL FACTS

A prolapsed cord occurs when a loop of the umbilical cord protrudes from the vaginal opening while the baby is still in the birth canal. It is life-threatening to the baby.

Most babies are born head-first but, on rare occasions, the baby is delivered feet- or buttocks-first. This is called a breech birth. In breech situations, support the body until the head delivers. Do not pull on the body.

on the umbilical cord, it may allow air to enter the baby's mouth and nose. You must maintain this position until the baby's head is delivered. Administer emergency oxygen to the mother if it is available. Summon more advanced medical personnel, if they have not already been contacted.

Limb Presentation

If the baby is delivered in an incomplete **breech,** or transverse lie (horizontal) position, the baby's foot (or feet), arm or shoulder will appear first. This is known as a limb presentation **(Fig. 24-16)**. If you encounter this, do *not* attempt to deliver the baby in the field. The mother should be transported to a medical facility. *Never* pull on the limb. Avoid even touching the limb, as this can stimulate the baby to try to take a breath, which can result in aspirating amniotic fluid.

A **cesarean section** will be needed to deliver the baby safely. Summon more advanced medical personnel, if they have not already been contacted. Administer emergency oxygen to the mother if it is available. Place her in a knee-chest position with her pelvis elevated. If she feels the need to push with contractions, have her pant, which can help ease the urge.

Multiple Births

Although most births involve only a single baby, a few will involve delivery of more than one. If the mother has had proper prenatal care, she will probably be aware that she is going to have more than one baby. Multiple births should be handled in the same manner as single births. The mother will have a separate set of contractions for each child being born. There may also be a separate placenta for each child, though this is not always the case. Keep in mind that the risk of hemorrhage following delivery is higher after giving birth to multiples.

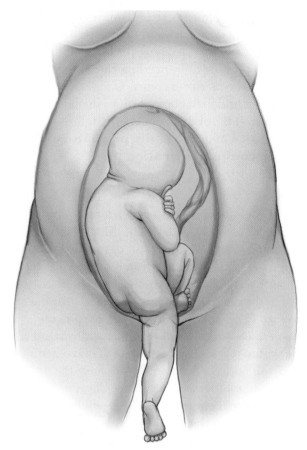

Fig. 24-16: Limb presentation

Premature Birth

When a baby is born before the end of 37 weeks of pregnancy, it is called a premature birth. Premature babies require special care because they are not fully developed. They are at increased risk for such complications as lung and breathing problems, infections and digestive difficulties. They are also more vulnerable to hypothermia.

Premature infants can typically be identified by their small, thin appearance and red, wrinkled skin. They also typically have a single crease along the sole of the foot; fuzzy, fine scalp hair; and ears that are not fully developed.

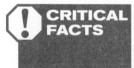

CRITICAL FACTS

If the baby is delivered in an incomplete breech, or transverse lie (horizontal) position, the baby's foot (or feet), arm or shoulder will appear first. This is known as a limb presentation. The mother must be transported to a medical facility. Never pull the limb. Avoid touching it.

Multiple births should be handled in the same manner as single births. The mother will have a separate set of contractions for each child being born.

When a baby is born before the end of 37 weeks of pregnancy, it is called a premature birth. Premature babies require special care because they are not fully developed.

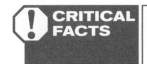

Meconium is the baby's first bowel movement. Amniotic fluid that is contaminated with meconium will be greenish or brownish yellow instead of clear. If this contaminated fluid is aspirated it can cause a blocked airway, respiratory distress, pneumonia and infection.

After the delivery of a premature baby, dry the infant thoroughly and wrap the baby in blankets, preferably warmed, or a plastic bubble-bag swaddle. Cover the head, leaving the face clear so the baby can breathe. Keep the baby in a warm place. Use a bulb syringe to gently suction away fluid from the baby's mouth and nose. Tie off the umbilical cord immediately, as a premature infant cannot tolerate even the smallest loss of blood. Administer emergency oxygen by blowing oxygen across (not directly into) the baby's face. Reduce the risk of infection by minimizing the number of people who handle the child. Do *not* let anyone breathe into the baby's face.

Meconium Aspiration

Meconium is the baby's first bowel movement. Amniotic fluid that is contaminated with meconium will be greenish or brownish yellow instead of clear. The presence of meconium-stained amniotic fluid is an indication that the baby experienced a period of oxygen deprivation (hypoxia), which causes the baby to have a bowel movement. The primary danger is that the baby will aspirate the contaminated fluid, which can result in complications including a blocked airway or respiratory distress, pneumonia and infection.

If you observe meconium staining in the amniotic fluid, it is crucial that you clear the mouth and nose before the baby takes the first breath. Suction the baby's mouth and nose with a bulb syringe or suction catheter as soon as the baby emerges from the birth canal. Avoid stimulating the baby in any way before clearing the mouth and nose, as this can induce the baby to try to take a breath. Do *not* squeeze the baby's chest or put your finger in the baby's mouth to try to prevent meconium aspiration.

Administer emergency oxygen to the baby if it is available. Summon more advanced medical personnel if they have not already been contacted. Keep the baby as warm and calm as possible and maintain the airway, if needed.

PUTTING IT ALL TOGETHER

Ideally, childbirth should occur in a controlled environment under the guidance of health care professionals trained in delivery. In a controlled environment, the necessary medical care is immediately available for mother and baby should any problem arise. However, unexpected deliveries do occur outside of the controlled environment and may require your assistance. By understanding the four stages of labor and knowing how to prepare the expectant mother for delivery, assist in the delivery and provide proper care for the mother and baby, you will be able to successfully assist in bringing a new child into the world.

YOU ARE THE EMERGENCY MEDICAL RESPONDER

While approaching the young woman who is in labor, the sister tells you that the patient is 26 years old. The pregnant woman is yelling, "The baby is coming!" She tells you that this will be her fourth child. What should you do?

Enrichment
More Complications During Pregnancy and Delivery

PLACENTA PREVIA

In most pregnancies, the placenta implants itself on the upper part of the uterine wall to establish its rich blood supply. In about one out of every 200 to 250 pregnancies, the placenta implants lower on the uterine wall, touching or covering the cervix, resulting in **placenta previa (Fig. 24-17)**. The condition can be–
- Marginal: The placenta touches the edge of the cervix.
- Partial: The placenta covers part of the cervix.
- Total or complete: The placenta covers the cervix completely.

The danger occurs if the placenta pulls away from the uterine wall, causing bleeding of oxygen-rich blood. Causes of the placenta tearing away include–
- Labor.
- Dilation of the cervix.
- Fetal movement.

The initial and only symptom of placenta previa is painless vaginal bleeding. To provide care, arrange for immediate transport. Elevate the patient's legs and maintain body temperature. If possible, administer emergency oxygen.

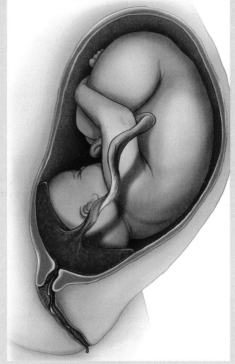

Fig. 24-17: Placenta previa

ABRUPTIO PLACENTAE

Abruptio placentae is a life-threatening emergency for both mother and child in which the placenta prematurely detaches from the uterus either partially or completely **(Fig. 24-18)**. It occurs in about one out of every 120 to 150 pregnancies and can occur at any time after 20 weeks gestation. The chance of its occurrence rises if it occurred in a previous pregnancy. Abruptio placentae can occur spontaneously or as a result of hypertension or maternal injury (trauma).

Symptoms of abruptio placentae, also called *placental abruption*, are–
- Abdominal pain.
- Back pain.
- Rapid uterine contractions.
- Uterine tenderness.
- Vaginal bleeding.

Bleeding may not be apparent at first, as blood accumulates between the placenta and uterine wall. Therefore, the first signs of abruptio placentae may be pain, abdominal rigidity and shock. To provide care, arrange for immediate transport. Monitor vital signs and treat for shock if necessary. Administer emergency oxygen, if available.

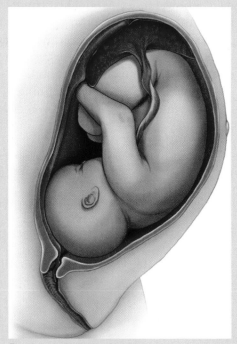

Fig. 24-18: Abruptio placentae

RUPTURED UTERUS

Rupture of the uterus is rare, but its occurrence is associated with a high incidence of infant fatality, reportedly as high as **65** percent. Maternal mortality associated with a ruptured uterus is significantly lower, but it can occur if significant time passes between the event and medical intervention.

The uterine wall, which thins during pregnancy, can rupture spontaneously or as the result of an abdominal trauma **(Fig. 24-19)**. Women who have had prior caesarian sections are at a higher risk of experiencing a ruptured uterus than women with first-time pregnancies or those who have delivered vaginally previously. Advanced maternal age is also a risk factor.

Signs and symptoms of a ruptured uterus are—

- Abdominal pain.
- Abnormal fetal heart pattern.
- Cessation of contractions.
- Deceleration of fetal heartbeat.
- Failure of labor to progress.
- Hyperstimulation of the uterus (excessive contractions).
- Signs of shock.
- Vaginal bleeding.

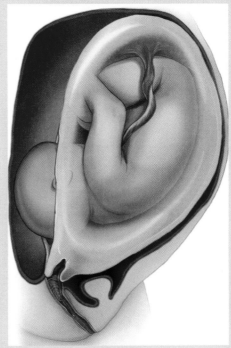

Fig. 24-19: Ruptured uterus

Once a uterine rupture is suspected, arrange for immediate transport. Stabilization of the mother and delivery of the fetus is imperative. As a rule, the time available for intervention is only between 10 and 37 minutes.

SHOULDER DYSTOCIA

Shoulder dystocia occurs when the fetus's shoulders are larger in width than the head. When the mother begins to deliver the baby, the head will emerge from the vagina, but a shoulder or both shoulders becomes caught between the maternal symphysis pubis (joint between the pubic bones) and the sacrum (base of the spine).

Other than a large fetus, often due to maternal diabetes, no risk factors for shoulder dystocia are recognized.

If the fetal head emerges from the vagina and then retracts, it is considered a symptom of shoulder dystocia. This is often called the "turtle sign." Shoulder dystocia has no other recognized symptoms. The danger with shoulder dystocia lies with the umbilical cord being compressed between the fetus and the maternal pelvis.

Do *not* apply excessive force, as this is unlikely to free the fetus and may cause injury. The HELPERR mnemonic is a tool used by health care providers that describes a set of maneuvers for managing shoulder dystocia during childbirth.

These maneuvers are only performed by a health care provider and are presented here for information only, as EMRs do not perform them:

- **H**elp: Request the appropriate personnel to respond.
- **E**valuate: Evaluate for episiotomy (incision between the vaginal opening and anus to prevent a more extensive vaginal tear during delivery will not release the shoulder on its own, as shoulder dystocia is a bone impaction).
- **L**egs: Maneuver the mother's legs in the McRoberts maneuver (repositions the baby).
- **P**ressure: Apply suprapubic pressure (making a fist, placing it just above the maternal pubic bone and pushing the fetal shoulder in one direction or the other).
- **E**nter: Enter maneuvers (internal rotation of the fetus).
- **R**emove: Remove the posterior arm from the birth canal.
- **R**oll: Roll the patient onto an all-fours position, which may dislodge the impaction; gravity may also assist.

25 Pediatrics

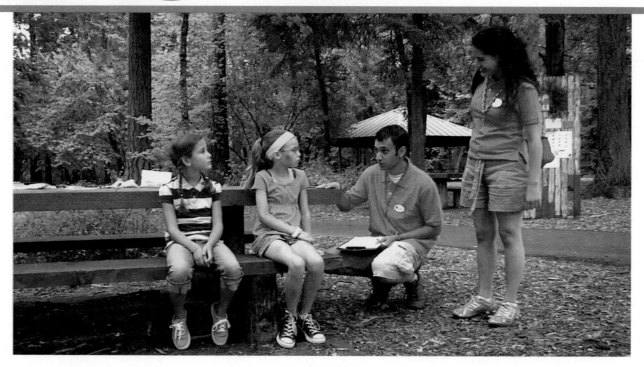

))) **YOU ARE THE EMERGENCY MEDICAL RESPONDER**

You are working as the camp health officer at a local summer camp when a young girl approaches you complaining that she has a rash. She says that she is allergic to certain things and may have come into contact with something that has now given her hives. How would you respond?

Key Terms

Adult: For the purpose of providing emergency medical care, anyone who appears to be approximately 12 years old or older.

Apparent life-threatening event (ALTE): A sudden event in infants under the age of 1 year, during which the infant experiences a combination of symptoms including apnea, change in color, change in muscle tone and coughing or gagging.

Child: For the purpose of providing emergency medical care, anyone who appears to be between the ages of about 1 year and about 12 years; when using an *automated external defibrillator* (AED), different age and weight criteria are used.

Child abuse: Action that results in the physical or psychological harm of a child; can be physical, sexual, verbal and/or emotional.

Child neglect: The most frequently reported type of abuse in which a parent or guardian fails to provide the necessary, age-appropriate care to a child; insufficient medical or emotional attention or respect given to a child.

Croup: A common upper airway virus that affects children under the age of 5.

Epidemiology: A branch of medicine that deals with the *incidence* (rate of occurrence) and *prevalence* (extent) of disease in populations.

Epiglottitis: A serious bacterial infection that causes severe swelling of the epiglottis, which can result in a blocked airway, causing respiratory failure in children; may be fatal.

Febrile seizure: Seizure activity brought on by an excessively high fever in a young child or an infant.

Fever: An elevated body temperature, beyond normal variation.

Infant: For the purpose of providing emergency medical care, anyone who appears to be younger than about 1 year of age.

Pediatric Assessment Triangle: A quick initial assessment of a child that involves observation of the child's appearance, breathing and skin.

Respiratory failure: Condition in which the respiratory system fails in oxygenation and/or carbon dioxide elimination; the respiratory system is beginning to shut down; the person may alternate between being agitated and sleepy.

Retraction: A visible sinking in of soft tissue between the ribs of a child or an infant.

Reye's syndrome: An illness brought on by high fever that affects the brain and other internal organs; can be caused by the use of aspirin in children and infants.

Seizure: Temporary abnormal electrical activity in the brain caused by injury, disease, fever, infection, metabolic disturbances or conditions that decrease oxygen levels.

Shaken baby syndrome: A type of abuse in which a young child has been shaken harshly, causing swelling of the brain and brain damage.

Status asthmaticus: A potentially fatal episode of asthma in which the patient does not respond to usual inhaled medications.

Sudden infant death syndrome (SIDS): The sudden death of an infant younger than 1 year that remains unexplained after the performance of a complete postmortem investigation, including an autopsy, an examination of the scene of death and a review of the care history.

Thready: Used to describe a pulse that is barely perceptible, often rapid and feels like a fine thread.

Learning Objectives

After reading this chapter, and completing the class activities, you will have the information needed to—

- Identify anatomical differences among adults, children and infants.
- Describe the general age groups for the purposes of emergency medical care.
- Describe the stages of child development.
- List the general considerations for assessing children and infants.
- Describe components of a pediatric assessment.

- Describe how to conduct a SAMPLE history for a pediatric patient.
- Identify common problems in pediatric patients.
- Describe common respiratory problems in children.
- Describe how to assess for and manage seizures in children.
- Describe considerations for children with special needs.

INTRODUCTION

In an emergency, you should be aware of the special needs and considerations of **children** and **infants**. Knowing these needs and considerations will help you better understand the nature of the emergency and provide appropriate care. A young child may be scared or nervous due to the circumstances of the emergency, because he or she is being assessed by a stranger, a combination of those reasons or some other reason. Being able to communicate with and reassure children and infants can be crucial to your ability to care for these patients effectively.

ANATOMICAL DIFFERENCES

It is important to be aware of the anatomical differences among **adults**, children and infants. The most significant of these differences involve the airway (**Fig. 25-1, A–B**).

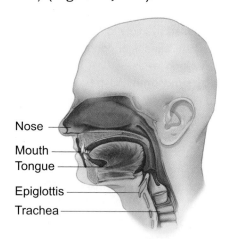

Nose
Mouth
Tongue
Epiglottis
Trachea

A

Nose
Mouth
Tongue
Epiglottis
B Trachea

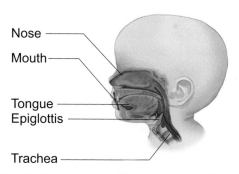

Fig. 25-1, A–B: The most significant anatomical differences between **(A)** adults and **(B)** children involve the airway and breathing.

Children and infants have proportionately larger tongues than do adults, so it is easier for the tongue to block the airway. Placing pressure under the chin, which can occur during the chin-lift or jaw-tilt maneuver, can cause the tongue to be pushed back and block the airway. Newborns and infants prefer to breathe through the nose and may *not* open their mouths when their nose is blocked, so they are more likely to develop respiratory distress if the nose is blocked.

Additionally, the epiglottis is much higher in children and infants than it is in adults. A newborn's trachea is also very narrow, only about 4 or 5 mm wide, so swelling, for example due to inhaling toxic fumes, can become life threatening very quickly.

Children and infants younger than age 5 also breathe at a rate two to three times faster than that of adults, and their breathing is shallower, as less volume and pressure are needed to ventilate the lungs.

Determining the Age Group of the Patient for the Purpose of Providing Emergency Medical Care

At times, care must be provided according to the age of the patient and it is not always easy to determine exact age. The American Red Cross follows established age categories for emergency care that are based on epidemiological patterns of injury including care needed, while at the same time being easy to recognize based on the patient's appearance.

In general, children and infants predominantly suffer respiratory emergencies, which, if untreated, can lead to cardiac emergencies. Adolescents and adults will often suffer primarily cardiac events. Lastly, an individual can generally look at a patient and determine if the patient is an adult, a child or an infant. At times, a small 13 month old may be categorized as an infant, or a small 13 year old as a child. However, the difference between the perceived age category and the actual age would not have any significant impact on care.

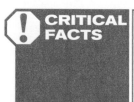

CRITICAL FACTS

It is important to be aware of the anatomical differences among adults, children and infants. The most significant of these differences involve the airway.

In general, children and infants predominantly suffer respiratory emergencies, which, if untreated, can lead to cardiac emergencies.

Anyone who appears younger than 1 year of age should be considered an infant; 1 to 12 years a child; and 12 and older an adult.

Additionally, the easy recognition of a perceived age category helps to provide appropriate care quickly, a benefit that far outweighs any age discrepancy.

Based on this physiological, epidemiological and recognition approach, the following general age groups have been developed:

- Infant—Anyone who appears to be younger than about 1 year of age.
- Child—Anyone who appears to be between the ages of about 1 year and about 12 years. For *automated external defibrillator* (AED) purposes, based on *U.S. Food and Drug Administration* (FDA) approval of pediatric-specific devices, a patient who is between the ages of 1 and 8 or weighs less than 55 pounds is considered a child. If precise age or weight is not known, the responder should use best judgment and *not* delay care to determine age.
- Adult—Anyone approximately 12 years old or older.

CHILD DEVELOPMENT
Infants (Birth to 1 Year)

Infants' inability to do anything for themselves and their inability to communicate where there may be pain or discomfort makes them among the most vulnerable of children and patients. After the first few weeks of birth, an infant can usually recognize a parent's or caregiver's voice. After a few months, facial recognition becomes possible. The quality of crying usually differs according to the cause, but the subtleties of the differences may only be recognized by the parents or caregivers. Crying could be triggered by hunger, the need for diapers to be changed, pain, fear or for unknown reasons.

Toddlers (1 to 3 Years)

Toddlers can readily recognize familiar faces and may be fearful of strangers **(Fig. 25-2, A)**. They may not be cooperative when

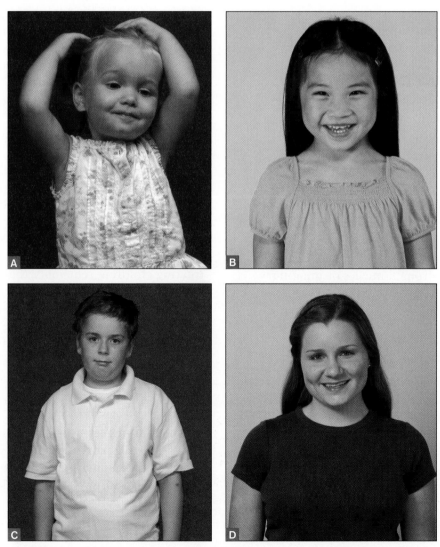

Fig. 25-2, A–D: **(A)** Toddler; **(B)** Preschooler; **(C)** School-aged child; **(D)** Teen

dealing with an unknown person, even if the parent or caregiver is in the room. Toddlers may also fear being separated from the people they know. Crying makes it difficult for them to communicate. Some toddlers relate well to stuffed animals, to help them calm down and demonstrate what the problem may be. When dealing with an unknown emergency with a toddler, keep in mind that toddlers' curiosity about the world around them makes poison ingestion a common injury.

Preschoolers (3 to 5 Years)

Preschoolers communicate their ideas more effectively than toddlers, but they may have difficulty with certain concepts (**Fig. 25-2, B**). They may have difficulty understanding complex sentences that contain more than one idea, so speak in simple terms. Children at this stage often feel that bad things are caused by their thoughts and behaviors. Their fears may seem out of proportion to the events. The sight of blood may be disturbing, but often a dressing or bandage can help calm the situation.

School Age Children (6 to 12 Years)

Children of school age have been exposed to more unfamiliar faces and are more likely to cooperate with strangers (**Fig. 25-2, C**). With reassurance from familiar faces (parents, caregivers, teachers), they are likely to understand the situation once it has been explained, and are able to cooperate with emergency responders. This age group is often fascinated with the topic of death and may have strong fantasies or imaginary ideas. Children of school age need continual reassurance.

Adolescents/Teens (13 to 18 Years)

The characteristics of adolescents and teens vary quite a bit from the beginning of the age group (age 13) to the end (age 18) (**Fig. 25-2, D**). Thirteen-year-olds are just leaving the school age group, and 18-year-olds are on the cusp of adulthood and already may have had to take on adult responsibilities. Generally, adolescents are more able to provide accurate information and

cooperate with emergency responders. However, they may be apt to fall into mass hysteria, in which multiple adolescents feel they are all experiencing the same problems or symptoms. This requires understanding and tolerance on behalf of the emergency rescuer. Generally, this group is quite modest and will require privacy. They are also aware of the potential for fatality or permanent disability and often fear they will experience this.

ASSESSING PEDIATRICS
General Considerations

Assessing an injured or sick child is similar to assessing an adult, with a few differences. Primary assessments on a conscious child should be done unobtrusively, so the child has time to get used to you and feel less threatened. Try to carry out as many of the components of the initial evaluation by careful observation, without touching the child or infant. Approach the parents or caregivers, if possible, as the child will see you communicating with them and subsequently may feel more comfortable with your exam and treatment. If appropriate, a parent or caregiver may hold the child during assessment and treatment.

Observe the young patient to assess for breathing, the presence of blood, movement and general appearance. Unless the child is agitated or upset, start the assessment using the head-to-toe approach. If the child is upset, the assessment can be done toe-to-head, which allows the patient to get used to you rather than have you in their face from the start. When treating children, remember that you are also treating their parents or caregivers as they, too, are likely to be scared or stressed. Reassess continuously as you wait for more advanced medical support to arrive. Document and report all your findings to more advanced medical personnel when they arrive.

Scene Size-Up

Begin observing the scene from the moment you arrive. The big picture will allow you to assess the situation and may give clues to other issues, such as **child abuse**. As usual, also assess the scene for personal safety.

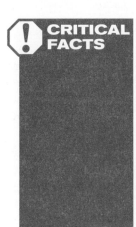
Assessing an injured or sick child is similar to assessing an adult, with a few differences. Primary assessments on a conscious child should be done unobtrusively, so the child has time to get used to you and feel less threatened. Try to carry out as many of the components of the initial evaluation by careful observation, without touching the child or infant.

Observe the young patient to assess for breathing, the presence of blood, movement and general appearance. Unless the child is agitated or upset, start the assessment using the head-to-toe approach.

The Pediatric Assessment Triangle is a quick initial assessment of a child that takes between 15 and 30 seconds and provides a picture of the severity of the child's or infant's illness or injury. This is done during size-up and before beginning the primary assessment. It does not require touching the patient, just looking and listening.

Be alert for any signs that may indicate poisoning (empty bottles, for example) and look for signs of child abuse. Are the adults responding in an appropriate manner? Are they appropriately concerned, or are they angry or indifferent? Does the child seem frightened of them and/or their reactions? Do the parents answer your questions directly? Is the environment safe for a child? While noting how the patient was found (position and location), keep in mind that the child may have been moved by well-meaning adults. Be sure to ask as part of your patient history. If you have confirmation that the patient has been moved, ask the adults where the child was and how the child was found.

Assessment
Pediatric Assessment Triangle

The **Pediatric Assessment Triangle** is a quick initial assessment of a child that takes between 15 and 30 seconds and provides a picture of the severity of the child's or infant's illness or injury. This is done during size-up and *before* beginning the primary assessment. It does *not* require touching the patient, just looking and listening.

You should observe three components in the child—appearance, work of breathing and skin:

- **Appearance:** Does the child appear to have normal muscle tone? Is the child crying, talking or moving about? Is the child able to interact with you or other adults in the area? Is the child able to make eye contact or be consoled?

- **Breathing:** Does the child appear to be breathing? Does breathing require great effort (flaring nostrils, indrawn area just below the throat or use of abdominal muscles)? Is the child leaning forward in an attempt to breathe? Is any noise coming from the child, such as wheezing or any other abnormal sound?

- **Skin (Circulation):** When looking at the child, is the skin pale, mottled or cyanotic (bluish)? Are any signs of trauma or bleeding present?

Equipment for Assessing and Caring for Children and Infants

As children come in all different sizes, so does the equipment used to assess them. A wide range of sizes should be available for assessing children, to provide optimal care.

Essential equipment and supplies include—

- *Bag-valve-mask resuscitators* (BVMs) with oxygen reservoirs.
- Oxygen masks.
- Nonrebreathing masks.
- Airway adjuncts.
- Bulb syringe.
- Portable suction unit with regulator.
- Suction catheters.
- Cervical immobilization devices.
- Backboard.
- Extremity splints.
- Stethoscope for pediatrics.
- Blood pressure cuffs.
- Thermal blankets.
- Water-soluble lubricant.

A new, clean stuffed animal and references for the Glasgow Coma Scale and Pediatric Trauma Score are also recommended.

Airway

An airway that is open, even if only partially open, will allow the child to cough, cry or breathe. Even with an open airway, the child should be observed closely for any change in status. A child whose airway becomes compromised or shows signs or symptoms of inadequate breathing or a lack of oxygen will need immediate care.

A child's airway can be blocked by anatomical or mechanical obstructions. For example, illness can cause constriction of the bronchi and upper airway as in **status asthmaticus** (asthma) or anaphylaxis (anatomical). Infection and trauma can also cause swelling and block the airway. Children are prone to airway obstruction caused by small objects as well as food (mechanical). Choking hazards among children include small objects such as coins, buttons, small toys and parts of toys and balloons, as well as certain food items. While hazardous for all children, these objects generally pose a larger threat to children under age 4.

If a solid object is blocking the child's upper airway, oxygen may not enter the lungs. This situation requires immediate care for a conscious choking child or infant—a combination of back blows and abdominal thrusts for a child, or back blows and chest thrusts for an infant. If secretions are blocking the airway, suctioning will help remove them. The suction may need to be repeated frequently to maintain an open airway, so the child should be monitored at all times.

Ventilation/Oxygenation

A child who is in respiratory distress may be agitated or drowsy. Agitation results from trying to get air; drowsiness is the result of insufficient oxygenation. The breathing effort increases in many cases, but as **respiratory failure** sets in, the breathing effort may decline considerably as the child weakens. Additionally, a combination can occur; the child may breathe with great effort for periods, followed by declining efforts as the child tires.

If the child is not breathing adequately or is not breathing at all, ventilation and/or oxygenation will be required (**Fig. 25-3**). Signs of the need for this assistance would be agitation or drowsiness, limp muscles, inability to respond and a pale or cyanotic appearance.

Circulation

Circulation in a child is similar to that of an adult, though the average child's pulse is more rapid than an adult's.

Observe the child for signs and symptoms of shock, which include restlessness, cold, clammy, pale or ashen skin; rapid or irregular breathing; falling blood pressure; altered mental status; rapid, weak or **thready** pulse; delayed capillary refill; and an absence of tears if the child or infant is crying. Place the child in the supine position (flat on the back).

A child who is in shock or is at risk of going into shock must be kept from getting chilled or overheated. Place a blanket over the child to help maintain the body temperature. Monitor the child closely for any changes in status.

Determining the Level of Consciousness

Using the AVPU scale, you can start to determine the child's *level of consciousness* (LOC). The AVPU scale is a mnemonic that

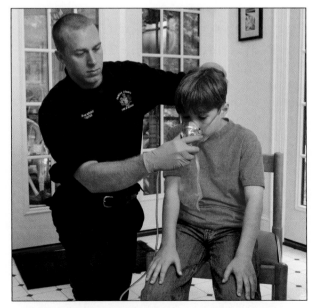

Fig. 25-3: If a child is not breathing adequately, give ventilations or administer emergency oxygen.

describes stages of awareness: **A**lert (the patient can respond to questions and is aware of the surroundings); **V**oice (the patient responds to verbal stimuli); **P**ain (the patient only responds to painful stimuli); and **U**nresponsive (the patient does *not* respond to *any* stimuli). The AVPU scale is covered more thoroughly in **Chapter 7**.

Another way to determine the LOC is pupil assessment, which involves checking to see if the pupils react to light. Shine a flashlight or penlight quickly into and then out of the child's eye. In a normal reaction, the pupil constricts in response to the light and then dilates again after the light is removed.

Movement is another good indication of LOC. Observe the child. A fully alert child will have spontaneous movements and as LOC diminishes so will the movement.

Exposure

Despite the need to keep the child covered if you are concerned about shock, you must be able to assess the child properly and thoroughly, barring any life-threatening situation. Check the child for any other injuries or signs of trauma. You do *not* need to uncover the child completely. You may remove the top part of the blanket to examine the upper body, cover the child and then remove the lower part of the blanket to examine the lower body.

Be swift and cover the child as quickly as possible. Because a large proportion of body heat is lost through the head and neck, cover the child's head to minimize the loss of body heat.

SAMPLE History

When taking a child's SAMPLE (signs and symptoms, allergies, medications, pertinent past medical history, last oral intake and events leading up to the incident) history, you will need the parents' or caregivers' cooperation **(Fig. 25-4)**. Encourage this cooperation by remaining respectful and polite during the conversation, even if the adults are difficult or if

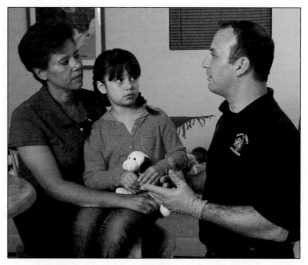

Fig. 25-4: When obtaining a SAMPLE history for a child, keep the child with the parent or caregiver.

you suspect child abuse or **child neglect**. Ask questions that require detailed answers, not yes-or-no questions. If the child is young but wants to participate, welcome this. An older child, particularly an adolescent, may want to speak with you privately. Keep this in mind if you must ask sensitive questions about topics such as sexual activity or drug use.

If you are not sure that the answers you receive are accurate or contain enough information, try asking the question in another manner, using different phrasing. Use feedback, repeating the answers as you make note of them, to be sure you heard correctly.

Symptoms and Duration

Ask the parents, caregivers, or child, if appropriate, about the symptoms, any changes (worsening or easing) and how long they have been present. While obtaining a patient history, inquire about—

- **Fever**.
- Unusual activity level.
- History of eating, drinking and urine output.
- History of vomiting, diarrhea and abdominal pain.

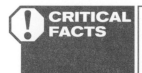

CRITICAL FACTS You will need the parents' or caregivers' cooperation while taking a child's SAMPLE history. Be respectful and polite, even if you suspect child abuse or neglect. Avoid asking yes-or-no questions. Allow a child to participate; older children may want to talk privately, especially if you must ask sensitive questions concerning sexual activity or drug use.

Allergies

Ask the parents, caregivers or child, if appropriate, if they have any allergies. While obtaining a patient history, inquire about allergies to—

- Medications.
- Food.
- Environmental elements, such as dust, pollen or bees.

Medications

Ask the parents or caregivers about medications the child might take. Does the child take any prescription medications or have the parents or caregivers given any over-the-counter medications recently? Does the child have any allergies to medications? Could the child have gotten into someone else's medications?

Pertinent Past Medical Problems or Chronic Illnesses

Ask the parents or caregivers if something like this has ever occurred before. If so, what caused it before and what happened in the long run? Does the child have any chronic illnesses, such as asthma or diabetes? Has the child been ill lately with any other type of illness?

Events Leading Up to the Injury or Illness

Ask the parents or caregivers what specifically was going on when the injury or illness was first noticed. What was the environment like (where did it happen)? What was the child doing? What was the child's reaction?

Physical Exam

Conducting a physical exam of a child or an infant requires some special handling. Try to have only one individual deal with the child, to reduce the anxiety of being handled by multiple strangers. If you can, crouch down to the child's eye level. Speak calmly and softly and maintain eye contact. Be gentle and *never* lose your temper. Involve people who are familiar to the child, if possible. For preschoolers, save frightening tools like stethoscopes until the child has had a chance to get used to you.

When examining a child, the standard procedure is to go from head to toe. For a very agitated child, however, the exam may be more successful if it is performed toe to head.

A head-to-toe exam involves the following components:

- Head: Look for bruising or swelling.
- Ears: Look for drainage suggestive of trauma or infection.
- Mouth: Look for loose teeth, identifiable odors or bleeding.
- Neck: Look for abnormal bruising.
- Chest and back: Look for bruises, injuries or rashes.
- Extremities: Look for deformities, swelling or pain on movement.

COMMON PROBLEMS IN PEDIATRIC PATIENTS

Certain problems are unique to children, such as specific kinds of injury and illness.

Airway Obstructions

Some of the most common airway problems you may encounter with small children and infants are airway obstructions. Airway obstructions may be categorized as either partial or complete. Signs of a partial airway obstruction in a child or an infant who is alert and sitting up include—

- Abnormal high-pitched musical sounds, crowing or noisy respirations.
- **Retraction**.
- Drooling.
- Frequent coughing.

Keep the child or infant in a position of comfort, possibly sitting on a parent's or caregiver's lap. The child can stay there while you administer emergency oxygen, if needed.

A complete airway obstruction is a life-threatening situation. A partial airway obstruction in a child or an infant who is showing signs of cyanosis should be treated as a complete airway obstruction. Signs of a complete airway obstruction include—

- Inability to cough, cry or speak.
- Cyanosis.
- Loss of consciousness.
- Altered mental status.

Care includes clearing the airway and attempting ventilation using the mouth-to-mask technique. For more information on clearing

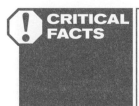

airway obstructions in children and infants, refer to **Chapter 11**.

Breathing Emergencies

Respiratory distress is apparent when the child or infant begins to experience difficulty breathing. If uncorrected, respiratory distress can lead to respiratory failure.

Anatomic and Physiological Differences in Children

Anatomical differences among adults, children and infants can change their susceptibility to respiratory difficulties and affect how to provide emergency care:

- In children and infants, the tongue is larger in relation to the space in the mouth than it is in adults. This can increase the risk of the tongue blocking the trachea.
- In children, the airway is smaller, resulting in more objects, such as different types of solid foods, being a choking hazard. Their smaller airway can make children more prone to developing infections or amassing liquid secretions. This also affects the choice of ventilation equipment used.
- In children, the trachea is not as long as it is in adults, so any attempt to open the airway by tilting the child's head too far back will result in blocking the airway.
- Children breathe using their diaphragm, so ensure nothing is pressing on the abdomen to prevent this. Also, if possible, allow the child to sit up.
- Young children and infants do *not* usually breathe through their mouth; they breathe through their nose. Ensure that the nose is as clear as possible for breathing.

Pathophysiology

The process of respiratory emergencies usually follows the pattern of respiratory distress, followed by respiratory failure, which is then followed by

respiratory arrest if emergency interventions are not attempted or are not successful.

Respiratory distress occurs when the child is having trouble breathing but is visibly able to breathe. A child in respiratory distress may be mentally alert and/or agitated. The patient's breathing effort is increased and the skin color may be normal or pale.

Respiratory distress preceding respiratory failure is characterized by:

- Infants: respiratory rate of more than 60 breaths per minute
- Children: respiratory rate of more than 30 breaths per minute
- Flaring of the nostrils
- Use of neck muscles and muscles between and below the margin of the ribs to aid in breathing
- Abnormal, high-pitched sounds when breathing
- Cyanosis
- Altered mental status
- Grunting

Respiratory failure occurs when the respiratory system is beginning to shut down. The child may be sleepy and lethargic, or may alternate between being agitated and sleepy. Muscle tone is generally limp, breathing is usually visible and breathing can decrease or alternate between increased and weak effort as the child becomes tired. The skin is usually pale, mottled or cyanotic.

Respiratory arrest occurs when the respiratory system shuts down. The child is unresponsive and completely limp. Signs of breathing may be slight, but are most likely absent, and the skin color is cyanotic.

The importance of recognizing early signs of respiratory distress cannot be emphasized enough. Early recognition of respiratory emergencies can make the difference between life and death. More information on the recognition and care of breathing emergencies can be found in **Chapters 10** and **11**.

Assessing Breathing Emergencies

The child's ability to breathe adequately must be assessed by checking the mental status, muscle tone, breathing movement, breathing effort and skin color. Once you have made your assessment, be sure to frequently perform follow-up assessments to note if there are any changes in the child's respiratory status.

Common Respiratory Problems in Children

Although many types of breathing problems can affect children, some will be seen by emergency responders more often than others, such as **croup**, **epiglottitis**, asthma and choking on an obstruction.

Croup is a common upper airway virus that affects children younger than 5. The airway constricts, limiting the passage of air, causing the child to produce an unusual sounding cough that can range from a high-pitched wheeze to a barking cough. Croup occurs most often during the evening and night hours.

A child with croup may progress quickly from respiratory distress to respiratory failure. Children with croup may benefit from humidified oxygen. If you are transporting the child to the hospital, you may see an improvement in the child once exposed to cool air outdoors.

Epiglottitis is a bacterial infection that causes severe swelling of the epiglottis. While it is extremely rare, the symptoms may be similar to croup; it is a more serious illness and can result in death if the airway is blocked completely.

If the child is older, you may see the *tripod position*, where the child is sitting up and leaning forward, perhaps with the chin thrust outward **(Fig. 25-5)**. Other signs are drooling, difficulty swallowing, voice changes and fever.

A child with epiglottitis can move from respiratory distress to respiratory failure very quickly without emergency care. With epiglottitis, keeping the child as calm as possible is vital. Do *not* examine the throat using a tongue depressor or place anything in the child's throat, as these can trigger a complete airway blockage.

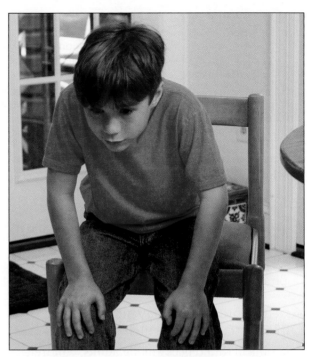

Fig. 25-5: An older child with epiglottitis may demonstrate the tripod position, in which the child sits up, leaning forward, possibly with the chin thrust outward.

Asthma is a common illness and can be triggered in many children by exposure to allergens. Air is drawn into the lungs, but as the bronchioles constrict during an asthma attack, they also may fill with mucus, blocking the air in the lungs from exiting. This blockage results in the characteristic wheeze when the patient exhales. Ask the parents or caregiver if the child is known to have asthma and, if so, if any rescue medications are available. If medications have been administered, find out what has been taken and how often up to the time of your arrival.

The status of a child with asthma can change very quickly, so constant monitoring is necessary. The typical signs of asthma include rapid respirations that take effort as respiratory distress develops, but the breathing may seem to become less labored. This does not indicate improvement, but rather deterioration in respiratory status.

Choking is a common emergency in young children, particularly once they become mobile and are able to explore on their own. Your interventions will be based on your assessments as to whether the child has a partial or complete airway obstruction.

Providing Care for Breathing Emergencies

Treatment of all respiratory emergencies is generally the same. Use equipment that is properly sized for the child, particularly if using an oxygen mask (**Fig. 25-6**). The mask should fit the child and should deliver the appropriate amount of oxygen. Monitor the airway and breathing continuously and arrange for transport as quickly as possible.

Circulatory Failure

As with adults, undetected and uncorrected circulatory failure in children and infants can cause cardiac arrest. Signs and symptoms of circulatory failure include—

- Increased heart rate (but can also be decreased).
- Unequal pulses (femoral compared with radial).
- Delayed capillary refill.
- Changes in mental status.

Unlike adults, children seldom initially suffer a cardiac emergency. Instead, they suffer a respiratory emergency that develops into a cardiac emergency. Motor-vehicle collisions, drowning, smoke inhalation, poisoning, airway obstruction and falls are all common causes of respiratory emergencies that can develop into a cardiac emergency. A cardiac emergency can also result from an acute respiratory condition, such as a severe asthma attack. *Always* be prepared for the possibility of circulatory failure when dealing with a respiratory emergency.

Care for circulatory failure includes identifying problems through assessment; assisting attempts to breathe by opening the airway, removing obstructions or providing ventilation; and observing for signs of cardiac arrest, performing CPR and using an AED. More information on the identification and care for circulatory failure can be found in **Chapter 13**.

Seizures

A **seizure** is temporary abnormal electrical activity in the brain caused by injury, disease, fever, infection, metabolic disturbances or conditions that decrease oxygen levels. A chronic condition, such as epilepsy, or an acute event may cause seizures.

In children, the most common type of seizure is a **febrile seizure**, which occurs with a rapidly rising or excessively high fever, higher than 103° F. Febrile seizures may have some or all of the following signs and symptoms:
- Sudden rise in body temperature
- Change in LOC
- Rhythmic jerking of the head and limbs
- Loss of bladder or bowel control
- Confusion
- Drowsiness
- Crying out
- Becoming rigid
- Holding the breath
- Rolling the eyes upward

Assessing Seizures

When obtaining a history from the parents or caregivers, you need to know several things to assess what type of seizure the child may be having and what may have caused it. Ask questions such as—
- Has the child ever had seizures before? If so, does the child have medications for them? If not, is there a family history of seizures?
- Does the child have diabetes? If so, what type of insulin/medication is being used and when

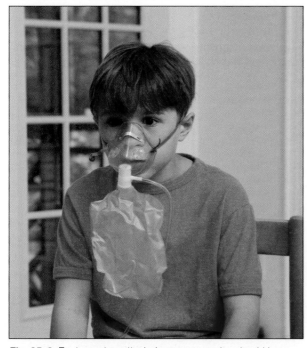

Fig. 25-6: Equipment, particularly oxygen masks, should be properly sized for the child so that it fits correctly.

was the last time it was given? Do the parents monitor the blood sugar level? If so, what was the child's blood sugar level when it was most recently monitored?

- Has the child begun taking any new medications lately? If the child takes medications, is it possible there may have been an overdose? Could the child have taken someone else's medication?
- Did the child have access to anything poisonous?
- Has the child had an injury, particularly a head trauma, recently?
- Has the child seemed sick or had a high fever, stiff neck or recent headache?
- What did the seizure look like? Did it involve the child's whole body, or only one half of the body? Did it start in one area and progress to the rest? Did the child fall when the seizure began and if so, was it possible the child's head struck an object or the floor?

Managing Seizures

The general principles of managing a seizure are to prevent injury, protect the child's airway and ensure that the airway is open after the seizure has ended. Call for more advanced medical personnel for a child or an infant who has had a seizure and for a young child or an infant who experienced a febrile seizure brought on by a high fever.

Do *not* put anything in the child's mouth and do *not* restrain the child. Ensure that the environment is as safe as possible to prevent injury to the child during the seizure by moving away any furniture or other objects.

After the seizure, ensure the child's airway is open and administer emergency oxygen if available. Suctioning may be necessary to remove excessive fluids. Also, after the seizure, assess the patient for any injuries that may have been sustained as a result of the seizure. If possible, position the child or infant on his or her side so that fluids (saliva, blood, vomit) can drain from the mouth.

Care for a child or an infant who experiences a febrile seizure is much the same as for any other seizure. Most febrile seizures last less than 5 minutes and are not life threatening. However, immediately after a febrile seizure it is important to cool the body if a fever is present.

See **Chapter 14** for more information on managing seizures.

Fever

Fever is defined as an elevated body temperature. It signifies a problem and, in a child or an infant, can indicate specific problems. Often these problems are not life threatening, but some can be. A high fever in a child often indicates some form of infection. In a young child, even a minor infection can result in a rather high fever, which is often defined as a temperature higher than 103° F. If a fever is present, call for more advanced medical help at once.

Your initial care for a child with a high fever is to gently cool the child. Never rush cooling down a child. If the fever has caused a febrile seizure, rapid cooling could bring on another seizure. Parents or caregivers often heavily dress children with fevers. Remove the excess clothing or blankets, and sponge the child with lukewarm water. Do *not* use an ice water bath or use rubbing alcohol to cool down the body. Both of these approaches are dangerous, and parents and caregivers should be discouraged from ever using them.

Do *not* give children or infants aspirin or products that contain aspirin when they show flu-like symptoms including fever, or if they may have a viral illness such as chicken pox, as this may result in an extremely serious medical condition called **Reye's syndrome**. Reye's syndrome is an illness that affects the brain and other internal organs. Ask the parents what medications they may have given the child so you can inform more advanced medical personnel.

Poisoning

Poisoning can cause many types of emergency calls, from seizures to cardiac arrest. It is the fifth leading cause of unintentional death in the United States for individuals between the ages of 1 and 24. Poisoning in young children is usually caused by the ingestion of household products that may be kept in the kitchen, bathroom or garage. Children may also take medications found in cupboards, on tables or even in visitors' purses or backpacks. Poisoning may also occur from swallowing solid objects, like batteries, particularly the watch-sized batteries found in many children's toys.

Shock

Shock is the body's reaction to a physical or emotional trauma in both adults and children. Physical trauma could include loss of blood. In small children, the loss of blood may be much more significant than in adolescents or adults. This adds to the increased risk of shock and the speed with which it may develop. Children can go into shock very quickly, regardless of the cause, and may go into cardiac arrest much faster than adults.

Causes of Shock in Children

In addition to trauma, shock may also be caused by infection. Infections can send the body into shock because of the body's reaction to the infection. The risk of shock increases with the severity and centrality of the infection.

Among children, the most common cause of shock is vomiting or diarrhea. As they lose fluid from the vomit and/or diarrhea, their body fluid volume becomes depleted and their blood pressure drops.

Assessing Shock

When assessing shock, watch the child's mental status, including any changes that have occurred since you arrived on the scene. Some children may experience a change in mental status so pronounced that it makes them unable to recognize their parents or caregivers. This altered mental status is a strong indicator that shock is developing quickly and may result in cardiac arrest.

Other signs and symptoms of shock include—
- Cold, clammy, pale or ashen skin, particularly in infants, as they are less capable of regulating body temperature.
- Rapid, weak or thready pulse.
- Rapid or irregular breathing.
- Lack of tears when crying.
- Low or lack of urine output.
- Falling blood pressure.

Providing Care for Shock

Lay the child flat if possible, but do not force it if the child is too agitated or upset. Constantly monitor the child's respiratory and circulatory status. Have equipment available should the child go into cardiac arrest.

Altered Mental Status

Altered mental status in children and infants is another medical condition you may encounter. This can be caused by low blood sugar, poisonings or overdoses, seizures, infections, trauma, decreased level of oxygen and the onset of shock. When assessing altered mental status, use the AVPU scale, which is covered more thoroughly in **Chapter 7**.

When arriving on the scene, determining the cause of the alteration in mental status right away is not essential. Your role is to support the patient by maintaining an open airway and administering emergency oxygen if it is available. Any information you can gather from the parents, caregivers or bystanders will help you care for the patient.

Trauma

Injury is the number-one cause of death for children in the United States. Many of these deaths are the result of motor-vehicle collisions. The greatest dangers to a child involved in a motor-vehicle crash are airway obstruction and bleeding. Ensure an open airway and control severe bleeding as quickly as possible. A relatively small amount of blood lost by an adult is a large amount for a child or an infant.

Because a child's head is large and heavy in proportion to the rest of the body, the head is the most frequently injured part of the child's body. A child injured as the result of force or a blow may also have sustained damage to the organs in the abdomen and chest. Because children have very soft, pliable ribs, such damage can cause severe internal bleeding. Care for a child with a chest injury involves keeping an open airway, assessing the chest for rise and fall and administering emergency oxygen if it is available.

In a car crash, a child only secured by a lap belt may have serious abdominal or spinal injuries. You may need to rely on bystanders' reports of what happened, as a severely injured child may not immediately show signs of injury.

Laws requiring children to ride in safety seats or wear safety belts have been enacted to stop some of the needless deaths of children associated with motor vehicle crashes. As a result, children's lives are being saved. However, you may have to check and care for an injured child or infant while the child is in a safety seat (**Fig. 25-7**). A safety seat does not normally pose any problems when checking a child or an infant. Leave the child or infant in the seat if the seat has not been damaged. If the child or infant is to be transported to a medical facility for examination, the child can often be safely secured in the safety seat for transport.

Care for extremity injuries in a child or an infant in the same way as for adults. When providing care for an injured child or infant, use equipment of the proper size. If equipment of the proper size is not available, manually stabilize extremity injuries until additional help arrives. Information on the general management of extremity injuries can be found in **Chapter 22**.

Try to comfort, calm and reassure the child and family members while waiting for additional *emergency medical services* (EMS) resources.

Child Abuse and Neglect

You may at some point encounter a situation involving an injured child in which you believe or have reason to suspect child abuse or neglect is involved.

Types of Abuse

Child abuse, or non-accidental trauma, is the physical, psychological or sexual assault of a child resulting in injury and emotional trauma. Child abuse involves an injury or pattern of injuries

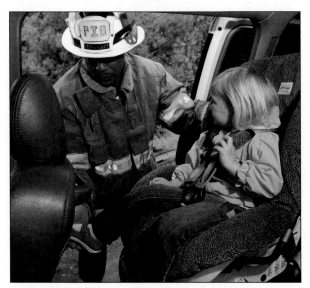

Fig. 25-7: If the safety seat has not been damaged, leave the child in it while you are checking and caring for the child.

that do *not* result from a mishap. Your might suspect child abuse if the child's injuries cannot be logically explained or a caregiver or parent gives an inconsistent or suspicious account of how the injuries occurred. Perpetrators of child abuse may often be evasive or volunteer very little information.

One type of abuse is **shaken baby syndrome**, which is the result of a young child being shaken harshly—hard enough to cause brain swelling and damage. Signs and symptoms of shaken baby syndrome include unconsciousness, lethargy/decreased muscle tone, extreme irritability, difficulty breathing, seizures, inability to lift head, inability of eyes to focus and decreased appetite.

Child neglect is insufficient attention given to or a lack of respect shown to a child who has a claim to that attention. Neglect is the most common type of child abuse reported. Signs and symptoms include—

- Lack of adult supervision.
- A child who appears underfed or malnourished.
- An unsafe living environment.
- Untreated chronic illness; for example, a child with asthma who has no medications available despite being issued a prescription.

Epidemiology of Child Abuse and Neglect

Epidemiology studies show that child abuse is not limited to a certain sector of society but may occur in any part. An estimated 500,000 to 4 million cases of child abuse occur every year, and thousands of these children die. Of all causes of death in children, it is the only one that has not decreased in the past 30 years.

Assessing Child Abuse and Neglect

Upon arriving on the scene, note anything in the child's history or at the scene that causes concern or suspicion of abuse or neglect. Watch the caregiver's behavior, which may be evasive; the caregiver (usually a parent) may not volunteer much information or may contradict information already given. Also observe for particular physical signs and symptoms:

- Injury that does not fit the description of what caused it

- Patterns of injury that include cigarette burns, whip marks and handprints (**Fig. 25-8, A–B**)
- Obvious or suspected fractures in a child younger than 2 years of age
- Any unexplained fractures
- Injuries in various stages of healing, especially bruises and burns (**Fig. 25-8, C**)
- Unexplained lacerations or abrasions, especially to the mouth, lips and eyes (**Fig. 25-8, D**)
- Injuries to the genitalia
- Pain when the child sits down
- More injuries than are common for a child of that age
- Repeated emergency calls to the same address

Managing Child Abuse and Neglect

When caring for a child who may have been abused, your first priority is to care for the child's injuries or illness. An abused child may be frightened, hysterical or withdrawn. Abused children may also be unwilling to talk about the incident in an attempt to protect the abuser or for self-protection. If you suspect abuse, explain your concerns to the responding police officers or *emergency medical technicians* (EMTs), if possible.

When answering a call where you suspect abuse, you must ensure your own safety. Do *not* place the child in the awkward position

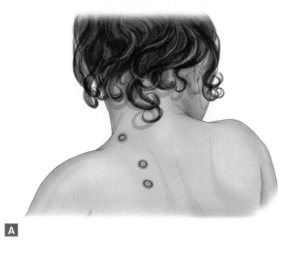

A

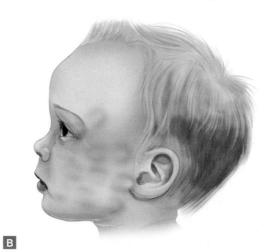

B

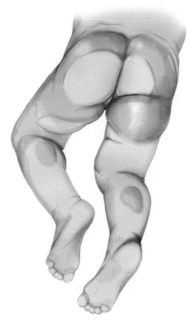

C

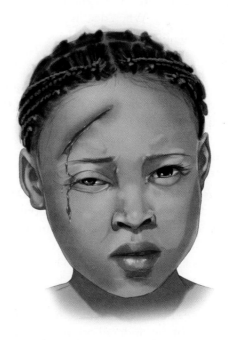

D

Fig. 25-8, A–D: When you arrive on the scene, observe for particular physical signs of child abuse or neglect. These include **(A)** cigarette burns, **(B)** handprints, **(C)** burns and **(D)** unexplained lacerations.

of having to tell you things that may cause tension with parents or caregivers. Focus on treating the child and making your assessments. *Never* confront the parents or caregivers about your suspicions, as this could put you and/or the child at risk. If you need to transport the child out of the environment, the parents' or caregivers' support is essential.

Legal Aspects of Child Abuse and Neglect

If you have reasonable cause to believe that abuse has occurred, you can report your suspicions to a community or state agency, such as the Department of Social Services, the Department of Children and Family Services or Child Protective Services. You may be afraid to report suspected child abuse because you do not wish to get involved or are afraid of getting sued.

You do *not* need to identify yourself when you report child abuse, although your report will have more credibility if you do. In some areas, certain professions are *legally obligated* to report suspicions of child abuse.

Documenting Child Abuse and Neglect

As with all emergency calls, you must document your observations and actions and the patient's response objectively. When dealing with suspected child abuse or child neglect, remain objective in your documentation. Do *not* write any supposition or theories. If there is later legal action, your notes may be used in court. Your notes have a better chance of being useful if they are thorough and objective.

Sudden Infant Death Syndrome

Sudden infant death syndrome (**SIDS**), which used to be called crib death, is the unexplained sudden death of an infant younger than 1, but it occurs most often between the ages of 4 weeks and 7 months. SIDS almost always occurs while the infant is sleeping. This condition does not seem to be linked to any disease. Because the cause or causes of SIDS are not yet understood, parents do not know if their child is at risk. SIDS is sometimes mistaken for child abuse because of

the unexplained death of an otherwise healthy child and the presence of bruise-like blotches that sometimes appear on the infant's body. However, SIDS is not related to child abuse. SIDS is also not believed to be hereditary, but it does tend to recur in families.

Epidemiology and Risk Factors

The rate of SIDS occurrence is significantly lower now than prior to 1992, when parents were first told to put infants to sleep on their back or side. Even so, unfortunately, SIDS still causes a significant number of deaths in infants younger than 1, and thousands of babies die of SIDS in the United States each year.

Parents should *not* leave pillows or blankets in the crib and should try to ensure that the infant is *not* exposed to any secondhand smoke. Babies who die of SIDS are most often reported to have been perfectly healthy, although some reports indicate some infants had a cold prior to their death.

Assessing and Managing SIDS

When called for a SIDS death, unless the infant is very obviously dead (rigor mortis has set in), attempt resuscitation with CPR as per infant protocols. Follow local EMS protocols for death in the field, and notify the appropriate authorities.

If possible, try to obtain the following information—

- When was the infant last checked on or put to bed and seen to be breathing?
- Who discovered the infant and what brought the person into the room (concern of infant sleeping too long, time to get up, etc.)?
- How was the infant lying in the crib, in what position?
- Was anything else in the crib?
- Were any other adults or children in the house while the infant was sleeping?
- What was the infant's state of health?
- Did the infant seem different, uncharacteristically quiet or cranky, for example, when last put in the crib?
- Did the infant have any illnesses or allergies?
- Was the infant given any medications?
- Were any medications or toxic substances nearby?
- How warm was the bedroom?

By the time the infant's condition is discovered, the infant will likely be in cardiac arrest. Ensure that someone has called more advanced medical personnel, or call for help yourself. Give the infant CPR until more advanced medical personnel take over.

Caregiver Support for SIDS

Because of the circumstances of the death, the parents and possibly siblings may be your patients as much as the infant. Shock can result from a severe emotional trauma, so observe the parents closely for signs and symptoms of shock.

When more advanced emergency personnel take over the infant's care, you can focus on the parents. Encourage them to accompany the infant. If they are concerned about leaving other children behind, see if a neighbor or friend is able to stay with their children.

Apparent Life-Threatening Events

An *apparent life-threatening event* (**ALTE**) is a sudden event in infants younger than 1, characterized by apnea, change in color, change in muscle tone and coughing or gagging. About half the time, ALTE is linked to an underlying digestive, neurologic or respiratory health problem, but it remains unexplained in half of cases. When linked to certain other conditions, ALTE is thought to be a risk factor for SIDS. At one time, it was believed these two conditions were more strongly linked and it was questioned whether ALTE was simply a "near-miss" case of SIDS, but experts no longer believe this is the case.

Considerations for Children with Special Needs

In addition to the more common problems any child may have, a child with special needs may have additional health concerns. When called to a scene with a child with special needs, the parents or caregivers can generally provide you with the most information, because they are the most familiar with the medical equipment the child may use. Pieces of equipment may include—

- Power wheelchairs.
- Ventilators.
- Communication systems.
- Feeding apparatus.

While making your assessments, the parents or caregivers can provide valuable insight into the problem. They may suspect a specific issue, or perhaps a similar situation occurred previously.

While assessing breathing and pulse, take into account that if a child is on a respirator or ventilator, the problem may not be with the child, but with the machine. You may need to manually give ventilations with a BVM or other device while the machine is being checked.

When caring for children, you depend on your assessment skills to determine the child's age and maturity level. When dealing with children who have special needs, the child's age and maturity level may not be as straightforward, depending on the child's disability. Do *not* assume a child's mental capacity if the child is unable to express thoughts or words. Ask the parents what the child is capable of understanding and speak directly to the child as you would to any other. Do *not* speak to the parents as if the child is not in the room.

THE EMERGENCY MEDICAL RESPONDER'S NEEDS

Dealing with emergency situations can be difficult for many *emergency medical responders* (EMRs). The difficulty can be compounded when the emergencies include children, particularly if they involve suspected child abuse or SIDS. The death of a child, especially if declared on the scene of an accident, can be very difficult for any rescuer.

While you are on scene, caring for the child and interacting with the parents, caregivers and/or bystanders, maintain a professional demeanor and control your emotions. This is easiest if you focus on the task at hand and *only* the task. However, once you are away from the scene, your professional "mask" may be removed as you deal with your own thoughts and emotions.

As a person, you are entitled to your own thoughts and emotions, be they anger, pain or sorrow. Feeling anxious and helpless is common and normal after such events. However, these feelings must be put in context so they do not overwhelm you and interfere with your professional and personal life.

Most emergency response teams have debriefing or defusing sessions available that allow responders to talk about what happened. More information on this topic can be found in **Chapter 2**.

PUTTING IT ALL TOGETHER

Caring for children is similar in many ways to caring for adults, but differences exist, both physical and emotional. Caring for a child often also means providing support and care to the parents or caregivers, who are often stressed and anxious.

Assessing breathing and pulse in children is, for the most part, the same as assessing the same things in adults. For both adults and children, breathing and pulse are your priority and must be assessed before all else. Although the airway must be patent in both adults and children, it is smaller and shorter in children, and their respirations are generally more rapid than those of an adult. When assessing circulation, a child who is bleeding may

go into shock more rapidly than an adult because of the lower quantity of blood circulating in a child's body.

Caring for children may also involve potentially anxiety-provoking situations, such as child abuse or neglect. If you suspect child abuse or neglect, you must perform your duties as a professional, and keep your personal feelings to yourself. You are not, however, helpless; you can report concerns of child abuse if you feel they are warranted.

Finally, as an EMR, you will likely face death on occasion, and dealing with a child's death may have an especially strong impact. Although you must remain professional while on the job, you also must recognize that—as a person—you have the right to feel upset, anxious, angry or any other emotion. Take care of yourself so that these emotions do not overcome you and affect your life.

YOU ARE THE EMERGENCY MEDICAL RESPONDER

As you continue to monitor the child's condition, you notice that the hives have spread beyond the affected area. What care should you provide?

26 Geriatrics and Special Needs Patients

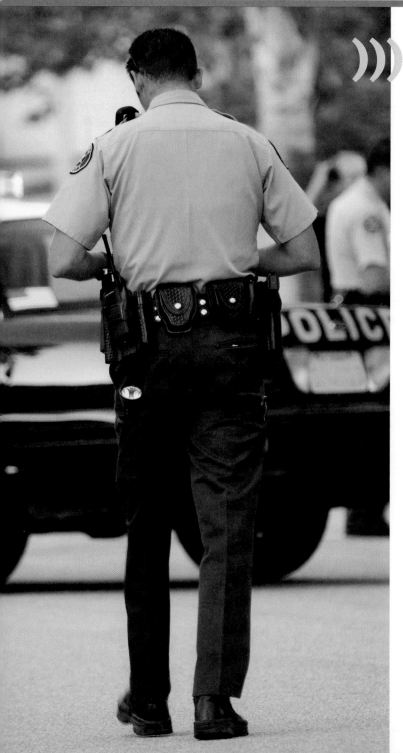

))) **YOU ARE THE EMERGENCY MEDICAL RESPONDER**

Your police unit responds to a scene where an elderly gentleman appears lost and disoriented. He does not know where he is, how he got there or how to get home. When you ask him what his name is, the gentleman cannot remember. How would you respond?

Key Terms

Alzheimer's disease: The most common type of dementia in older people, in which thought, memory and language are impaired.

Asperger syndrome: A disorder on the autism spectrum; those with Asperger syndrome have a milder form of the disorder.

Autism spectrum disorders (ASD): A group of disorders characterized by some degree of impairment in communication and social interaction as well as repetitive behaviors.

Bereavement care: Care provided to families during the period of grief and mourning surrounding a death.

Catastrophic reaction: A reaction a person experiences when the person has become overwhelmed; signs include screaming, throwing objects and striking out.

Chronic diseases: Diseases that occur gradually and continue over a long period of time.

Cognitive impairment: Impairment of thinking abilities including memory, judgment, reasoning, problem solving and decision making.

Deafness: The loss of the ability to hear from one or both ears; can be mild, moderate, severe or profound and can be inherited, occur at birth or be acquired at a later point in life, due to illness, medication, noise exposure or injury.

Dementia: A collection of symptoms caused by any of several disorders of the brain; characterized by significantly impaired intellectual functioning that interferes with normal activities and relationships.

Edema: Swelling in body tissues caused by fluid accumulation.

Hard of hearing: A degree of hearing loss that is mild enough to allow the person to continue to rely on hearing for communication.

Hospice care: Care provided in the final months of life to a terminally ill patient.

Mental illness: A range of medical conditions that affect a person's mood or ability to think, feel, relate to others and function in everyday activities.

Service animal: A guide dog, signal dog or other animal individually trained to provide assistance to a person with a disability.

Sundowning: A symptom of Alzheimer's disease in which the person becomes increasingly restless or confused as late afternoon or evening approaches.

Learning Objectives

After reading this chapter, and completing the class activities, you will have the information needed to—

- Describe physical and mental differences that are important in geriatric patients.
- Describe how to assess a geriatric patient.
- Describe how to provide care for a geriatric patient.
- Describe common problems in geriatric patients.
- List the types of elder abuse.
- List risk factors for elder abuse.
- List signs and behaviors of elder abuse.
- Identify and describe chronic diseases and disabilities.
- Describe considerations for providing care to special needs patients.

INTRODUCTION

When responding to elderly patients, remember that patience, kindness and respect will help you care for the patient in the most effective manner. Misconceptions about geriatric patients, such as that they are all weak or sickly, **hard of hearing** and have difficulty learning new things, can often lead to elderly people being treated like children and not like responsible adults. Explaining the steps you are taking to treat and care for them, and using the same kind and respectful manner you would use with younger adult patients, will prove to be successful with geriatric patients.

This chapter will provide you with the information needed to assist geriatric patients and identify and deal with any special needs they may have, such as **dementia**, including **Alzheimer's disease**.

You will also learn about patients with special needs, such as those with **mental illness**, intellectual disabilities and other special needs, such as visual impairment or **deafness**. Special needs also exist for the physically challenged, as well as for those suffering from **chronic diseases**. In this section, you will learn about important factors to take into account when caring for patients with conditions such as arthritis, cancer, cerebral palsy and multiple sclerosis.

GERIATRIC PATIENTS

The geriatric population, those aged 65 years and older, is the fastest-growing age group in the United States. Because people are living longer, older people make up a large proportion of the population and, thus, make up a greater segment of those requiring care. Geriatric patients are, in many ways, no different from younger adult patients, but everyone undergoes some changes in their physical and mental health as they age, and these changes need to be considered when providing care (**Fig. 26-1**).

Physical and Mental Differences to Consider in Geriatrics

As people age, normal changes in physical and mental functioning occur. These changes occur

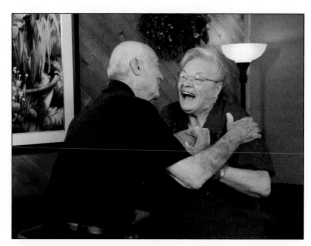
Fig. 26-1: The geriatric population includes those aged 65 years and older.

in all body systems, including nervous, digestive, respiratory, circulatory, musculoskeletal, integumentary, genitourinary and endocrine.

Sensory Changes in the Elderly

Aging patients often have decreased sharpness of the senses, and this loss of sensory awareness brings possible risks that are unique to this age group.

Vision

Because vision in the elderly may be poor due to problems such as decreased night and peripheral vision, farsightedness, cataracts and decreased tolerance to glare, accidents are more likely to occur. Misreading instructions for medication, falls and motor-vehicle crashes are common among geriatric patients, and may be due, in part, to vision problems (**Fig. 26-2**).

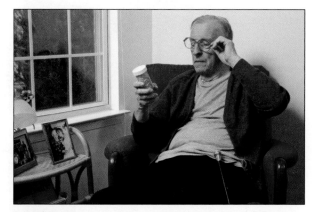
Fig. 26-2: Poor vision, common in the elderly, may result in an increased likelihood for misreading medication instructions.

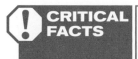
CRITICAL FACTS

As people age, normal changes in physical and mental functioning occur. These changes occur in all body systems, including nervous, digestive, respiratory, circulatory, musculoskeletal, integumentary, genitourinary and endocrine.

Hearing

The ability to hear gradually diminishes with age, especially for higher frequency sounds. Hearing loss can be an indirect cause of injury; for example, an elderly patient might have trouble hearing a warning alarm or siren.

Sense of Touch and Pain

Diminished pain sensation can also prove dangerous for elderly patients, as they may not be aware of an injury or of the seriousness of an injury.

Diminished Taste and Smell

A decrease in sense of taste and/or smell can lead to health problems such as poor nutrition, decreased appetite and even food poisoning, if an elderly person is unable to detect that food has gone bad. A decrease in the ability to smell can also be a safety concern, as odors such as natural gas, propane or gasoline may not be easily detected.

Heart/Blood Vessels

Aging causes the heart to work harder. The heart muscle thickens and becomes less elastic, and arteries stiffen, which makes it harder for blood to flow through them.

Over the years, plaque can build up within the arteries and restrict or block blood flow in a condition called *atherosclerosis*. Blood clots can also form and further restrict blood flow, factors which can lead to heart attack or stroke **(Fig. 26-3)**.

Heart failure also develops when the heart cannot pump enough blood to meet the body's demand. Valve problems, including narrowing or leaking of the aortic or mitral valve, are also common in the elderly.

Arrhythmias are usually categorized according to the affected part of the heart—the atrial (upper) part, or the ventricular (lower) part of the heart—as well as by the change in rhythm. An aneurysm is a widening or ballooning out of a major artery that develops in the aorta or one of the other major arteries in the chest or abdomen. Aneurysms are common in older adults, especially those with high blood pressure or coronary artery disease.

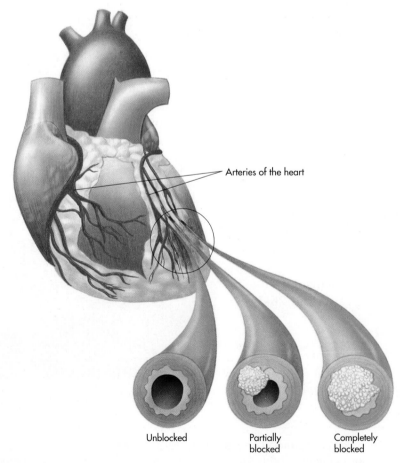

Arteries of the heart

Unblocked   Partially blocked   Completely blocked

Fig. 26-3: Buildup of fatty materials on the inner walls of the arteries reduces blood flow to the heart muscle and may cause a heart attack.

Lungs and Breathing

Aging also affects the lungs, which become stiffer and less elastic, shrinking the airways and weakening the chest muscles. This causes the total flow of air into and out of the lungs to decrease, and increases the chances of developing breathing problems. Older people are also more prone to lung infections, such as pneumonia, due to changes in the lungs and immune system.

Stomach and Intestines

With aging, the digestive tract becomes stiffer, and the contractions which allow food to move effectively through the digestive system decrease. Elderly people may also suffer from conditions and diseases, such as hardening of the arteries and diabetes, which can upset the function of the intestines and lead to symptoms and complications. Medications commonly prescribed for older adults can also cause problems in the digestive tract. Problems in various digestive organs can cause different symptoms, such as difficulty swallowing, stomachache, nausea, diarrhea and constipation. This often affects appetite and nutrition, leading to fatigue and weight loss.

Nervous System

The majority of middle-aged and older adults retain their abilities to learn, remember and solve problems. However, **cognitive impairment**, exhibited by memory loss and other problems, such as issues with perception, balance, coordination, reasoning, judgment and sleep, can occur and are *not* a normal part of aging. They can be the result of reversible causes, such as acute illness, or the side effects of medication. Cognitive impairment also can be the result of certain neurological disorders including a range of dementias. Some changes also may be due to clinical depression, which is more common in the elderly.

Muscles and Bones

Problems of the musculoskeletal system are common in older adults and can range from minor sprains or inflammation to fractures, arthritis or cancer. Bones become less dense over time, especially in women, and this can lead to fractures. Musculoskeletal problems can also lead to a more sedentary lifestyle and the inactivity itself can lead to a further decline in function.

Other

Other common health issues for geriatric patients include urinary problems, skin diseases, decreased ability to fight off illness and nutritional problems.

Assessing and Caring for the Geriatric Patient

Assessing the Geriatric Patient

When assessing a geriatric patient, follow the same care and procedures, including checking breathing and pulse, as you would for a younger adult. However, you should keep the following points in mind when providing care for the elderly.

Patients who appear untidy and uncared for may not be taking good care of themselves and might have been neglectful in tending to their own medical needs. Whenever possible, speak to the patient's family or caregivers to identify the patient's usual behavioral patterns and whether the patient is behaving normally or has changed in response to an emergency.

When speaking with geriatric patients, speak a little more slowly and clearly, and allow time to ensure they understand, unless the situation appears urgent. Speak to the patient at eye level, and turn lights on to make it easier for the patient to see you (**Fig. 26-4**).

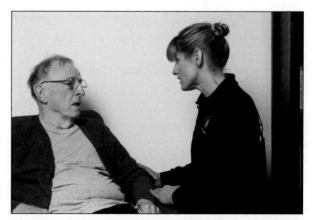

Fig. 26-4: Speak with geriatric patients at eye level, and speak slowly and clearly, allowing time to ensure they understand.

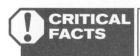
CRITICAL FACTS When assessing a geriatric patient, follow the same care and procedures, including checking breathing and pulse, as you would for a younger adult.

When obtaining the SAMPLE history from the patient, consider the following:

- The patient may become tired easily.
- You will need to clearly explain what you are doing before beginning the examination.
- The patient may downplay symptoms due to fear of institutionalization or losing independence.
- It may be difficult to assess peripheral pulses.
- Some signs and symptoms you observe may be a part of normal aging; distinguish these from any that may be related to the emergency.

Due to many factors, including diminished senses, an elderly patient may not show severe symptoms, even if very ill. Continue to reassess the patient's condition, as it may deteriorate quickly.

Some older patients may be participants in the Vial of Life program, which was designed to allow patients to provide medical information to *emergency medical services* (EMS) personnel. The Vial of Life kit is offered to patients across North America and is kept on the patient's refrigerator to alert responders to the patient's health conditions, medications and any other medical information the patient wishes to supply (**Fig. 26-5**). The kit includes a form, a plastic bag to store the form and decals to inform responders that the information is available. One decal is kept on the patient's front door and the other is on the bag. The kit is ideal for a situation in which a patient is unresponsive, home alone and unable to provide vital information. Check the patient's door and refrigerator to see if the patient is a participant in the program.

Caring for the Geriatric Patient

Some key considerations exist in the care of a geriatric patient:

- Explain everything you are doing, calmly and slowly.
- Handle the patient's skin with special care, as it can tear easily.

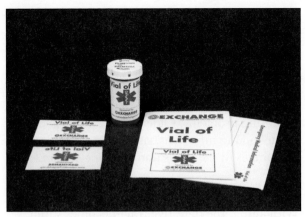

Fig. 26-5: Vial of Life kit

- If the patient is responsive and a stroke is suspected, the patient may have difficulty chewing, swallowing and clearing the airway of secretions.
- Dentures and other dental devices can cause airway obstruction.
- If artificial ventilation is required and the patient is wearing dentures, it may be easier to leave the dentures in place.
- If it is difficult to tilt the patient's head back due to conditions such as a curvature of the spine, perform a jaw-thrust (without head extension) maneuver.
- Blood-thinning medications and aspirin may make any bleeding more difficult to control.
- If the patient's mental status changes and the patient is unable to maintain the airway, consider inserting an *oropharyngeal airway* (OPA). OPAs should *only* be used on unconscious, unresponsive patients with *no* gag reflex.
- Be prepared to assist with ventilation, but do *not* apply too much pressure, as this could result in chest injury.
- Continue to re-evaluate during transport.

Consider the following conditions when positioning a patient for transport:

- If the patient is responsive and able to breathe, place the patient in the Fowler's position (**Fig. 26-6**).

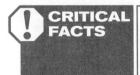

CRITICAL FACTS There are several considerations when caring for a geriatric patient. These include working calmly, slowly and with extra care; being aware of dentures and how to deal with them; being aware of blood-thinning medications and aspirin; and knowing what care procedures are appropriate for a geriatric patient, such as being aware of the amount of pressure you use when assisting with ventilation to avoid chest injury.

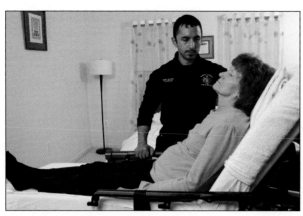

Fig. 26-6: Place the patient in the Fowler's position for transport if he or she is responsive and breathing.

- If the patient has an altered mental status and you cannot protect the airway, place the patient on his or her side or in the modified *high arm in endangered spine* (H.A.IN.E.S.) recovery position.
- If a spinal injury is suspected, a patient with a curvature of the spine could be injured if placed on a backboard. Use blankets for immobilization.
- Unresponsive patients should be immobilized as a precaution.

Common Problems in the Geriatric Patient

Dementia

Geriatric patients can become confused when their cognitive functions decrease. Confusion is a symptom of memory loss, and can be a sign of cognitive impairment. Some types of cognitive impairment are chronic and cannot be reversed; these are referred to as dementias. Dementia is a set of symptoms characterized by problems with memory, reasoning, orientation and personal care. A patient with dementia may behave oddly and become anxious or aggressive. As people with dementia become increasingly unaware of their surroundings, they ultimately become unable to perform normal tasks. About 50 percent of all people admitted to nursing homes suffer from some type of dementia.

Dementia is not caused by stress or a crisis, but often during a time of crisis others may notice something is wrong, as the person becomes increasingly confused. Dementia is not a normal part of growing older, but it is estimated that about 6 to 10 percent of people aged 65 years or older have dementia and about 30 percent of people 85 or older develop it.

Alzheimer's Disease

Alzheimer's disease is the most common type of dementia among older people. Those with the disease have the same basic needs as other patients. Witnessing a patient behaving dysfunctionally can be frustrating, but try to focus on the patient and that person's attempts to tell you something is wrong. Your job is to find out what the patient is trying to communicate, so that you can provide appropriate care.

A person with Alzheimer's disease may demonstrate some common patterns such as—

- Putting up a social facade by pretending not to know or remember a certain situation.
- Pacing and wandering.
- Rummaging and hoarding.
- Extreme **catastrophic reactions**, such as screaming, throwing objects or striking out.
- **Sundowning** (restlessness and confusion in the evening).
- Speaking nonsense.
- Hallucinating or believing things that are not true.
- Exhibiting depression, anger or suspicion.

If you know how to respond to these behaviors, you can provide better care and treat the patient with dignity and respect. If you encounter a patient who is walking aimlessly and then walking away, ask if you may walk with the person, and use this as a way to guide the patient back to the appropriate place. Talk to the patient and listen carefully to what the patient has to say. Take steps to prevent the patient from leaving.

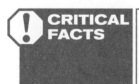

CRITICAL FACTS

Geriatric patients can become confused when their cognitive functions decrease. Confusion is a symptom of memory loss, and can be a sign of cognitive impairment. Some types of cognitive impairment are chronic and cannot be reversed; these are referred to as dementias.

Alzheimer's disease is the most common type of dementia among older people.

In the case of a catastrophic reaction, reassure the patient that you are not going to cause any harm and that you also will not allow the person to hurt anyone. Let the patient know the limits by saying something such as, "It's not okay to hit someone."

A person with Alzheimer's disease may become increasingly restless or confused as late afternoon or evening approaches, becoming more demanding, upset, suspicious or disoriented. This type of behavior is called sundowning, and is common in people with Alzheimer's disease. These patients may exhibit the following types of behavior:

- Restlessness, anxiety
- Worried expression
- Reluctance to enter the person's own room
- Reluctance to enter brightly lighted areas
- Crying
- Wringing hands
- Pushing others away
- Gritting teeth
- Taking off clothing

These behaviors may represent real physical needs, such as needing to use the bathroom or being hungry, uncomfortable or in pain. Responding in a kind, gentle manner will help calm the patient so you can discover what the problems are.

Elder Abuse

Elder abuse occurs when someone does something that harms or threatens the health and welfare of an elderly person, or when a caregiver fails to provide adequate care for an elderly person.

Research suggests that 4 percent of adults older than 65 are subjected to elder mistreatment in the United States. This mistreatment can occur within the family, in formal care settings or in the community or society at large. Elder abuse within the family is often the result of a caregiver being overwhelmed or not knowing what is needed when providing care for an elderly person. Reluctance to provide care can also lead to mistreatment. Mistreatment in a formal care setting is often attributable to staff who have not had adequate training in providing direct patient care.

Elder abuse can include—
- Physical abuse.
- Emotional abuse.
- Neglect (intentional or unintentional).
- Financial exploitation.
- Abandonment.
- Any combination of the above.

Risk factors for elder abuse include—
- Mental impairment in the dependent person or caregiver (or both).
- Isolation of the dependent person or the caregiver (or both).
- Inadequate living arrangements for the dependent person.
- Inability to perform daily functions.
- Frailty.
- Family conflict.
- Family history of abusive behavior, alcohol or drug abuse, mental illness or intellectual disability.
- Stressful family events.
- Poverty.
- Financial stress, especially related to health care needs.

In situations where frail or debilitated older people cannot help themselves at all, they may need more care than the caregiver is able to provide. Mentally ill people who hit, spit or scream can cause stress to the caregiver, causing the caregiver to respond with some form of elder mistreatment.

Watch for visible signs and certain behaviors by either the elderly patient or the caregiver that

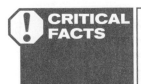
CRITICAL FACTS

Elder abuse takes many forms: physical, emotional, neglect, financial exploitation, abandonment or any combination of these.

Risk factors of elder abuse include mental impairment or isolation of the patient and/or caregiver, inadequate living situation, inability to perform daily functions, frailty, family conflict, abuse or stress or history of these, poverty and financial stress.

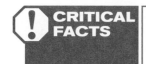

may provide clues that elder abuse has occurred. Some signs that may raise suspicion of elder abuse include—

- A person who is frequently left alone.
- A history of frequent trips to the emergency room.
- Old and new fractures or bruises, especially bruises on both sides of the inner arms and thighs.
- Repeated falls.
- Unexplained hair loss, skin rashes, irritation or skin ulceration.
- Inappropriate dress.
- Malnourishment.
- Lack of energy or spirit.
- Poor hygiene.
- Reports of the patient being left in unsafe situations or having an inability to get needed medication.

Maintain a proper perspective if you suspect an abusive situation. Do *not* confront the suspected abuser. Take note of any inconsistencies between the reports received from the patient and the suspected abuser. Follow local protocols in relation to elder abuse and the legal obligations to report suspected elder abuse. Document your findings as per local protocols and report your suspicions to the hospital upon arrival.

PATIENTS WITH SPECIAL NEEDS

Mental Illness

Mental illness is a broad term that describes a range of medical conditions that affect a person's mood or ability to think, feel, relate to others and function in everyday activities. About one-quarter of Americans suffer from a diagnosable mental disorder in a given year, though some of these are temporary conditions. About 6 percent of Americans suffer from serious mental illnesses, such as schizophrenia, major depression, panic disorder, bipolar disorder or personality disorder, although many are treatable with medication and psychosocial treatment.

The National Institute of Mental Health describes several types of mental illnesses:

- Mood disorders; for example, major depression and bipolar disorder
- Schizophrenia
- Anxiety disorders; for example, panic disorder, obsessive-compulsive disorder and post-traumatic stress disorder
- Eating disorders
- *Attention-deficit/hyperactivity disorder* (ADHD)
- Autism
- Alzheimer's disease

Intellectual Disabilities

Patients with an intellectual disability have a significantly below-average score on a test of mental ability or intelligence. Their ability to function in areas of daily life, such as communication, self-care and getting along in social situations and school activities, is also limited. Different degrees of intellectual disability exist, and a person's level can be defined by the *intelligence quotient* (IQ), or on how dependent the person is on others to perform daily needs.

Down Syndrome

Down syndrome is a genetic condition that results from having an extra copy of chromosome 21. Both mental and physical symptoms will be evident, although the symptoms can range from mild to severe. People with Down syndrome have mild-to-moderate intellectual impairment. Additionally, other health problems, such as heart disease, dementia, hearing loss and problems with the intestines, eyes, thyroid and skeleton, are common in people with Down syndrome. People with this syndrome share characteristic facial features, such as flattened facial features, small head, upward-slanting eyes that are unusual for the child's ethnic group, unusually shaped ears and a protruding tongue. It is not uncommon for people with Down syndrome to live productive lives well into adulthood.

Visually Impaired

When a person is visually impaired, the eyesight cannot always be corrected to a "normal" level. Types of visual impairments include a loss of visual acuity, where the eye does not see objects as clearly as normal, or a loss of visual field, where the eye cannot see as wide an area as normal without moving the eyes or turning the head.

When approaching patients, look for signs of visual impairment, such as glasses or a white cane. When approaching someone you know has a visual impairment, announce that you are approaching, who you are and why you are there so that the patient is not frightened. Ask if the person can see. Keep in mind that some blind patients are able to use other senses to compensate for their lack of sight. Especially at an accident scene, these patients may find the unfamiliar sights and sounds disorienting and may be frightened. Explain what is happening at the scene, what the sounds and smells are and what may happen at the scene such as additional loud sounds caused by equipment or traffic.

If a patient wears glasses, try to find them at the scene or in the home. This is especially important for elderly patients, who may try to hide the fact they are visually impaired. As with all patients, reassure them, explain what you are doing and use a gentle touch to keep them calm. Explain what is happening at each step so the patient feels more in control. Nearly two-thirds of children with visual impairment also have one or more other disabilities, such as intellectual disability, cerebral palsy, deafness or epilepsy. Children with more severe visual impairment are more likely than children with milder visual impairment to have additional disabilities.

Deaf and Hard of Hearing

Deafness is the loss of the ability to hear from one or both ears. It can be inherited, occur at birth or be acquired at a later point in life due to illness, medication, noise exposure or injury. The severity of the deafness can be mild, moderate, severe or profound. Two main types of deafness exist, and they are defined by the location of the problem. A *conductive* hearing loss occurs when there is a problem with the outer or middle ear; a *sensorineural* hearing loss is due to a problem with the inner ear and possibly the nerve that goes from the ear to the brain. Some people have both types of deafness.

The term "deaf" describes someone who is unable to hear well enough to rely on hearing as a means of communication. The term "**hard of hearing**" can be used to describe people who have a less severe hearing loss and are still able to rely on their hearing for communication.

Hearing loss is a disability that may not be immediately obvious to you when approaching a patient. Be certain a patient can hear you, especially when treating geriatric patients. Identify yourself, and speak slowly and clearly, but do not shout. Ask if the patient can hear you. Position yourself so the patient can hear you better by facing the patient; some patients who are hard of hearing can read lips. You can also try speaking directly into the person's ear. If possible, turn off background noise, such as a television or radio. If this does not work, write down your questions.

Physically Challenged

A person who is physically challenged may have been born with the condition or may have acquired it later in life. The person may have a general diminished ability to move due to illness or injury, and may use a mobility aid, such as a walker or wheelchair (**Fig. 26-7, A–B**). If you are aware that someone is physically challenged, ask what help the patient needs, for example to transfer from one surface to another (bed to chair) or to walk.

Traumatic Brain Injury

Someone who has suffered a traumatic brain injury may have been involved in a motor vehicle collision, suffered a fall or been the victim of an assault. Someone who has survived a traumatic brain injury may have permanent cognitive and physical problems. Cognitive impairment often includes difficulty with attention, memory, judgment, reasoning, problem solving and decision making. Physical problems can range from mild to severe and may result in the person moving slowly or relying on a mobility aid, such as a walker or wheelchair.

Chronic Diseases and Disabilities

Illnesses that occur gradually and continue over a long period of time are referred to as chronic conditions. Often, a chronic condition lasts

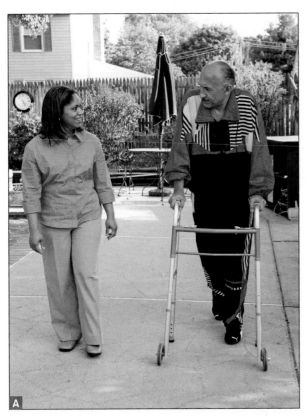

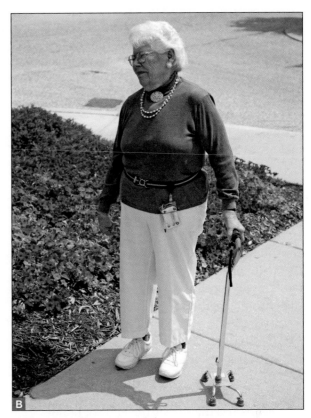

Fig. 26-7, A–B: A person who is physically challenged may use a mobility aid, such as **(A)** a walker or **(B)** a cane.

Service Animals

A **service animal** is any guide dog, signal dog or other animal individually trained to provide assistance to an individual with a disability. These animals are considered service animals under the *Americans with Disabilities Act* (ADA), whether or not they have been licensed or certified by a state or local government.

Service dogs perform some of the functions and tasks that the individual with a disability cannot perform independently. These dogs receive special training to help assist patients with many different types of disabilities, such as visual impairment, limited mobility, balance problems, autism, seizures or other medical problems like low blood sugar or psychiatric disabilities. Services include retrieving objects, pulling wheelchairs, opening and closing doors, turning light switches off and on, barking when help is needed, finding another person, leading the person to the handler, assisting with balance and counterbalance, providing deep pressure and many other individual tasks.

A service animal is not a pet and can be identified by either a backpack or special harness. By law, service animals *must* be allowed into most establishments. EMRs should not handle the service animal unless absolutely required. *Never* separate the patient from the service animal, as this could cause stress, agitation and anxiety to both parties which can complicate patient care. It could also become a safety issue.

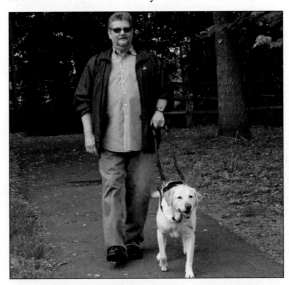

A service animal has been individually trained to provide assistance to an individual with a disability. Never separate an individual from his or her service animal.

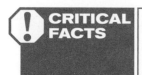

Illnesses that occur gradually and continue over a long period of time (even lifetime) are referred to as chronic conditions. Chronic conditions include heart disease, diabetes and arthritis. Patients with some chronic conditions, such as multiple sclerosis, can live for years with few symptoms and then suddenly experience a flare-up with many symptoms appearing at once.

throughout the person's life. Chronic conditions include heart disease, diabetes and arthritis. Patients with some chronic conditions, such as multiple sclerosis, can live for years with few symptoms and then suddenly experience a flare-up with many symptoms appearing at once. In such an acute phase, the patient will often consult a physician and, following treatment, the acute phase may be resolved. However, the patient will continue to live with the effects of the chronic condition.

Arthritis

Arthritis is a condition that causes joints to become inflamed, swollen, stiff and painful. A few or many joints may be affected as the smooth tissues that cover the ends of bones become rough or wear away, causing painful friction between bones upon movement. Because of this friction, tissues around the joints swell, leading to stiffness, which makes normal movement difficult.

When providing care for a patient with arthritis, keep the following in mind:

- Assure the patient that you are aware that movement is painful, and that you are there to help.
- *Never* move a joint that is painful, red or swollen.
- Handle the patient's joints carefully, supporting the areas above and below the joint when you move them.

Cancer

Cancer is the abnormal growth of new cells that can spread and crowd out or destroy other body tissues in the form of a malignant tumor, which is a solid mass or a growth of abnormal cells that can grow anywhere in the body. Malignant tumors can spread to other parts of the body, growing quickly and invading and destroying other body tissue.

Typically, cancer is treated according to the type and location of the cancer, and whether or not it has spread. The three most common approaches to treatment are surgery, chemotherapy and radiation. Common side effects of chemotherapy include nausea, diarrhea, loss of hair and extremely dry skin. Many people will experience skin burns, fatigue and possibly nausea and vomiting with radiation treatment and others may experience hair loss as a result of the radiation treatment.

When providing care for a person being treated for cancer, infection control is important because chemotherapy and radiation affect a person's immune system. Strict hand washing guidelines and standard precautions must be taken. *Never* provide care for a patient who is receiving cancer treatment if you have a cold or flu.

A patient receiving chemotherapy or radiation treatment may feel tired. Skin changes and rashes from some drugs or burns from radiation treatment are common, so be gentle.

Cerebral Palsy

Cerebral palsy is the name given to a group of disorders affecting a person's ability to move and maintain balance and posture. It does not get worse over time, although symptoms can change over a patient's lifetime.

Cerebral palsy causes damage to the part of the brain that controls the amount of resistance to movement in a muscle (muscle tone), which allows you to keep your body in specific postures or positions.

Cystic Fibrosis

Cystic fibrosis (CF) is an inherited disease of the mucus and sweat glands, affecting the lungs, pancreas, liver, intestines, sinuses and sex organs. CF causes mucus to become thick and sticky, blocking the airways. This makes it easy for bacteria to grow, which leads to repeated serious lung infections. These infections can cause serious damage to the lungs. Mucus can also block tubes, or ducts, in the pancreas, so that digestive enzymes cannot reach the small intestine. Without these, the intestines cannot absorb fats and proteins fully.

The most common symptoms of CF include—

- Frequent coughing that brings up thick sputum, or phlegm.
- Frequent bouts of bronchitis and pneumonia that can lead to inflammation and permanent lung damage.
- Salty-tasting skin.
- Dehydration.
- Infertility (mostly in men).
- Ongoing diarrhea or bulky, foul-smelling and greasy stools.
- Huge appetite but poor weight gain and growth.
- Stomach pain and discomfort caused by gas.

Multiple Sclerosis

Multiple sclerosis (MS) is a chronic disease that destroys the coating on nerve cells in the brain and spinal cord, interfering with the nerves' ability to communicate with each other. MS is more common in females than in males, and the onset typically occurs as early as the teen years and as late as age 50. Symptoms usually appear and disappear over a period of years and can include—

- Feelings of numbness, tingling and burning.
- Overwhelming fatigue at all times.
- Vision problems.
- Insomnia.
- Speech problems.
- Bowel and bladder problems.
- Fits of anger or crying.
- Paralysis.
- Forgetfulness and slowness in understanding.
- **Edema** and cold feet due to lack of circulation.

When treating patients with MS, help them focus on what they *can* do.

Muscular Dystrophy

Muscular dystrophy is a group of genetic disorders in which patients suffer progressive weakness and degeneration of the muscles. About a quarter of a million children and adults are living with the disease in the United States. In the most common form, *Duchenne muscular dystrophy*, the disease begins in early childhood; in other forms, it begins later in life. People with muscular dystrophy may have mild-to-

severe muscle weakness, depending on the type. Although the disorder primarily affects the skeletal muscles—the muscles that allow you to move—some types of muscular dystrophy affect cardiac muscles. In the later stages of the disease, patients with muscular dystrophy often develop respiratory problems and may require assisted ventilation.

Autism

Autism Spectrum Disorders (**ASD**) are a range of developmental disorders, including autism at the more severe end of the spectrum and **Asperger syndrome** at the less severe end. The diagnosis of autism seems to have become more common in recent years. The Centers for Disease Control and Prevention report that the rate of ASD is 3.4 per 1,000 in children between 3 and 10 years of age. Males are 3 to 4 times more likely to have ASD than females.

Children with ASD have deficits in social interaction and communication, and exhibit repetitive behaviors and interests. Some may also have sensory disturbances. People with these disorders interpret the world only through verbal reasoning.

Children with autism exhibit unusual behaviors that are usually noticed first by the parents. A baby may seem unresponsive to people or focus intently on one item for long periods of time. However, symptoms can also appear in older children who have been developing normally. A normal child who has shown affection and spoken as a toddler can become silent, withdrawn, self-abusive or indifferent to social overtures.

Remember that patients with autism might not look at you directly and physical touch may be disturbing to them. Avoid interpreting these mannerisms or responses as being unsociable. When communicating with patients with autism, it may help to use verbal explanations of emotions.

Hospice Care

Hospice care is the care provided to a terminally ill patient in the final 6 months of life, consisting of a group of caregivers who offer medical, mental, physical, social, economic and spiritual support. Central to the hospice way of thinking are the ideas that the dying person is an individual who should not be separated from the family or support system and that dying is a normal and expected part of the life cycle. The family is encouraged and trained to participate in the care.

The focus of hospice care is on keeping the person as comfortable and pain-free as possible, because the fear of pain greatly contributes to the person's stress, as well as that of the family and caregivers. The emphasis is not on curing the illness, but rather on providing physical, emotional, social and spiritual comfort to the dying person. The hospice philosophy also provides practical assistance, emotional support and **bereavement care** to the dying person's family. Pain relief is administered without the use of needles, using oral medications, pain relieving patches and pills that can be given between the cheek and gums.

Emergency medical responders (EMRs) are usually not required during hospice care. However, you may sometimes be called in by a family member or other caregiver when, for example, a patient becomes short of breath. You may be required to attend to a patient who has made special arrangements regarding his or her treatment or care in an emergency, such as the patient's wishes regarding resuscitation. You must understand the type of hospice you are being called to and any living wills or advance directives that may be in place. You may require official forms such as *Do Not Resuscitate* (DNR) Orders as confirmation regarding a living will.

PUTTING IT ALL TOGETHER

In this chapter, you have learned the importance of treating all patients with respect, regardless of age, health condition, mental status or physical ability. You have learned about common issues the elderly may face and how to deal with challenges such as hearing loss, loss of sensory acuity and other health conditions. You are now aware of the different types of dementias you may encounter with elderly patients, including Alzheimer's disease, and the importance of recognizing that not all elderly patients have diminished cognitive abilities.

Along with the challenges the elderly face, you have also learned about dealing with different chronic illnesses and the importance of dealing with patients on an individual basis in accordance with their specific symptoms and difficulties. All patients require clear communication and respect during assessment and treatment.

YOU ARE THE EMERGENCY MEDICAL RESPONDER

As you continue your care, the man begins to remember small bits of information, but still does not remember where he lives or where he is. He becomes agitated at the help being provided, saying he does not need any help. How should you continue to provide care for the patient?

UNIT

8

EMS OPERATIONS

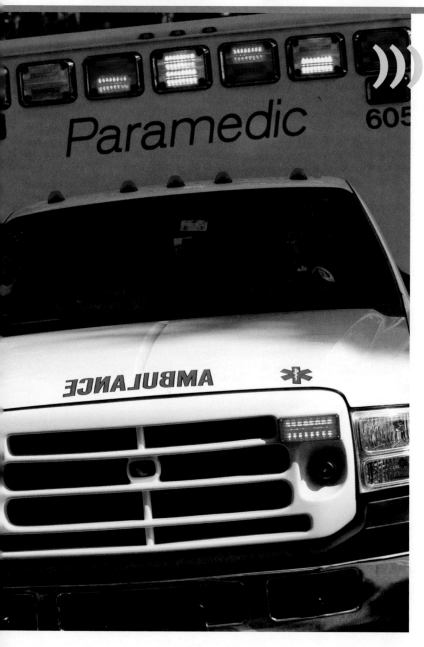

27

EMS Support and Operations

))) YOU ARE THE EMERGENCY MEDICAL RESPONDER

You are an *emergency medical responder* (EMR) approaching the scene of a two-car collision at a busy intersection. It is rush hour and traffic is heavy. One of the involved cars is situated on the median strip, and the other is off the road on the shoulder, just past the intersection. There are multiple occupants in each vehicle. How would you respond? What should you consider when you size-up the scene?

Key Terms

Air medical transport: A type of transport to a medical facility or between medical facilities by helicopter or fixed-wing aircraft.

Audible warning devices: Devices in an emergency vehicle to warn oncoming and side traffic of the vehicle's approach; includes both sirens and air horns.

Emergency medical dispatcher (EMD): A telecommunicator who has received special training for triaging a request for medical service and allocating appropriate resources to the scene of an incident, and for providing prearrival medical instructions to patients or bystanders before more advanced medical personnel arrive.

Jump kit: A bag or box containing equipment used by the *emergency medical responder* (EMR) when responding to a medical emergency; includes items such as resuscitation masks and airway adjuncts, gloves, blood pressure cuffs and bandages.

Landing zone (LZ): A term from military jargon used to describe any area where an aircraft, such as an air medical helicopter, can land safely.

Packaging: The process of getting a patient ready to be transferred safely from the scene to an ambulance or a helicopter.

Transferring: The responsibility of transporting a patient to an ambulance, as well as transferring information about the patient and incident to advanced medical personnel who take over care.

Trauma alert criteria: An assessment system used by *emergency medical services* (EMS) providers to rapidly identify those patients determined to have sustained severe injuries that warrant immediate evacuation for specialized medical treatment; based on several factors including status of airway, breathing and circulation; Glasgow Coma Scale score; certain types of injuries present; and the patient's age; separate criteria for pediatric and adult patients.

Visual warning devices: Warning lights in an emergency vehicle that, used together with audible warning devices, alert other drivers of the vehicle's approach.

Learning Objectives

After reading this chapter, and completing the class activities, you will have the information needed to—

- Describe the roles of traditional and non-traditional *emergency medical responders* (EMRs).
- Explain all phases of an *emergency medical services* (EMS) response and associated responsibilities of an EMR.
- Identify the basic equipment used by an EMR.
- Define air medical transport and the criteria for when it should be requested.

- Discuss safety issues related to air medical transport and *landing zones* (LZs).
- Discuss emergency vehicle safety and other safety issues during response.
- Identify and describe high-risk situations.
- Summarize patient care issues in the ambulance.

INTRODUCTION

In earlier chapters, you learned how to care for persons who are injured or ill. Although these skills are important for *emergency medical responders* (EMRs) to learn, certain non-medical operational skills are just as important. In this chapter, you will learn about *emergency medical services* (EMS) support and operations, including the phases of an ambulance or other transport vehicle call and air medical response. As an EMR, you may never be involved in all of these situations but, as a functioning part of the EMS system, you should have a brief overview of some of the aspects of out-of-hospital care.

ROLES OF THE EMR IN THE EMS SYSTEM

The term EMR can mean different things to different people. In general, EMRs are individuals who have been trained to provide a minimum standard of care according to the current national scope of practice and EMS educational standards. While EMRs may function as regular members of an ambulance crew in some states, in other states and areas they have other roles. There are also several types of EMRs, ranging from those who stabilize and transport patients to those who can provide prehospital medical care in the field, but do not transport.

Traditional EMRs

When we talk about traditional EMRs, we generally refer to people who function within the 9-1-1 system. These traditional EMRs are usually affiliated with a service, such as EMS systems, law enforcement, fire rescue, search and rescue or sometimes lifeguarding and ski patrol. Another area in emergency medical response is *hazardous material* (HAZMAT) or *hazardous waste operations and emergency response* (HAZWOPER).

Non-Traditional EMRs

Non-traditional EMRs have had the same training as traditional EMRs but work in less traditional settings. These people include athletic trainers, park rangers, trip leaders and others. You also find these EMRs working as members of industrial *medical emergency response teams* (MERT), or those involved in rope rescue, specialized trench rescue or confined space rescue. Any EMR, traditional or non-traditional, should be familiar with the EMS system and his or her role in it.

PHASES OF A RESPONSE

A typical EMS response has nine phases. They are —

1. Preparation for an emergency call.
2. Dispatch.
3. En-route to the scene.
4. Arrival at the scene and patient contact.
5. **Transferring** the patient to the ambulance.
6. En-route to the receiving facility.
7. Arrival at the receiving facility.
8. Clear medical facility.
9. Available for next emergency call.

Phase 1: Preparation for an Emergency Call

To be ready to respond to a scene, it is important to spend time preparing yourself, your equipment and your vehicle. As an EMR, you have a responsibility to keep yourself physically fit and mentally prepared for the challenges of responding to an emergency. Part of preparing for the call involves the initial training you receive as an EMR. It is important to remember that the end of your EMR training is the beginning of having a duty to respond to emergencies. You have a responsibility to continue your training through refresher and continuing education programs. Some EMRs take more advanced training to become *emergency medical technicians* (EMTs).

In preparing to respond to an emergency, you should have basic medical equipment on hand. **Jump kits** come in a variety of sizes and shapes and are commercially available. The contents may be regulated by a certifying agency or by your unit. In either case, be familiar with the contents and layout of the jump kits used by your unit or organization.

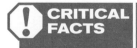 **CRITICAL FACTS** A typical EMS response has nine phases, from preparation for an emergency call to availability for the next emergency call.

In some areas, EMRs work in a system in which they may be involved in transporting the patient to the receiving facility. If this is the case, the EMR will have to prepare and inspect the ambulance or transport vehicle before every shift. Local EMS systems and state regulations determine what equipment and supplies must be in the vehicle and any vehicle safety and readiness inspections required.

In other areas or circumstances, EMRs may be the only emergency personnel responding to a scene. You should review state and local policies, rules and regulations regarding the minimum staffing requirements in your area.

Phase 2: Dispatch

In many areas of the country, a communications center/*public safety answering point* (PSAP) has a central access number such as 9-1-1 for ambulance, police or fire rescue personnel. Specially trained personnel, known as ***emergency medical dispatchers* (EMDs)**, often staff these communications centers, and are available on a 24-hour basis. They assist by obtaining the caller's location and information critical to dispatching the appropriate personnel and equipment. They are specially trained to help the caller care for patients until emergency personnel arrive.

During the call, the EMD will ask the caller specific questions that will determine the appropriate emergency personnel to dispatch. The EMD will ask the nature of the emergency and the *mechanism of injury* (MOI) or nature of the illness. The EMD will ask for the caller's name, location and call-back number. Additional information, such as the exact location of the patient (e.g., second floor, back apartment), number of patients and the severity of the injuries, can be relayed to those responding to the emergency after the initial dispatch has been issued. Also, the EMD will obtain information from the caller relating to unusual situations, conditions or problems at the scene. This will ensure that the appropriate personnel arrive at the scene as quickly and safely as possible. In cases of possible cardiac arrest, the EMD will ask if an *automated external defibrillator* (AED) is available and being used.

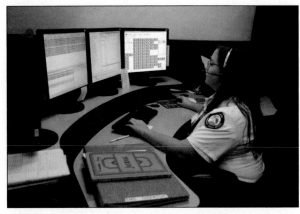

Fig. 27-1: A call taker in a communications center processes information from the caller and relays it to the EMD, then stays on the phone to provide further information as the situation unfolds.

A call taker is used by most communications centers that handle many calls. The call taker processes the information from the caller and provides the EMD information. The information is then transferred to the dispatcher, who transmits the data to the appropriate units. The call taker stays on the phone, providing prearrival information and gathering further information as the situation unfolds (**Fig. 27-1**). Environments in which a call taker and dispatcher perform identical functions include rural areas or a communications center with a minimal call load.

Phase 3: En-Route to the Scene

To help a patient, you must be able to reach the scene safely. The most important skill to use at this time is common sense. Walk with purpose—do *not* run—to any emergency scene or your vehicle. Pacing yourself allows you to think clearly, survey the area and plan for arrival at the scene. It also reduces the risk of injuries from tripping and falling.

If you are in a vehicle, whether a personal or emergency vehicle, you must always use a safety belt. Some areas require all personnel working in the EMS system to attend an emergency vehicle operator-training program. If you function in an EMS system that requires response in a private vehicle, become aware of the state and local laws and regulations that govern operation of private vehicles as emergency vehicles in that area. In all cases, when responding to an emergency,

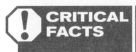

CRITICAL FACTS

In many areas of the country, a communications center/PSAP has a central access number such as 9-1-1 for ambulance, police or fire rescue personnel.

EMRs should use appropriate driving behavior, including consideration for the safety of others. Emergency response to the scene does not exempt any emergency personnel from traffic laws. The driver must know the traffic laws that govern the use of lights, sirens and intersection procedures.

Phase 4: Arrival at the Scene and Patient Contact

In this phase of response, you should be slow and cautious in your approach (**Fig. 27-2**). If you have access to the appropriate communications equipment, notify the EMD of your arrival. As you enter the area, size-up the scene and situation. If the scene is not safe, notify dispatch to send personnel from the agencies necessary to make it safe. Never endanger your life or the life of anyone else responding or already at the scene.

When approaching the scene, follow standard precautions before making any contact with the patient. Use gloves, gown, mask and protective eyewear when appropriate. Be sure to ask yourself critical questions. Is the scene safe? Are there any hazards to the rescuers or the patients? Look up, look down and look all around. What was the MOI or nature of illness? How many patients are there? Do you need any additional help?

Safety issues may necessitate assistance from law enforcement with crowd control. Assess as much as possible from inside your vehicle. Ensure your vehicle can leave the scene quickly if needed. For example, have your vehicle pointing toward the exit of a dead-end street, so you do not waste time leaving a dangerous situation.

There may be local protocols for when you should leave your vehicle given certain circumstances. If protocols indicate you should

wait for law enforcement personnel to arrive, do not exit the vehicle before their arrival.

After the scene size-up has been completed, primary, secondary and ongoing patient assessments will begin. Additionally, history taking, including baseline vital signs and initial care, will be provided to stabilize the patient(s) prior to transport.

Phase 5: Transferring the Patient to the Ambulance

Though transport is not a traditional role for an EMR, at times you may be part of the ambulance crew or be asked to help transfer a patient to the ambulance (**Fig. 27-3**). By the time the ambulance arrives, you may have completed the primary assessment, the physical exam, the patient's history and begun care. You may have recorded the vital signs and started **packaging** the patient for transfer. Packaging refers to getting the patient ready for transport, and moving the patient onto the stretcher to support the patient during transport. Transferring the patient means more than moving the patient to the ambulance. You also have a responsibility to transfer information about the patient and the incident to more advanced medical personnel who take over care.

Phase 6: En-Route to the Receiving Facility

Once the patient is loaded into the ambulance, all personnel should wear safety belts or safety restraints. The communications center is notified and the crew member in charge of caring for the patient determines whether the trip to the receiving facility will be fast, at a normal speed or slow (**Fig. 27-4**).

The transport crew members provide ongoing medical care and psychological support

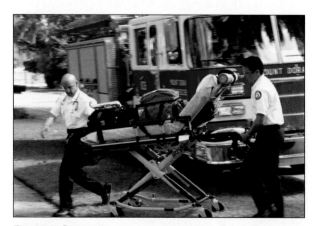

Fig. 27-2: Size-up the scene to ensure your safety before approaching patients. *Courtesy of Ted Crites.*

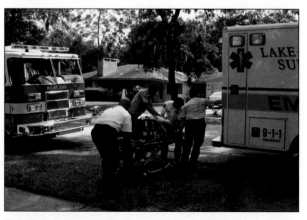

Fig. 27-3: At times, you may be asked to help transfer a patient to the ambulance. *Courtesy of Terry Georgia.*

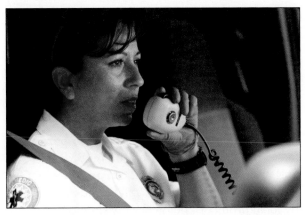

Fig. 27-4: Once the patient is loaded into the ambulance, notify the communications center.

for the patient until arrival at the hospital. They may ask additional questions, document the history and care of the patient and continue to monitor vital signs.

As soon as possible, the transport crew notifies the receiving facility about the patient and the expected time of arrival. The receiving facility is informed if there are any changes in the patient's status or condition. The driver may have to adjust the driving speed to meet what the crew member in charge says about the patient's needs.

Phase 7: Arrival at the Receiving Facility

During this phase, transport crew members transfer the patient to the care of the nurses and doctors at the receiving facility (**Fig. 27-5**). Crew members never leave patients unattended during a call or during the transfer of care. At the hospital, crew members give information about the scene and the patient. They also complete whatever documentation is necessary to meet local and state standards and their organization's protocols. If necessary,

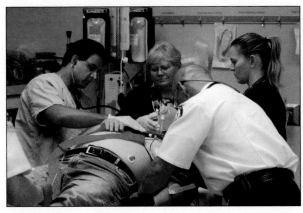

Fig. 27-5: Upon arrival at the hospital, the patient is in the care of the nurses and doctors.

crew members begin some of the post-run responsibilities such as exchanging or restocking medical supplies. The cleaning of the ambulance is also performed during this phase. Personnel should wear gloves and follow local procedures for disposal of soiled linen and supplies. The ambulance stretcher should be cleaned and made ready for the next call. Members of the crew should wash their hands thoroughly after every response.

Phases 8 and 9: Clear Medical Facility and Available for Call

When returning to the station (phase 8), the operator of the vehicle should notify the communications center. During the ride back to the station, personnel should take the opportunity to review details of the run and discuss how things could have been done differently or more efficiently. The ride back provides opportunities for crew members to air concerns or diffuse any stress that may have developed during the response. Doing these things helps the crew to prepare physically and emotionally for the next response.

In the last phase of response (phase 9), the emergency vehicle should be refueled if necessary and any repairs or adjustments should be made (**Fig. 27-6**). Fuel tanks should never be allowed

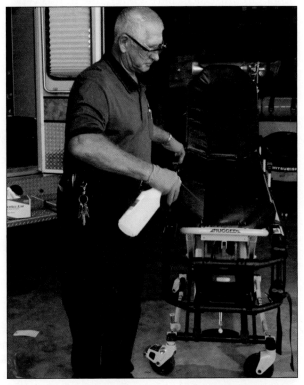

Fig. 27-6: Once back at the station, the emergency vehicle and equipment are prepared for the next response. *Courtesy of Terry Georgia.*

to get below half full. If necessary, restock any disposable items in the vehicle's medical supplies. Reports and any unfinished paperwork should be completed and the communications center should be notified that the unit is back in service and ready for another call. Always follow local procedures established by your service or organization.

Once back at the station, crew members should also prepare themselves for the next response. Preparation may include removing and laundering contaminated clothing as soon as possible. Uniforms or clothing soiled with the patient's blood or body fluids should not be taken home to be laundered; they should be laundered by a laundry service that deals with contaminated clothing or as specified in the organization's protocols.

AIR MEDICAL TRANSPORT CONSIDERATIONS

In certain situations, it is sometimes best for the patient to be transported to the receiving medical facility by helicopter (**Fig. 27-7**). This type of transport enables severely injured or ill persons to be transported quickly to specialty centers and large treatment facilities. Geography and other circumstances play a large role in this type of transport decision, and emergency personnel should follow local and state protocols.

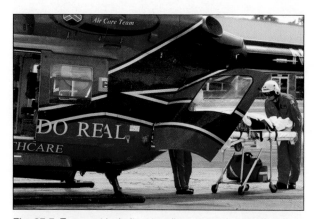

Fig. 27-7: Transport by helicopter allows severely injured or ill patients to be transported quickly. *Courtesy of Ted Crites.*

When to Request Air Medical Transport

In most situations where **air medical transport** is requested it is needed because one or more patients is in critical condition. During air medical operations you must always keep the safety of everyone present the top priority.

Trauma alerts and air medical transport may be required for a number of different MOIs and natures of illness. Specific **trauma alert criteria** vary from state to state and are driven by local protocols, but generally should be followed in emergency calls that include—

- A vehicle rollover with an unrestrained passenger(s).
- A situation involving a motorcycle in which the driver is thrown at a speed greater than 20 *miles per hour* (mph). Helmet laws vary and may be an additional factor if a rider was not wearing a helmet, even if the motorcycle was traveling at a slower speed.
- A situation where there are multiple injured or ill people.
- A pedestrian struck at greater than 10 mph and, in some instances, greater than 5 mph based on a patient's age or physical condition.
- A fall from a height greater than about 15 feet, with age or the presence of a long bone fracture being possible added factors.
- Critical stroke and cardiac alert patients, if ground transport by ambulance exceeds 45 minutes to the receiving facility.
- Critical trauma patients, who should be transported by air transport if ambulance transport to the trauma center exceeds 30 minutes.

The distance to be traveled and the time it will take to transport the patient(s) must be considered. Patients with conditions that are time-critical include those with chest or abdominal injuries with signs of respiratory shock or distress; patients in shock or experiencing an acute stroke; patients who have sustained any serious injury and show altered vital signs; patients with head injuries with altered mental status; and those patients

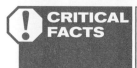
CRITICAL FACTS

Helicopters can be the best transportation choice when dealing with severely injured or ill persons who need quick transport to specialty centers or large treatment facilities. Geography and circumstances play a role in the decision, and local and state protocols should always be followed.

with a penetrating injury or in any other situation where time is obviously critical (such as a severe poisoning [e.g., carbon monoxide], heart attack, stroke or amputation).

Requesting air medical transport is reasonable when—

- It will take more than 30 minutes by ambulance to transport the patient to a trauma center.
- It will take longer to transport the patient to a trauma center by ambulance than by air transport.
- The patient's transport will be delayed by more than 30 minutes because of the need for extrication.
- The patient will require rapid transport to a specialty center. This could include a burn center or pediatric, comprehensive stroke or trauma center.

Advantages

In some situations, you may need to request air transport for your patient because he or she is unstable and the length of time for ground transport would lower the chances of survival. If the helicopter is carrying a medical crew, air transport allows for quicker access to more advanced emergency care. The medical crews on air transport are highly trained and can include nurses, paramedics and/or physicians. There is also specialized equipment that the medical crews are trained to use, including monitoring devices, intubation and advanced airway equipment and chest decompression kits. Collisions or crashes that occur off-road or in remote areas may not be accessible by road vehicles; use of a helicopter allows for patient evacuation. Another advantage of using air transport is that many large hospital centers and trauma centers have helipads to allow for helicopter landings.

Disadvantages

Helicopter transport is affected by weather conditions. If conditions are unfavorable, such as high winds or low visibility, the patient cannot be transported. The altitude available for a safe rescue may be vital in determining whether the rescue is feasible. If there is not enough room for the helicopter to hover or land safely, the rescue is not possible. There may be airspeed restrictions imposed by air control authorities in certain designated areas that could impede the aircraft's

arrival at the receiving medical facility. Another possible disadvantage is that helicopter size varies considerably, depending on the model. Smaller helicopters may not be able to accommodate patients and rescuers, as well as necessary equipment. Landing in mountainous terrain or among forested areas can be very difficult for a helicopter pilot. The area must be safe and there must be a viable landing site. Air transport is also significantly more costly than ground transportation.

Activation

Air medical activation must follow local and state guidelines. There are also state statutes, which vary across the country. It is essential that you review your state's protocols for activation of the *helicopter emergency medical system* (HEMS). In addition, rules vary according to institution, locale and state. There are also ordinance standards for each city, county and/or district. However, resources should be consistent with the standards developed by the Commission for the Accreditation of Medical Transport Systems.

Indications for Patient Transport

In general, air medical transport is used for several reasons including medical (e.g., stroke or cardiac alert) and trauma. With these types of emergencies, time is of the essence. This type of transport may be needed in situations involving spinal injuries, burns, organ procurement, high-risk obstetrics and premature babies. Helicopters are also used in the field in search and rescue missions. They are able to cover more terrain than land vehicles and can be used to rescue patients from inaccessible locations.

Considerations with Air Medical Transport

Types

There are two main types of air medical transport, rotorcraft and fixed-wing. Rotorcrafts (e.g., helicopters) are used to get into areas that are not accessible to any other type of rescue craft. Their maneuverability allows them to move up and down and side-to-side as needed, allowing for special rescue procedures such as hoisting. Fixed-wing crafts (e.g., planes, jets) are used to transport over long distances, usually between medical facilities.

Weather

Weather plays a significant role in the use of aircraft for rescue and transport. Pilots must have a minimum amount of visibility, and air temperature affects the altitude at which the helicopter can hover.

Space and Load

The amount of space available in a helicopter depends on the type of helicopter and its maximum takeoff and landing weights. When calculating space, rescuers must take into account how many patients require transport, the rescuers who must accompany the patient(s) and any essential life-saving equipment. In calculating weight, the pilot must take into account not only the passengers and equipment, but the fuel load as well.

Control Systems

Flying helicopters is an extremely demanding task because of their complex function. The pilot must coordinate the lift of the vehicle with the forward or side-to-side movement, if any, or the altitude and air temperature if attempting to hover. Because of the design of the vehicle, the pilot cannot see below the helicopter, which is why guidance is always needed.

Landing Zones

Choosing a safe **landing zone** (**LZ**) for a helicopter is paramount (**Fig. 27-8**). The pilot cannot see the area directly below the aircraft and must be guided. The pilot must also have a visual reference point at all times. Ideal conditions for LZs include—

- A minimum 10,000-square-foot area (100 feet by 100 feet). Some pilots prefer a rectangular landing area to allow for a 45-degree approach. Some aircraft may need a larger area.
- Flat land.
- Firm land. Avoid dusty ground or powdery snow if possible, as these conditions can impair vision as the helicopter rotors churn up the wind. Also, loose rocks can become dangerous projectiles when a helicopter lands or takes off. There is no guarantee that ice on a body of water would ever be strong enough for a helicopter landing.
- An area clear of any obstacles, such as trees or utility poles.
- An area clear of any type of vehicular traffic or pedestrians.

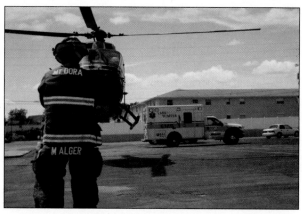

Fig. 27-8: A safe landing zone is paramount to the safety of a helicopter transport.

One person should be in charge of the LZ, coordinating the scene. To prevent distraction or confusion, this is the only person who should be communicating with the pilot. The coordinator should ensure that the LZ is well marked with cones or a flameless light source in all four corners. Nighttime landings can be guided with vehicle lights or any other *nonflame* light source, but the lights should always remain at ground level, never directed toward the pilot.

To help with the helicopter landing, the coordinator should be protected with a fastened helmet, hearing and eye protection, long sleeves and pants. The coordinator is then stationed outside the landing perimeter; usually with his or her back to the wind unless the pilot instructs an alternate landing approach. If possible, people should also be stationed at the left and the right outside the landing perimeter. Any bystanders not involved in the landing should be kept a minimum of 200 feet away from the site.

Patient Transfer
Interacting with Flight Personnel

If you are transferring a patient to the care of flight personnel, you will have to provide all the information you have obtained about the situation. This includes patient history, injury or illness history, presentation of the patient when you came upon the scene, any changes while waiting for the helicopter and status and vital signs (**Fig. 27-9**).

Patient Packaging and Preparation

Preparation for transport may include securing the patient's airway, immobilizing, splinting and the completion of emergency care procedures

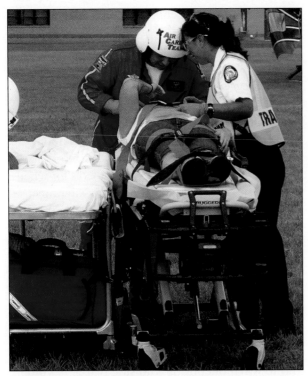

Fig. 27-9: Provide all information on a patient to flight personnel. *Courtesy of Ted Crites.*

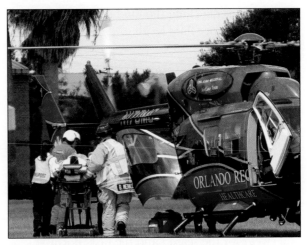

Fig. 27-10: Tail rotors are dangerous. Approach only if given permission by the pilot and only from the front or side so the pilot sees you. *Courtesy of Ted Crites.*

necessary for safely transferring a patient from the scene to an ambulance or helicopter.

Scene Safety

It is essential that no loose objects be allowed within the LZ. They may become projectiles, causing damage or injury. Objects such as medical equipment, linens or sheets and bags and other loose objects can become airborne from the rotary winds (rotor wash), and may strike the rotor blades or get sucked up into engine intakes causing a breakdown or injuries. Secure everything that can be secured and move anything else as far away as possible from the LZ. If the land is sandy or dusty, it should be wet down to limit the amount of dirt and dust churned up by the rotor wash.

Only those personnel who must approach the aircraft should be permitted within the LZ, and only after the pilot has signaled that it is safe to approach. *Make eye contact with the pilot* to confirm your permission to approach, and *maintain* eye contact until you have arrived at the door of the helicopter.

Tail rotors are very dangerous and a person assigned as a tail rotor guard may be posted to prevent people from coming near or approaching the aircraft from the rear. Allow the medical crew from the aircraft to approach you instead. Approaching from the front or side allows the pilot to see the responders (**Fig. 27-10**).

Your posture should be crouched over somewhat and, if there is an incline of any sort, you must approach from the lowest point and always from the side or front, never the rear. Even if approaching from the side, you must remain in the pilot's view. You should not be wearing a hat of any type; only a fastened helmet is permitted. Do not wear billowing clothing. If carrying equipment, such as an IV pole, this must be kept low and parallel to the ground so it does not get struck by the blades.

Special Tactics

Responders may be called to participate in rescues using mechanical hoists or *special insertion and extrication* (SPIE) lines. Because these rescuers have special training, your role would be to ensure that the area is as safe as possible for the specialty team.

EMERGENCY VEHICLE SAFETY

Apparatus Preparedness

Part of being prepared to respond to emergencies is being able to depend on your equipment and transportation. This means performing regular daily checks, more often if the situation warrants it. While checking for adequate tire inflation, also check the tires for wear and tear as well as anything unusual, like nails or debris in the tire. Ensure that warning devices (lights, siren, horn) are in working order.

Check with your employer and/or state regarding checklists for required vehicle maintenance. Such checklists should include items such as checking the fluid circulation system and wiper fluid levels.

Equipment Preparedness

You should also ensure that the appropriate safety equipment is available and in working order. *Personal protective equipment* (PPE) must be in full working condition for you to do your job effectively and safely. Depending on what is required in your situation, PPE may include helmets, work gloves, steel-tipped boots and structural firefighting protective clothing. It also includes protective eyewear, hearing protection, appropriate outerwear for the season and the task, portable radio and body armor if considered necessary.

Rescues often take place in the dark or in inclement weather, where visibility may be poor. It is important for you to wear reflective clothing, ideally a reflective safety vest, but reflective tape on your clothing and other gear also works well (**Fig. 27-11**).

Safety Issues During Response

During a response, safety is paramount. All personnel must be properly seated and use safety belts. All equipment in the cab area, rear of ambulance and any compartment areas should be appropriately secured.

Consideration of Use of Lights and Sirens

Emergency response to a scene does *not* exempt any emergency personnel from traffic laws. It

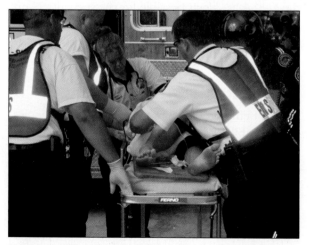

Fig. 27-11: Wear reflective clothing, such as a safety vest, or reflective tape to increase your visibility during rescues, especially when it is dark or in inclement weather. *Courtesy of Captain Phil Kleinberg, EMT-P, Lake-Sumter EMS.*

is the drivers' responsibility to make sure they know the traffic laws that govern the use of lights, sirens and intersection procedures.

Risk/Benefit Analysis

Use of lights and sirens is becoming increasingly questioned in emergency rescue services. Numerous studies have been conducted about the effectiveness versus the safety aspect of the practice. Learn your agency's protocols for when the patient's condition and situation warrants use of lights and sirens.

Audible Warning Devices

Audible warning devices include both the siren and the air horn. You should be familiar with your agency's requirements concerning the use of both.

The purpose of using your siren is to warn traffic in front of you that you are approaching and to warn oncoming and side traffic of your presence. It is also used to ask for the right of way. Because today's vehicles are better insulated from outside noise and because many drivers and passengers listen to loud music or have loud conversations inside, do *not* assume they can hear you approach. The outside environment may also be noisy and affect their ability to hear a siren. Alternatively, they may hear you but not fully realize from which direction you are coming. If you feel that your siren was not heard, do *not* come up behind a vehicle and turn your siren on suddenly, as this may startle the driver and cause a crash. Also, be aware that the siren can have an effect on you in the ambulance. There can be a hypnotizing effect that may make you pay less attention to your surroundings and your driving.

Your air horn can be used to clear traffic in a single situation, like an intersection. Like the siren, do *not* use the air horn behind or close to another vehicle as it may startle the driver into losing control. Do *not* use it continuously, but it can be used with or without your siren, depending on what the local and state laws are for your area.

Visual Warning Devices

Using **visual warning devices**, such as warning lights and emergency lights, depends on local and state laws. It is highly recommended that you do *not* use emergency lights without your siren; they should be used together or not at all. Headlights should be on, day or night, but high beams should *not* be used as emergency lights as they can blind oncoming drivers, as well as drivers in front of you through their rearview mirror.

If using a siren and/or lights, many drivers choose to turn them off a few blocks before the destination to avoid attracting attention.

Respond with Due Regard

Rescue vehicle drivers should obey traffic laws, be careful at intersections and only drive in emergency mode when lights and sirens are employed. Factors such as weather, road conditions and traffic must be taken into consideration when making driving decisions.

High-Risk Situations

Intersections

Collisions at intersections can occur when the rescue driver has a green light and does not expect a driver to run a late yellow light or a red light, or when a pedestrian or cyclist may be crossing and not be visible to the driver due to other vehicles. Slow down and come to a complete stop at intersections and ensure that all drivers are aware of your presence before proceeding. Another dangerous situation arises when more than one emergency vehicle is responding, either in the same direction or from different directions. Ensure that all emergency vehicles are obvious to all motorists and to people around the intersections, so they know to expect more than one emergency vehicle.

Highway Access

Always use caution when entering roads or highways. Be especially careful when using the shoulder in rush hour or gridlock situations. Follow the rules of the road and do not assume other drivers are aware of your presence. State laws differ in regards to how other drivers should respond when emergency vehicles are approaching. For example, some states require that drivers pull to the right to allow the emergency vehicle to pass without a problem, while other states do not require drivers to pull to the right. Know your state's laws to ensure your safety and the safety of those around you.

Speed Considerations

You should only travel at increased speed, beyond posted speed limits, when using lights and sirens, and only if permitted by local and state laws. If driving at a high speed, weather and road conditions must also be taken into consideration and extra caution should be taken when going around curves, going over hills, going down hills, turning corners and braking.

Driving Distractions

Be sure to eliminate all possible distractions, as your ability to concentrate and drive safely is of utmost importance. Typical distracting factors include mobile computers, *Global Positioning Systems* (GPSs), mobile radios, vehicle stereo, wireless devices and eating and drinking.

Inclement Weather

Driving in inclement weather can make emergency response more stressful. Be sure to leave extra distance between you and the car in front of you—especially on wet pavement, which usually requires double the normal distance to ensure enough braking room. If driving on ice or snow, count on about five times the normal distance needed.

Most drivers are aware of the risk of skidding on ice, but hydroplaning—riding on a film of water—is a very real risk in rain. If you do begin to hydroplane, corrective actions are similar to those of skidding on ice: take your foot off the accelerator and, unless you have an *anti-lock braking system* (ABS), pump the brake gently. Do *not* try to turn out of the hydroplane.

When driving in fog or any other situation where vision is greatly diminished, you must slow down; do *not* brake suddenly in case someone is following too closely behind you. Use your headlights, but not your high beams. If legal in your locale or state, use your four-way flashers/ hazard lights if driving slower than the posted limit. If about to use your brake, warn those behind you by tapping your brake, activating your brake lights.

Aggressive Drivers

Aggressive drivers can be found anywhere, at any time. They have less concern for other drivers and are generally frustrated. An aggressive driver is someone who not only threatens other drivers verbally or with gestures, but who also ignores traffic laws such as running stop signs and red lights, making unsafe lane changes, weaving in and out of traffic and tailgating other drivers. Aggressive drivers may disregard ambulances and other emergency vehicles. Be cautious when confronted with an aggressive driver and do not react to the driver's behavior or actions. Back off if needed and do not assume an aggressive driver will obey the rules of the road. When encountering an aggressive driver, notify law enforcement immediately. Obtain a tag number and vehicle description, if it is safe to do so.

Unpaved Roadways

Unpaved roadways such as dirt roads or gravel-covered surfaces can pose unsafe driving conditions that include marginal traction; muddy, slick conditions during rainy weather; and uneven surfaces. Always drive with extra caution on unpaved roads and never drive faster than conditions safely permit when driving on any road surface.

Responding Alone

In many traffic-related emergencies requiring fire rescue units to respond, they will position their larger vehicles in such a way as to protect the scene and allow for emergency care. When responding alone, or when you are first on scene, be especially careful when approaching and when exiting your vehicle. Check your mirrors, look back for traffic and open your door slowly especially if it opens toward traffic. Wear proper reflective gear. Request assistance from law enforcement personnel to assist with traffic control.

Fatigue

There may be times when an EMS vehicle driver feels sleepy while driving, especially on long transports. This may be especially true on longer shifts. Avoid caffeine and sugar; they may provide energy in the short term, but cause a rebound drop in energy a few hours later, which can make you feel even more sleepy as well as disturb sleep. Fresh air is a better alternative, as is 10 minutes of deep breathing. Open the vehicle's window or get out of the vehicle if you can for a few minutes. Stretching also helps. If you take prescribed medications that cause sleepiness and impair

your ability to perform your job safely, seek help and avoid driving when the medication is interfering. If you are using antihistamines, choose ones that cause less drowsiness.

360-Degree Assessment

When approaching an emergency, dangers can be present all around you. Be sure to scan up, down and behind you as well as looking forward and side-to-side as you size-up the scene (**Fig. 27-12**). This will help you more thoroughly assess the entire situation.

Downed Electrical Lines

When a vehicle is in contact with an electrical wire, consider the wire energized (live) until you know otherwise. Water is an effective conductor of electricity, so be especially careful of downed electrical wires in a wet or rainy environment. When you arrive at the scene, your first priority is to ensure your safety and that of others in the immediate area. A safety area should be established at a point twice the length of the span (distance between the poles) of the wire (**Fig. 27-13**). Attempt to reach and move patients *only* after the power company has been notified and has secured any electrical current from reaching downed wires or cables. Tell occupants inside an involved vehicle to *remain in the vehicle*. If needed, you may be able to give them instructions on how to provide some basic first aid care for any injured patients in the vehicle until they can be safely reached by professional rescuers. Do *not* attempt to deal with any electrical hazards unless

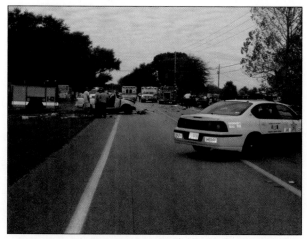

Fig. 27-12: Dangers or unsafe conditions can be present all around you. Assess the scene from all angles. *Courtesy of Captain Phil Kleinberg, EMT-P, Lake-Sumter EMS.*

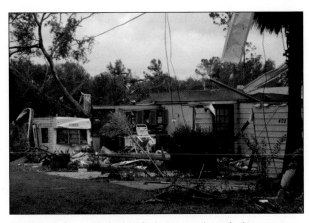

Fig. 27-13: Downed electrical wires are extremely dangerous and require that a safety area is established. *Courtesy of Captain Phil Kleinberg, EMT-P, Lake-Sumter EMS.*

you are specifically trained to do so and have the proper equipment. Once the current has been shut down, the vehicle can be safely approached.

Leaking Fuel or Fluids

Check to see if there is any fuel or fluid leaking from the vehicle. Check for a source that could ignite a fire. If there is a source, the fire department must be notified if you have not done so already.

Smoke or Fire

If smoke or fire is present, the fire department must be notified if you have not already done so. If you attempt a rescue, approach the vehicle from the side only, to lessen the risk should explosion occur.

Broken Glass

Broken glass from windows or windshields can be anywhere on the scene. If it poses a risk and cannot be avoided, covering it may reduce the chances of injury.

Trapped or Ejected Patients

As you size-up the scene, check for trapped patients. If a patient is trapped in a vehicle, the fire and rescue department may have specialized extrication equipment to help get the patient safely out of the vehicle. Also, look around the area to see if any patients were ejected from the vehicle upon impact.

Mechanism of Injury/Nature of Illness

As you approach the patient, consider the MOI or nature of illness. Doing so involves trying to find out what happened. Look around the scene for clues as to what caused the emergency and the extent of the damage. Consider the force that may have been involved in creating an injury. This will cause you to think about the possible type and extent of the patient's injuries. Take in the whole picture. How a motor vehicle is crushed or nearby objects such as shattered glass, a fallen ladder or a spilled medicine container may suggest what happened. If the victim is unconscious, considering the MOI or nature of illness may be the only way you can determine what happened.

Patient Care in the Ambulance

All personnel, including the driver and others riding in or on the ambulance must be properly seated and secured with safety belts for their own safety as well as for the safety of others in the vehicle, unless they are moving about for essential tasks in the patient compartment (**Fig. 27-14**). Do not remove your safety belt just before arrival to save time, as research shows the last few minutes of the emergency response drive are the most dangerous to team members.

If safety belts must be removed while you are in the patient compartment to provide care to the patient, precautions must be taken regarding how you position yourself and how you move. Always hold on to something secure inside the compartment when moving about unsecured.

Patients should *always* be properly secured while in the patient compartment. All stretcher straps are to be appropriately in place and tightened.

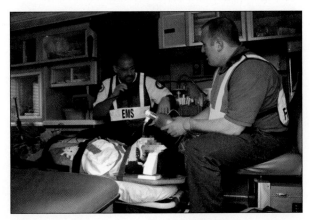

Fig. 27-14: Patients in an ambulance should always be properly secured, and all personnel should be cautious when moving to provide care. *Courtesy of Captain Phil Kleinberg, EMT-P, Lake-Sumter EMS.*

Patient care in the ambulance can be hazardous because of the movement necessary by the rescuer. While remaining as safe as possible, the rescuer must be able to carry out certain procedures. Check the protocols in your local area or state regarding which procedures these might be, as they may require that the ambulance not be in motion at that time.

Move deliberately and slowly, keeping your feet well placed, shoulder width apart, on the floor to maintain stability. Rescuers should practice the idea that three of five essential body parts should be safely "hugging" the ambulance at all times. The five body parts are the two hands, two feet and backside, which should be seated as much as possible during ambulance movement. If you hook your foot around the stretcher bar as you are seated, this gives an extra measure of safety and security.

CPR may be necessary en-route to the hospital. This requires extra care for the rescuer. Maintain balance as much as possible and have the driver call out if any bumpy areas (e.g., railroad tracks or potholes) or severe turns are coming up, so that you may brace yourself.

While performing CPR, spread your feet to shoulder width to maintain a more secure stance and bend your knees to lower your center of gravity. If possible, have someone help you by holding on to your belt to stabilize you. That other person should be secured with a seat belt.

Securing Equipment

All moveable equipment in the cab must be secured for your safety. In the event of a motor-vehicle collision, all unsecured items have the potential of becoming life-threatening projectiles. This includes personal items left on the dashboard, such as pens and notebooks.

Unless using a piece of equipment, it must be securely stored to prevent injury in the case of a sudden stop, swerve or motor-vehicle crash. This includes everything from heavier monitoring equipment and AEDs to lighter clipboards and cups.

LEAVING THE SCENE

Before you leave the scene, ensure all hazards have been mitigated. Pick up and dispose of all equipment and trash properly. All used sharps must be placed in a closed, puncture-resistant, leak-proof, tamper-proof biohazard sharps container. All contaminated clothing, products or material must be placed in a biohazard container. All containers must be stored in a safe manner and, if leakage occurs, they must be placed in a second leak-proof container. Check with your local and state laws about proper disposal of these contaminated items.

All reusable equipment must be collected from the scene for cleaning and restocking. All disposable equipment must be discarded in appropriate containers and replaced with new equipment after the emergency.

Turn the scene over to the appropriate authority prior to leaving. There may be situations when EMRs must turn over care of their patient to other emergency personnel, including law enforcement, fire suppression, highway department and other personnel. The names of the initial responders should be given to the crew taking over care and should be recorded on the prehospital care report for any possible follow ups. While generally one only transfers care to a higher-level certified emergency responder, there may be situations that necessitate turning over care to a lower certified rescuer. For example, in a *multi-casualty incident* (MCI), responders may be required to move on to the next patient for assessment, leaving the patient with a lower certified rescuer, after an appropriate briefing.

EMS EQUIPMENT

Maintaining equipment readiness is essential. If you are involved in transporting patients to the receiving facility, you will have to prepare and inspect the ambulance before every shift. Local EMS systems and state regulations determine what equipment and supplies must be in the vehicle.

Jump Kit

In preparing to respond to an emergency, you should have basic medical equipment on hand. Always have a jump kit fully stocked and ready to go should an emergency occur (**Fig. 27-15**). Do not overfill the jump kit, but minimum supplies should include—

- Airways (oral).
- Suction equipment.
- Artificial ventilation devices (e.g., resuscitation mask or *bag-valve-mask resuscitator* [BVM]).
- Basic wound supplies (e.g. dressings and bandages).

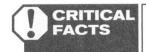
Other supplies to include are—
- PPE, such as gloves, protective eyewear, masks and face shields.
- Maps.
- Scissors.
- Blood pressure cuff.
- Stethoscope.
- Flashlight.
- Note pad and pen.
- Hand sanitizer.
- Any other equipment required by local or state standards.

PUTTING IT ALL TOGETHER

EMRs are individuals who have been trained to a minimum standard of care according to the current national scope of practice and EMS educational standards. They may function in traditional roles as regular members of an ambulance crew in some states, while in others they may work in non-traditional settings as trip leaders or athletic trainers. There are also several types of EMRs, including those with additional training who are able to transport patients as well as provide advanced, prehospital medical care.

A typical EMS response has nine phases: preparation for an emergency call, dispatch, en-route to the scene, arrival at the scene, transferring the patient to the ambulance, en-route to the receiving facility, arrival at the receiving facility, en-route to the station and post-run.

In certain situations, it may be best for patients to be transported to a medical facility by air. This method enables severely injured or ill persons to be transported quickly to specialty centers and large treatment facilities. Geography and other circumstances play a large role in this type of transport decision, and emergency personnel should follow local and state protocols.

To be prepared to answer emergencies, EMRs must be able to depend on their equipment and transportation. This means performing regular checks of the vehicle's tires and audible and visual warning devices to make sure everything is in working order, and ensuring that all necessary equipment and supplies are on hand.

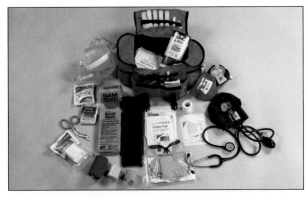

Fig. 27-15: Jump kit

YOU ARE THE EMERGENCY MEDICAL RESPONDER

Additional fire rescue, police and EMS units arrive. You see that one of the occupants of the vehicle that is on the shoulder of the road apparently was not wearing a seat belt, was ejected from the vehicle and is not moving. The driver of the car on the median strip is conscious, but because of traffic you cannot get to that vehicle. What are some safety considerations and issues with this situation? With heavy traffic backing up in all directions, and one patient with severe trauma, what transport options should be considered?

Enrichment
Operational Safety and Security Measures

PERSONNEL

The beginning of each shift should involve a briefing, either in person or through written notes, about any issues involving crew safety. These issues could involve personal threats against the unit or specific rescuers or be general threats. Security measures should have been discussed previously in training and reviewed as needed.

VEHICLES

The threat of stolen vehicles is very real. Under no circumstances should an ambulance or rescue vehicle be left running or unattended with the key in the ignition.

All vehicles must be monitored, whether in- or out-of-service. Any vehicles that are no longer to be used for emergency or rescue purposes must be stripped of all emergency equipment, lights, sirens and markings.

All use of ambulances and rescue vehicles must be tracked to avoid unauthorized use. If ambulances or rescue vehicles need repair or servicing outside of authorized areas, they must be secured in such a way that they cannot be used by unauthorized personnel.

28

Access and Extrication

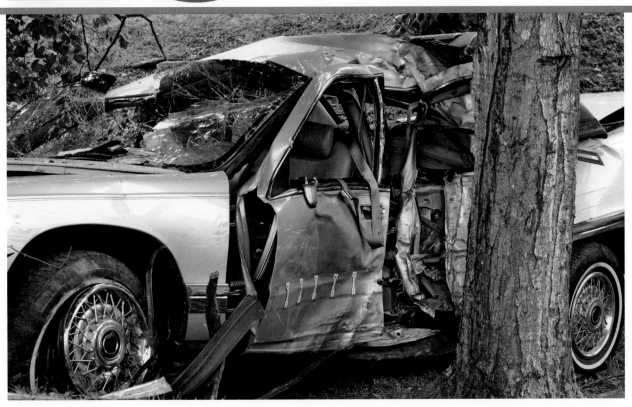

))) **YOU ARE THE EMERGENCY MEDICAL RESPONDER**

You are an *emergency medical responder* (EMR) and a member of a rural volunteer rescue squad. There has been a motor-vehicle crash on a main county road in which the driver apparently lost control of his car on a curve and struck a large tree. There is major damage to the car's front end. The driver (and sole occupant) most likely impacted the steering wheel with his upper body. He appears to be pinned. Fire rescue personnel are on scene. As you size-up the scene you notice that fluids are leaking from the vehicle and there is a steady flow of traffic on the road; the car is tilted along the shoulder. What potential safety issues should be considered? How might your ability to provide emergency medical care be affected by this situation?

Key Terms

Access: Reaching a patient who is trapped in a motor vehicle or a dangerous situation, for the purpose of extrication and providing medical care.

Complex access: In an extrication, the process of using specialized tools or equipment to gain access to the patient.

Cribbing: A system using wood or supports, arranged diagonally to a vehicle's frame, to safely prop it up, creating a stable environment.

Extrication: The safe and appropriate removal of a patient trapped in a motor vehicle or a dangerous situation.

"Rule of thumb": A guideline for positioning oneself far enough away from a scene involving *hazardous material* (HAZMAT): one's thumb, pointing up at arm's length, should cover the hazardous area from one's view.

Simple access: In an extrication, the process of getting to the patient without the use of equipment.

Vehicle stabilization: Steps taken to stabilize a motor vehicle in place so that it cannot move and cause further harm to patients or responders.

Learning Objectives

After reading this chapter, and completing the class activities, you will have the information needed to—

- Have a basic understanding of access and extrication.
- Explain the role of the *emergency medical responder* (EMR) in an extrication operation.
- List basic extrication equipment.
- Describe basic personal protective equipment used in extrication operations.
- Describe steps necessary to ensure patient safety during extrication.
- List the reasons for controlling traffic at an emergency scene.

- Describe unique hazards that may exist at an emergency scene.
- Define *hazardous material* (HAZMAT).
- List basic safety procedures associated with a HAZMAT situation.
- Describe the importance of vehicle stability.
- List the general steps to stabilize a vehicle.
- Know the difference between simple access and complex access.
- Know how to provide care to patients who require extrication at the scene.

INTRODUCTION

One of your primary responsibilities as an *emergency medical responder* (EMR) is to provide care for an injured or ill patient. Sometimes, however, providing care is not possible because you cannot reach the patient. One example is a situation in which someone is able to call 9-1-1 or the local emergency number for help but is unable to unlock the door of a home or office to let rescuers inside. This situation also occurs in a large number of motor-vehicle collisions, with locked or crushed vehicle doors, tightly rolled up windows or unstable vehicles. In other instances, fire, water, fuel leaks or other elements may prevent you from reaching the patient.

In these cases, you must immediately think of how you can safely gain **access** to the patient. If you cannot reach the patient, you cannot provide medical care. Always remember, when attempting to reach someone, your safety is the most important consideration. Protect yourself and the patient by doing only what you are trained to do, using equipment you are trained to use and wearing clothing appropriate for the situation. Items such as helmets, face shields, protective eyewear and heavy-duty gloves will help keep you safe as you attempt to gain access to a trapped patient. Simple tools can also be helpful.

FUNDAMENTALS OF EXTRICATION AND RESCUE OPERATIONS

Role of the EMR

Extrication is the safe and appropriate removal of a patient trapped in a motor vehicle or a dangerous situation. At times, an EMR may be called upon to help care for someone in this type of situation. It will be your role to administer the necessary care to the patient before extrication and ensure that the patient is removed in a way that minimizes further injury. Providing care for the patient may come before the extrication process; however, in many instances, patient care will occur simultaneously with the extrication process. During any extrication, it is critical that those providing medical care and those who are performing extrication are in constant communication with each other to maintain safety and avoid aggravating the patient's injuries or causing further pain.

Although fire rescue workers, *emergency medical technicians* (EMTs) and other specially trained personnel will perform most extrication procedures, when EMRs are involved in this type of rescue they should work closely with other rescuers to protect the patient. A chain of command should also be established to ensure that the scene is well managed and the patient's care remains a priority.

Additional Resources

Basic extrication equipment includes crowbars, screwdrivers, chisels, hammers, pliers, work gloves and goggles, wrenches, shovels, car jacks, tire irons, knives and ropes or chains.

Many emergency scenes draw crowds of onlookers and individuals wishing to help. Law enforcement personnel will play a major role in helping to secure the scene and control the crowd while the extrication is in progress.

Also, consider the need for specialists to handle or help control any hazards present. This could include representatives from utility providers, such as the natural gas company or the power company, or could include *hazardous material* (HAZMAT) responders. HAZMAT responders provide medical care and extrication of patients from a *hot zone* (area with the highest degree of danger in a HAZMAT emergency scene), where potentially hazardous chemical spills are involved. In the case of fuel spills or other potential hazards associated with extrication, the fire department may deploy a charged hose line to protect the scene, the patient and rescue personnel.

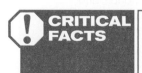

CRITICAL FACTS

Extrication is the safe and appropriate removal of a patient trapped in a motor vehicle or a dangerous situation.

Basic extrication equipment includes crowbars, screwdrivers, chisels, hammers, pliers, work gloves and goggles, wrenches, shovels, car jacks, tire irons, knives and ropes or chains.

Depending on the severity of the injuries and location of the scene, patient transportation by an air medical service may be required. Other activities, such as patient decontamination, may be required prior to transport by ground ambulance or other ground transport vehicle or by air medical services.

Scene Safety
Personal Safety

The first priority for all EMRs is their own safety. All personnel involved at the scene should wear protective clothing and follow guidelines set up by state and local protocols. The *National Fire Protection Association* (NFPA) and the *Occupational Safety and Health Administration* (OSHA) have guidelines to follow when considering the purchase of safety clothing. At a minimum, when responding to a motor-vehicle collision or other extrication situation, EMRs should have the following equipment:

- Protective helmet with chin strap
- Protective eyewear
- Puncture- and flame-resistant outerwear (turnout gear)
- Heavy, protective gloves
- Boots with steel toes and insoles

As with any emergency, begin by sizing up the scene to see if it is safe. If it is not safe, determine whether you can make it safe so you can attempt to gain access to the patient. Well-intentioned EMRs and others are injured or killed each year while attempting to help patients involved in motor-vehicle collisions. Such unfortunate instances are preventable by taking adequate measures to make the scene safe before trying to gain access and provide care.

Patient Safety

Once you have obtained safe access to a trapped patient, provide the same care you would to any trauma patient. Ensure you stabilize the cervical spine, complete the primary assessment and provide critical interventions as necessary. Patients will require protection from the debris created by the extrication process. Cover patients with tarps or blankets to protect them from broken glass, sharp metal and other hazards, including the environment. Lessen their fears by explaining what you will do and any noise that may occur in the process. Establishing a rapport with patients will help them focus on your support and listen to your instructions and guidance throughout the extrication. Asking patients if they are prepared as each step takes place will also help them feel more in control of the situation and less panicked or frightened.

It is also important to continue to monitor patients throughout the process and, if their condition changes, immediately inform the rescue crew of any growing danger.

Caution bystanders in the area to stay away from the scene. Their presence can cause additional confusion and increase the risk of injury.

Stabilize and immobilize the patient's spine, if possible, before removing the patient from the vehicle (**Fig. 28-1**). The only time in which an urgent move without spinal support should be considered is in the case of urgency, when there

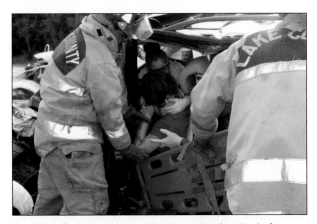

Fig. 28-1: Stabilize and immobilize the patient's spine before removing him or her from the vehicle. *Courtesy of Captain Phil Kleinberg, EMT-P, Lake-Sumter EMS.*

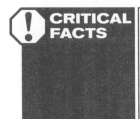
CRITICAL FACTS

Protective clothing is essential on the scene. Follow state and local protocols and familiarize yourself with guidelines put forth by NFPA and OSHA. Minimum equipment when dealing with collisions and extrications includes protective helmets and eyewear, turnout gear, protective gloves and boots with steel toes and insoles.

Once you have obtained safe access to a trapped patient, provide the same care you would to any trauma patient. Ensure you stabilize the cervical spine, complete the primary assessment and provide critical interventions as necessary.

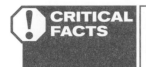

CRITICAL FACTS | Blocking is a positioning technique that creates a physical barrier between the work area and traffic flowing toward the emergency scene. It creates a safer environment and provides an optimal position for patient loading.

is an immediate threat to life from fire or other critical situation.

Scene and Traffic Control

There are several important reasons to control traffic at the scene: to protect the scene from further potential collisions, prevent injury to the rescue team, ensure minimal disruption and allow emergency vehicles to reach the scene. On arrival, request the assistance of additional law enforcement and fire services personnel to help control the scene and assign a scene safety officer.

Emergency vehicles should be placed in optimal positions for safety and for easy patient loading. *Blocking* is a technique of positioning fire apparatus, such as large engines, at an angle to traffic lanes (**Fig. 28-2**). This creates a physical barrier between the work area and traffic flowing toward the emergency scene. The scene should be protected with the first-arriving apparatus; block off at least one additional lane. Ambulances should park within the "shadow" created by the larger apparatus. The apparatus should also "block to the right" or "block to the left," so as not to obstruct the loading doors of ambulances. The ambulance patient loading area should be facing away from the closest lane of moving traffic. All patient loading into ambulances is carried out from within the protected work zone that is created by the positioning of the other rescue apparatus.

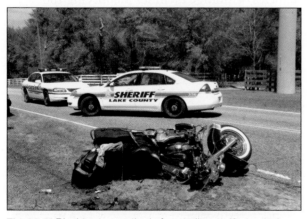

Fig. 28-2: Blocking is a method of controlling traffic in which emergency vehicles are positioned to create a physical barrier between the emergency scene and the flow of traffic. *Courtesy of Captain Phil Kleinberg, EMT-P, Lake-Sumter EMS.*

Establish advance warning for vehicles, by using traffic cones or flares. Place these at 10–15-foot intervals, to create a safe zone in a radius of at least 50 feet around the scene. If using flares, be sure there are no fluid leaks.

Unique Hazards

Alternative-Fueled (Hybrid) Vehicles

It is important to understand the differences between gasoline- and alternative-fueled vehicles, especially hybrid vehicles. Many people are concerned about the risk of electrocution. Following safety precautions and the manufacturer's recommendations reduces the risk of injury to rescuers and vehicle occupants.

As with any conventional vehicle, removing the ignition key and disconnecting the battery will disable a hybrid's high-voltage controller. Keep in mind that some hybrid vehicles do not have an ignition key, but do have an on/off switch that must be pressed before disconnecting the battery. However, some models may remain "live" for up to 10 minutes after the vehicle is shut off or disabled. Rescuers must always follow the manufacturer's emergency response guidelines for the specific make and model of the vehicle.

One important difference is that a hybrid vehicle can remain silent and still be operational if the collision is minor and/or did not activate any of the collision sensors. Therefore, it is essential that rescuers *chock* or block the wheels to prevent the vehicle from moving under power or by gravity. Be careful not to place **cribbing** under any high-voltage (usually *orange* in color) cabling.

Hybrid automobile manufacturers publish *Emergency Response Guides* (ERGs) for each model of hybrid vehicle they produce. Rescuers should be familiar with the safety procedures provided in these resources.

Undeployed Vehicle Safety Devices

In some collisions, air bags may not have deployed, and may present a hazard during extrication. The force of a deploying air bag can turn access and extrication tools into destructive missiles that can cause serious injury to rescuers and patients. Air bags can be found in several locations throughout a vehicle and can number as many as a dozen separate units depending on the vehicle make and model. If a patient is pinned directly behind an undeployed air bag, both battery cables should be disconnected, following established safety protocols. Ideally, wait for deactivation of the system before attempting to extricate the patient. Do not mechanically cut through or displace the steering column until after deactivation of the system. Do not cut or drill into the air bag module. Also, do not apply heat to the area of the steering wheel hub, as an undeployed air bag inflates in a normal manner if the chemicals sealed inside the air bag module reach a temperature above 350° F.

HAZMAT

As an EMR, you may find yourself involved in a situation in which there are chemical or other harmful or toxic substances. EMRs must be trained to quickly identify such situations and access specially trained personnel to deal with the situation.

A *hazardous material* is any chemical substance or material that can pose a threat to the health, safety and property of an individual. A HAZMAT incident is any situation that deals with the release of hazardous material. When dealing with a HAZMAT situation, work within a structured system that provides guidance in managing this type of scene **(Fig. 28-3)**.

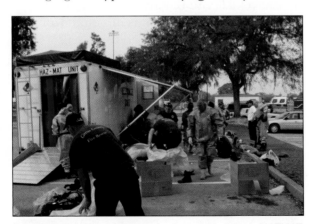

Fig. 28-3: Unless you have received special training in HAZMAT handling, stay away from the area. *Courtesy of Captain Phil Kleinberg, EMT-P, Lake-Sumter EMS.*

Unless you have received special training in HAZMAT handling and have the necessary equipment to do so without danger, stay well away from the area or in the designated *cold zone* (support area in the outer perimeter of a HAZMAT emergency scene). While en-route to a potential HAZMAT scene, obtain as much prearrival information as possible from dispatch. Stay out of low areas where vapors and liquids may collect and stay upwind and uphill of the scene. Be alert for wind changes that could cause vapors to blow toward you. Do not attempt to be a hero. It is common for responding ambulance crews approaching the scene to recognize a HAZMAT placard and immediately move to a safe area and summon more advanced help. When approaching the scene, use binoculars from a safe distance to look for potential hazards and to obtain the placard number. Refer to the *Emergency Response Guidebook* for detailed information.

Many fire departments have specially trained HAZMAT teams to handle incidents involving these materials. While awaiting help, keep people away from the danger zone. One easy method to determine the danger zone area is called "**rule of thumb**." The "rule of thumb" states that, to be safe, position yourself far enough away from the scene that your thumb, pointing up at arm's length, covers the hazardous area from your view.

When approaching any scene, be aware of dangers involving chemicals. Whether a motor-vehicle collision or an industrial emergency is involved, you should be able to recognize clues that indicate the presence of hazardous material. These include signs (placards) on vehicles or storage facilities identifying the presence of these materials, evidence of spilled liquids or solids, unusual odors, clouds of vapor and leaking containers.

VEHICLE STABILIZATION

Any movement of the vehicle during patient care or extrication can prove dangerous or even deadly to patients with severe spinal injuries, or could result in injury to the rescue team. Local fire department and rescue squad personnel

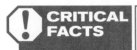

CRITICAL FACTS | A hazardous material is any chemical substance or material that can pose a threat to the health, safety and property of an individual.

specially trained in **vehicle stabilization** and extrication will respond to the scene when requested.

To make the scene as safe as possible, it is important to ensure that the motor vehicle is stable. You can assume a vehicle is *unstable* if—

- It is positioned on a tilted surface.
- It is stacked on top of another vehicle, even partly.
- It is on a slippery surface.
- It is overturned or on its side.

Stabilizing an upright vehicle is a relatively simple task. Placing blocks or wedges against the wheels of the vehicle will greatly reduce the chance of the vehicle moving. This process is called chocking (**Fig. 28-4**). You can use items such as rocks, logs, wooden blocks and spare tires. If a strong rope or chain is available, attach it to the frame of the car and then secure it to strong anchor points, such as large trees, guardrails or another vehicle. Letting the air out of the car's tires also reduces the possibility of movement.

To stabilize a vehicle, take the following steps:
- Put the vehicle in "park," or in gear (if a manual transmission).
- Set the parking brake.

- Turn off the vehicle ignition and remove the key.
- If there are no patients in the seats, move the seats back and roll down the windows.
- Disconnect the battery or power source.
- Identify and avoid hazardous vehicle safety components such as seatbelt pretensioners, undeployed air bags, integrated child booster seats and a *lower anchors and tethers for children* (LATCH) system.

Depending on the condition and positioning of the vehicle, further steps must be taken to ensure the vehicle cannot fall or roll. *Cribbing* is a system that creates a stable environment for the vehicle. It uses wood or supports, arranged diagonally to the vehicle's frame, to safely prop up a vehicle (**Fig. 28-5**). Cribbing should not be used under tires because it tends to cause rolling. There should never be more than 1–2 inches between the cribbing and vehicle.

For vehicles remaining upright, use blocks or wedges to prevent rolling. When possible, position

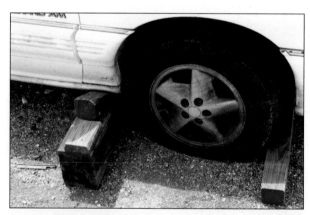

Fig. 28-4: Chocking. *Courtesy of Ted Crites.*

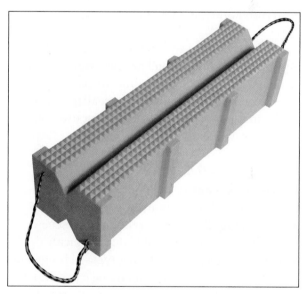

Fig. 28-5: 6" x 7" x 24" super crib with lanyards. *Courtesy of Turtle Plastics.*

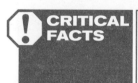

CRITICAL FACTS

A vehicle should be considered unstable if it is on a tilted or slippery surface, completely or partly on top of another vehicle, or overturned or on its side.

To stabilize a vehicle, take the following steps:
- Put the vehicle in "park," or in gear (if a manual transmission).
- Set the parking brake.
- Turn off the vehicle ignition and remove the key.
- If there are no patients in the seats, move the seats back and roll down the windows.
- Disconnect the battery or power source.
- Identify and avoid hazardous vehicle safety components.

the wheels against the curb. The tire valve stem may also be cut so the car rests safely on its rims. The rims should also be chocked as a precaution.

Overturned vehicles must have a solid object such as a wheel chock, timber, spare tire or cribbing between the roof and roadway. A jack can be used to angle the vehicle against the object. Hook a chain to the axle and loop the chain to a tree or post.

GAINING ACCESS

Simple Access

The term **simple access** describes the process of getting to a patient without the use of equipment. Although simple access does not require the use of equipment, the EMR should remember to wear protective equipment and use standard precautions as appropriate. Methods of simple access include—

- Trying to open each door.
- Trying to open the windows.
- Having the patient(s) unlock the doors or open and roll down the windows.

When you arrive on the scene, if specialized equipment and personnel are necessary to access patients call to have these units dispatched. If after accessing the patients you realize that the additional personnel and equipment are not necessary, you can easily cancel them.

Complex Access

Complex access describes the process of using specialized tools or equipment to gain access to a patient (**Fig. 28-6**). Several types of rescue training courses are available that deal with vehicle and ropes rescue. Other types of programs provide training in trench, high-angle and water rescue. As an EMR, you may encounter situations in which you will use basic equipment and techniques to gain access to a patient.

Tools

There are different types of extrication tools used to access patients (**Fig. 28-7**). Hand tools might

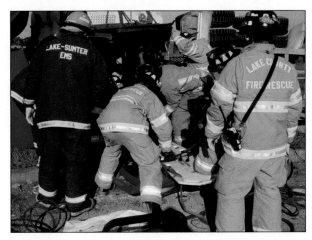

Fig. 28-6: Complex access requires the use of specialized tools or equipment to gain access to a patient. *Courtesy of Captain Phil Kleinberg, EMT-P, Lake-Sumter EMS.*

include a "come-along," a ratcheting cable device used for pulling. Pneumatic tools might include air bags, which can be used to aid with lifting.

The most commonly used extrication tool is the power hydraulic tool, such as the Hurst Jaws of Life®. This tool uses anywhere from 20,000–40,000 *pounds per square inch* (psi) to spread apart metal, and is most commonly used to remove the doors from a vehicle. However, it can also be beneficial for crushing and pulling or pushing the dash area forward. Hydraulic tools, such as a jack, may also be used to lift the vehicle.

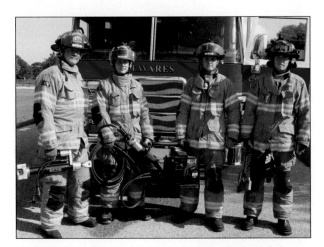

Fig. 28-7: Extrication tools, used to access patients, include hand tools, pneumatic tools, hydraulic tools, cutters and rams. *Courtesy of Ted Crites.*

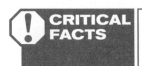

CRITICAL FACTS The term simple access describes the process of getting to a patient without the use of equipment. Complex access describes the process of using specialized tools or equipment to gain access to a patient.

Other frequently used tools are cutters, which can employ 30,000–60,000 psi. Cutters do as their name suggests—cut. Most often, they are used to cut the posts that hold up the roof of a motor vehicle. There are also hydraulic tools that combine cutters and jaws into one tool.

A third type of extrication tool is the ram, which uses its force to spread. This is in similar fashion to the action of a jaws tool but with a much straighter and wider spread. Often the ram is used to push the dash area away from the front passenger compartment of a vehicle.

EXTRICATION
Role of the EMR

During extrication, your first priority is your own safety. Contact the communications center immediately and request that fire and law enforcement personnel respond to the scene. Information regarding number of vehicles, number of patients and the presence of any hazardous substances is very important.

Wearing the proper equipment is essential to ensure your safety; however, this is not enough in the case of some accident scenes. Ensure the scene is safe before approaching a patient. Once the scene is secure and the vehicle stable, attempt to reach the patient and complete the primary assessment. Together with other rescue personnel, establish a chain of command to ensure the utmost safety and care for patients and rescue team members.

Extrication Tools

It is important to be prepared in case the local rescue squad cannot make it to the scene as quickly as necessary. In these situations, the following tools and equipment are key to assisting in the safe extrication of a patient as quickly as possible:
- Hammer
- Screwdriver
- Chisel
- Crowbar
- Pliers
- Work gloves and goggles
- Shovel
- Tire irons
- Wrenches
- Knives, including linoleum knives
- Car jacks
- Ropes or chains

Extricating the Patient

Extricating the patient is a task carried out by specially trained personnel. Of primary concern is preventing further harm to the patient. The most important factor in achieving this is proper training of personnel, so that everyone is familiar with extrication procedures and team members communicate effectively.

Every extrication is different and some can be quite complex. In some situations, the patient may be trapped in the car seat or partially trapped under the seat. When this happens, it may be possible to alleviate the situation by using the car's seat adjustment lever. If this is insufficient, the seat can be taken out by removing the nuts securing the seat or by forcing the seat using portable rams, spreaders or come-alongs. This latter option may involve rough movement, which may not be a viable option, depending on the patient's condition.

Providing Care

It is important to have a sufficiently large number of skilled personnel available during extrication, as there are multiple tasks to look after at the same time. Always try to move the device, not the patient, during extrication. At all times, maintain manual cervical spine stabilization. Use the path of least resistance when making decisions regarding equipment and moving the patient.

Once you have gained access to the patient, follow procedures for suspected head, neck and spinal injuries. Complete the primary assessment and provide the appropriate care.

Stay with the patient at all times and continually monitor his or her condition. If it

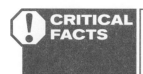

CRITICAL FACTS

Extricating the patient is a task reserved for specially trained personnel. Preventing further harm to the patient is a primary concern in extrication.

Be sure to stay with the extricated patient at all times. Continually monitor his or her condition.

worsens, communicate this to the rest of the team members, as they may wish to change the method to a more rapid type of extrication.

PUTTING IT ALL TOGETHER

There are times when an EMR may not be able to provide immediate care for an injured or ill person because the EMR cannot reach the person. This can happen as a result of motor-vehicle collisions, fire, water or other elements.

While fire rescue personnel and others have special training and equipment, an EMR may be called upon to assist in vehicle extrication. Vehicle extrication involves multiple steps—stabilizing the vehicle, attempting to gain access to patients inside the vehicle and, if unable to do so, carrying out the steps involved in extricating the patients from the vehicle in the safest manner possible.

All steps in the vehicle extrication process require specialized training and must be carried out by a team of rescue personnel. During the procedure, it is critical that EMRs take steps to ensure their own safety. Sadly, some EMRs and others are injured or killed each year when struck by an oncoming vehicle while attempting to help patients involved in motor-vehicle collisions. Be sure to take adequate measures to make the scene safe before trying to gain access and provide care. When providing care, rescuers should take steps to protect the patient's head, neck and spine.

 YOU ARE THE EMERGENCY MEDICAL RESPONDER

As you perform the primary assessment, the patient complains of numbness and tingling in his hands. What type of injury do you suspect the patient may have and what other steps would you take as you provide care for this patient?

29

Hazardous Materials Emergencies

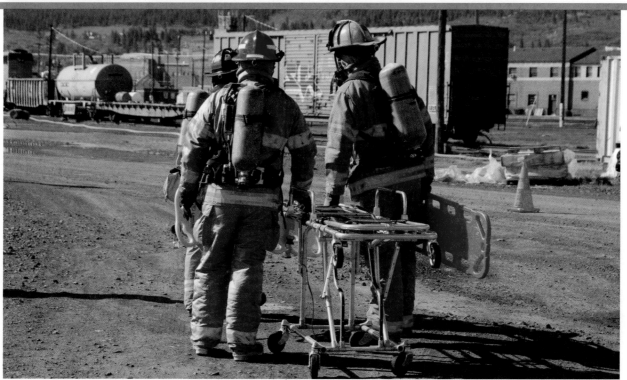

You are the first *emergency medical responder* (EMR) to arrive at the scene of a freight train derailment. According to the train's placards and signage, several of the cars are carrying liquefied chlorine gas, at least two cars are leaking and there is a yellowish cloud hanging low over the area. The winds are light, about 5 to 10 *miles per hour* (mph) and are coming from the northeast. Would you know how to respond? What would you do?

Key Terms

Cold zone: Also called the *support zone*, this area is the outer perimeter of the zones most directly affected by an emergency involving hazardous materials.

Emergency Response Guidebook: A resource available from the U.S. *Department of Transportation* (DOT) to help identify hazardous materials and appropriate care for those exposed to them.

Flammability: The degree to which a substance may ignite.

Hazardous materials (HAZMAT) incident: Any situation that deals with the unplanned release of hazardous materials.

Hot zone: Also called the *exclusion zone*, this is the area in which the most danger exists from a HAZMAT incident.

Material Safety Data Sheet (MSDS): A sheet (provided by the manufacturer) that identifies the substance, physical properties and any associated hazards for a given material (e.g., fire, explosion and health hazards), as well as emergency first aid.

Reactivity: The degree to which a substance may react when exposed to other substances.

Shipping papers: Documents drivers must carry by law when transporting hazardous materials; list the names, possible associated dangers and four-digit identification numbers of the substances.

Staging area: Location established where resources can be placed while awaiting tactical assignment.

Toxicity: The degree to which a substance is poisonous or toxic.

Warm zone: Also called the *contamination reduction zone*; the area immediately outside the hot zone.

Learning Objectives

After reading this chapter, and completing the class activities, you will have the information needed to—

- Define *hazardous materials* (HAZMAT).
- Describe the basic response to a HAZMAT incident.
- Know where to find available resources regarding training and response to HAZMAT incidents.
- Have a basic understanding of placards and the *Emergency Response Guidebook*.
- List basic *personal protective equipment* (PPE) necessary for responding to a HAZMAT incident.
- Know other resources available to respond to HAZMAT incidents.
- Understand the principles of decontamination and providing care during a HAZMAT incident.

INTRODUCTION

As an *emergency medical responder* (EMR), you may find yourself involved in a situation in which there are chemical or other harmful or toxic substances. EMRs must be trained to quickly identify such situations and activate specially trained personnel to deal with them.

The possibility of being involved in a ***hazardous materials* (HAZMAT) incident** should be an everyday concern of all personnel involved in the *emergency medical services* (EMS) system. Most people think that a HAZMAT incident only involves train and truck crashes, but hazardous materials can also be found in the home, school, industry and various public places. Whenever there is any leaking or spilling of chemicals, the potential of a HAZMAT incident exists.

HAZARDOUS MATERIALS
What Are Hazardous Materials?

Hazardous materials are everywhere. A *hazardous material* (HAZMAT) is any chemical substance or material that can pose a threat to the health, safety and property of an individual **(Fig. 29-1)**. These materials include wastes, chemicals and other dangerous products, including explosives, poisonous gases, corrosives, radioactive materials, compressed gases, oxidizers and flammable solids and liquids. For example, hospitals may have radioactive materials if they practice nuclear medicine. Farms and lawn and garden companies stock fertilizers, insecticides and pesticides. Various waste products from any number of manufacturers may also be considered toxic or hazardous.

If you work as part of an EMS system, you should participate in a First Responder/ Emergency Medical Responder Awareness Level Hazardous Materials training program. This program provides training in recognizing a HAZMAT incident and how to approach it safely.

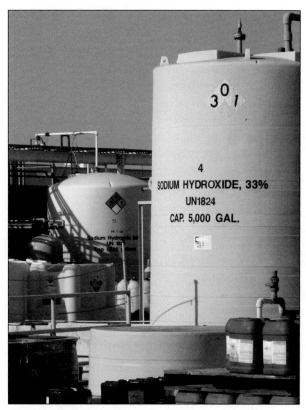

Fig. 29-1: Any chemical substance or material that poses a health, safety or property threat is a hazardous material. *Courtesy of Captain Phil Kleinberg, EMT-P, Lake-Sumter EMS.*

Terms you should familiarize yourself with when dealing with a HAZMAT incident include—

- **Flammability**. The degree to which a substance may ignite.
- HAZMAT. Any chemical substance or material that can pose a threat or risk to life, health, safety or property if not properly handled or contained.
- ***Material Safety Data Sheets* (MSDS)**. Sheets (provided by the manufacturer) that identify the substance, physical properties and any associated hazards for a given material (e.g. fire, explosion and health hazards), as well as emergency first aid.
- **Reactivity**. The degree to which a substance may react when exposed to other substances.
- **Shipping papers**. Documents drivers must carry by law when transporting hazardous materials; the papers list the names, associated

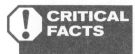

A HAZMAT is any chemical substance or material that can pose a threat to the health, safety and property of an individual.

dangers and four-digit identification numbers of the substances.

- **Staging area**. The location established where resources can be placed while awaiting tactical assignment.
- **Toxicity**. The degree to which a substance is poisonous or toxic.

Identifying Hazardous Materials
Resources

Several books available from the *U.S. Department of Transportation* (DOT) help identify hazardous materials and appropriate care procedures. The ***Emergency Response Guidebook*** is one such reference book (**Fig. 29-2**). The guidebook is available in English and Spanish and can be downloaded to pocket PCs and PDAs for easy and quick access to information on handling hazardous materials. The *Chemical Transportation Emergency Center* (CHEMTREC) can provide further

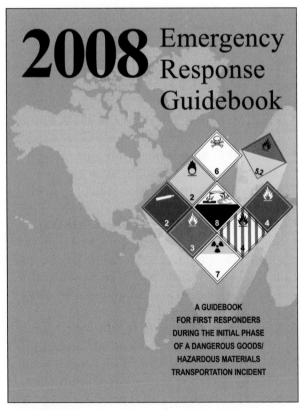

Fig. 29-2: Several books available from the DOT, such as the *Emergency Response Guidebook*, help identify hazardous materials and appropriate care procedures.

information and guidance on hazardous materials. The CHEMTREC 24-Hour HAZMAT Communications Center toll-free phone number is **1-800-262-8200**.

CAMEO® is an online library of more than 6000 data sheets containing response-related information and recommendations for hazardous materials that are commonly transported, used and/or stored in the United States. It is designed to plan for and respond to chemical emergencies and was developed by the *Environmental Protection Agency's* (EPA's) *Office of Emergency Management* (OEM) and the *National Oceanic and Atmospheric Administration's* (NOAA's) *Office of Response and Restoration* (OR&R).

The *National Institute for Occupational Safety and Health* (NIOSH) is the federal agency responsible for conducting research and making recommendations for the prevention of work-related injury and illness. NIOSH provides free resources on various chemicals and also publishes a pocket guide to chemical hazards.

Regulatory Requirements

EMRs should review the *Occupational Safety and Health Administration* (OSHA) and EPA safety guidelines as well as the *National Fire Protection Association* (NFPA) HAZMAT requirements for EMS providers.

Placards and Shipping Papers

Placards, or signs, are required by federal law to be placed on any vehicles that contain specific quantities of hazardous materials. In addition, manufacturers and others associated with the production and distribution of these materials are required by law to display the appropriate placard. Placards often clearly identify the danger of the substance. Terms such as "explosive," "flammable," "corrosive" and "radioactive" are frequently used. Universally recognized symbols are also used. **Figure 29-3** shows some common labels and placards for identifying hazardous materials. Shipping papers, also called *manifests* or *waybills*, are a means of identifying hazardous substances being transported from one location to another.

HAZMAT INCIDENTS

A HAZMAT incident is any situation that deals with the release of hazardous material. When dealing with a HAZMAT incident, you work within a structured system that provides guidance in managing this type of scene.

Preparing for a HAZMAT Incident and Activating the Plan

Establishing command at a HAZMAT incident may be your responsibility as an EMR. The following steps should be taken in preparation for the worst-case scenarios developing at the scene:

- Establish a clear chain of command.
- A single command officer must be assigned to maintain control of the situation and to make decisions at every stage of the rescue. The rescue team must be aware of who is in command and when decision-making powers are transferred to another officer.
- Establish a system of communication that is accessible and familiar to all rescuers.
- Establish a receiving facility that is as close to the scene as possible and that is able to receive and handle the number of patients and continued decontamination processes required.

Once the plan has been established, the EMR must stay in command until relieved by someone higher in the chain of command. The following information must be transferred to the new command officer:

- Nature of the substance and problems
- Identity of the hazardous materials
- Kind of containers and their condition
- Weather conditions, especially wind direction
- Time since the emergency occurred
- Stage of the rescue and what steps are already in place

- Number of patients involved
- Possibility of additional patients

Recognizing a HAZMAT Incident

When approaching any scene, you should be aware of dangers involving chemicals. Whether a motor-vehicle collision or an industrial emergency, you should be able to recognize clues that indicate the presence of hazardous materials (**Fig. 29-4**). These include—

- Signs (placards) on vehicles or storage facilities.
- Spilled liquids or solids.
- Unusual odors.
- Clouds of vapor, including colored vapor.
- Smoking or burning materials.
- Boiling or spattering of materials.
- Unusual condition of containers (e.g., unexpected peeling or deterioration).
- Leaking containers with possible frost near the leak.

Also, observe for clues of possible terrorism. In some cases, such as a nuclear attack or explosion, the possibility that a terrorist attack has taken place will be more obvious. However, when dealing with a chemical or biological attack, it may be more difficult to confirm your suspicions. There are some general clues you can use when approaching a disaster scene:

- When called to an incident at well-populated areas such as airports, subways, government buildings, schools or large public gatherings, always use caution and suspect the possibility that terrorism exists.
- When called to a scene where numerous patients are suffering from an unidentifiable illness, the possibility you are entering a potentially dangerous environment is also high.
- When called to a scene where animals in the area are dead or appear incapacitated, the possibility of chemical exposure may exist.

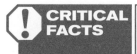 **CRITICAL FACTS** Indications of the presence of hazardous materials include placards; spilled, splattered or boiling materials; unusual odors; vapor clouds; and containers that are leaking, in deteriorating condition or are otherwise atypical.

TABLE OF PLACARDS AND INITIAL

USE THIS TABLE ONLY IF MATERIALS CANNOT BE SPECIFICALLY IDENTIFIED BY

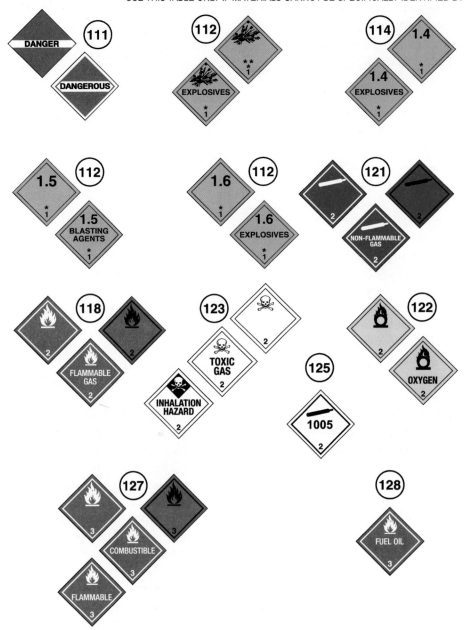

Fig. 29-3: Universally recognized symbols are used to identify the dangers of hazardous materials.

This includes the presence of odors resembling those of bitter almonds, peaches, mustard, freshly cut grass, garlic or pungent or sweet odors.

Unfortunately, in those cases where biological agents have been released, it is not always obvious there is danger. Pathogens can enter a person's system and not be evident until symptoms become evident, sometimes days after exposure. Often it becomes difficult to contain the spread of an outbreak, particularly through the community of caregivers who may be infected in the vicinity of the attack.

When called to a HAZMAT incident, it may be your responsibility as an EMR to help lay the groundwork for the rescue scene. As a responder you should—

- Be able to identify the unsafe materials and the scene as a HAZMAT incident.

RESPONSE GUIDE TO USE ON-SCENE
USING THE SHIPPING DOCUMENT, NUMBERED PLACARD, OR ORANGE PANEL NUMBER

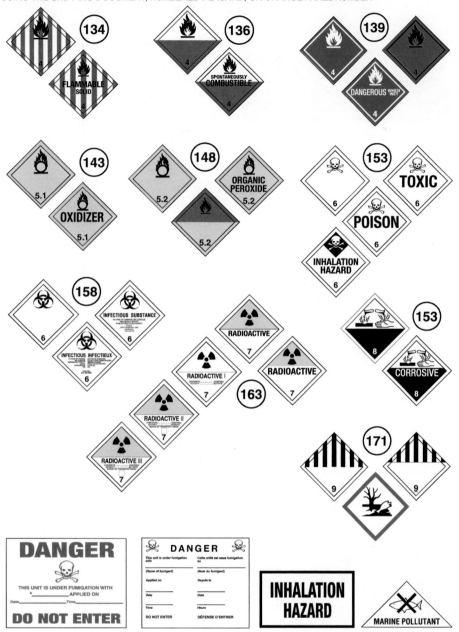

Fig. 29-3: Universally recognized symbols are used to identify the dangers of hazardous materials.

- Help establish or assign a safe location to position yourself and the rescue team.
- Always approach a suspected or real HAZMAT incident from upwind and uphill.
- Help establish the command and control zones as well as a medical treatment area.
- Always ask yourself—
  - What has been done?
  - What is being done?
  - What actions need to be taken next?

Identifying the Hazardous Substance

Once a HAZMAT incident has been identified, and you are in a safe position, try to identify the hazardous substances and the seriousness of the incident. Look for placards; NFPA numbers; warning signs like "flammable," "explosive," "corrosive" or "radioactive"; shipping papers; or areas where materials or containers are held or

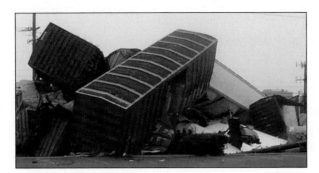

Fig. 29-4: Unusual placement or conditions and leaking containers are indications of the presence of hazardous materials. *Courtesy of Capt. Tony Duran, Los Angeles County Fire Department.*

stored (**Fig. 29-5**). By law, any business holding materials considered hazardous must have permits to hold or contain those materials. Containers should be identified in order to assess the danger level of leaks or further contamination. Containers can include—

- Rooms, buildings or outside areas.
- Above-ground tanks and vats.
- Individual containers, cartons and packages.

As already mentioned, placards will identify the exact substances in question. When dealing with a vehicular incident, shipping papers will be held by the driver as reference to the substances involved.

When in doubt, remember that the Emergency Response Guidebook, CHEMTREC, Cameo

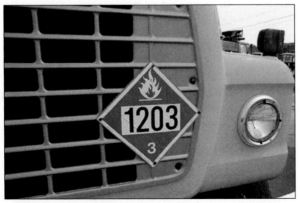

Fig. 29-5: By law, specific types of placards must indicate the presence of hazardous materials.

and NIOSH resources are available to you as well. The HAZMAT team ultimately will be responsible for identifying the substance, but in your role as an EMR you could be able to provide the initial identification. If arriving on the scene, collect the information and report to dispatch.

SCENE SAFETY AND PERSONAL PROTECTIVE EQUIPMENT

Unless you have received special training in handling hazardous materials and have the necessary equipment to do so without danger, you should stay well away from the area. While en-route to a potential HAZMAT incident, obtain as much prearrival information as possible from dispatch. When on the scene, stay out of low areas where vapors and liquids may collect, and always stay upwind and uphill of the scene. Be alert for wind changes that could cause vapors to blow toward you and other rescuers. Do not attempt to be a hero. It is not uncommon for responding ambulance crews approaching the scene to recognize a HAZMAT placard and immediately move to a safe area and summon more advanced help.

Many fire departments have specially trained teams to handle incidents involving hazardous materials. While awaiting help, you may be tasked to keep people away from the danger zone.

Especially in the case of radiation exposure, the following safety precautions must be taken to ensure scene safety:

- From a distance, survey the area for the radiation symbol on vehicles, buildings or containers.
- Determine the source of the radiation without moving closer to the scene.
- Position your vehicle upwind and uphill of the leak.
- Do not park near liquid spills or containers that may be cracked or leaking.
- Be aware of the possibility of contamination from other substances.

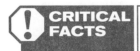 **CRITICAL FACTS** Stay away from a HAZMAT scene unless you are properly trained and have the proper equipment.

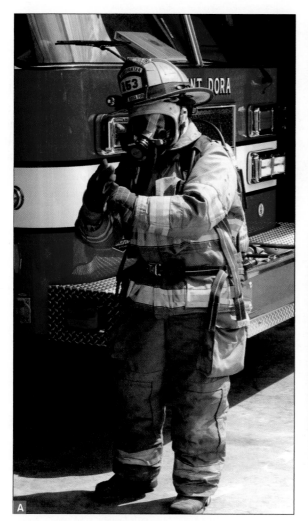
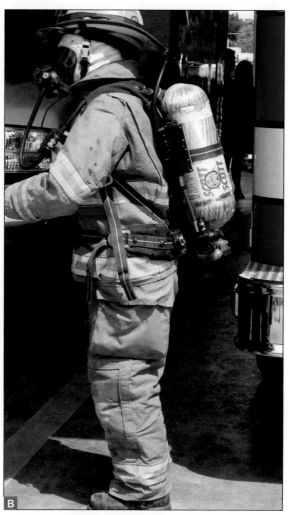

Fig. 29-6, A–B: **(A)** Protective clothing and **(B)** a SCBA can help protect you in cases of radiation. *Courtesy of Ted Crites.*

- When radiation is suspected, immediately don a positive-pressure *self-contained breathing apparatus* (SCBA) and protective clothing **(Fig. 29-6, A-B)**. Seal off all openings with duct tape. Wear double gloves and two pairs of paper shoe covers under heavy rubber boots.
- If radiation is suspected, do not attempt a rescue. Radiation cannot be felt, smelled or heard. EMRs could be exposed to lethal doses without any immediate signs or symptoms.

For your own personal protection consider—
- The time you have been exposed to the radiation source.

- The distance between you and the source.
- The density of your protective clothing.
- The amount of radioactive material you and the patient have been exposed to.

Whenever possible, remove yourself and the patient from the contaminated area or the contaminated material from the patient. The longer the time, the closer the distance and the more materials you are exposed to, the worse the situation and the more protection you will require to decrease your risk of exposure.

Some hazardous materials, such as natural gas, are flammable and can cause an explosion.

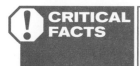

CRITICAL FACTS

If you must work near a radiation source, think about your personal protection and well as your patient's. Consider how much time you have spent near the source, the distance between you and the source, the density of your PPE and the amount of radioactive material you and the patient are exposed to.

Even turning on a light switch or using a telephone or radio may create a spark that sets off an explosion. When you call for help, use a telephone or radio well away from the scene.

In certain situations, you may come across *methamphetamine* (meth) labs. Meth labs are very hazardous due to inhalation hazards and the possibility of absorption of dangerous compounds to all exposed. An even greater hazard is the instability and highly explosive nature of these labs. Meth labs can be set up in homes, trailers and even the trunks of cars. Even a small electrical spark, such as the flick of a light switch, near the types of compounds found in these locations could cause a significant explosion. Always use caution if you suspect that there might be a meth lab at the location you are attempting to access.

Establishing Safety Zones

To decrease the risk of the HAZMAT incident expanding, it is necessary to establish a safety zone. Three control zones are created in these situations, including (**Fig. 29-7**)—

- The **hot zone** or exclusion zone. This is the area in which the most danger exists. Entry is only allowed with the proper PPE. The only reason to be inside the

hot zone is for rescue, treatment for any conditions that are life threatening and initial decontamination.
- The **warm zone** or contamination reduction zone. This is the area immediately outside the hot zone. PPE is necessary here as well. This is where complete decontamination of the patient takes place. The purpose of this zone is for life-saving emergency care—for example, airway management and immobilization.
- The **cold zone** or support zone. This the outer perimeter; entry into this area is not permitted unless all contaminated PPE and equipment are removed.

Entry into these zones is established by the amount of training a responder or member of the rescue team has completed. The warm and hot zones can only be entered by those who have received OSHA *Hazardous Waste Operations and Emergency Response* (HAZWOPER) training at the first responder awareness level and who are dressed in appropriate PPE and SCBA.

CONTAMINATION AND DECONTAMINATION
Contamination and Routes of Exposure

A patient may have suffered from contamination via several possible routes, including topical (through the skin), respiratory (inhaled), gastrointestinal (ingested) or parenteral (*intramuscular* [IM], *intravenous* [IV] or *subcutaneous* [sub-Q]). Potential signs and symptoms for each are as follows:

- Cardiovascular: Abnormally rapid heart rhythms, specifically in the lower chambers of the heart (ventricular arrhythmias), including rapid or irregular heartbeats. Both are life threatening. Blood pressure lower than 90/60 mmHg (hypotension).
- Respiratory: Swelling and/or fluid accumulation in the lungs (acute pulmonary edema) or larynx (laryngeal edema), which can lead to impaired gas exchange and respiratory failure. Abnormal contraction of the smooth muscle of the bronchi, causing an acute narrowing and obstruction

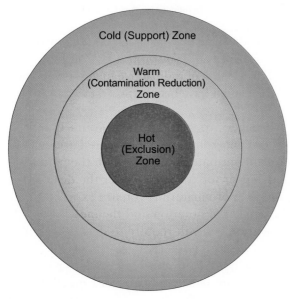

Fig. 29-7: In HAZMAT situations, three control zones are designated, from most to least dangerous: hot, warm and cold.

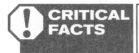

CRITICAL FACTS In HAZMAT situations, three control zones are designated, from most to least dangerous: hot, warm and cold.

HAZMAT–Recognition, Identification and Determination

Hazardous materials are often present at accident sites and in emergency settings. An EMR who is first on scene to a possible hazardous materials spill should follow these three steps: recognition, identification and determination.

The first and most basic issue is *recognition* of the presence of a hazardous material. Prompt recognition and awareness of hazardous materials is very important to the safety of the public and for the safety of the responders. Contact dispatch and report specific details of the scene.

Once the presence of a hazardous material has been determined, its specific identity and characteristics can be established. This is known as *identification*. The EMR should relay information regarding placard colors and numbers, and any label information. Shipping papers that include MSDSs will also help to indentify the hazardous material(s).

Determination of the extent of involvement a hazardous material plays in an incident is necessary to determine if it is responsible for injuries or damage at the scene of the incident. Often, hazardous materials may be present but pose no immediate, serious threat.

It cannot be overemphasized that until it has been determined that hazardous materials are not responsible for injuries or damage at an incident, EMRs should take every precaution to protect themselves and the public from exposure.

of the respiratory airway (bronchospasm) or a high-pitched, whistling breathing caused by a blockage in the throat or larynx (stridor), cough, dyspnea and chest pain. Respiratory symptoms may be delayed.

- Central nervous system: Stupor, lethargy, coma and the possibility of seizures.
- *Gastrointestinal* (GI): GI bleeding due to liquefaction necrosis (irreversible death of cells) of the GI tract.
- Eye: Vapor contamination can result in chemical conjunctivitis. Necrosis and blindness can result from exposure to liquids and anhydrous (ammonia) gas.

Decontamination

There are several methods of decontamination, including gross, dilution, absorption, neutralization and isolation/disposal. Initial, or "gross" decontamination, is performed as the person enters the warm zone. Any immediate life-threatening conditions are addressed during this stage. Soap and copious amounts of water are used and any clothing, equipment and tools must be left in the hot zone **(Fig. 29-8)**.

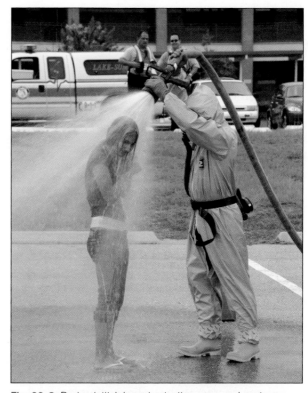

Fig. 29-8: During initial decontamination, soap and copious amounts of water are used to address any immediate life-threatening situations. *Courtesy of Captain Phil Kleinberg, EMT-P, Lake-Sumter EMS.*

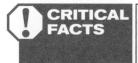
CRITICAL FACTS

There are several possible routes of exposure and contamination, including topical, respiratory, gastrointestinal and parenteral.

There are several methods of decontamination, including gross, dilution, absorption, neutralization and isolation/disposal.

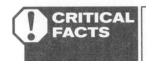

CRITICAL FACTS | When assessing and treating a patient in a HAZMAT incident, it is important to concentrate on the life-threatening signs and symptoms as opposed to strictly dealing with the contamination and exposure itself.

At this point, a primary assessment is carried out. *Dilution* refers to the method of reducing the concentration of a contaminant to a safe level. *Isolation/disposal* refers to the method of decontamination in which contaminated equipment and materials are bagged or covered and set aside, usually for subsequent shipment to an approved landfill for disposal. *Absorption* is the process of using material that will absorb and hold contaminants such as corrosive and liquid chemicals. *Neutralization* involves chemically altering a substance to render it harmless or make it less harmful.

Emergency Medical Treatment
Establishing a Location

Establishing a clear perimeter between zones is of critical importance to prevent the spread of contamination. When selecting the location for the command post and staging area, it is necessary to position support equipment upwind and uphill of the hot zone. Equipment that may be required during the rescue process should be kept in the staging areas beyond the crowd control line. Access to the different zones must be safely controlled, limiting access as much as possible.

Providing Care

When you arrive at the scene, park upwind and uphill from the scene at a safe distance. Keep bystanders and any other unnecessary people away from the scene. Isolate the scene and establish hot, warm and cold zones, keeping people out of areas accordingly. Do not enter these zones unless trained to an OSHA HAZWOPER first responder awareness level or higher, and have appropriate PPE and SCBA. Avoid any contact with the hazardous material. If there is no risk to EMS personnel, HAZMAT teams should move patients to a safe zone.

Determine the number of patients involved in the incident and evaluate the need for additional resources. Follow safety practices that minimize your exposure and that of other people at the scene.

When assessing and treating a patient in a HAZMAT incident, it is important to concentrate on the life-threatening signs and symptoms as opposed to strictly dealing with the contamination and exposure itself. Removing the patient from a scene involving hazardous materials should be done as quickly as possible to decrease exposure. Assessment and management of the patient should then be carried out as you would normally. When radiation is a concern, contact the Poison Control Center at 1-800-222-1222 or consult with medical direction.

PUTTING IT ALL TOGETHER

Hazardous materials are everywhere around us and there is always a possibility of a HAZMAT incident. As an EMR, you may find yourself involved in a situation in which there are chemical or other harmful or toxic substances. EMRs must be trained to quickly identify such situations and activate specially trained personnel to deal with the situation.

A HAZMAT incident is one in which dangerous chemicals have somehow been released and pose a threat to life. When dealing with a HAZMAT incident, work within a structured system that provides guidance in managing this type of scene.

There are several resources available to assist you in identifying hazardous materials and the steps involved in providing care. In a HAZMAT incident, your priorities are to protect the safety of rescuers and patients at the scene by providing care and assisting with decontamination. Planning for HAZMAT incidents is essential for an effective response.

)))) YOU ARE THE EMERGENCY MEDICAL RESPONDER

Since you recognize the scene as a HAZMAT incident, what questions should you ask yourself immediately? What initial actions should you take and why?

30

Incident Command and Multiple-Casualty Incidents

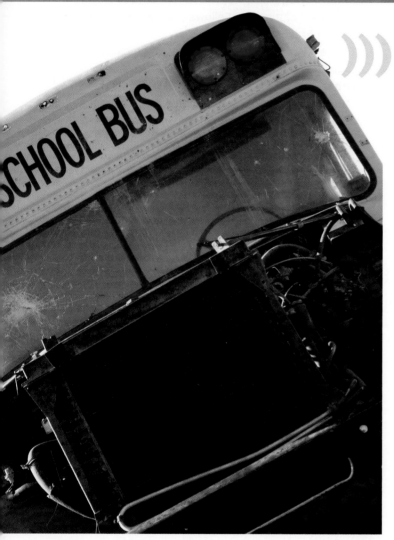

))) **YOU ARE THE EMERGENCY MEDICAL RESPONDER**

A school bus carrying 30 students is involved in a collision and is severely damaged near the front of the bus. The students are scared and some are injured. People are starting to crowd around the area, and the local fire department already is on scene. As an *emergency medical responder* (EMR) on scene, what should you do?

Key Terms

Deceased/non-salvageable/expectant (Black):
A triage category of those involved in a *multiple-(or mass-) casualty incident* (MCI) who are obviously dead or who have suffered non-life-sustaining injuries.

Delayed care (Yellow): A triage category of those involved in an MCI with an injury, but whose chances of survival will not be reduced by a delay.

Immediate care (Red): A triage category of those involved in an MCI whose needs require urgent life-saving care.

Incident command system (ICS): A standardized, on-scene, all-hazards incident management approach that allows for the integration of facilities, equipment, personnel, procedures and communications operating within a common organizational structure; enables a coordinated response among various jurisdictions and functional agencies, both public and private; and establishes common processes for planning and managing resources.

Multiple- (or mass-) casualty incident (MCI):
An incident that generates more patients than available resources can manage using routine procedures.

National Response Framework (NRF): The guiding principles that enable all response partners to prepare for and provide a unified national response to disasters and emergencies—from the smallest incident to the largest catastrophe. The *Framework* establishes a comprehensive, national, all-hazards approach to domestic incident response.

Simple Triage and Rapid Transport (START): A method of triage that allows quick assessment and prioritization of injured people.

Triage: A method of sorting patients into categories based on the urgency of their need for care.

Triage tags: A system of identifying patients during an MCI; different colored tags signify different levels of urgency for care.

Walking wounded (Green): A triage category of those involved in an MCI who are able to walk by themselves to a designated area to await care.

Learning Objectives

After reading this chapter, you will have the information needed to—

- Describe the purpose of the *National Response Framework* (NRF).
- Describe the purpose and functional positions of the *incident command system* (ICS).
- Explain the role of the *emergency medical responder* (EMR) in the ICS.
- Define multiple-casualty incidents.

- Explain the principles of triage.
- Conduct a triage assessment.
- Understand different triage systems and pediatric variations.
- Understand the stressors associated with *multiple-casualty incidents* (MCIs).

INTRODUCTION

As an *emergency medical responder* (EMR), you are likely to be required to assist with an emergency with multiple victims, and to do so you need a plan of action to enable you to rapidly determine what additional resources are needed and how best to manage them. During a serious incident, you may be on the scene for 15 minutes or longer before adequate resources are available to care for a large number of injured people.

Management of an appropriate initial response can eliminate potential problems for arriving personnel and possibly save the lives of several injured people. To accomplish this, you must be able to make the scene safe for you and others to work, delegate responsibilities to others, manage available resources, identify and care for the patients most in need of care and relinquish command as more highly trained and qualified personnel arrive.

NATIONAL INCIDENT MANAGEMENT SYSTEM

"The *National Incident Management System* (NIMS) provides a systematic, proactive approach to guide departments and agencies at all levels of government, nongovernmental organizations and the private sector to work seamlessly to prevent, protect against, respond to, recover from and mitigate the effects of incidents, regardless of cause, size, location or complexity, in order to reduce the loss of life and property and harm to the environment." *(Source: femagov)*

"NIMS works hand in hand with the ***National Response Framework*** (NRF). NIMS provides the template for the management of incidents, while the NRF provides the structure and mechanisms for national-level policy for incident management." *(Source: femagov)*

The National Response Framework

The NRF (or *Framework*) is a guide to how the nation conducts all-hazards response. It is built upon scalable, flexible and adaptable coordinating structures to align key roles and responsibilities *across the nation*. It describes specific authorities and best practices for managing incidents that range from the serious but purely local, to large-scale terrorist attacks or catastrophic natural disasters.

Incident Command System

To effectively manage an emergency situation and to provide appropriate care, an ***incident command system*** (**ICS**) must be established, organizing who is responsible for overall direction, the roles of other participants and the resources required. Although the ICS is capable of providing a management structure for incidents both large and small, it is scalable based on incident requirements. Establishing the ICS is particularly important in a ***multiple- (or mass-) casualty incident*** (**MCI**), to effectively manage many resources.

The ICS is a management system, originally developed in California to help manage the process of fighting forest fires, that has since evolved into an all-hazards incident management system. It has proven especially effective as a strategy in emergencies involving multiple patients because of its ability to manage many functions and resources.

To understand the ICS, think of it as an organization composed of rescuers working together to achieve a common goal. The *incident commander* (IC), through delegated authority of a local government, is tasked with the responsibility of establishing the incident objectives and managing resources. The IC supervises these resources utilizing the ICS.

EMS Roles in the ICS

In any emergency, the first responder on the scene becomes the incident commander. The incident commander is responsible for assessing the situation, deciding what calls to make and what tasks need to be done and assigning the tasks to

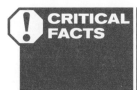

CRITICAL FACTS

As an EMR, you are likely to be required to assist with an emergency with multiple victims, and to do so you need a plan of action to enable you to rapidly determine what additional resources are needed and how best to manage them.

The ICS is a management system, originally developed in California to help manage the process of fighting forest fires, that has since evolved into an all-hazards incident management system.

In any emergency, the first responder on the scene becomes the incident commander. The incident commander is responsible for assessing the situation, deciding what calls to make and what tasks need to be done and assigning the tasks to appropriate personnel.

If you are first on the scene and the senior EMR on the scene, you are the incident commander until someone more experienced arrives. As incident commander, it is your responsibility to identify a scene as an MCI, assess the scene safety and determine if any action is required to secure the scene. If you are *not* the incident commander, it is your job to fit in wherever you are needed.

appropriate personnel (**Fig. 30-1**). The rescuer who assumes the role as incident commander remains in that role until a more senior or experienced person arrives on the scene and assumes command, or until the incident is over.

When transitioning command to a more senior person, the outgoing incident commander must ensure that everything necessary has been done before leaving the scene or accepting another assignment.

If the incident is small and contained, it is likely that one person in the incident commander role may handle all aspects of directing care. However, in situations with multiple casualties and/or events, the incident commander must delegate a variety of roles to other rescuers. While not all of these functional positions may be necessary, these are the ones most often required—the larger the incident, the more functional positions are required:

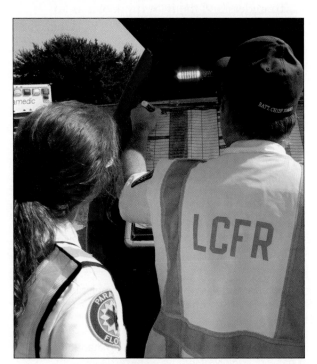

Fig. 30-1: In an emergency, the first responder on the scene becomes the incident commander. *Courtesy of Ted Crites.*

- The triage officer supervises the initial **triage**, tagging and moving of patients to designated treatment areas.
- The treatment officer sets up a treatment area and supervises medical care, ensuring triage order is maintained and changes the order if patients deteriorate and become eligible for a higher triage category.
- The transportation officer arranges for ambulances or other transport vehicles while tracking priority, identity and destination of all injured or ill people leaving the scene.
- The staging officer releases and distributes resources as needed to the incident and works to avoid transportation gridlock.
- The safety officer maintains scene safety by identifying potential dangers and taking action to prevent them from causing injury to all involved.

Other roles that may need to be filled include—
- Supply.
- Mobile command/communications.
- Extrication.
- Rehabilitation.
- Morgue.
- Logistics.

The Role of the Emergency Medical Responder

Your role as an EMR is to fit into the team wherever you are assigned. If you are first on the scene, you may find yourself acting as incident commander until someone more experienced arrives. If you are with a partner or co-worker, the most senior takes on the role of incident commander. Your responsibility is to identify if this is an MCI and assess the scene's safety to determine if any action must be taken to secure the scene to prevent further injury.

After assessing safety, as incident commander, you must account for the number of patients, including those who may not appear to be injured, determine whether anyone needs rescuing (extrication), determine the number of ambulances required and indicate the number of functional positions and extra personnel required. You must also ensure access to areas to stage resources and make note of any situations that may affect the scene, including weather, difficulty accessing the site and the terrain.

You must be easily identifiable as the incident commander to prevent confusion. Determine local protocols in effect for identifying yourself as the officer-in-charge and your vehicle as the initial command post (vests or a green light on the command vehicle are common procedures). Be sure to report all issues and necessary information—do not go into detail during radio transmission. This is the time for short, concise, accurate and pertinent bits of information.

When someone with more experience or seniority relieves you, be sure to relay all important and pertinent information verbally, including what has been recorded. The person taking over will need to know information such as when the incident began, when you arrived on the scene, how many people are injured, how many people are acting as rescuers, any potential dangers, what has been done since the beginning of the rescue and objectives that need to be accomplished.

If you arrive on the scene *after* someone has already taken command, identify yourself to the incident commander and report to the staging officer. You will then be tasked to a detail where you are most needed, based on your experience and capability. This could be assisting medical personnel, aiding in crowd or traffic control, helping to maintain scene security or helping to establish temporary shelter. By using the ICS in numerous emergencies, the tasks of reaching, caring for and transporting injured or ill people are performed more effectively, thereby saving more lives. Since there are variations in the plan for managing MCIs with ICS throughout the country, you should become familiar with the MCI plan for your location.

MULTIPLE-CASUALTY INCIDENTS

An MCI is an incident which generates more patients than available resources can manage using routine procedures. As the term implies, an MCI refers to a situation involving two or more people. You are most likely to encounter MCIs involving injury to small numbers of people, such as a motor-vehicle crash involving the driver and a passenger. But MCIs can also be large-scale events, such as those caused by natural disasters or those from materials/structures made by humans. Examples include—

- Transportation accidents.
- Flood.
- Fire.
- Explosion.
- Structure collapse.
- Train derailment (**Fig. 30-2, A-B**).

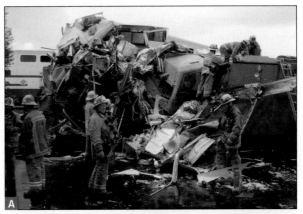

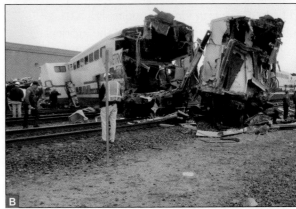

Fig. 30-2, A–B: Large-scale events involving human-made structures or materials, such as a train derailment, can result in an MCI. *Courtesy of Capt. Tony Duran, Los Angeles County Fire Department.*

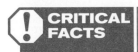
CRITICAL FACTS An MCI is an incident which generates more patients than available resources can manage using routine procedures.

- Airliner crash.
- *Hazardous materials* (HAZMAT) incidents.
- Earthquake.
- Tornado (**Fig. 30-3**).
- Hurricane.

Some incidents can result in hundreds or even thousands of injured or ill people. Whether small or large scale, MCIs can strain the resources of a local community. Coping effectively with an MCI requires a plan that enables you to acquire and manage additional personnel, equipment and supplies.

TRIAGE

In an MCI, you must modify your assessment skills and technique for checking injured or ill people. This requires you to understand the priorities of treatment and transportation. It also requires you to accept death and dying because some patients, such as those in cardiac arrest who would normally receive CPR and be a high priority, will be beyond your ability to help in this situation.

To identify which patients require urgent care in an MCI, you use a process known as triage. Triage is a French term derived from "trier," meaning "to sort," and was first used to refer to the sorting and treatment of those injured in battle.

The Triage Officer

The first step is to identify and assign a triage officer. This is a responsibility of the incident commander. The triage officer is an integral position of the ICS in MCI management. If you are the only person on the scene, the role falls on you until you receive help. The triage officer remains in that role until all patients are triaged and until relieved or reassigned by the IC. The triage officer determines the requirements for additional resources (to perform triage), performs triage of all patients and assigns personnel and equipment to the highest priority patients in the triage area.

Primary and Secondary Triage

Primary triage is used on the scene to rapidly categorize the condition of patients. When performing your first assessment, note the approximate number and location of patients and what the transportation needs are going to be, such as stretchers, litters or special extrication equipment.

Keep in mind that these are just primary assessments and patients may be re-triaged later; their status may change accordingly. Using the methods outlined by your locality, ensure that all patients have the appropriate color tape or card attached in a visible fashion. According to *Simple Triage and Rapid Transport* (**START**) principles, it should take no longer than 30 seconds per patient to do your assessment and tagging.

Patient status can change quickly. If it is necessary and there is time and space, a secondary triage may be performed after the primary triage (**Fig. 30-4**). This is often performed after patients are moved to the treatment area or at a funnel point just before they enter the treatment area. If the status of a patient changes, leave the first tag in place

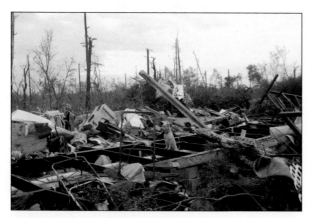

Fig. 30-3: Natural disasters, such as tornadoes, can result in MCIs. *Courtesy of Captain Phil Kleinberg, EMT-P, Lake-Sumter EMS.*

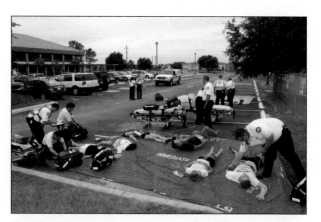

Fig. 30-4: Triage is used on the scene to rapidly categorize the condition of patients. *Courtesy of Captain Phil Kleinberg, EMT-P, Lake-Sumter EMS.*

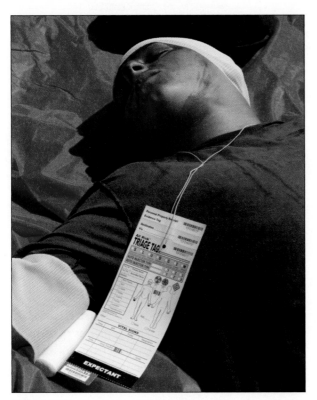

Fig. 30-5: Triage tags are used to note the status of patients in an MCI. *Courtesy of Terry Georgia.*

and draw a bold line through it. Then, add the second, most up-to-date assessment tag.

Note that slots on tags do not necessarily need to be completely filled out at once. As new information becomes available, add that information to the **triage tag** (**Fig. 30-5**).

Triage Tagging Systems

There are a variety of triage tags you may use or encounter in a triage area. Because large disasters can bring rescuers in from a wide area, internationally understood methods of communication are essential. Thus, the colors green, red, yellow and black are commonly used for the triage tagging system.

The *METTAG™* patient identification system uses symbols, rather than words, to allow rescuers to quickly identify patient status (**Fig. 30-6**). The *rabbit* means urgent, the *turtle* means can be delayed, the *ambulance with a bold line through it* means that no urgent transport is needed and a *shovel and cross* symbol is used for the dead.

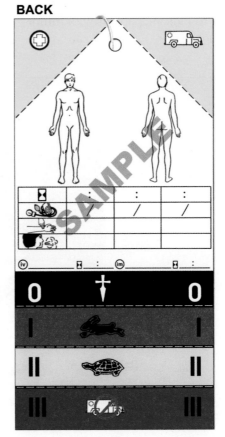

Fig. 30-6: The METTAG™ patient identification system uses symbols rather than words to allow rescuers to quickly identify patient status.

Another option is the *Smart Tag*™, adopted by certain U.S. cities and states (**Fig. 30-7**). This tag features a folding design for ease of use.

Additionally many states have adopted the START tag or adaptations of it. Some states choose to customize their tag designs, while some response systems simply use colored flagging tape (**Fig. 30-8**).

The START System

The **START** system is a simple way to quickly assess and prioritize injured or ill people. It requires you to check only three items: breathing, circulation and *level of consciousness* (LOC) (**Fig. 30-9**). As you check these items, classify injured or ill people into one of four levels that reflect the severity of their injury or illness and the need for care. These levels are "minor/ **walking wounded**," "delayed," "immediate" and "deceased/non-salvageable." Some advanced triage systems also include a fifth category, "hold," to indicate patients with minor injuries who do not require a doctor's care.

Ambulatory (Walking Wounded)

The first step is to sort those who can walk on their own, the ambulatory or walking wounded (Green). To do this, use a public address (PA) method if possible. Get their attention and direct these patients to move on their own to a designated area. This allows you to find out quickly who is not in grave danger and clears the emergency area of those who do not need to be there. Ambulatory patients are tagged as Green.

Immediate

The first of the other categories is **immediate care (Red)**. This categorization means that the patient needs immediate care and transport to a medical facility. Patients are considered immediate if they are unconscious or cannot follow simple commands, require active airway management, have a respiratory rate of greater than 30, have a delayed (more than 2 seconds) capillary refill or absent radial pulse or require bleeding control for severe hemorrhage from major blood vessels. Immediate patients are tagged Red.

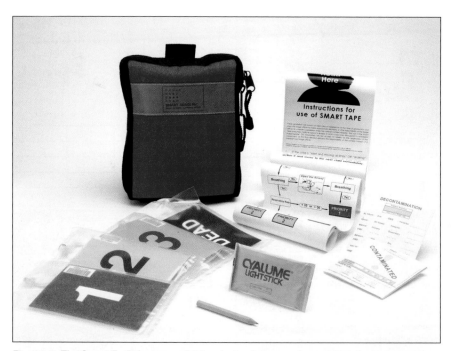

Fig. 30-7: The Smart Tag™ features a folding design for ease of use. *All intellectual property rights of the items shown in this image are the property of TSG Associates LLP. Written permission is required before use by any third party.*

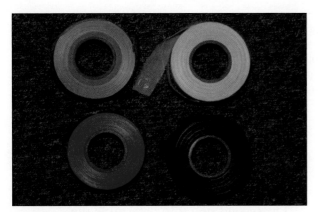

Fig. 30-8: Some states choose to customize their tag designs, while some response systems use colored flagging tape. *Courtesy of Captain Phil Kleinberg, EMT-P, Lake-Sumter EMS.*

Delayed

The second category is **delayed care (Yellow)**, meaning patients who may be suffering severe injuries but a delay in their treatment will not reduce their chance of survival. Those tagged delayed are non-ambulatory and are breathing, have a pulse and their LOC is within normal limits. While they do not have life-threatening injuries, they may have back injuries with or without spinal cord damage, major or multiple bone or joint injuries or burns without airway problems. However, the following types of burns need immediate, advanced care: flame burns that occurred in a confined space; burns covering more than one body part; burns to the head, neck, hands, feet or genitals; any partial-thickness or full-thickness burns to a child or an older adult; or burns resulting from chemicals, explosions or electricity. Delayed patients are tagged Yellow.

Deceased

The third category, **deceased/non-salvageable/expectant (Black)**, is assigned to those individuals who are obviously dead or who have mortal injuries. Patients who are not breathing and who fail to breathe after attempts to open and clear the airway (even if they have a pulse) are classified as deceased/non-salvageable/expectant. This classification also applies to obvious mortal injuries such as decapitation. Deceased patients are tagged Black.

Hold

Some advanced triage systems also include a hold category, to indicate patients with minor injuries who do not require a doctor's care, such

START Triage

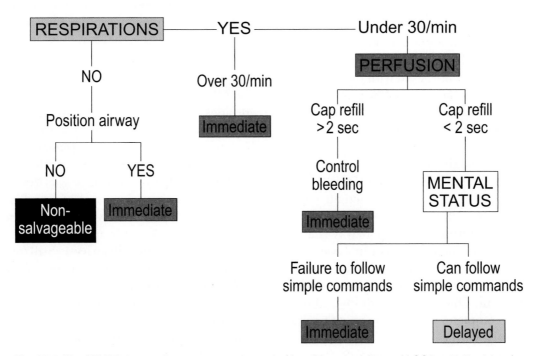

Fig. 30-9: The START triage system uses an assessment of breathing, circulation and LOC to prioritize injured or ill patients.

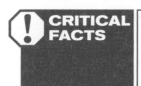
as minor painful, swollen, deformed extremities or minor soft tissue injuries. These patients may be tagged White and dismissed, with a recommendation to obtain basic first aid care at home or elsewhere.

Assessment in Triage

The START system is a popular method that is simple and depends on condition-based classification. You determine the different levels by assessing four aspects that can be recalled with the acronym ARPM. ARPM stands for—

- Ability to get up and walk (ambulatory).
- Respiratory status.
- Perfusion status.
- Mental status.

Once ambulatory patients are out of the area, you will need to check respiratory status of the remaining patients. If there are no respirations, clear the mouth of any foreign objects and make sure the airway is open. If there are still no respirations and the patient does not begin breathing independently, even with the airway open, the patient is classified as "deceased/non-salvageable." There is no need to check the pulse. Place the appropriate tag on the patient and move on.

If the patient begins to breathe independently when you open the airway, classify the patient as needing immediate care and tag appropriately. Any individual who needs help maintaining an open airway is a high priority. Position the patient in a way that will maintain an open airway, place the appropriate tag on the person and move on to the next patient. Once triage of all injured or ill people is complete, you may be able to come back and assist with care.

If the patient is breathing when you arrive, check the rate of the patient's breathing.

Someone breathing more than 30 times a minute should be classified as immediate care.

The second step is to determine the perfusion status. This is done by checking capillary refill and radial pulse, with the pulse being the more reliable measure, as capillary refill is dependent on multiple factors. If you cannot find the radial pulse in either arm, then the patient's blood pressure is substantially low. Control any severe bleeding by using direct pressure and applying a bandage. Classify the person as requiring immediate care and move on to the next patient.

The third step is to determine the patient's LOC, by using the *AVPU* (Alert, Voice, Pain, Unresponsive) scale. A patient who is alert and responds appropriately to verbal stimuli is classified as delayed care. This patient has some injury that prevents him or her from moving to safety, but the condition is not life threatening. Someone who remains unconscious and responds only to painful stimuli or responds inappropriately to verbal stimuli is classified as immediate care.

Other Methods of Triage

Besides the START triage system, there are others, such as the *Sort-Assess-Lifesaving Interventions-Treatment and/or Transport* (SALT) Mass Casualty Triage (**Fig. 30-10**). The SALT Mass Casualty Triage was developed using all existing triage systems, and is meant for all patients involved, even special populations and children. It sorts patients into three priorities: Priority 1: Still/obvious life threat; Priority 2: Waving/purposeful movement; and Priority 3: Walking. It then goes on to include individual assessments, beginning with limited, rapid *life-saving interventions* (LSI), such as controlling severe bleeding; opening and clearing the airway; or giving 2 ventilations if the patient is a child,

SALT Mass Casualty Triage

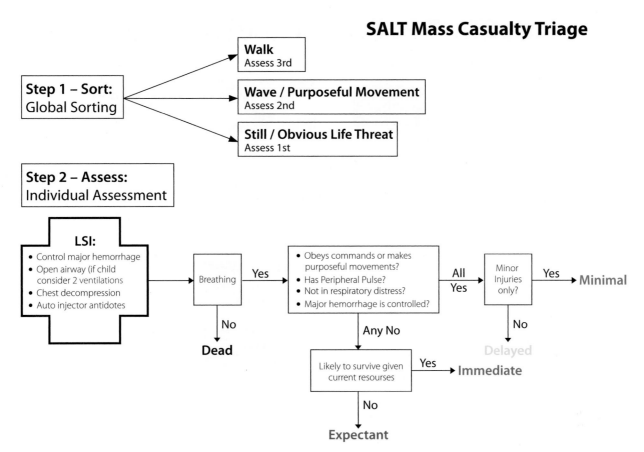

Fig. 30-10: The SALT Mass Casualty Triage system sorts patients into three priorities: still/obvious life threat, waving/purposeful movement and walking.

chest compressions or auto-injector antidotes. At this point, you would prioritize patients for treatment and/or transport by assigning them to one of five categories: Immediate, Expectant, Delayed, Minimal or Dead.

Pediatric Considerations

JumpSTART Pediatric Triage

An emergency that involves children must be handled differently from the way you would an emergency with adults. The psychological differences between adults and children could cause errors in tagging children. The *JumpSTART* triage method should be used on anyone who appears to be a child, regardless of actual chronological age, but is not done on infants younger than 12 months old **(Fig. 30-11)**.

Using the same START steps outlined previously, you would assess whether the child is ambulatory, the respiratory status, whether there is any major bleeding and the mental status.

Children who are ambulatory should be tagged accordingly and escorted to the proper area; do *not* send them alone. Children who are breathing must be monitored for the rate. It should be between 15 and 45 breaths per minute. If it is any lower or higher, or if they begin breathing spontaneously after you open the airway, they should be tagged as immediate care. A child who does *not* breathe after the airway has been cleared and does *not* have a peripheral pulse should be tagged as deceased/non-salvageable. However, if a pulse is present, even if there is no breathing after the airway is cleared, you should give 5 ventilations before determining the child's status.

For circulation, or perfusion, check the child's peripheral pulse. If there is none present, the child should be tagged immediate care. Finally, for mental status, see if the child responds to your voice. Code the child as delayed care if there is no response to all stimuli. If the child does respond to pain but only with sounds, the tag should be for immediate care.

JumpSTART Pediatric MCI Triage©

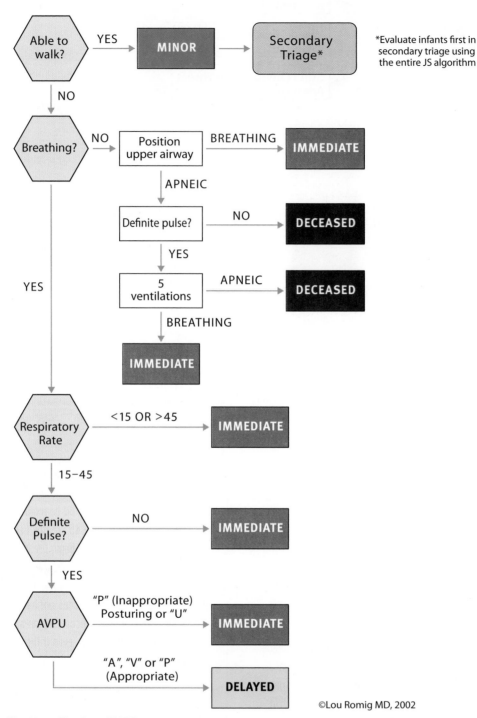

*Evaluate infants first in secondary triage using the entire JS algorithm

©Lou Romig MD, 2002

Fig. 30-11: The JumpSTART triage method, used on children older than 12 months of age, uses the same START steps to assess children.

Treatment

Following triage, patients must be processed through the treatment area (**Fig. 30-12**). The treatment officer is appointed by the IC and is responsible for identifying a treatment area of sufficient space and with adequate ingress and egress for ambulances. The treatment officer ensures the appropriate

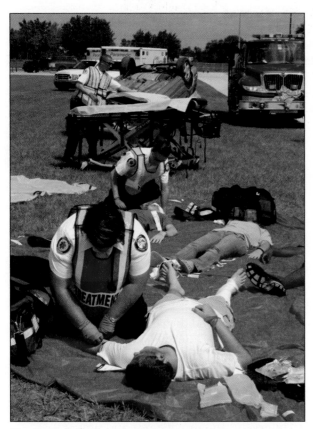
Fig. 30-12: Following triage, patients are processed through the treatment area, where patients are cared for, re-triaged or transported according to need. *Courtesy of Terry Georgia.*

medical care of all patients, directs re-triage if indicated and communicates with the transportation officer regarding the transportation of the patients and appropriate destination hospital requirements (trauma center consideration) in the correct order, according to triage. Patients tagged as immediate have priority and should be treated to correct any life-threatening conditions. They should be transported by the most appropriate means to the various hospitals according to the local MCI plan.

While patients are waiting for transport, they should be continually monitored for changes in status. For example, it is always possible that a patient tagged as delayed may experience deterioration in condition and need to be tagged as immediate.

Staging

The staging officer should be one of the first officers assigned by the IC. It is important that

the staging officer establish an area suitable to park multiple units in an organized fashion. This officer must maintain accountability of all units assigned for immediate release to the transportation officer.

Transportation

The transportation officer is assigned by the IC. The major responsibility of the transportation officer is patient accountability. This is a documentation-rich position and aide(s) are often required based on the scope and complexity of the incident. The transportation officer communicates with receiving hospitals, units assigned by the staging officer, the staging officer and the treatment officer. The transportation officer is responsible for assigning patients to ambulances, helicopters and buses, assigning destination hospitals and maintaining patient tracking records.

The ambulances, helicopters and buses will be instructed which hospital is accepting their patient or patients. They then radio ahead to the hospital, notifying hospital personnel of their impending arrival. This is the time when appropriate advance information is given, such as the injuries involved and estimated time of arrival.

Once all the immediate and delayed patients have been transported, the ambulatory patients also may be transported. Essential emergency equipment and EMRs should be on the transport, in case a patient deteriorates from ambulatory to delayed, or even immediate, care.

STRESS AT AN MCI
Patient Stress

The impact of an MCI can reach far beyond visible injuries. The stress of living through such an event can result in cognitive, emotional, physical and behavioral responses. Some may occur right away, others may only appear days after the event.

Patient stress can be the result of individual injuries, but also concern over loved ones who may have been involved in the MCI

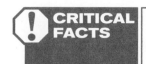
Communication is a vital link to manage an MCI smoothly. However, if you find yourself in a situation where communication is not ideal, remember that your first priority is your patients and the care you are there to provide. Do *not* let the frustration of difficulties with communication affect your work.

(**Fig. 30-13**). Not knowing what is happening is very stressful and frightening, and can interfere with the physical care of the patient.

Some people are at greater risk of severe stress reactions. Children may react strongly, experiencing extreme fears of further harm. Elderly patients and those who already suffer from health problems, either physical or emotional, may also be at increased risk.

Responder Stress

After each call, there should be opportunity to discuss how the call went, as well as any feelings or issues that may have resulted. This is particularly important following an MCI, which can often seem overwhelming and difficult to handle. Trained counselors may help lead the discussion and reduce the risk of post-traumatic stress.

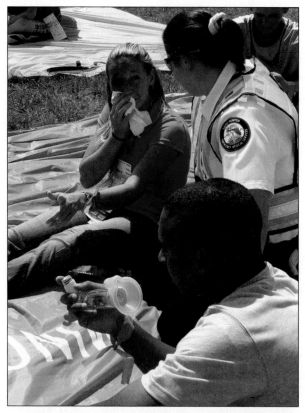

Fig. 30-13: Patient stress can be the result of individual injuries or concern over loved ones. *Courtesy of Ted Crites.*

Reducing stress *during* the MCI is also important. This can be done by ensuring that rescuers know exactly what is expected of them. If they do not understand their roles or duties, frustration and stress may result. If rescuers are in roles that match their specific strengths, this helps in reducing stress.

Ensure that rescuers get adequate rest, according to the protocols for your organization. Rest and down time are essential, regardless of the situation. This time can be used for the rescuers to eat and drink (no alcohol), close their eyes or talk. If possible, counselors on the scene can help at this point.

Keep an eye on the rescuers. Even though they may feel they are coping well, if you are on the lookout for exhaustion or stress, you may be able to intervene and provide rest and support.

Encourage rescuers to talk among themselves, though their conversation must be kept professional to avoid misunderstandings from other workers or the patients.

Following the MCI, debriefing is a vital part of the process. Allowing rescuers to go over their role in the MCI and the outcome allows for release of stress and learning opportunities for future events.

Managing and Reducing Stress

Whenever possible, reunite family members. The goal is to reduce their stress and fear, but this can also be helpful for rescuers, since family members can provide missing information and can support each other.

Limit the information that may be getting out of the scene. Only designated authorities should be speaking to members of the media, and those rescuers who are working on the scene should not discuss individual patients with anyone other than immediate family members who are on hand.

Be honest. Tell patients what is happening in terms they can understand. Limit the use of official or medical language, as it can seem confusing and frightening if misunderstood.

If possible, for those who are able, assign tasks to help others. This can help reduce stress and make them feel useful. If patients are reluctant to receive help, encourage them to accept it, so that perhaps they may return the favor at some point by helping someone else.

Encourage questions and discussion. Fear of the unknown is often worse than reality. Be careful not to offer false hope; if you cannot answer a question, say so and see if you can determine the answer from the right sources.

COMMUNICATION

Communication is a vital link in the smooth running of an MCI. However, it is important that rescuers understand that communication is not always as smooth and effective as would be desired. If you find yourself in a situation where communication is not ideal, remember that your first priority is your patients and the care you are there to provide. Do *not* let the frustration of difficulties with communication affect your work.

To help communication run smoothly, remember to always speak as clearly as possible—do not rush your speech—because being asked to repeat or being misunderstood can cause a delay in care or transport. Use simple, clear language. Use communication tools such as radio communications only when necessary, so as not to clutter the airwaves. For obvious reasons, face-to-face communication is usually the easiest means of communication.

PUTTING IT ALL TOGETHER

As an EMR, you may need to assist with an emergency involving multiple people. To do so effectively requires a plan of action so that you can rapidly determine what additional resources are needed and how best to use them. An appropriate initial response can eliminate potential problems for arriving personnel and possibly save the lives of several injured people. You will need to be able to make the scene safe for you and others to work, delegate responsibilities to others, manage available resources, identify and care for the patients most in need of care and relinquish command as more highly trained personnel arrive.

MCIs can be stressful and challenging for EMRs. By following set protocols for establishing priority care, confusion can be minimized for both responders and patients.

The two most important issues to remember are assessment and communication. For patients in an MCI, your assessments differ from those of one-on-one situations. In an MCI, you must be able to provide care to as many patients as possible, so you must focus on those who can be saved or helped.

Communication between you and your colleagues is vital in maintaining control of the situation, minimizing stress and providing quality care. Communication with the patients and their loved ones will help keep them from panicking and help them listen to instructions.

Finally, equally important to caring for your patients is caring for yourself. Be sure that you and your colleagues get enough rest and support during and after the MCI.

YOU ARE THE EMERGENCY MEDICAL RESPONDER

A number of students from the bus are yelling at you to help them, and one of the firefighters asks you to come over and check the coach, whose pain in his abdomen and chest seems to be getting worse. What should you do?

31 Response to Disasters and Terrorism

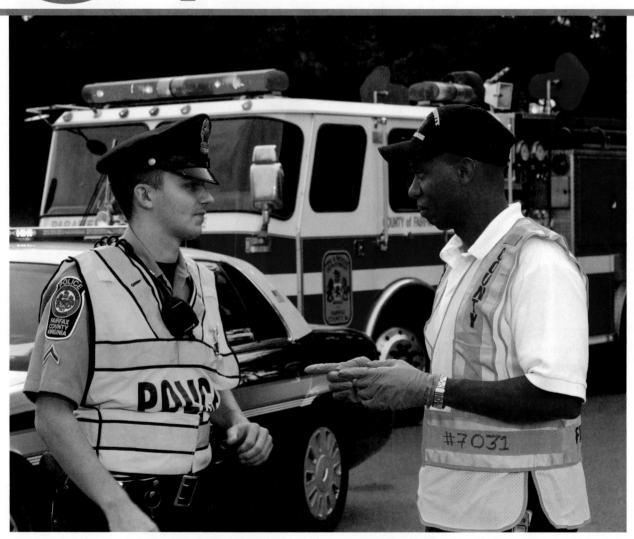

))) YOU ARE THE EMERGENCY MEDICAL RESPONDER

You are an emergency medical responder dispatched to the scene of an explosion. On arrival you are staged with other emergency vehicles one block away. You are told that police suspect that a building was targeted by an extremist group and it is thought there were no injuries from the blast. What should concern you at this time? How would you respond? What should you consider when you size-up the scene?

Key Terms

All-hazards approach: An approach to disaster readiness that involves the capability of responding to any type of disaster with a range of equipment and resources.

Asymptomatic: A situation in which a patient has no symptoms.

Atropine: An anticholinergic drug with multiple effects; used in antidotes to counteract the effects of nerve agents and to counter the effects of organophosphate (chemical compounds found in many common insecticides and used to produce toxic nerve agents, such as sarin) poisoning.

Bioterrorism: The deliberate release of agents typically found in nature, such as viruses, bacteria and other pathogens, to cause illness or death in people, animals or plants.

Blast lung: Sometimes referred to as *lung blast*; the most common fatal primary blast injury, describing damage to the lungs caused by the over-pressurization wave from high-order explosives.

B NICE: An acronym for the five main types of terrorist weapons: biological contamination, nuclear detonation, incendiary fires, toxic chemical release and conventional explosions.

CBRNE: The current acronym used by the Department of Homeland Security to describe the main types of weapons of mass destruction: chemical, biological, radiological/nuclear and explosive.

DuoDote™: A type of kit with pre-measured doses of antidote used to counteract the effects of nerve agents.

High-order explosives (HE): Explosives such as TNT, nitroglycerin, etc., that produce a defining supersonic over-pressurization shockwave.

Incendiary weapons: Devices designed to burn at extremely high temperatures, such as napalm and white phosphorus; mostly designed to be used against equipment, though some (e.g. napalm) are designed to be used against people.

Low-order explosives (LE): Explosives such as pipe bombs, gunpowder, etc., that create a subsonic explosion.

Mark I™ Kit: A type of kit with pre-measured doses of antidote to counteract the effects of nerve agents.

Morbidity: Illness; effects of a condition or disease.

Mortality: Death due to a certain condition or disease.

Nerve agents: Toxic chemical warfare agents that interrupt the chemical function of nerves.

Pralidoxime chloride (Protopam Chloride; 2-PAM Cl): A drug contained in antidote kits used to counteract the effects of nerve agents, commonly called *2-PAM chloride*.

Primary effects: In referring to explosive and incendiary devices, the effects of the impact of the over-pressurization wave from HE on body surfaces.

Secondary effects: In referring to explosive and incendiary devices, the impact of flying debris and bomb fragments against any body part.

Tertiary effects: The results of individuals being thrown by the blast wind caused by explosive and incendiary devices; can involve any body part.

WMDs: Weapons of mass destruction.

Learning Objectives

After reading this chapter, and completing the class activities, you will have the information needed to—

- Have a basic understanding of *emergency medical services* (EMS) operations during terrorist, public health, *weapon of mass destruction* (WMD) and disaster emergencies.
- Describe the *National Incident Management System* (NIMS) and the *National Response Framework* (NRF).
- Discuss basic elements of preparation and planning for disaster and *chemical, biological, radiological/nuclear and explosive* (CBRNE)/WMD response.
- Describe general steps of disaster response.
- Describe general steps of a CBRNE/WMD response.
- List different types of WMDs.

- Describe the roles of *emergency medical responders* (EMRs) during a natural, human-caused or biological disaster.
- Describe how to provide emergency medical care during disaster or CBRNE/WMD response.
- Identify the basic equipment needed by EMRs for a CBRNE/WMD response.
- List the steps to provide self-care and peer care in response to nerve agent poisoning.
- Discuss preparedness and planning considerations for a pandemic influenza public health disaster *(Enrichment)*.
- Discuss the need for personal preparedness *(Enrichment)*.

INTRODUCTION

The reality of potential terrorist attacks has grown progressively since the Oklahoma City bombing in 1995, but nothing has ever shown more powerfully or more poignantly how quickly a terrorist attack can take place, and how devastating its effects, than the September 11, 2001, attacks on the World Trade Center and the Pentagon.

Terrorism is not a new phenomenon. The United States has witnessed a number of acts of terrorism over the years: the 1985 hijacking of the Achille Lauro cruise ship; the bombing of Pan Am flight 103 over Lockerbie, Scotland in 1988; the 1993 World Trade Center bombing; the 1998 bombings of U.S. embassies in several East African countries; and the USS Cole suicide bombing in 2000 in Yemen, to name a few.

Not all disasters that have affected U.S. citizens were caused by terrorists. Some of the more destructive are natural disasters, such as hurricanes, floods, earthquakes, wildland fires and tornadoes. Disasters can also be the result of outbreaks of communicable diseases/pandemics or contamination of food or water supply. Biological disasters can result from naturally occurring outbreaks or because of **bioterrorism**.

With the growing threat of natural, biological and human-caused disasters, the knowledge of how to deal with such tragedies is just as important to rescuers as any other rescue call you may receive. The goal of this chapter is to ensure you are able to deal successfully with such events through careful preparation, ensuring safety for yourself and others and understanding the nature of and appropriate response to disasters.

PREPARING FOR DISASTERS AND TERRORIST INCIDENTS

Preparedness for disasters and terrorist incidents involves many different agencies working together in a coordinated effort, to meet a common goal. This is true at the local level, with police, fire, *emergency medical services* (EMS) personnel, public health, transportation and other town or county agencies; it is also true of organizations at the regional, federal and private levels.

The organizational structure and roles each of these agencies plays in disaster response are ultimately coordinated at the federal level by the *Federal Emergency Management Agency* (FEMA). FEMA coordinates the response to and recovery from disasters in the United States when the disaster is large enough to overwhelm local and state resources. FEMA also works collaboratively with other organizations such as state and local emergency management agencies and federal agencies and emergency response organizations such as the American Red Cross.

In 2008, FEMA developed and introduced the *National Response Framework* (NRF), which guides all organizations involved in disaster management on how to respond to disasters and emergencies. The NRF identifies the *National Disaster Medical System* (NDMS) as the system to augment the nation's medical response capabilities.

The NDMS is a system that supports federal agencies in managing and coordinating medical response to major emergencies and disasters. One responsibility of the NDMS is to oversee several different types of disaster medical teams, including *Disaster Medical Assistance Teams* (DMATs). DMATs are groups of professional and paraprofessional medical as well as administrative and logistical personnel who provide medical care during a disaster.

INCIDENT MANAGEMENT

The *National Incident Management System* (NIMS) is a comprehensive national framework for managing incidents. It outlines the structures for response activities for command and management. NIMS provides a consistent, nationwide response at all levels: federal, state,

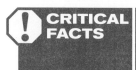
CRITICAL FACTS — Preparedness for disasters and terrorist incidents involves many different agencies working together in a coordinated effort to meet a common goal. In 2008, FEMA introduced the NRF, which guides all disaster management organizations in proper response. The NDMS is the system that augments the nation's medical response capabilities.

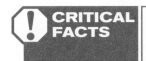

NIMS is a comprehensive national framework for managing incidents. It outlines the structures for response activities for command and management. NIMS provides a consistent, nationwide response.

tribal and local governments; the private sector; and *nongovernmental organizations* (NGOs). With this structure, agencies at all levels can work together in a consistent manner, to respond to incidents of any type or size.

NIMS provides a core set of common concepts, principles, terminology and technologies in these areas:

- *Incident command system* (ICS)
- *Multiagency coordination system* (MACS)
- Unified command
- Training
- Identification and management of resources
- Mutual aid and assistance
- Situational awareness
- Qualifications and certification
- Collection, tracking and reporting of incident information
- Crisis action planning
- Exercises

One of these components, the ICS, is a management system that allows effective incident management by bringing together facilities, equipment, personnel, procedures and communications within a single organizational structure, so that everyone involved in a disaster has an understanding of their roles and is able to respond effectively and efficiently. This system is used by all levels of government, as well as many NGOs and private organizations.

Incident command is structured in five main functional areas:

- Command
- Operations
- Planning
- Logistics
- Finance/administration

Among other roles within the ICS is the incident commander, who is responsible for all activities including resources and operations at the incident site. The incident commander also delegates duties to other responding staff. (See **Chapter 30** for further information about the ICS.) All *emergency medical responders* (EMRs) are

Warning Systems and Disaster Communications Systems

During a disaster, one of the most critical aspects of response is the capability to communicate information about the disaster to the public. The *Emergency Alert System* (EAS) is a nationwide public warning system to alert and warn the public. It requires all broadcasters (cable television systems, wireless cable systems, satellite radio services, etc.) to direct the communications to the president, to be able to address the American public during a national emergency. State and local authorities may also use the system for critical emergency information such as *America's Missing: Broadcast Emergency Response* (AMBER) alerts and weather information targeted to a specific area.

Once the president has been informed, as well as other officials at the federal, state and local levels, the public is made aware of the disaster. The EAS is administered by the *Department of Homeland Security* (DHS) through the *Federal Emergency Management Agency* (FEMA) and the *National Oceanic and Atmospheric Administration's National Weather Service* (NWS). It is regulated through the *Federal Communications Commission* (FCC).

Once communications reach those authorized in the federal government, national alerts and warnings to the public are communicated through the EAS to state and local governments, so that emergency management officials can alert the public at the local level and mobilize the necessary responding agencies.

required by *Homeland Security Presidential Directive-5* (HSPD-5) to complete specific ICS training. For more information please visit *http://training.fema.gov/IS/crslist.asp*.

Also within the structure of NIMS are 15 *emergency support functions* (ESFs), mechanisms for grouping the functions most frequently used to provide emergency management support during emergency/disaster incidents and planned events. Following is a list of the ESFs:

- ESF #1 - Transportation: Aviation/airspace management and control; transportation safety; restoration/recovery of transportation infrastructure; movement restrictions; damage and impact assessment
- ESF #2 - Communications: Coordination with telecommunications and information technology industries; restoration and repair of telecommunications infrastructure; protection, restoration and sustainment of national cyber and information technology resources; oversight of communications within the federal incident management and response structures
- ESF #3 – Public Works and Engineering: Infrastructure protection and emergency repair; infrastructure restoration; engineering services and construction management; emergency contracting support for life-saving and life-sustaining services including water supplies
- ESF #4 – Firefighting: Coordination of federal firefighting activities; support to wildland, rural and urban firefighting operations
- ESF #5 – Emergency Management: Coordination of incident management and response efforts; issuance of mission assignments; resource and human capital; incident action planning; financial management
- ESF #6 – Mass Care, Emergency Assistance, Housing and Human Services: Mass care; emergency assistance; disaster housing; human services
- ESF #7 - Logistics Management and Resource Support: Comprehensive, national incident logistics planning, management and sustainment capability; resource support (facility space, office equipment and supplies, contracting services, etc.)
- ESF #8 – Public Health and Medical Services: Public health; medical; mental health services; mass fatality management
- ESF #9 – Search and Rescue: Life-saving assistance; search and rescue operations

- ESF #10 – Oil and Hazardous Materials Response: Oil and hazardous materials (chemical, biological, radiological, etc.) response; environmental short- and long-term cleanup
- ESF #11 – Agriculture and Natural Resources: Nutrition assistance; animal and plant disease and pest response; food safety and security; natural and cultural resources and historic properties protection and restoration; safety and well-being of household pets
- ESF #12 – Energy: Energy infrastructure assessment, repair and restoration; energy industry utilities coordination; energy forecast
- ESF #13 – Public Safety and Security: Facility and resource security; security planning and technical resource assistance; public safety and security support; support for access, traffic and crowd control
- ESF #14 – Long-Term Community Recovery: Social and economic community impact assessment; long-term community recovery assistance to states, local governments and the private sector; analysis and review of mitigation program implementation
- ESF #15 – External Affairs: Emergency public information and protective action guidance; media and community relations; congressional and international affairs; tribal and insular affairs

EMRs typically are supported by ESF #8 (Public Health and Medical Services) but may also coordinate with ESFs #4 and #9 (Firefighting and Search and Rescue), depending on the complexity of the incident or event. The American Red Cross is the primary agency for ESF #6 (Mass Care, Emergency Assistance, Housing and Human Services). It also acts as a support agency for ESFs #3, 5, 8, 11, 14 and 15, and as a cooperating agency for several of the support and incidents annexes (components of individual ESFs).

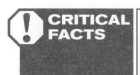 **CRITICAL FACTS**

If you are the first responder on the scene of a disaster, you may be called upon to assume a leadership role. If someone else has assumed this role, it is your responsibility to assist the leader or assume another role. It may be triaging patients, providing medical care, providing patient reception at staging facilities or preparing patients for evacuation.

THE ROLE OF THE EMERGENCY MEDICAL RESPONDER

At the scene of a disaster, if you are the first responder on the scene, you may be called upon to assume a leadership role. If someone else has assumed this role, it is your responsibility to assist the leader or assume another role, usually in triaging patients, providing medical care, providing patient reception at staging facilities or preparing patients for evacuation (**Fig. 31-1**).

Upon arriving on the scene, assess for scene hazards, the number of patients, patient priorities, the need for extrication, the number of ambulances or other transport vehicles needed and any other factors that affect the scene, as well as the need for resources and where to stage those resources. Radio your report with a request for any additional resources needed and then set up functions to accommodate resources as they arrive, including staging, supply, extrication, triage, treatment, transportation and rehab.

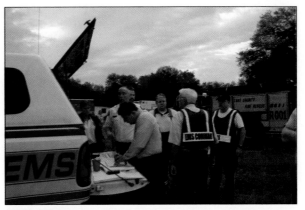

Fig. 31-1: If you are the first responder on the scene, you may have to assume a leadership role. *Courtesy of Captain Phil Kleinberg, EMT-P, Lake-Sumter EMS.*

DISASTER RESPONSE

Responding to a disaster call may prove to be the most challenging and mentally stressful scene you ever attend. Every incident is different and it is impossible to cover all of the specific steps and considerations for a specific scene. You will need to be prepared to address various issues and precautions simultaneously. The types of disasters

Mutual Aid

Mutual aid is a formal agreement among emergency responders to lend assistance across the various jurisdictions of public services such as fire departments, EMS operations and law enforcement during an emergency situation or disaster that exceeds local resources. Aid must be requested. The following general information must be supplied by the requesting community:
- A description of the personnel, equipment and other resources required
- The estimated length of time resources may be required
- The areas of experience, training and abilities of the personnel, and the capabilities of the equipment to be furnished

The person, service or agency receiving the request must then let the community in which the disaster took place know the estimated time when assistance can arrive at the designated location, as well as the names of the people designated as supervisory personnel.

The following rules will apply during the rescue efforts:
- The personnel and equipment of the assisting team are under the direction and control of the requesting community while at the disaster site.
- Emergency personnel continue under the command and control of their regular leaders, but the organizational units come under the operational control of the emergency services authorities of the community receiving assistance. The receiving party is responsible for informing the responding party when their services will no longer be required.
- All equipment and personnel provided by the assisting team while at the site of an emergency remain under the control and direction of its own designated representative, who can remove any or all equipment or personnel from the site at any time the representative deems it appropriate.
- An assisting team's priority lies with its own jurisdiction, and the team must continue to offer reasonable protection and services. Therefore, the assisting team has the right to withdraw any and all aid provided, after giving the disaster area notification of the need to do so.

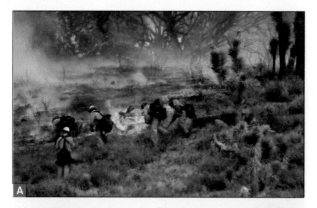
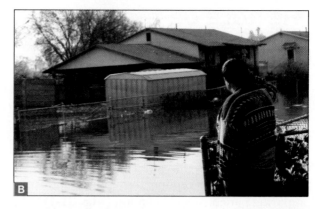
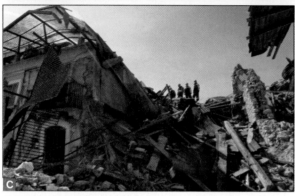
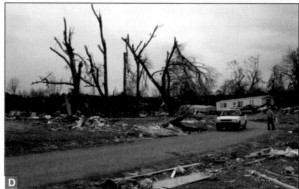

Fig. 31-2, A–D: Natural disasters, such as **(A)** wildland fire (*courtesy of Jeff Zimmerman, Zimmerman Media LLC*), **(B)** flood (*courtesy of Robert Baker*), **(C)** earthquake (*courtesy of Chris Helgren*) or **(D)** tornado (*courtesy of Joseph Songer*), can leave entire communities incapacitated and large numbers of people seriously injured.

you may respond to are varied, but fall into three main categories: natural disasters, human-caused disasters and biological disasters.

Natural Disasters

The devastating effects of natural disasters have been felt worldwide. Damage caused by earthquakes, hurricanes/tropical storms, landslides, thunderstorms, tsunamis, winter storms, tornadoes, heat waves, floods, wildfires and volcanic eruptions can leave entire communities completely incapacitated, with large numbers of people seriously injured **(Fig. 31-2, A-D)**. Massive infrastructure damage may occur, resulting in entire communities seeking shelter, food and other assistance.

Human-Caused Disasters

Human-caused disasters include terrorist attacks using chemical, biological, radiological/nuclear and explosive weapons; fire (residential or environmental); *hazardous materials* (HAZMAT) incidents; as well as large-scale *multiple-casualty incidents* (MCIs) such as transportation mishaps **(Fig. 31-3)**.

Biological Disasters

Biological disasters are not just the creative writing of science fiction. One need only look back at the flu epidemic of 1918 to be reminded of how real they are. In that epidemic, as many as 600,000 Americans lost their lives, as did some 40 million people worldwide. We have a lot more knowledge about dealing with a biological disaster today, but as we are warned by the World Health Organization, other epidemics such as

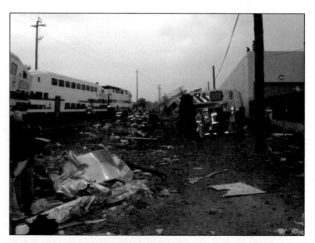

Fig. 31-3: Human-caused disasters. *Courtesy of Capt. Tony Duran, Los Angeles County Fire Department.*

Evacuations

In the case where a disaster has been predicted, such as a wildland fire, hurricane or flood, steps must be taken to evacuate a community. State emergency management offices have the authority to order and implement evacuations. The keys to a successful evacuation are communication and organization to avoid panic and the possibility of injury to people and property. Therefore, alerts regarding the evacuation must be made often and with clarity to residents who are affected by the need to leave their homes. There may be some who will not believe the level of danger the impending disaster may have on them or their property, and who may wish to remain in their homes. This reaction is normal, but it is imperative to maintain communication with these people and convince them of the level of danger they will face if they remain.

Evacuation warnings should communicate the following points:

- The nature of the disaster and the estimated time until it will impact the area
- The level of devastation the disaster is expected to cause, to help convince people to leave
- The routes assigned as safe for their evacuation
- The appropriate destinations where food, shelter and water are available

All possible means of communication should be used, including radio, television, loudspeakers, public address systems in buildings, etc. Again, the sense of urgency and clarity are the deciding factors for whether people choose to flee or not.

---

the avian flu or the next flu pandemic could be only months away (**Fig. 31-4**). Outbreaks of communicable diseases/pandemics, as well as contamination of food or water supply by pathogens, are all very real possibilities. In addition to the threat of naturally occurring outbreaks, biological disasters can also be the result of bioterrorism.

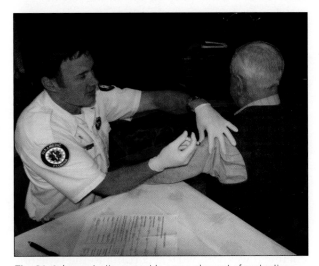

Fig. 31-4: Immunizations provide some element of protection against biological disasters. *Courtesy of Captain Phil Kleinberg, EMT-P, Lake-Sumter EMS.*

EMS Operations During Terrorist Attacks, Public Health Emergencies, WMD Incidents and Disaster Events

In any kind of large-scale disaster, it is important to use an **all-hazards approach**, which means being prepared with the equipment and resources needed to respond to many different types of disasters.

Regardless of the type of disaster, until you are aware of the specific hazards involved, distance yourself from the scene and only approach when it is safe to do so. Continue to monitor the scene, as there may be secondary explosions, for example, or traps meant to injure and possibly kill rescuers. If you are arriving on the scene of an armed attack, communicate immediately with law enforcement.

Initiate incident command or, if it has already been initiated, expand as assigned and communicate your findings to the ICS. Within the ICS, the necessary emergency services are called and responsibility for different sections can be assigned to the appropriate personnel as they arrive.

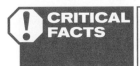

CRITICAL FACTS

In any kind of large-scale disaster, it is important to use an all-hazards approach, which means being prepared with the equipment and resources needed to respond to many different types of disasters.

Establish a perimeter around the area in order to protect yourself and other rescuers as well as the public from injury. If you are at the scene of a terrorist incident, establish an escape plan and a mobilization point. Designate the role of incident safety officer and assess command post security.

WMDS (CHEMICAL, BIOLOGICAL, RADIOLOGICAL/NUCLEAR AND EXPLOSIVE INCIDENTS)

Terrorism has been around for many years, yet the threat of terrorism is something increasingly on the minds of Americans in recent years. The FBI defines terrorism according to the U.S. *Code of Federal Regulations* (CFR):

> "Terrorism includes the unlawful use of force and violence against persons or property to intimidate or coerce a government, the civilian population, or any segment thereof, in furtherance of political or social objectives."

While these terrible crimes seem senseless, the terrorists who commit them have specific goals they are trying to achieve. They seek to incite fear, confusion and panic, as well as to inflict destruction on both physical and political infrastructure, and through these actions cause intimidation to those in authority and others. Terrorists may be motivated to inflict such destruction and fear for different reasons, including political and religious beliefs, environmental causes, racial bias or a desire for revenge.

When terrorists strike, their most likely weapons of choice are guns and explosives, as these are relatively inexpensive, easy to obtain and use and easy to transport. Less often, they may turn to *weapons of mass destruction* (**WMDs**), which, by their nature, cause widespread fear and destruction.

EMRs need to be aware of public reaction when faced with WMDs. While this type of weapon is used less frequently, their power lies in their ability to inflict significant fear and panic.

WMDs are commonly classified by the acronym **CBRNE**:

- Chemical
- Biological
- Radiological/Nuclear
- Explosives

This terminology is used by the Department of Homeland Security and understood internationally. Another system of classifying WMDs is **B NICE**, which stands for biological, nuclear, incendiary, chemical and explosive. This system of classification is similar to CBRNE, but it includes **incendiary weapons** (e.g., napalm, magnesium, phosphorous, etc.) as a separate type, whereas these devices are included under the term "explosives" under CBRNE. The terms are, in general, used interchangeably.

Chemical Weapons

A chemical emergency occurs when a hazardous chemical has been released and the release has the potential for harming people's health. In the case of a terrorist attack, the chemicals are released with the deliberate purpose of causing harm.

Chemical agents are difficult to turn into weapons, as they disperse easily in open environments. This can reduce their destructive power. However, the public perceives chemical weapons as highly effective, thus terrorists achieve their goal. The other major characteristic of chemical agents is that they affect the body quickly, with symptoms often appearing immediately, which is different from the impact of biological or nuclear agents, which may not occur until days after the event.

Providing Care

Steps to provide care for patients exposed to chemical weapons vary according to the type of

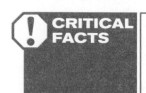

CRITICAL FACTS

The FBI defines terrorism as "the unlawful use of force and violence against persons or property to intimidate or coerce a government, the civilian population, or any segment thereof, in furtherance of political or social objectives."

There are four classifications of WMDs: Chemical, Biological, Radiological/Nuclear and Explosives. The common acronym for these classifications is CBRNE.

chemical. This is one of the great challenges in responding to a chemical incident; symptoms are not always obvious, and identifying the substance is not always possible.

If you are unable to identify the chemical, prepare yourself for the worst-case possibilities concerning toxicity when selecting *personal protective equipment* (PPE) and decontamination procedures. Assess the patient for traditional challenges such as airway and circulation concerns, and check for obvious symptoms such as neuromuscular, dermatological and vascular findings. If necessary, maintain cervical manual stabilization and apply a cervical collar and a backboard. Administer emergency oxygen as required and assist ventilation with a *bag-valve-mask resuscitator* (BVM) if necessary.

Prior to transportation, report the patient's condition, treatment and estimated time of arrival to the base station and receiving medical facility. If a chemical has been ingested, have several towels and open plastic bags ready to quickly clean up and isolate the patient's toxic vomit. Consult with the base station physician or regional poison control center for advice regarding triage of multiple patients. **Asymptomatic** patients who are discharged should be advised to seek medical care promptly if symptoms develop.

Chemical agents can be categorized into five types: **nerve agents**, blister agents, blood agents, pulmonary agents and incapacitating agents.

Nerve Agents

Nerve agents, such as *tabun* (GA) and *methylphosphonothioic acid* (VX), are particularly toxic chemical agents that disrupt the chemical recovery phase following a neuromuscular signal. Nerve agents are liquid when at normal temperatures but turn into a combination vapor/liquid when dispersed. They are usually odorless, although they may smell like fruit or fish.

Symptoms vary depending on the dose. A strong dose can cause death within minutes, if inhaled or absorbed into the skin. Signs and symptoms include runny nose, watery eyes, twitching, pinpoint pupils, painful eyes, blurred vision, drooling, excessive sweating, coughing, weakness, drowsiness, headache, nausea, vomiting, abdominal pain, slow or fast heart rate, abnormally high or low blood pressure and more. Exposure causes irritation or severe damage to the eyes and respiratory tract, and may cause redness or severe blistering of the skin with larger doses. The blisters are similar to those caused by second-degree burns. These signs do not appear immediately but arise after several hours or a day, depending on the dose.

When a patient has been exposed to a nerve agent, in general the priorities are to decontaminate, ventilate (expose to fresh air), administer antidotes, administer valium (to prevent seizures) and provide supportive therapy. Depending on the type of agent, different antidotes are available.

Blister Agents

Blister agents, also called *vesicants*, include *sulfur mustard* (HD) and *phosgene oxime* (CX). These agents cause the skin and mucous membranes to form blisters on contact. Sulfur mustard can sometimes be detected by its odor of garlic, onions or horseradish, but it can be difficult to detect because the smell is faint.

When exposed to sulfur mustard, either in liquid or vapor form, patients experience irritation or severe damage to the eyes and respiratory tract. Sulfur mustard may cause redness or severe blistering of the skin with larger doses. As with the blisters from nerve agents, these blisters resemble second-degree burns. Also, as with nerve agents, signs appear from several hours to a day after exposure, depending on the dose. If the patient has had a significant exposure, there may also be systemic effects that cause damage to bone marrow and the epithelial lining of the *gastrointestinal* (GI) tract.

There are no known antidotes or treatments for exposure to blister agents; treatment of both the blisters and respiratory effects is supportive and nonspecific. Care includes decontamination by discarding contaminated clothing, and cleaning equipment with soap, water and diluted bleach (0.5-1.0 percent). Do *not* use bleach on patients.

"Blood" Agents

Blood agents, such as cyanide, attack the body's cellular metabolism. They do not actually affect the blood, as was once thought, but disrupt cellular respiration. Cyanide can enter the body by being ingested, injected or inhaled, but not by being absorbed into the skin. Despite its devastating effects, if it dissipates into the air, it rapidly becomes harmless. Cyanide can be recognized by its odor of bitter almonds, though not everyone is able to detect it.

Cyanide's effect of poisoning the cells prevents them from taking up oxygen, which in turn leads to asphyxia and cyanosis (blue tinge to the skin caused by a lack of oxygen). Cyanide is a quick-acting agent, and can cause death within 5 to 8 minutes if the exposure is severe.

Treatment for cyanide poisoning is by antidote, using a *Cyanokit®* (hydroxocobalamin), sodium nitrite or sodium thiosulfate, all of which must be administered immediately and intravenously.

Pulmonary Agents

Pulmonary agents include *phosgene* (CG), which causes lung injury by forming *hydrochloric acid* (HCl) when it contacts mucous membranes, thereby irritating and damaging lung tissue. When phosgene explodes, it turns into a colorless, watery vapor with a smell that has been described as that of new-mown hay.

Signs and symptoms are severe illness and even death from pulmonary edema and acute respiratory distress syndrome.

There is no specific antidote for phosgene. The only way to provide care is to remove the person from the agent and resuscitate. EMRs should take measures to protect themselves in a situation where phosgene may be present, by using a chemical protective mask with a charcoal canister.

Incapacitating Agents

An incapacitating agent is defined by the *Department of Defense* (DOD) as "an agent that produces temporary physiological or mental effects, or both, which will render individuals incapable of concerted effort in the performance of their assigned duties" (***Source:*** *University of Albany*).

These agents, which include MACE, tear gas and pepper spray, contain a hallucinogenic agent, *3-quinuclidinyl benzilate*, also referred to as *BZ* or *QNB*. They are usually nonlethal and generally not used by terrorists, but may be used, for example, by law enforcement authorities to control a violent crowd. The BZ may be dispersed as a fine aerosol or dissolved in *dimethyl sulfoxide* (DMSO) and absorbed into the skin.

Effects may be delayed for 30 minutes to 24 hours. There are both peripheral (external) and systemic (throughout the body) effects. Peripheral effects include pupil dilation, dry mouth and skin, and flushing of the skin, particularly the face and neck. Symptoms may appear similar to those seen in someone exposed to certain nerve agents and then treated with an excess of **atropine**. Systemic effects include disturbances to consciousness, delusions and hallucinations, impaired memory and poor judgment, disorientation and ataxia (uncoordinated gait or manner of walking). Overall, effects depend on the dose and may last for up to 4 days.

Monitor the patient who has been incapacitated by one of these agents and take precautions to prevent yourself from being exposed.

Biological Weapons

Bioterrorism is the deliberate release of agents typically found in nature, such as viruses, bacteria or other pathogens (agents), for the purpose of causing illness, disease or death in people, animals or plants. Often these agents can be changed, increasing their potency and making them resistant to current medications, or even increasing their ability to be spread into the environment.

Types of Biological Agents/ Diseases

There are many diseases and biological agents that have been determined to be a threat. These are categorized into three groups according to their level of threat, from highest to lowest:

Class A biological agents/diseases include anthrax, plague, smallpox, tularemia, viral hemorrhagic fevers (e.g., *Ebola*) and botulism. These agents and diseases pose the greatest threat to public health and national security, as they can be easily spread from person to person and result in high **mortality** (death) rates.

Class B biological agents/diseases include brucellosis, Q fever, glanders, alphaviruses, food pathogens (e.g., *Salmonella, Shigella, E coli*), water pathogens (e.g., *Vibrio cholerae* and *Cryptosporidium*), Ricin toxin, *staphylococcal enterotoxin B* and epsilon toxin of *Clostridium perfringens*. This class of agents poses a moderate level of risk, as they are moderately easy to spread and result in moderate **morbidity** (illness) rates and low mortality rates.

Class C biological agents/diseases are those considered to be emerging infectious diseases, such as hanta virus, Nipah virus, yellow fever, multi-drug-resistant tuberculosis and tick-borne viruses. These agents have the potential to be engineered for mass dissemination. They are easy to spread and have the potential for high mortality and morbidity rates.

When a bioterrorism event has occurred, often there is a single suspected case of an uncommon disease or there are single or multiple suspected cases of a common disease or syndrome that do not respond to treatment as expected. Clusters of a similar illness may occur in the same timeframe in different locales. There may be unusual clinical, geographical, seasonal or temporal presentations of a disease and/or unusual transmission routes; an unexplained increase in the incidence of an endemic disease; or an unusual illness that affects a large, disparate population or is unusual for a population or age group. You may see an unusual pattern of illness or death among animals or humans, or a sudden increase in non-specific illnesses such as pneumonia, bleeding disorders, unexplained rashes and mucosal or skin irritation (particularly in adults), neuromuscular symptoms (such as muscle weakness and paralysis) or diarrhea.

For most of these diseases/agents, patients initially experience flu-like symptoms such as fever, aches and listlessness or fatigue.

Providing Care

While the early signs and symptoms may be similar for different diseases/agents, treatment will depend on the nature of the agent. For example, those caused by a virus *cannot* be treated with antibiotics, while those caused by a bacterium may be treated with antibiotics.

Often, though, when these illnesses/diseases are caused by a terrorist act, you will not know the cause right away. While it is essential to take steps to recognize the specific agent, provide supportive care right away, including assessing the patient for traditional challenges such as airway and circulation concerns, and checking for obvious symptoms such as neuromuscular, dermatological and vascular findings. Once examined by a physician, the patient will likely be given specific antibiotics or antitoxins. Immunizations may also be given as a preventative measure for certain agents.

Although most biological agents are not highly contagious, a few are, so it is essential to isolate the patient, protect yourself with the proper PPE and use standard exposure control procedures

including *high efficiency particulate air* (HEPA) filter mask and gloves (**Fig. 31-5**).

Radiological/Nuclear Weapons

The effects of a nuclear weapon detonation depend on the yield and success of the detonation. For example, a poorly maintained or manufactured bomb might produce no explosion, yet still spread radioactive material. Or the device could have a partial nuclear detonation, which would have a much greater impact than, for example, the explosive that destroyed the Oklahoma City Federal Building in 1995.

The detonation of a nuclear device, regardless of size, could prove catastrophic. A nuclear explosion has several damaging effects, caused by the air blast, heat, ionizing radiation, ground shock and secondary radiation.

There are four types of radiation exposure. These include patients who—

1. Received a significant dose from an external source, including large radiation sources over a short period of time, or smaller radioactive sources over a long period of time.
2. Received internal contamination from inhalation and/or ingestion of radioactive material.
3. Have external contamination of the body surface and/or clothing by liquids or particles.
4. Were exposed through a combination of the above.

In general, determining that someone has been exposed to radiation can be difficult. However, acute radiation syndrome follows a predictable pattern that unfolds over several

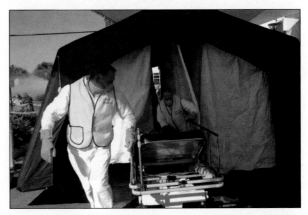

Fig. 31-5: Always protect yourself from hazards by employing appropriate PPE and using standard exposure control procedures. *Courtesy of Captain Phil Kleinberg, EMT-P, Lake-Sumter EMS.*

days or weeks after substantial exposure or catastrophic events. Patients may present individually over a longer period of time after exposure to unknown radiation sources. Specific symptoms of concern, especially following a 2- to 3-week period with nausea and vomiting, are thermal burn-like skin lesions without documented heat exposure, a tendency to bleed (nosebleeds, gingival (gum) bleeding, bruising) and hair loss. Symptom clusters, as delayed effects after radiation exposure, include headache, fatigue, weakness, partial- and full-thickness skin damage, hair loss, ulceration, anorexia, nausea, vomiting, diarrhea, reduced levels of white blood cells, bruising and infections.

Providing Care

Assess and treat life-threatening injuries immediately. Move patients away from the hot zone (the area in which the most danger exists) using proper patient transfer techniques to prevent further injury (**Fig. 31-6**). Stay within the controlled zone if contamination is suspected.

Expose wounds and cover with sterile dressings, decontaminating open wounds as required. Patients should be monitored at the control line for possible contamination only after they are medically stable. Remove contaminated clothing only if removal can be accomplished without causing further injury.

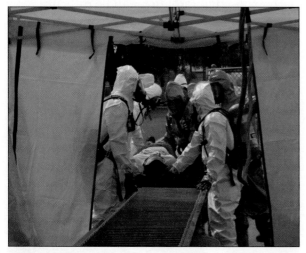

Fig. 31-6: When providing care in a situation of radiation exposure, move patients away from the hot zone using proper patient transfer techniques. *Courtesy of Captain Phil Kleinberg, EMT-P, Lake-Sumter EMS.*

Contaminated patients who do not have life-threatening or serious injuries may be decontaminated on site, starting with the removal of their clothing. Do not remove patients from a backboard if one was used when packaging for transport.

It is essential to use standard precautions to help prevent the spread of contamination from injured patients to yourself or other emergency personnel. Notify proper authorities and the hospital of all pertinent information about patients and the scene. Ask for any special instructions the hospital may have, such as using an entrance other than the routine emergency department entrance for the purposes of radiological contamination control.

Explosives and Incendiary Weapons

Traditional weapons and explosives still present a very real threat for use in terrorist attacks on the United States. As an EMR, understanding the unique types of injuries associated with explosives is imperative to ensure appropriate treatment and handling of patients at a blast site.

There are two major types of explosives:

- *High-order explosives* (**HE**), e.g., TNT, C-4, Semtex, nitroglycerin, dynamite and *ammonium nitrate fuel oil* (ANFO), which produce a defining supersonic over-pressurization shock wave
- *Low-order explosives* (**LE**), including pipe bombs, gunpowder and most pure petroleum-based bombs such as Molotov cocktails or aircraft improvised as guided missiles, which create a subsonic explosion

Blasts can also be caused by explosive and incendiary (fire) bombs, which are characterized based on their source. Manufactured weapons are military issued, mass produced and quality tested, and are exclusively HE. Improvised weapons are produced in small quantities, or use a device outside its intended purpose, such as converting a commercial aircraft into a guided missile.

There are three basic mechanisms of blast injury:

- **Primary effects** are unique to HE, and result from the impact of the over-pressurization wave on body surfaces. The most common injuries are to the lungs, GI tract, eye, head and middle ear

- **Secondary effects** are caused by flying debris and bomb fragments; any body part may be affected
- **Tertiary effects** may occur from individuals being thrown by the blast wind, and also can involve any body part

Injury patterns will depend on whether you are dealing with HE or LE blasts as well as on the position of the body when the blast occurs. Patients who are standing or lying perpendicular to the blast will suffer greater injuries compared with those who are lying directly toward or away from the blast.

Lung injuries include **blast lung**, the most common fatal primary blast injury. Blast lung is caused by the HE over-pressurization wave. Middle ear injury most commonly includes tympanic membrane (eardrum) perforation. Abdominal injuries include bowel perforation, hemorrhage, mesenteric shear injuries, solid organ lacerations and testicular rupture. Injuries to the head include concussion or *mild traumatic brain injury* (MTBI). Other injuries include air embolism, compartment syndrome, rhabdomyolysis (skeletal muscle tissue damage) and acute renal failure. Also consider the possibility of exposure to inhaled toxins and poisonings (e.g., *carbon monoxide* [CO], *cyanide* [CN], *methemoglobin* [MetHgb]) in both industrial and criminal explosions. Wounds can also be contaminated, as with tetanus.

Providing Care

After performing a preliminary evaluation and establishing scene safety, EMRs should initiate rescues of severely injured and/or trapped patients, evacuate ambulatory patients, perform triage and treat life-threatening injuries. Leave fatalities and their surroundings undisturbed, and avoid disturbing areas not directly involved in rescue activities. Initiate documentation of the scene as soon as conditions permit. The site of a bomb blast is a crime scene and, as an EMR, although your primary responsibility is to rescue living people and provide treatment for life-threatening injuries, it is also important to preserve evidence and avoid disturbing areas not directly involved in the rescue activities, including those areas containing fatalities.

RESPONSE TO A CBRNE WMD INCIDENT
Preparation

Planning for a WMD incident involves several aspects of preparation, including medical direction, personal preparation, equipment, transportation and communications.

Medical direction will be provided on a massive scale during a WMD incident. Your EMS system needs to include a larger number of care providers from within your region as well as medical control systems from different areas. Disrupted communications systems can make it difficult to activate and summon appropriate medical services; therefore, preparing emergency measures as standing orders is the most effective manner in which to activate a plan. This leaves communication channels available for scene updates, incoming patient reports and the essential communications required in extraordinary circumstances.

In all WMD case scenarios, the massive numbers of rescuers involved could lead to scene confusion. It is imperative, especially in cases where interagency coordination is required, that all levels of support services define their respective roles and responsibilities at the scene and are managed by the ICS. Regional pre-planning, coordination and rehearsal are recommended in order to ensure all involved services are familiar with their roles and arrive at the scene prepared to perform those services without conflict or delay. Planning must include an assessment of hazards, exposure potential, respiratory protection needs, entry conditions, exit routes and decontamination strategies.

The types of weapons used at a CBRNE incident cover a broad spectrum of dangers, including the possibility of exposure to pathogens, chemicals and radiation. Because of this, it is important for EMRs to understand the threats at the scene and why it is critical to take proper precautions first. For example, it is critical to have necessary antidotes ready if there is a risk of exposure to nerve agents.

Equipment and Supplies

Inventory of equipment and supplies will vary depending on the type of WMD used in an attack. In order to be able to respond as quickly as possible with the appropriate equipment, medications and personnel, lists of locations of traditional storage areas must be kept and remain accessible to neighboring communities, to allow the dispatch center to quickly access the resources regionally, statewide or nationwide.

In a large-scale incident, it is necessary to rely on other services to supply the proper equipment and, in most cases, knowledge, to CBRNE calls. Nerve agents require large amounts of certain drugs as well as ventilators. If you are called to the site of a chemical incident, you may require specialized PPE such as *self-contained breathing apparatus* (SCBA) or HAZMAT suits. If you are responding to the scene of a large explosion, you may require heavy rescue equipment, search and rescue units, devices for electronic detection and trained search dogs. The proper protocols and procedures regarding mutual assistance set-ups and the deployment of equipment must be followed in accordance with your community's plan.

Arrival on Scene

On-site incident management allows responders to work together as effectively as possible. As a rescuer, the responsibility for preparing the site for rescue efforts may fall on you. If you are among the first to arrive on the scene of a WMD incident, your speedy and accurate assessment of the scene and the actions you take to establish incident command as quickly and efficiently as possible are the most important steps you can take in saving lives and helping the injured. Your instincts as an EMR will be to help patients first. However, your scene size-up to measure the scope of the disaster, and the information you collect to identify the appropriate resources, are your first priorities.

When approaching the scene, consider the time since the incident, your distance from it and any necessary shielding. Remember, EMRs may be targets, so you must be wary of potential secondary attacks.

Provide an initial on-scene report to dispatch, with a description of the incident along with the need for specialized resources, initial actions taken, number of injured and the nature and quantity of additional resources required.

Look for outward signs and characteristics of terrorist incidents, such as mass casualties presenting with identical symptoms that have

Search and Rescue

A variety of specialized services can be used when a search and rescue mission is required following a disaster. This may include building collapse, avalanche or ships lost at sea.

Search and rescue capabilities include distress monitoring, communications, location of distressed personnel, coordination and execution of rescue operations including extrication or evacuation, along with the provisioning of medical assistance and civilian services through the use of public and private resources to assist persons and property in potential or actual distress.

Emergency support function #9 (ESF #9) provides the following specialized search and rescue services during incidents or potential incidents requiring a coordinated federal response:

- *Structure Collapse* (Urban) *Search and Rescue* (US&R)
- Waterborne Search and Rescue
- Inland/Wilderness Search and Rescue
- Aeronautical Search and Rescue

no identifiable cause. Attempt to identify the weapon used by looking for outward signs of the use of WMDs, such as strange odors like bitter almond, peaches or fresh-cut grass. Consider the necessary protective actions according to the type of weapons: CBRNE.

Determine the number of people involved and implement local protocols for mass casualty incidents as necessary. As part of your assessment, evaluate the need for additional resources. Evaluate and alter plans as necessary, including consideration of changing weather and a change to incidents occurring at the site such as secondary attacks or injuries to rescuers.

Scene Safety

Identifying the weapon involved is a major part of responding to a WMD scene. Once you are aware of the hazards you are responding to, you can protect yourself, fellow rescuers and the public effectively.

Approach the scene from upwind and uphill if chemical, biological or nuclear weapons are suspected. Avoid confined spaces where chemical or biological agents may be trapped due to poor ventilation. Be suspicious of a potential terrorist attack when called to a well-populated area, as these are typical targets for attacks.

The possibility that secondary devices may have been planted at the scene is a real and serious threat to the teams responding to a CBRNE call. With this is mind, as with all calls, your own safety must be your top priority. Remain aware of the dangers to your health when you are entering a scene and while you are offering assistance to patients. Establishing what substances have been released, how and where, will help to best ascertain the proper PPE required, procedures to follow and the appropriate patient treatment.

Unlike other EMS calls, if terrorists are involved, it is possible they will try to sabotage your efforts to respond. Therefore, hospital facilities must take security measures to limit the traffic in and out of the area, setting safe perimeters around the hospital and allowing access only to those with proper authorization. Secondary devices may be used by terrorists to keep EMRs from responding, making it advisable for all units and agencies involved to be familiar with and able to operate under the ICS.

Ascertain the proper PPE needed to enter the scene, using an all-hazards safety approach. If you are approaching a patient who is suspected of having a communicable disease, make sure to use a HEPA or N-95 mask, gloves, eye protection and gown for personal protection. This information must also be conveyed to the medical facility to which the patient is being transported, so that they may prepare for appropriate isolation.

Providing Care

As you provide care, make sure to keep patients informed of your actions, and protect them from further harm. Be alert to specific signs and symptoms associated with the different types of weapons. Because of the potentially large numbers of patients who will need care in a short space of time, you may quickly be in a situation where the ratio of patients to providers is much higher than you are accustomed to.

In the case of mass casualties at a CBRNE scene, there are multiple scenarios with which you may be faced. Each scenario, be it chemical, biological, radiation/nuclear or explosive, will require a different approach to treatment, potential for contamination and other considerations. Treating patients at such a scene is different from any other scene to which you may be called.

Written protocols will address the signs and symptoms associated with each type of WMD and instruct you on the recommended treatment. You must understand the danger each presents and then follow the recommended precautions before entering the scene, as well as how to provide care during and following the response.

You may find that the types of injuries and patients you encounter are similar in nature, due to the effects of the incident. Massive soft tissue wounds and burns are common injuries resulting from explosions or nuclear ignition. Medications may be required to treat patients who have been affected by chemical dispersal.

You may also face unique patient care challenges you would not normally encounter in other emergency situations. For example, you may need to administer high-dose atropine for nerve agents. Also different from usual routines is that patients may remain in your care for much longer than you are used to, and you may need to address their overall needs (nutrition, hydration and personal hygiene).

You may also find it especially difficult to attend to so many patients who are expected to die. While this may not be unusual for EMRs, the difference in the WMD situation is that you may be with patients longer and witness their conditions worsening to the point of death in front of you, without being able to do anything to prevent their deaths. When patients die, you also need to provide isolation and storage until other, living patients have been evacuated from the area.

When carrying out triage, the concept of "greater good" applies. This means that you must treat everyone according to their injury or illness, and not according to who they are; this includes terrorists or criminals.

PROVIDING SELF-CARE AND PEER CARE FOR NERVE AGENTS

Poisoning by Nerve Agents

Nerve agents are the most toxic of chemical agents and are hazardous in both their liquid and vapor states. They are potent enough to cause death within minutes after exposure. The clinical effects from nerve agent exposure are caused by excess *acetylcholine*, a chemical in the brain.

The initial effects of exposure to a nerve agent depend on the dose and route. The routes include inhalation via gas, absorption through the skin and ingestion from liquids or food. The dose and amount of exposure to the agent work together to cause varying effects.

Nerve Agents—Liquid

Exposure to a small droplet of liquid on the skin may produce few physical findings, whereas a large amount causes effects within minutes. Sweating, blanching (whitening of the skin) and occasional muscle twitching at the site may be present soon after exposure of a small amount, but may no longer be present at the onset of GI effects. Signs of a large amount of exposure are the same as after vapor exposure, and appear within minutes. Commonly there is an asymptomatic period of 1 to 30 minutes before symptoms appear, including loss of consciousness, seizure activity, apnea (periods when breathing stops) and muscular flaccidity (loss of tone). Effects can be delayed for as long as 18 hours after contact with small amounts, and are initially GI-related and not life threatening. Generally, the longer symptoms are delayed, the less likely it is that effects from exposure are severe.

Nerve Agents—Vapor

Effects from nerve agent vapor begin within seconds to several minutes after exposure. After exposure to a very low amount of vapor, miosis (constriction of the pupil of the eye) and other effects may not begin for several minutes, and miosis may not end for 15 to 30 minutes after the patient is removed from the vapor. Effects may continue to progress for a period of time, but usually not for more than minutes after exposure stops. The effects caused by a mild vapor exposure may be easily confused with an upper respiratory illness or even allergies. Miosis, if present, will help to distinguish these. Likewise, GI symptoms from another illness may be confused with those from nerve agent effects.

When assessing someone who has been exposed to a nerve agent, there are several potential findings from which to deduce required treatment. Triage as "immediate" if the patient is unconscious, convulsing, breathing with difficulty or has apnea, and is possibly flaccid. Consider a patient "expectant" if the patient shows all of the above symptoms, but has no pulse or blood pressure and is therefore not expected to survive. Categorize as "minimal" a patient who is walking, talking, breathing and whose circulation is intact. Consider the person "delayed" if further medical observation, large amounts of antidotes or artificial ventilation is required after triage.

Providing Care

Ventilation is required when patients demonstrate obvious symptoms. In this situation, remove secretions, maintain an open airway, use artificial ventilation if necessary and possible, and repeat atropine immediately as directed.

The means of ventilation depends on the equipment available at the scene. As these patients generally experience bronchoconstriction and lots of secretions, expect high airway resistance (50–70 cm of water), which make initial ventilation difficult. Expect a noticeable decrease in resistance after atropine has been administered. Secretions may thicken with atropine and may make ventilation efforts difficult. If this occurs, frequent suctioning is required for up to 3 hours.

Patients whose skin or clothing is contaminated with a liquid nerve agent can contaminate you by direct contact or through off-gasing vapor. Decontamination of the skin is not required after exposure to vapor alone, but clothing should be removed because it may contain "trapped" vapor.

Atropine and *pralidoxime chloride* (**Protopam Chloride; 2-PAM Cl**) are antidotes for nerve agent toxicity. Pralidoxime must be administered within a short time— between minutes and a few hours following exposure (depending on the specific agent) to be effective.

When the nerve agent has been ingested, exposure may continue for some time, due to slow absorption from the lower bowel, which can result in fatal relapses despite what appears to be an initial improvement. Continued medical monitoring and transport are mandatory for patients who have ingested a nerve agent.

Decontamination is critical for skin exposure, and should be done with standard decontamination procedures. Patient monitoring should be directed to the same signs and symptoms as with all nerve agent exposures. Keep a record of any medications used.

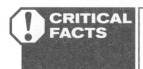

CRITICAL FACTS If you or a peer show signs or symptoms that indicate the presence of nerve agent poisoning, and if you are authorized to do so by medical direction, administer a nerve agent auto-injector kit.

Nerve Agent Antidote Auto-Injector Kit

There are currently two main nerve agent antidote kits: the Mark I™ and the Duo Dote™. Mark I™ Kits are auto-injectors that provide simple, accurate drug administration of a premeasured, controlled dose of medication used to relieve, counteract or reverse the effects of poisons or drugs such as nerve agents.

In 2007, the U.S. Food and Drug Administration approved another nerve agent antidote kit, **DuoDote™**, for use by trained EMS personnel to treat civilians exposed to nerve agents. It contains both atropine and 2-PAM chloride in one auto-injector syringe. The Mark I™ is being phased out and replaced by the **DuoDote™**.

The two drugs contained in both the Duo Dote™ and Mark I™ Kit are atropine and 2-PAM chloride. Atropine increases heart rate, dries secretions, decreases gastric upset and dilates pupils. 2-PAM chloride reverses some effects of nerve agent poisoning such as muscle twitching and difficulty breathing.

If you or a peer show signs or symptoms that indicate the presence of nerve agent poisoning, and if you are authorized to do so by medical direction, administer a nerve agent auto-injector kit. If you self-administer the antidote and there is no improvement in 10 minutes, look for a fellow EMR or caregiver at the site to assist in evaluating your condition before further antidote is given. If you are severely ill (e.g., gasping respirations, twitching, etc.), a fellow caregiver should administer the antidote immediately.

Always follow medical direction and the manufacturer's instructions for use of any nerve agent antidote auto-injector.

Administration of DuoDote™ Kit

1. Tear open the plastic pouch at any of the notches.
2. Remove the DuoDote™ Auto-Injector from the pouch.
3. Place the DuoDote™ Auto-Injector in your writing hand.
4. Firmly grasp the center of the DuoDote™ Auto-Injector with the *green* tip (needle end) pointing down. Do *not* touch the green end.
5. Pull off the *gray* safety release.
6. Quickly and firmly push the green tip straight down (at a 90-degree angle) against the mid-outer thigh. The DuoDote™ Auto-Injector can inject through clothing, but pockets must be empty.
7. Continue to push firmly until you feel the DuoDote™ Auto-Injector trigger.
8. Remove the DuoDote™ Auto-Injector from the thigh and look at the *green* tip. If the needle is *not* visible, the injection has not been made. Check to be sure the *gray* safety release has been removed, and repeat from step 4. You must press hard enough to ensure that the injection has been made.
9. Push the needle against a hard surface to bend the needle back against the DuoDote™ Auto-Injector.
10. Put the used DuoDote™ Auto-Injector back into the plastic pouch. Keep the DuoDote™ Auto-Injector with the patient.

PUTTING IT ALL TOGETHER

One of the most challenging roles for an EMR is to be called to respond to a disaster, whether an intentional one such as a terrorist attack, possibly using WMDs, or a manmade disaster like a hurricane. The only way to respond to such catastrophic events is to be properly trained and prepared to respond.

WMDs can be divided into five major categories, collectively referred to as *CBRNE*: chemical, biological, radiological/nuclear and explosive. Each of these types of weapons has unique characteristics in the nature of the damage it can inflict, the hazards with which they are associated, the signs and symptoms of exposure and the specific care required to help people involved in the disaster.

In any wide-scale disaster such as these, it is critical to be prepared with sufficient appropriately trained personnel, equipment and supplies, communication systems and the appropriate protocols, so that all personnel know what to do.

It is important to understand the nature of nerve agents, how they enter the body and the signs and symptoms they produce. In the event of exposure to poisoning by a nerve agent, you may be required to provide self-care or care to a peer.

YOU ARE THE EMERGENCY MEDICAL RESPONDER

There is some question about the cause of the explosion but police strongly suspect that it was a terrorist act using a WMD, most likely a high-order explosive. While waiting at the staging area you notice a large trash bag near a dumpster in close proximity to staged apparatus. You should be alert for what other types of situations and how would you react upon their discovery?

Enrichment
Preparing for a Public Health Disaster—Pandemic Flu

Pandemic influenza (or pandemic flu) is virulent human influenza A virus that causes a global outbreak of serious illness in humans. As there is little natural immunity, the disease spreads easily and is sustainable from person to person. In situations where the fatality rate is higher than expected during a normal flu season, this type of influenza virus can seriously impact the nation, affecting and even halting its health care delivery system, transportation system, economy and social structure.

As an EMR, your services are in high demand during a public health disaster. Yet you and your unit may be faced with some of the same challenges many businesses and organizations do during such times, such as increased employee absenteeism, disruption of supply chains and increased rates of illness and death. Both 9-1-1 systems and EMS personnel are well integrated into the nation's pandemic influenza planning, and response is essential to the nation's health and safety in the event of a pandemic.

The National Strategy for Pandemic Influenza identifies responsibilities for federal, state and local governments as well as non-governmental organizations, businesses and individuals, and is built on three pillars:

- Preparedness and communication: Acts taken before a pandemic to ensure preparedness, and the communication and coordination of roles and responsibilities to all levels of government, segments of society and individuals.
- Surveillance and detection: Domestic and international systems set up to detect the earliest warning possible to protect the population.
- Response and containment: Actions to limit the spread of the outbreak and to mitigate the health, social and economic impacts of a pandemic.

Both EMS and 9-1-1 system planning for pandemic influenza should be carried out in the context of the following phases of pandemic influenza identified by the *World Health Organization* (WHO) and the U.S. government:
- Early detection
- Treatment with antiviral medications
- The use of infection control measures to prevent transmission
- Vaccination

Interventions used to help contain the spread of the virus include the following:
- Treatment with influenza antiviral medications and isolation of all persons with confirmed or probable pandemic influenza
- Voluntary home quarantine of members of households with confirmed or probable influenza case(s)
- Dismissal of students from school and school-based activities, and closure of childcare programs, coupled with protecting children and teenagers through social distancing in the community
- Use of social distancing measures to reduce contact between adults in the community and workplace, including cancellation of large public gatherings and alteration of workplace environments and schedules to offer a healthy workplace without disrupting essential services.

Disease surveillance plays an important role in pandemic influenza mitigation, and both EMS and 9-1-1 systems play a large part in maintaining and collecting patient information such as fever, reporting updated information on an emerging pathogen (e.g., during the SARS epidemic, questions pertaining to foreign travel were pertinent) and identifying probable signs and symptoms of an emerging viral strain.

Enrichment
Personal Preparedness

In a disaster or emergency situation, EMRs are likely to be concerned with the well-being of their own families and friends. It is important for their own reassurance, and for the purposes of educating the public, that rescuers understand how to prepare on an individual basis for disasters. The American Red Cross suggests three basic steps to prepare to respond to a disaster or life-threatening emergency:

1. Get a kit.
2. Make a plan.
3. Be informed.

GET A KIT

When assembling or restocking your kit, store at least 3 days' worth of food, water and supplies in an easy-to-carry preparedness kit. Keep extra supplies on hand at home in case you cannot leave the affected area. Keep your kit where it is easily accessible. Remember to check your kit every 6 months and replace expired or outdated items.

Whether you purchase an official Red Cross preparedness kit or assemble your own, you should include what you need to provide comfort for everyday scrapes or life-threatening emergencies. A standard preparedness kit should include water, food, medications, radio, first aid kit, personal documents, contact information, map, money, clothing, sanitary supplies, pet supplies and tools.

MAKE A PLAN

When preparing for a disaster, always talk with your family, plan and learn how and when to turn off utilities and use life-saving tools such as fire extinguishers. Tell everyone where emergency information and supplies are stored. Provide copies of the family's preparedness plan to each member of the family. Ensure that information is always up to date, and practice evacuations, following the routes outlined in your plan. Identify alternative routes and make sure to include pets in your evacuation plans.

As an element of your preparedness plan, choose an out-of-area contact to call in case of an emergency. Tell all family and friends that this out-of-area contact is the person they should all phone to relay messages. Your contact should live far enough away that the person will not be affected by the disaster. You should also predetermine two meeting places, to save time and minimize confusion: 1) right outside your home; e.g. in cases such as a home fire and 2) outside your neighborhood or town, for when you cannot return home or you must evacuate.

BE INFORMED

In addition to preparing a kit and making a plan you should also know different ways to get informed, including ways you and your family would get information during a disaster or emergency, learning about the disasters that may occur in your area by knowing your region and learning first aid from your local Red Cross chapter. Visit the Be Red Cross Ready website (*redcross.org*) for further information.

32 Special Operations

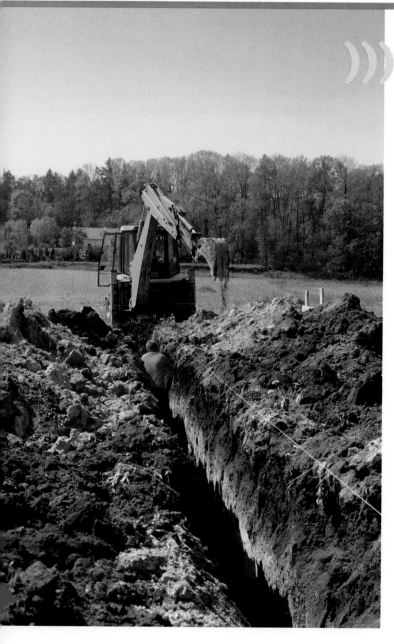

))) YOU ARE THE EMERGENCY MEDICAL RESPONDER

You are the *emergency medical responder* (EMR) at the scene of a construction site cave-in. On arrival, you find a man who was working in an open trench that has collapsed around him to mid-chest level. How would you respond? What are your immediate concerns?

Key Terms

Confined space: Any space with limited access that is not intended for continuous human occupancy; has limited or restricted means of entry or exit.

Distressed swimmer: A swimmer showing anxiety or panic; often identified as a swimmer who has gone beyond his or her swimming abilities.

Drowning: An event in which a victim experiences respiratory impairment due to submersion in water. Drowning may or may not result in death.

Drowning victim–active: Someone who is vertical in the water but has no supporting kick, is unable to move forward and cannot call out for help.

Drowning victim–passive: Someone who is not moving and is floating either face-up or face-down, on or near the surface of the water, or is submerged.

Litter: A portable stretcher used to carry a patient over rough terrain.

Non-swimming rescues and assists: Rescues and assists that can be performed from a pool deck, pier or shoreline by reaching, using an extremity or object, by throwing a floating object or by standing in the water to provide either of these assists; performed instead of swimming out to the person in distress.

Rappelling: The act of descending (as from a cliff) by sliding down a rope passed under one thigh, across the body and over the opposite shoulder or through a special friction device.

Reaching assist: A method of rescuing someone in the water by using an object to extend the rescuer's reach or by reaching with an arm or leg.

Throwing assist: A method of rescuing someone in the water by throwing the person a floating object, with or without a line attached.

Wading assist: A method of rescuing someone in the water by wading out to the person in distress.

Learning Objectives

After reading this chapter, and completing the class activities, you will have the information needed to—

- Have a basic understanding of specialized rescue units.
- Recognize signals of distressed swimmers or drowning victims.
- Be familiar with non-swimming rescues and assists.
- Have a basic understanding of special rescue situations such as ice rescues, hazardous terrain, confined space rescues, cave-ins, crime scenes, fireground operations and special events.

INTRODUCTION

As an *emergency medical responder* (EMR), you may be involved in rescues that find you in some precarious and dangerous situations. These situations will require special operations units to assist in the rescue efforts. These units may include—

- The Tactical *Emergency Medical Services* (EMS) Unit: for situations such as hostage barricades, active shooters, high-risk warrants and other situations requiring a tactical response team.
- The *Hazardous Materials* (HAZMAT) EMS Response Unit: for situations involving *weapons of mass destruction* (WMD) and HAZMAT incidents, to provide EMS care to patients in the warm zone, the area immediately outside the hot zone (the area in which the most danger exists).
- The Fire Rehabilitation Unit: to provide "rest, rehydration, nourishment and medical evaluation to members (firefighters) who are involved in extended or extreme incident scene operations" (***Source:*** *NFPA 1584*).
- The Disaster/*Multiple-Casualty Incident* (MCI) Response Unit: to support rescuers at MCIs, major incidents and those responding to other disasters with basic MCI equipment such as caches of backboards, splinting equipment, wound care supplies and IV administration supplies. Equipment also may include multi-patient oxygen delivery systems. This unit also provides services for managing large-scale or special rescue situations.
- The *Search and Rescue* (SAR) Unit: to support search and rescue operations.
- The Specialized Vehicle Response Unit: to support operations involving all-terrain response vehicles required for difficult-to-reach or hazardous terrains.

Water Rescue

Some people who drown never intended to be in the water. They may have simply slipped in and did not know what to do. **Drowning** is the fifth most common cause of death from unintentional injury in the United States, but rises to second among those 1 to 14 years of age. Children less than 5 years of age and young adults from ages 15 to 24 have the highest rates of drowning. Children with seizure disorders are *four times* more likely to drown than those without such disorders. Males are *four times* more likely to drown than females.

Younger children can drown at any moment, even in as little as an *inch* of water. Most young children drown in home pools. But, children can also drown in many other types of water settings, including drainage canals, irrigation ditches and even bathtubs, large buckets and toilets.

Alcohol and water do not mix. Drinking alcohol in, on or around water is dangerous. The U.S. Coast Guard reports that more than half of boating-related drowning deaths involve alcohol.

Being able to recognize that an individual is having trouble in the water may help save that person's life. Most people who are drowning cannot or do not call for help. They spend their energy trying to keep their mouth and nose above the water to breathe. They might slip under water quickly and never resurface. There are two kinds of water emergency situations—a swimmer in distress and a drowning person.

A **distressed swimmer** may be too tired to get to shore or to the side of the pool, but is able to stay afloat and breathe and may be calling for help (**Fig. 32-1**). The person may be floating, treading water or clinging to an object or a line for support. Someone who is trying to swim but making little or no forward progress may be in distress. Without assistance, a person in distress may lose the ability to float and begin to drown.

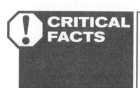
CRITICAL FACTS

Drowning is the fifth most common cause of death from unintentional injury in the United States, but rises to second among those 1 to 14 years of age. A victim may have never intended on even being in the water.

———

Younger children can drown at any moment, even in as little as an inch of water. Most young children drown in home pools. Children less than 5 years of age and young adults from ages 15 to 24 have the highest rates of drowning.

———

Most people who are drowning spend their energy trying to keep their mouth and nose above the water. Recognizing someone who seems to be having trouble in the water, but is not calling out for help, may help save his or her life.

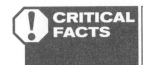
There are three types of water-related victims: a distressed swimmer who is too tired to continue but afloat; a drowning victim who is active, vertical but not moving forward; and a drowning victim who is passive, floating or submerged and not moving.

Only those trained in swimming rescues should enter the water to assist with drowning emergencies. For your safety, look for a lifeguard before attempting a rescue, have the appropriate safety equipment, call for help immediately if you do not have that equipment and only swim out if you have the proper training, skills and equipment.

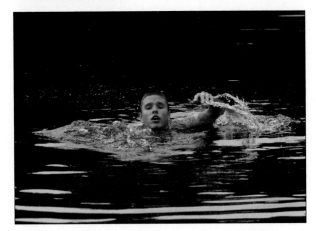

Fig. 32-1: A distressed swimmer is able to stay afloat and breathe, but may be too tired to get to shore or to the side of the pool.

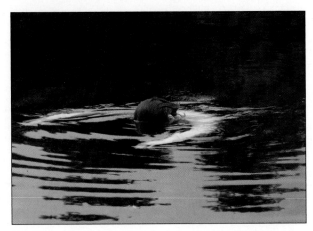

Fig. 32-2: A drowning victim who is passive is not moving and will be floating face-up or face-down on or near the surface of the water or may be submerged.

A **drowning victim—active** could be at the surface or sinking. He or she could also be positioned vertically in the water and leaning back slightly. This victim is unlikely to have a supporting kick or the ability to move forward. The person's arms are at the sides, pressing down in an attempt to keep the mouth and nose above water to breathe. All energy is going into the struggle to breathe, and the person cannot call out for help.

A **drowning victim—passive** may have a limp body or convulsive-like movements. He or she could be floating face-up or face-down on or near the surface, or may be submerged (**Fig. 32-2**). **Table 32-1** shows characteristics of drowning persons.

You should not attempt a swimming rescue unless you are trained to do so. Following these steps will help to reduce your risk of drowning:

- Look for a lifeguard to help before attempting a rescue.
- Make sure you have appropriate equipment for your own safety and that of the drowning person's.
- Call for help immediately if proper equipment is not available.
- Never swim out to a person unless you have the proper training, skills and equipment.

To be prepared for an aquatic emergency, it is important to understand the environment. Pay attention to the potential hazards that exist and the conditions of the water. Familiarize yourself with the common recreational activities in your area and the potential hazards. Consider the age, ability and physical challenges of participants in those activities and learn what kinds of local water incidents and injuries are common in your area.

As in any emergency situation, proceed safely. Make sure the scene is safe. If the person is in the water, decide first whether help is needed in order for the person to get out, and then act based on your training. Look for anyone else who may be in trouble. Look for bystanders who can call for help or help you provide first aid.

During the emergency situation, your preparation will allow you to respond quickly; you may only have seconds to act. Your first goal is to stay safe. Rushing into the water to help someone may put you at risk of drowning, too. Once you ensure your own safety, your goal is to help get the person out of the water. If the person is *unconscious*, send someone to call for more advanced medical personnel while you start the rescue. If the person is *conscious*, first get the person out of the water and then determine whether more advanced medical personnel are needed.

Table 32-1:

Behaviors of Distressed Swimmers and Drowning Victims Compared with Swimmers

	SWIMMER	DISTRESSED SWIMMER	DROWNING VICTIM — ACTIVE	DROWNING VICTIM — PASSIVE
Breathing	Rhythmic breathing	Can continue breathing and might call for help	Struggles to breathe; cannot call out for help	Is not breathing
Arm and Leg Action	Relatively coordinated	Floating, sculling or treading water; might wave for help	Holds arms to sides, alternately moving up and pressing down; has no supporting kick	None
Body Position	Horizontal	Horizontal, vertical or diagonal, depending on means of support	Vertical	Horizontal or vertical; face up, face down or submerged
Locomotion (ability to move from place to place)	Recognizable	Makes little or no forward progress; less and less able to support self	None; has only 20 to 60 seconds before submerging	None

You can help a person in trouble in the water by using **reaching assists**, **throwing assists** or **wading assists**. Whenever possible, start the rescue by talking to the person. Let the person know help is coming. If noise is a problem or if the person is too far away to hear you, use nonverbal communication strategies. Tell the person what to do to help with the rescue, such as grasping a line, ring buoy or other object that floats. Ask the individual to move toward you, such as by using the back float with slight leg movements or small strokes. Some people reach safety by themselves with the calm and encouraging assistance of someone calling to them.

Non-swimming rescues and assists include—

- Reaching Assists. Firmly brace yourself on a pool deck, pier or shoreline and reach out to the person with any object that will extend your reach, such as a pole, oar or paddle, tree branch, shirt, belt or towel (**Fig. 32-3**). If no equipment is available, you can still perform a reaching assist by lying down and extending your arm or leg for the person to grab.

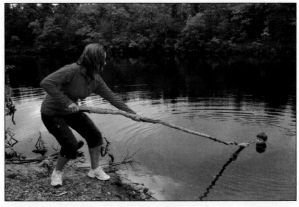

Fig. 32-3: To perform a reaching assist, firmly brace yourself on solid ground and reach out to the person in need of help with an item that will extend your reach.

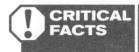 **CRITICAL FACTS** Non-swimming rescues and assists include reaching, throwing and wading assists. The distance of the victim and the conditions of the water will dictate which method is best.

- Throwing Assists. An effective way to rescue someone beyond your reach is to throw a floating object with a line attached out to the person (**Fig. 32-4**). Once the person grasps the object, pull the individual to safety. Throwing equipment includes heaving lines, ring buoys, throw bags or any floating object available, such as a picnic jug, small cooler, buoyant cushion, kickboard or extra life jacket.
- Wading Assists. If the water is safe and shallow enough (not over your chest), you can wade in to reach the person. If a current or soft or unknown bottom makes wading dangerous, do *not* go in the water. If possible, wear a life jacket and take something with you to extend your reach such as a ring buoy, buoyant cushion, kickboard, life jacket, tree branch, pole, air mattress, plastic cooler, picnic jug, paddle or water exercise belt.

When the emergency is over, you may need to assist with follow-up procedures that may include—
- Confirming and documenting witness interviews.
- Reporting the incident to the appropriate individuals.
- Filling out proper report forms to document injuries for use in court or for insurance purposes.

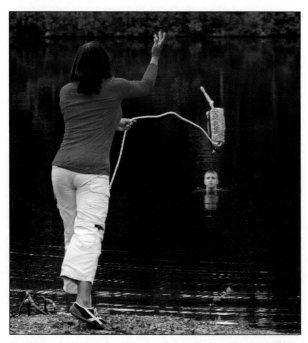

Fig. 32-4: To perform a throwing assist, throw a floating object with a line out to a person in need of help and pull the individual to safety once they have grasped the object.

- Contacting the patient's family or guardian.
- Dealing with the media.
- Debriefing.
- Assessing what happened and evaluating the actions taken.

Critical incident stress may follow an incident in which a serious injury or death occurs. The stress of the experience may overcome your ability to cope, and some effects of critical incident stress may appear right away while others may follow days, weeks or even months after the incident. Consider seeking professional help in these cases to prevent posttraumatic stress disorder.

Ice Rescue

In icy water, a person's body temperature begins to drop almost as soon as the body hits the water. The body loses heat in water *32 times* faster than it does in the air. Swallowing water accelerates this cooling. As the body's core temperature drops, the metabolic rate drops. Activity in the cells comes to almost a standstill, and the person requires very little oxygen. Any oxygen left in the blood is diverted from other parts of the body to the brain and heart.

If a person falls through the ice, do *not* go onto the ice to attempt a rescue, as it may be too thin to support you. It is your responsibility as a rescuer to call for an ice rescue team immediately. In the case of a drowning person, always attempt to rescue the person using reaching and throwing assists (**Fig. 32-5**). Continue talking to the person until the ice rescue team arrives. If you are able to pull the person from the water, provide care for hypothermia.

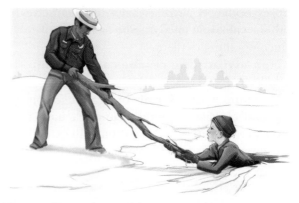

Fig. 32-5: Use reaching and throwing assists to rescue a drowning person who has fallen through the ice.

HAZARDOUS TERRAIN

Nature can offer many challenges to the EMR when faced with a rescue in hazardous terrain. Whether it is challenging weather conditions or dangerous, rough terrain, special procedures must be in place to help provide safety for both the rescuer and patient (**Fig. 32-6**).

One of the challenges you may face is evacuating a patient from a dangerous area where the terrain is rough and difficult to maneuver over. The most common equipment used for this type of rescue is the **litter**, or portable stretcher. Part of the challenge offered by rough terrain evacuation is that it takes 18–20 people to carry a patient over 1 mile of rough terrain. This is why teams must be selected in groups of four, and to ensure equal balance of the litter, team members should be as close in height as possible. The reason 18 to 20 people are required is to ensure no one on the team overtires. After a

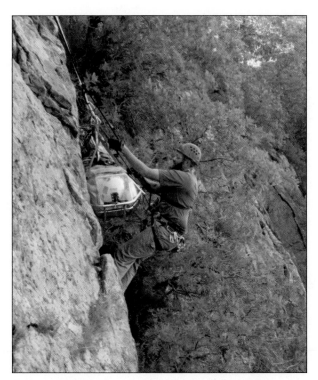

Fig. 32-6: A rescue in hazardous terrain poses many challenges. *Courtesy of University of Utah, Remote Rescue Training*

short distance, teams should rotate positions, changing sides and positions after each progression. It is then advised that teams alternate, giving each team a chance to rest. This will ensure a safe rescue, without anyone becoming exhausted and unable to complete the evacuation.

Another factor during a hazardous terrain rescue is the position of the patient in relation to the terrain: the more drastic the angle of the terrain, the more risky the rescue. To avoid dropping the patient or falling during the rescue, a rope system can be used to lift or lower the patient on the litter. A high-angle rescue, such as from a cliff, gorge or side of a building, would entail lifting or lowering a patient with these ropes. In severe cases, a high-angle rescue team may be required. These scenarios may include—

- A slope of more than 40 degrees.
- Terrain below and around the slope that poses serious danger for slips and falls.
- Terrain that requires rescue teams to approach and evacuate using a secured rope (**rappelling**).

In the case of a low-angle rescue, a rope may *not* be required. These scenarios would include situations where—

- The slope is less than 40 degrees.
- Approaching or evacuating the patient, hands are *not* required to provide balance.
- Accidental slips or falls would *not* prove life threatening or result in serious injury.

As with any emergency scene, it is your responsibility as a rescuer to assess the situation and call for the proper rescue team. While waiting for the team to arrive, follow proper procedures, including assessment of the patient as appropriate.

CONFINED SPACE

Any space with limited access that is not intended for continuous human occupancy is considered

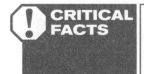

CRITICAL FACTS

Any space with limited access that is not intended for continuous human occupancy is considered a confined space. Rescues in confined spaces are usually for falls, explosions, asphyxia, medical problems or machinery entrapment. Confined spaces may be at ground level, above ground or below ground.

a **confined space** (**Fig. 32-7**). Rescues in confined spaces are usually for falls, explosions, asphyxia, medical problems or machinery entrapment. Confined spaces may be at ground level, above ground or below ground.

Silos used to store agricultural materials are often designed to limit oxygen and, therefore, present the hazard of poisonous gases caused by fermentation as well as the danger of engulfment by the contained product in the silo. Grain bins and grain elevators pose the same dangers as silos.

Low oxygen levels in these spaces pose a significant risk, as do poisonous gases such as carbon monoxide, hydrogen sulfide and carbon dioxide. Atmospheres containing other gases also may be explosive.

Below-ground confined spaces, such as underground vaults or utility vaults for water, sewers or electrical power, also can pose situations in which poisonous gases may be present. Electrical vaults pose the added danger of possible electrocution. Wells, culverts and cisterns containing water may also present a high risk of drowning.

Upon arrival at the scene, determine the nature of the emergency and find out if there are any permits for the site so that you can determine the type of work being done. Without entering the site, try to determine how many workers are involved and whether there are any hazards present. Next, call for a specialized rescue team and establish a safe perimeter around the area, preventing anyone from entering. Do *not* enter the scene unless you are sure it is safe. When able, assist in the rescue and offer medical assistance if appropriate.

There are specific safety precautions dictated by the *Occupational Safety and Health Administration* (OSHA). These guidelines are intended to protect workers who must access confined spaces to perform specific jobs. These safety precautions include requirements for proper ventilation and monitoring for poisonous gases, safely locked electrical systems, dissipated stored energy and disconnected pipes. They also address the use of appropriate respiratory protection for rescuers, including *self-contained breathing apparatus* (SCBA) or *supplied air breathing apparatus* (SABA).

Cave-Ins

Cave-ins from a trench are associated with particular risk. To prevent cave-ins, OSHA has rules about shoring or making a "trench box" in any trench deeper than 5 feet, to prevent walls from giving way. If a worker is involved in a cave-in, the person may be buried either completely or partially. If a second worker jumps in to save that person, the rescuer may cause a secondary collapse and become buried as well.

It is easy to underestimate the danger of being covered in soil, but it weighs about 100 pounds per cubic yard. Buried under only 2 feet of soil may mean a worker is under about 1000 pounds of weight, which can cause respiratory problems if the soil is covering the person's chest. It is imperative to call a specialized trench team for rescue at a cave-in. Do *not* let anyone enter the trench or the area immediately around it; once there has been a cave-in, the likelihood of a secondary one is increased.

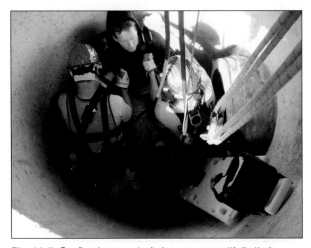

Fig. 32-7: Confined spaces include any space with limited access that is not intended for continuous human occupancy. *Courtesy of Chief Carle L. Bishop, Clermont Fire Department.*

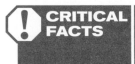

CRITICAL FACTS Cave-ins from a trench are associated with particular risk. To prevent cave-ins, OSHA has rules about shoring or making a "trench box" in any trench deeper than 5 feet, to prevent walls from giving way.

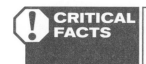

CRITICAL FACTS

Law enforcement officers are in charge of a crime scene. It is your responsibility to keep in mind the importance of maintaining the integrity of evidence that can be compromised or destroyed when you enter a crime scene.

CRIME SCENE

Law enforcement officers are in charge of a crime scene. It is your responsibility to keep in mind the importance of maintaining the integrity of evidence that can be compromised or destroyed when you enter a crime scene. *Always* consult with police officers before disturbing items that may be evidence of a crime. You must take precautions to avoid disturbing crime scene evidence (e.g., weapons, bloodstains, vehicles, skid marks) or other evidence that can be vital to investigators to reconstruct the crime or accident scene. It is also important not to introduce evidence *into* a crime scene. In all such cases, direction will be provided from the officer in charge and EMRs should *not* take action without permission from law enforcement that it is clear for you to enter, usually with an appropriate escort.

There are four types of crime scene situations you may be called to:

- A closed access to an unsecured crime scene means that a hazard still exists, such as in a hostage situation, when the suspect(s) is still on the scene or environmental hazards are still present.
- A limited-access crime scene means that critical evidence could be destroyed or compromised on the scene and that hazards may still be present, including environmental hazards.
- An open-access crime scene still has evidence to be collected. However, personnel have access to the entire area. It is still necessary to consult with police before disturbing anything, as critical evidence could still be destroyed or compromised.
- A cold crime scene no longer has evidential concerns or hazards present.

As a rescuer, when you arrive at a scene where criminal activity is suspected, take the following steps:

- Notify law enforcement personnel if they are not already at the scene.

- Take precautions *not* to remove or disturb anything at the scene unless it is absolutely necessary to perform critical patient care.
- Document any situations in which you need to disturb the scene in the interest of patient care.
- In situations where sexual assault is suspected or alleged by the patient, notify law enforcement personnel and do *not* allow the patient to wash, shower or change clothing.
- When removing clothing following gunshot wounds, stabbing or other assaults, if at all possible, do *not* cut clothing through or near the bullet or stab wound holes.
- Allow bloody clothing to dry.
- Avoid allowing blood or debris to contaminate another area or clothing.
- Do *not* roll clothes up in a ball.
- *Never* put wet or bloody clothes in plastic bags.
- Handle clothing as little and as carefully as possible, as powder flakes from gunshot wounds may be present and this may decrease the value of powder-deposit examination.
- Consider bagging the patient's hands if the situation permits.
- Minimize the introduction of evidence into a crime scene. Communicate with law enforcement concerning any items you left behind (such as medical supplies) and if you disturbed anything (such as moving furniture to access a patient).
- Yield to the primary investigative agency on the scene.

FIREGROUND OPERATIONS

Any fire can be dangerous. Make sure that the local fire department has been summoned. Only firefighters, who are highly trained and use equipment that protects them against fire and smoke, should approach a fire. Do *not* let others approach. Gather information to help the responding fire and EMS units. Find out the possible number of people trapped, their location, the fire's cause and whether any explosives or chemicals are present. Give this information to emergency personnel when they arrive. If you are not trained to fight fires or lack the necessary equipment, follow these basic guidelines:

- Do *not* approach a burning vehicle.
- *Never* enter a burning or smoke-filled building.
- If you are in a building that is on fire, *always* check doors before opening them. If a door is hot to the touch, do *not* open it.
- Since smoke and fumes rise, stay close to the floor (**Fig. 32-8**).
- *Never* use an elevator in a building that may be burning.

As with a crime scene situation and law enforcement personnel, fireground operations always yield to the fire services department to lead and coordinate operations.

Fire departments are uniquely equipped to simultaneously address patients' needs at a fire, including—

- Physical rescue of patients.
- Protection from the dangers posed by a fire.
- Creation of a safe physical environment.

As always, scene safety is the primary objective at every fire rescue. The rapid response times of the fire department offer a crucial advantage to fire-related emergency situations. Most fire departments are equipped with automated defibrillators. They are also equipped to perform rapid multi-faceted response, rapid identification and triage to the appropriate facility.

SPECIAL EVENTS AND STANDBY

You may be assigned to a special event or be on standby in case there is a need for emergency medical attention. Such events could include major sporting events like the Super Bowl or concerts, large-scale conventions or other national security events (**Fig. 32-9**). The following general guidelines are for awareness purposes and may vary by state or EMS jurisdiction.

An individual, agency or organization may submit a request for an EMS team to be present at a special event by providing a plan outlining the following information to the appropriate agency:

- The nature of the event and its location, length and anticipated attendance
- The sponsor of the event
- The qualifications of the special event supervisory physician and the special event EMS incident commander, as well as their names
- The number of emergency medical personnel involved and their qualifications
- The type and quantity of emergency medical vehicles, equipment and supplies required, in accordance with the anticipated number of participants or spectators
- A description of the on-site treatment facilities, including maps of the special event site

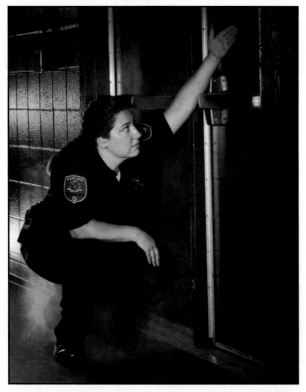

Fig. 32-8: If in a burning or smoke-filled building, check all doors before opening them. If a door is hot to the touch, do not open it. Stay close to the floor.

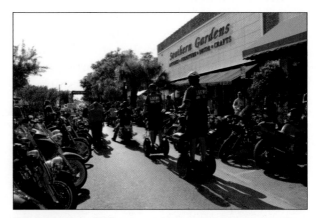

Fig. 32-9: As an EMR, you may be assigned to be on standby at a special event in case there is a need for emergency medical attention. *Courtesy of Captain Phil Kleinberg, EMT-P, Lake-Sumter EMS.*

- The level of care to be provided: *basic life support* (BLS), *advanced life support* (ALS) or both
- Patient transfer protocols and agreements
- A description of the special event emergency medical communications capabilities
- Plans for educating event attendees regarding EMS system access, specific hazards or severe weather
- Measures that will be taken to coordinate EMS care for the special event with local emergency services and public safety agencies

A special event EMS incident commander must be assigned at a special event to supervise the EMS team during the event. The director's responsibilities include—
- Preparation of the plan.
- Management of the delivery of special event EMS care.
- Ensuring implementation and coordination of details contained in the special event EMS plan.

The special event EMS incident commander must be experienced in the administration and management of prehospital care at the BLS or ALS level. This person must possess experience in the medical supervision of prehospital care at the BLS or ALS level.

The required staff, qualifications and equipment for a special event are as follows:
- Special event emergency medical staff shall be certified at BLS or ALS levels.
- The number of staffed, licensed ambulances or other transport vehicles required to be stationed on-site are as follows:
  - One ambulance for known or expected populations of 5000 to 25,000 participants
  - Two ambulances for more than 25,000 but less than 55,000 participants
  - Three ambulances for more than 55,000 participants
  - Personnel must be available to care for special event spectators or participants within 10 minutes of notification of the need for emergency care.
  - EMS personnel must be currently certified at the ambulance attendant, emergency medical responder, *emergency medical technician* (EMT), advanced EMT, paramedic or health care professional level.

A special event where more than 25,000 participants or spectators are expected requires an on-site treatment facility, providing protection from weather or other elements to ensure patient safety and comfort. Beds and equipment for at least four simultaneous patients must be provided for evaluation and treatment, with adequate lighting and ventilation. A special event EMS system must also have on-site communication capabilities, to ensure uniform access to care for patients in need of EMS care; on-site coordination of the activities of EMS personnel; communication with existing community *public safety answering points* (PSAPs); and interface with other involved public safety agencies. Receiving facilities and ambulances providing emergency transportation must also be ensured.

The sponsoring agency is responsible for the implementation of the plan and must ensure participants and spectators are aware of the following:
- The location of EMS providers at the special event
- How to obtain emergency medical care at the special event
- The procedure in the case of specific hazards or serious changing conditions, such as severe weather

PUTTING IT ALL TOGETHER

As with all calls, the main focus of a special operations situation is to remember your safety and the safety of the patient. Calling the proper service to assist in the rescue will contribute to the success of the rescue efforts.

Use reaching and throwing assists when attempting to retrieve a patient from water. Remember *never* to enter fast-moving water and to tether yourself or any rescue craft you may be using in the rescue attempts. Watch for signs of a distressed swimmer and an actively or a passively drowning victim when sizing up the scene. When attempting ice rescues, remember the dangers thin ice can pose and the added consideration of how hypothermia can affect a person's ability to grasp rescue equipment.

Confined space situations pose different dangers during a rescue. The presence of gases, engulfment and possible drowning or electrocution can all be factors, depending on the nature of the space.

The physical demands of litter rescue from hazardous terrain can require as many as 20 rescuers to ensure the safe evacuation of a patient. The slope of the area can also pose challenges and, in high-angle situations, a special team is required to evacuate patients.

When approaching a crime scene, remember that law enforcement personnel on the scene are in charge. *Always* obtain permission to enter the scene and, when attending to victims of a crime, ensure that the scene is left as undisturbed as possible. If you are first on the scene, call for assistance and attend to the patient as best you can.

Management of fireground operations must be passed on to the fire rescue team. *Never* enter a burning structure or vehicle. *Always* call for the fire department when danger of fire exists, or whenever a team has not already been called.

Finally, when attending a special event, remember to receive direction from the special event EMS director and keep in mind that a special event emergency supervisory physician will be present to assist in case of a serious medical emergency. The number of staffed, licensed ambulance requirements stationed on-site is dictated by the number of spectators or participants at the event.

YOU ARE THE EMERGENCY MEDICAL RESPONDER

You find that the patient is conscious but appears to be in respiratory distress from the compression of the soil surrounding him. What are your treatment priorities? What kind of additional support will you need, and what are some special safety considerations you must consider in order to rescue this patient?

Glossary

Abandonment: Ending the care of an injured or ill person without obtaining that patient's consent or without ensuring that someone with equal or greater training will continue care.

Abrasion: The most common type of open wound; characterized by skin that has been rubbed or scraped away.

Abruptio placentae: Placental abruption; a life-threatening emergency that occurs when the placenta detaches from the uterus.

Absence seizures: A type of generalized seizure in which there are minimal or no movements; patient may appear to have a blank stare; also known as petit mal or non-convulsive seizures.

Absorbed poison: A poison that enters the body through the skin.

Access: Reaching a patient who is trapped in a motor vehicle or a dangerous situation, for the purpose of extrication and providing medical care.

Acute: Having a rapid and severe onset, then quickly subsiding.

Acute abdomen: The sudden onset of severe abdominal pain that may be related to one of many medical conditions or a specific injury to the abdomen.

Acute coronary syndrome (ACS): Term that describes a range of clinical conditions, including unstable angina, that are due to insufficient blood supply to the heart muscle resulting from *coronary heart disease* (CHD).

Acute myocardial ischemia: An episode of chest pain due to reduced blood flow to the heart muscle.

Adaptive immunity: The type of protection from disease that the body develops throughout a lifetime as a person is exposed to diseases or immunized against them.

Addiction: The compulsive need to use a substance; stopping use would cause the user to suffer mental, physical and emotional distress.

Adult: For the purpose of providing emergency medical care, anyone who appears to be approximately 12 years old or older.

Adult respiratory distress syndrome (ARDS): A lung condition in which trauma to the lungs leads to inflammation, accumulation of fluid in the alveolar air sacs, low blood oxygen and respiratory distress.

Advance directive: A written instruction, signed by the patient and a physician, that documents a patient's wishes if the patient is unable to communicate his or her wishes.

Advanced emergency medical technician (AEMT): A person trained in emergency care, with the additional training to allow insertion of IVs, administration of medications, performance of advanced airway procedures, and setting up and assessing of *electrocardiograms* (ECGs or EKGs); formerly referred to as EMT-Intermediate.

Agonal gasp: Isolated or infrequent gasping in the absence of other breathing in an unconscious person; can occur after the heart has stopped beating. Agonal gasps are not breathing.

AIDS: A disease of the immune system caused by infection with HIV.

Air medical transport: A type of transport to a medical facility or between medical facilities by helicopter or fixed-wing aircraft.

Air splint: A hollow, inflatable splint for immobilizing a part of the body.

Airway: The pathway for air from the mouth and nose through the pharynx, larynx and trachea and into the lungs.

Airway adjunct: A mechanical device used to help keep the tongue from obstructing the airway; can be either nasal or oral.

All-hazards approach: An approach to disaster readiness that involves the capability of responding to any type of disaster with a range of equipment and resources.

Altered mental status: A disturbance in a patient's *level of consciousness* (LOC) including confusion and delirium; causes include injury, infection, poison, drug abuse and fluid/electrolyte imbalance.

Alzheimer's disease: The most common type of dementia in older people, in which thought, memory and language are impaired.

Amniotic fluid: The fluid in the amniotic sac; surrounds and protects the fetus.

Amniotic sac: "Bag of waters"; sac that encloses the fetus during pregnancy and bursts during the birthing process.

Amputation: The complete removal or severing of an external body part.

Anabolic steroid: A drug sometimes used by athletes to enhance performance and increase muscle mass; also has medical use in stimulating weight gain for people unable to gain weight naturally.

Anaphylaxis: A form of distributive shock caused by an often sudden severe allergic reaction, in which air passages may swell and restrict breathing; also referred to as *anaphylactic shock*.

Anatomic splint: A splint formed by supporting an injured part of the body with an uninjured, neighboring body part; for example, splinting one finger against another; also called a *self-splint*.

Anatomy: The study of structures, including gross anatomy (structures that can be seen with the naked eye) and microscopic anatomy (structures seen under the microscope).

Aneurysm: An abnormal bulging of an artery due to weakness in the blood vessel; may occur in the aorta (main artery of the heart), brain, leg or other location.

Angina pectoris: Pain in the chest that comes and goes at different times; caused by a lack of oxygen reaching the heart; can be stable (occurring under exertion or stress) or unstable (occurring at rest, without reason).

Angulation: An angular deformity in a fractured bone.

Ankle drag: A method of moving a patient by grasping the patient's ankles; also known as the foot drag.

Antibodies: A type of protein found in blood or other bodily fluids; used by the immune system to identify and neutralize pathogens, such as bacteria and viruses.

Antidote: A substance that counteracts and neutralizes the effects of a poison.

Antihistamine: A type of drug taken to treat allergic reactions.

Anti-inflammatory drug: A type of drug taken to reduce inflammation or swelling.

Antivenin: A substance used to counteract the poisonous effects of venom.

Anxiety disorder: A condition in which normal anxiety becomes excessive and can prevent people from functioning normally; types include generalized anxiety disorder, obsessive-compulsive disorder, panic disorder, post-traumatic stress disorder, phobias and social-anxiety disorder.

APGAR score: A mnemonic that describes five measures used to assess the newborn: Appearance, Pulse, Grimace, Activity and Respiration.

Aphasia: A disorder characterized by difficulty or inability to produce or understand language, caused by injury to the areas of the brain that control language.

Apnea: A condition that causes breathing to stop periodically or be significantly reduced.

Apparent life-threatening event (ALTE): A sudden event in infants under the age of 1 year, during which the infant experiences a combination of symptoms including apnea, change in color, change in muscle tone and coughing or gagging.

Applied ethics: The use of ethics in decision making; applying ethical values.

Arrhythmia: Disturbance in the regular rhythmic beating of the heart.

Arterial gas embolism: A condition in which air bubbles enter the bloodstream and subsequently travel to the brain; results from a rapid ascent from deep water, which expands air in the lungs too quickly.

Arteries: Large blood vessels that carry oxygen-rich blood from the heart to all parts of the body, except for the pulmonary arteries, which carry oxygen-poor blood from the heart to the lungs.

Artificial ventilation: A mechanical means used to assist breathing, such as with a *bag-valve-mask resuscitator* (BVM) or resuscitation mask.

Asperger syndrome: A disorder on the autism spectrum; those with Asperger syndrome have a milder form of the disorder.

Aspiration: To take, suck or inhale blood, vomit, saliva or other foreign material into the lungs.

Assault: A crime that occurs when a person tries to physically harm another in a way that makes the person under attack feel immediately threatened.

Asthma: An ongoing condition in which the airways swell; the air passages can become constricted or blocked when affected by various triggers.

Asthma attack: The sudden worsening of asthma signs and symptoms, caused by inflammation of the airways and the tightening of muscles around the airways of a person with asthma, making breathing difficult.

Asthma trigger: Anything that sets off an asthma attack, such as animal dander, dust, smoke, exercise, stress or medications.

Asymptomatic: A situation in which a patient has no symptoms.

Asystole: A condition where the heart has stopped generating electrical activity.

Atherosclerosis: A condition in which deposits of plaque, including cholesterol (a fatty substance made by the liver and found in foods containing animal or animal products) build up on the inner walls of the arteries, causing them to harden and narrow, reducing the amount of blood that can flow through; develops gradually and can go undetected for many years.

Atrial fibrillation: Irregular and fast electrical discharges of the heart that lead to an irregular heart beat; the most common type of abnormal cardiac rhythm.

Atrioventricular (AV) node: A cluster of cells in the center of the heart, between the atria and ventricles; serves as a relay to slow down the signal received from the *sinoatrial* (SA) node before it passes through to the ventricles.

Atropine: An anticholinergic drug with multiple effects; used in antidotes to counteract the effects of nerve agents and to counter the effects of organophosphate (chemical compounds found in many common insecticides and used to produce toxic nerve agents, such as sarin) poisoning.

Audible warning devices: Devices in an emergency vehicle to warn oncoming and side traffic of the vehicle's approach; includes both sirens and air horns.

Aura phase: The first stage of a generalized seizure, during which the patient experiences perceptual disturbances, often visual or olfactory in nature.

Auscultation: Listening to sounds within the body, typically through a stethoscope.

Autism spectrum disorders (ASD): A group of disorders characterized by some degree of impairment in communication and social interaction as well as repetitive behaviors.

Automated external defibrillator (AED): A portable electronic device that analyzes the heart's electrical rhythm and, if necessary, can deliver an electrical shock to a person in cardiac arrest.

AVPU: Mnemonic describing the four levels of patient response: Alert, Verbal, Painful and Unresponsive.

Avulsion: An injury in which a portion of the skin, and sometimes other soft tissue, is partially or completely torn away.

B NICE: An acronym for the five main types of terrorist weapons: biological contamination, nuclear detonation, incendiary fires, toxic chemical release and conventional explosions.

Backboard: A piece of equipment used to immobilize a patient's head, neck and spine during transport.

Bacteria: One-celled organisms that can cause infection; a common type of pathogen.

Bag-valve-mask resuscitator (BVM): A hand-held breathing device consisting of a self-inflating bag, a one-way valve and a face mask; can be used with or without emergency oxygen.

Bandage: Material used to wrap or cover a part of the body; commonly used to hold a dressing or splint in place.

Bandage compress: A thick gauze dressing attached to a gauze bandage.

Barotrauma: Injury sustained because of pressure differences between areas of the body and the surrounding environment; most commonly occurs in air travel and scuba diving.

Battery: A crime that occurs when there is unlawful touching of a person without the person's consent.

Behavior: How people conduct themselves or respond to their environment.

Behavioral emergency: A situation in which a person exhibits abnormal behavior that is unacceptable or intolerable, for example violence to oneself or others.

Bereavement care: Care provided to families during the period of grief and mourning surrounding a death.

Binder: A cloth wrapped around a patient to securely hold the arm against the patient's chest to add stability; also called a *swathe*.

Biohazard: A biological agent that presents a hazard to the health or well-being of those exposed.

Bioterrorism: The deliberate release of agents typically found in nature, such as viruses, bacteria and other pathogens, to cause illness or death in people, animals or plants.

Bipolar disorder: A brain disorder that causes abnormal, severe shifts in mood, energy and a person's ability to function; the person swings from the extreme lows of depression to the highs of mania; also called manic-depressive disorder.

Birth canal: The passageway from the uterus to the outside of the body through which a baby passes during birth.

Blanket drag: A method of moving a patient, using a blanket, in an emergency situation where equipment is limited and the patient is suspected of having a head, neck or spinal injury.

Blast injury: An injury caused by an explosion; may occur because of the energy released, the debris or the impact of the person falling against an object or the ground.

Blast lung: Sometimes referred to as *lung blast*; the most common fatal primary blast injury, describing damage to the lungs caused by the over-pressurization wave from high-order explosives.

Bleeding: The loss of blood from arteries, veins or capillaries.

Blood glucose level (BGL): The level of glucose circulating in the blood; measured using a glucometer.

Blood pressure (BP): The force exerted by blood against the blood vessel walls as it travels throughout the body.

Blood volume: The total amount of blood circulating within the body.

Bloodborne: Used to describe a substance carried in the blood (e.g., bloodborne pathogens are pathogens carried through the blood).

Bloodborne pathogens: Germs that may be present in human blood or other body fluids that can cause disease in humans.

Bloody show: Thick discharge from the vagina that occurs during labor as the mucous plug (mucus with pink or light red streaks) is expelled; often signifies the onset of labor.

Blunt trauma: An injury in which a person is struck by or falls against a blunt object such as a steering wheel or dashboard, resulting in an injury that does not penetrate the body, may not be evident and may be more widespread and serious than suspected.

Body mechanics: The field of physiology that studies muscular actions and the function of the muscles in maintaining posture.

Body substance isolation (BSI) precautions: Protective measures to prevent exposure to communicable diseases; defines all body fluids and substances as infectious.

Body system: A group of organs and other structures that works together to carry out specific functions.

Bone: A dense, hard tissue that forms the skeleton.

Brachial artery: The main artery of the upper arm; runs from the shoulder down to the bend of the elbow.

Braxton Hicks contractions: False labor; irregular contractions of the uterus that do not intensify or become more frequent as genuine labor contractions do.

Breathing emergency: An emergency in which breathing is impaired; can become life threatening; also called a *respiratory emergency*.

Breathing rate: Term used to describe the number of breaths per minute.

Breech birth: The delivery of a baby's feet or buttocks first.

Bulb syringe: Small nasal syringe to remove secretions from the newborn's mouth and nose.

Burn: An injury to the skin or other body tissues caused by heat, chemicals, electricity or radiation.

Cannabis products: Substances such as marijuana and hashish that are derived from the *Cannabis sativa* plant; can produce feelings of elation, distorted perceptions of time and space, and impaired motor coordination and judgment.

Capillaries: Tiny blood vessels linking arteries and veins that transfer oxygen and other nutrients from the blood to all body cells and remove waste products.

Capillary refill: A technique for estimating how the body is reacting to injury or illness by checking the ability of the capillaries to refill with blood.

Carbon monoxide (CO): An odorless, colorless, toxic gas produced as a byproduct of combustion.

Cardiac arrest: A condition in which the heart has stopped or beats too irregularly or weakly to pump blood effectively.

Cardiac Chain of Survival: A set of four critical steps in responding to a cardiac emergency: early recognition and access to the *emergency medical services* (EMS) system, early CPR, early defibrillation and early advanced medical care.

Cardiac muscle: A specialized type of muscle found in the heart.

Cardiogenic shock: The result of the heart being unable to supply adequate blood circulation to the vital organs, resulting in an inadequate supply of nutrients; caused by trauma or disease.

Cardiopulmonary resuscitation (CPR): A technique that combines chest compressions and ventilations to circulate blood containing oxygen to the brain and other vital organs for a person whose heart and breathing have stopped.

Cardiovascular disease: A disease affecting the heart and blood vessels.

Carotid artery: The major artery located on either side of the neck that supplies blood to the brain.

Catastrophic reaction: A reaction a person experiences when the person has become overwhelmed; signs include screaming, throwing objects and striking out.

CBRNE: The current acronym used by the Department of Homeland Security to describe the main types of weapons of mass destruction: chemical, biological, radiological/ nuclear and explosive.

Cells: The basic units that combine to form all living tissue.

Cerebrospinal fluid: A clear fluid that flows within the ventricles of the brain and around the brain and spinal cord.

Certification: Credentialing at the local level; usually entails completing a probationary period and updating and/or recertification to cover changing knowledge and skills.

Cervical collar: A commercially produced rigid device that is positioned around the neck to limit movement of the head and neck; also called a *C-collar*.

Cervix: The lower, narrow part of the uterus (womb) that forms a canal that opens into the vagina, which leads to the outside of the body; upper part of the birth canal.

Cesarean section: C-section; delivery of a baby through an incision in the mother's belly and uterus.

Chemical burn: A burn caused by strong, caustic chemicals damaging the skin.

Chest compressions: A technique used in CPR, in which external pressure is placed on the chest to increase the level of pressure in the chest cavity and cause the blood to circulate through the arteries.

Chest tube: A tube surgically inserted into the chest to drain blood, fluid or air, and to allow the lungs to expand.

Chief complaint: A brief description, usually in the patient's own words, of why EMS personnel were called to the scene.

Child: For the purpose of providing emergency medical care, anyone who appears to be between the ages of about 1 year and about 12 years; when using an AED, different age and weight criteria are used.

Child abuse: Action that results in the physical or psychological harm of a child; can be physical, sexual, verbal and/or emotional.

Child neglect: The most frequently reported type of abuse in which a parent or guardian fails to provide the necessary, age-appropriate care to a child; insufficient medical or emotional attention or respect given to a child.

Chocking: The use of items such as wooden blocks placed against the wheels of a vehicle to help stabilize it.

Cholesterol: A fatty substance made by the liver and found in foods containing animal or animal products; diets high in cholesterol contribute to the risk of heart disease.

Chronic: Persistent over a long period of time.

Chronic diseases: Diseases that occur gradually and continue over a long period of time.

Chronic obstructive pulmonary disease (COPD): A progressive lung disease in which the patient has difficulty breathing because of damage to the lungs; airways become obstructed and the alveolar sacs lose their ability to fill with air.

Circulatory system: A group of organs and other structures that carries oxygen-rich blood and other nutrients throughout the body and removes waste.

Circumferential splint: A type of splint that surrounds or encircles an injured body part.

Clinical depression: A mood disorder in which feelings of sadness, loss, anger or frustration interfere with everyday life for an extended period of time.

Clonic phase: The third phase of a generalized seizure, during which the patient experiences the seizure itself.

Closed fracture: A type of fracture in which the skin over the broken bone is intact.

Closed wound: A wound in which soft tissue damage occurs beneath the skin and the skin is not broken.

Clothes drag: A type of emergency move that uses the patient's clothing; used for a patient suspected of having a head, neck or spinal injury.

Clotting: The process by which blood thickens at a wound site to seal an opening in a blood vessel and stop bleeding.

Cognitive impairment: Impairment of thinking abilities including memory, judgment, reasoning, problem solving and decision making.

Cold zone: Also called the *support zone*, this area is the outer perimeter of the zones most directly affected by an emergency involving hazardous materials.

Commotio cordis: Sudden cardiac arrest from a blunt, non-penetrating blow to the chest, of which the basis is *ventricular fibrillation* (V-fib) triggered by chest wall impact immediately over the heart.

Communications center (dispatch): The point of contact between the public and responders (also known as a *9-1-1 call center* or *Public Service Answering Point* [PSAP]); responsible for taking basic information from callers and dispatching the appropriate personnel; in some communities may also provide prearrival instructions to the 9-1-1 caller.

Compartment syndrome: Condition in which there is swelling and an increase in pressure within a limited space that presses on and compromises blood vessels, nerves and tendons that run through that limited space; usually involves the leg, forearm, arm, thigh, shoulder or buttock.

Competence: The patient's ability to understand the *emergency medical responder's* (EMR's) questions and the implications of decisions made.

Complex access: In an extrication, the process of using specialized tools or equipment to gain access to the patient.

Complex partial seizures: A type of partial seizure in which the patient may experience an altered mental status or be unresponsive.

Concussion: A temporary loss of brain function caused by a blow to the head.

Conduction: One of the ways the body loses or gains heat; occurs when the skin is in contact with something with a lower or higher temperature.

Confidentiality: Protection of a patient's privacy by not revealing any personal patient information except to law enforcement personnel or EMS personnel caring for the patient.

Confined space: Any space with limited access that is not intended for continuous human occupancy; has limited or restricted means of entry or exit.

Congestive heart failure: A chronic condition in which the heart no longer pumps blood effectively throughout the body.

Consent: Permission to provide care; given by an injured or ill person to a responder.

Contraction: During labor, the rhythmic tightening and relaxing of muscles of the uterus.

Contusion: An injury to the soft tissues that results in blood vessel damage (usually to capillaries) and leakage of blood into the surrounding tissues; caused when blood vessels are damaged or broken as the result of a blow to the skin, resulting in swelling and a reddish-purple discoloration on the skin; commonly referred to as a bruise.

Convection: One of the ways the body loses or gains heat; occurs when air moves over the skin and carries away or increases heat.

Core temperature: The temperature inside the body.

Coronary heart disease (CHD): A disease in which cholesterol and plaque build up on the inner walls of the arteries that supply blood to the heart; also called *coronary artery disease* (CAD).

CPR breathing barrier: Devices that allow for artificial ventilations without direct mouth-to-mouth contact; includes resuscitation masks and BVMs.

Crackles: An abnormal fine, crackling breath sound on inhalation that may be a sign of fluid in the lungs; also known as *rales*.

Cravat: A folded triangular bandage used to hold splints in place.

Crepitus: A grating or popping sound under the skin that can be due to a number of causes, including two pieces of bone rubbing against each other.

Cribbing: A system using wood or supports, arranged diagonally to a vehicle's frame, to safely prop it up, creating a stable environment.

Cricoid: A solid ring of cartilage just below and behind the thyroid cartilage.

Critical burn: Any burn that is potentially life threatening, disabling or disfiguring; a burn requiring advanced medical care.

Critical incident stress: Stress triggered by involvement in a serious or traumatic incident.

Croup: A common upper airway virus that affects children under the age of 5.

Crowning: The phase during labor when the baby's head is visible at the opening of the vagina.

Crush injury: An injury to a body part, often an extremity, caused by a high degree of pressure; may result in serious damage to underlying tissues and cause bleeding, bruising, fracture, laceration and compartment syndrome.

Cyanosis: A condition in which the patient's skin, nail beds and mucous membranes appear a bluish or grayish color because of insufficient levels of oxygen in the blood.

Cyanotic: Showing bluish discoloration of the skin, nailbeds and mucous membranes due to insufficient levels of oxygen in the blood.

DCAP-BTLS: A mnemonic to help remember the components of a rapid trauma assessment; the initials stand for deformities, contusions, abrasions, punctures/penetrations, burns, tenderness, lacerations and swelling.

Deadspace: The areas within the respiratory system between the pharynx and the alveoli that contains a small amount of air that does not reach the alveoli.

Deafness: The loss of the ability to hear from one or both ears; can be mild, moderate, severe or profound and can be inherited, occur at birth or be acquired at a later point in life, due to illness, medication, noise exposure or injury.

Debriefing: A method of helping people cope with exposure to serious or traumatic incidents by discussing the emotional impact of the event.

Deceased/non-salvageable/expectant (Black): A triage category of those involved in a *multiple-(or mass-) casualty incident* (MCI) who are obviously dead or who have suffered non-life-sustaining injuries.

Decompression sickness: A sometimes fatal disorder caused by the release of gas bubbles into body tissue; also known as *"the bends"*; occurs when scuba divers ascend too rapidly, without allowing sufficient time for gases to exit body tissues and be removed through exhalation.

Defibrillation: An electrical shock that disrupts the electrical activity of the heart long enough to allow the heart to spontaneously develop an effective rhythm on its own.

Defusing: Similar to a debriefing but shorter and less formal; a method of discussing a serious or traumatic event soon afterward; done to help people cope.

Dehydration: Inadequate fluids in the body's tissues.

Delayed care (Yellow): A triage category of those involved in a MCI with an injury, but whose chances of survival will not be reduced by a delay.

Dementia: A collection of symptoms caused by any of several disorders of the brain; characterized by significantly impaired intellectual functioning that interferes with normal activities and relationships.

Dependency: The desire or need to continually use a substance.

Depressant: A substance that affects the central nervous system and slows down physical and mental activity; can be used to treat anxiety, tension and high blood pressure.

Dermis: The deeper layer of the skin; contains the nerves, sweat glands, oil glands and blood vessels.

Designer drugs: Potent and illegal street drugs formed from a medicinal substance whose drug composition has been modified (designed).

Detailed physical exam: An in-depth head-to-toe physical exam; takes more time than the rapid assessment and is only done when time and the patient's condition allow.

Diabetes: A disease in which there are high levels of blood glucose due to defects in insulin production, insulin action or both.

Diabetic coma: A life-threatening complication of diabetes in which very high blood sugar causes the patient to become unconscious.

Diabetic emergency: A situation in which a person becomes ill because of an imbalance of insulin and sugar in the bloodstream.

Diabetic ketoacidosis (DKA): An accumulation of organic acids and ketones (waste products) in the blood; occurs when there is inadequate insulin and high blood sugar levels.

Diastolic blood pressure: The force exerted against the arteries when the heart is between contractions, or at rest.

Digestive system: A group of organs and other structures that digests food and eliminates wastes.

Dilation: The process of enlargement or stretching; during delivery, refers to the opening of the cervix to allow the baby to be born.

Dilation: The process of enlargement, stretching or expansion; used to describe blood vessels.

Direct carry: A method of moving a patient from a bed to a stretcher or vice-versa; performed by two responders.

Direct contact: Mode of transmission of pathogens that occurs through directly touching infected blood or body fluid, or other agents such as chemicals, drugs or toxins.

Direct force: A force that causes injury at the point of impact.

Direct ground lift: A non-emergency method of lifting a patient directly from the ground; performed by several responders.

Direct medical control: A type of medical direction, also called "on-line," "base-station," "immediate" or "concurrent medical control"; under this type of medical direction the physician speaks directly with emergency care providers at the scene of an emergency.

Direct pressure: Pressure applied on a wound to control bleeding.

Disease-causing agent: A pathogen or germ that can cause disease or illness (e.g., a bacterium or virus).

Dislocation: The displacement of a bone from its normal position at a joint.

Dispatch: Personnel trained in taking critical information from emergency callers and relaying it to the appropriate rescue personnel.

Distressed swimmer: A swimmer showing anxiety or panic; often identified as a swimmer who has gone beyond his or her swimming abilities.

Distributive shock: A type of shock caused by inadequate distribution of blood, either in the blood vessels or throughout the body, leading to inadequate volumes of blood returning to the heart.

Do no harm: The principle that people who intervene to help others must do their best to ensure their actions will do no harm to the patient.

Do not resuscitate (DNR) order: A type of advance directive that protects a patient's right to refuse efforts for resuscitation; also known as a *do not attempt resuscitation* (DNAR) order.

DOTS: A mnemonic to help remember what to look for during the physical exam; the initials stand for deformities, open injuries, tenderness and swelling.

Draw sheet: A method of moving a patient from a bed to a stretcher or vice-versa by using the stretcher's bottom sheet.

Dressing: A pad placed directly over a wound to absorb blood and other body fluids and to prevent infection.

Droplet transmission: Mode of transmission of pathogens that occurs when a person inhales droplets from an infected person's cough or sneeze; also known as respiratory droplet transmission.

Dropping: "Engagement" or "lightening"; when the baby drops into a lower position and is engaged in the mother's pelvis; usually takes place a few weeks before labor begins.

Drowning: An event in which a victim experiences respiratory impairment due to submersion in water. Drowning may or may not result in death.

Drowning victim—active: Someone who is vertical in the water but has no supporting kick, is unable to move forward and cannot call out for help.

Drowning victim—passive: Someone who is not moving and is floating either face-up or face-down, on or near the surface of the water, or is submerged.

Drug: Any substance, other than food, intended to affect the functions of the body.

DuoDote™: A type of kit with pre-measured doses of antidote used to counteract the effects of nerve agents.

Durable power of attorney for health care: A legal document that expresses a patient's specific wishes regarding his or her health care; also empowers an individual, usually a relative or friend, to speak on behalf of the patient should he or she become seriously injured or ill and unable to speak for him- or herself.

Duty to act: A legal responsibility of some individuals to provide a reasonable standard of emergency care.

Echo method: A communication technique in which the listener repeats orders word for word to ensure the message was heard and understood accurately.

Eclampsia: A complication during pregnancy in which the patient has convulsions or seizures associated with high blood pressure.

Ectopic pregnancy: A pregnancy outside of the uterus; most often occurs in the fallopian tubes.

Edema: Swelling in body tissues caused by fluid accumulation.

Elastic bandage: A bandage designed to keep continuous pressure on a body part; also called an *elastic wrap*.

Elder abuse: Action that results in the physical or psychological harm of an elderly person; can be physical, sexual, verbal and/or emotional, usually on someone who is disabled or frail.

Elder neglect: A type of abuse in which a caregiver fails to provide the necessary care to an elderly person.

Electrical burn: A burn caused by contact with an electrical source, which allows an electrical current to pass through the body.

Electrocardiogram (ECG or EKG): A test that measures and records the electrical activity of the heart.

Electrolytes: Substances that are electrically conductive in solution and are essential to the regulation of nerve and muscle function and fluid balance throughout the body; include sodium, potassium, chloride, calcium and phosphate.

Embolism: A blockage in an artery or a vein caused by a blood clot or fragment of plaque that travels through the blood vessels until it gets stuck, preventing blood flow.

Embryo: The term used to describe the early stage of development in the uterus, from fertilization to the beginning of the third month.

Emergency medical dispatcher (EMD): A telecommunicator who has received special training for triaging a request for medical service and allocating appropriate resources to the scene of an incident, and for providing prearrival medical instructions to patients or bystanders before more advanced medical personnel arrive.

Emergency medical responder (EMR): A person trained in emergency medical care who may be called on to provide such care as a routine part of the job, paid or volunteer; often the first trained professional to respond to emergencies; formerly called "first responder."

Emergency medical services (EMS) system: A network of community resources and medical personnel that provides emergency medical care to people who are injured or suddenly fall ill.

Emergency medical technician (EMT): Someone who has successfully completed a state-approved EMT training program; EMTs take over care from EMRs and work on stabilizing and preparing the patient for transport; formerly referred to as EMT-Basic.

Emergency oxygen: Oxygen delivered to a patient from an oxygen cylinder through a delivery device; can be given to a nonbreathing or breathing patient who is not receiving adequate oxygen from the environment.

Emergency Response Guidebook: A resource available from the U.S. *Department of Transportation* (DOT) to help identify hazardous materials and appropriate care for those exposed to them.

Emphysema: A chronic, degenerative lung disease in which there is damage to the alveoli.

Endocrine system: A group of organs and other structures that regulates and coordinates the activities of other systems by producing chemicals (hormones) that influence tissue activity.

Engineering controls: Control measures that eliminate, isolate or remove a hazard from the workplace; things used in the workplace to help reduce the risk of an exposure.

Epidemiology: A branch of medicine that deals with the incidence (rate of occurrence) and prevalence (extent) of disease in populations.

Epidermis: The outer layer of the skin; provides a barrier to bacteria and other organisms that can cause infection.

Epiglottitis: A serious bacterial infection that causes severe swelling of the epiglottis, which can result in a blocked airway, causing respiratory failure in children; may be fatal.

Epilepsy: A brain disorder characterized by recurrent seizures.

Ethics: A branch of philosophy concerned with the set of moral principles a person holds about what is right and wrong.

Evaporation: One of the ways the body loses heat; occurs when the body is wet and the moisture evaporates, cooling the skin.

Evisceration: A severe injury that causes the abdominal organs to protrude through the wound.

Exposure: An instance in which someone is exposed to a pathogen or has contact with blood or body fluids or objects in the environment that contain disease-causing agents.

Exposure control plan: Plan in the workplace that outlines the employer's protective measures to eliminate or minimize employee exposure incidents.

Expressed consent: Permission to receive emergency care granted by a competent adult either verbally, nonverbally or through gestures.

External bleeding: Bleeding on the outside of the body; often, visible bleeding.

Extremity: A limb of the body; *upper extremity* is the arm; *lower extremity* is the leg.

Extremity lift: A two-responder, non-emergency lift in which one responder supports the patient's arms and the other the patient's legs.

Extrication: The safe and appropriate removal of a patient trapped in a motor vehicle or a dangerous situation.

Fainting: Temporary loss of consciousness; usually related to temporary insufficient blood flow to the brain; also known as *syncope*, "blacking out" or "passing out."

FAST: An acronym to help remember the symptoms of stroke; stands for **F**ace, **A**rm, **S**peech and **T**ime.

Febrile seizure: Seizure activity brought on by an excessively high fever in a young child or an infant.

Fetal monitoring: A variety of tests used to measure fetal stress, either internally or externally.

Fetus: The term used to describe the stage of development in the uterus after the embryo stage, beginning at the start of the third month.

Fever: An elevated body temperature, beyond normal variation.

Finger sweep: A method of clearing the mouth of foreign material that presents a risk of blocking the airway or being aspirated into the lungs.

Firefighter's carry: A type of carry during which the patient is supported over the responder's shoulders.

Firefighter's drag: A method of moving a patient in which the patient is bound to the responder's neck and held underneath the responder; the responder moves the patient by crawling.

Flail chest: A serious injury in which multiple rib fractures result in a loose section of ribs that does not move normally with the rest of the chest during breathing and often moves in the *opposite* direction.

Flammability: The degree to which a substance may ignite.

Flowmeter: A device used to regulate, in *liters per minute* (LPM), the amount of oxygen administered to a patient.

Focused medical assessment: A physical exam on a *medical* patient, focused only on the area of the chief complaint, e.g., the chest in a patient complaining of chest pain.

Focused trauma assessment: A physical exam on a *trauma* patient, focused only on an isolated area with a known injury such as a hand with an obvious laceration.

Foreign body airway obstruction (FBAO): The presence of foreign matter, such as food, that obstructs the airway.

Fracture: A break or disruption in bone tissue.

Free diving: An extreme sport in which divers compete under water without any underwater breathing apparatus.

Frostbite: A condition in which body tissues freeze; most commonly occurs in the fingers, toes, ears and nose.

Full-thickness burn: A burn injury involving all layers of skin and underlying tissues; skin may be brown or charred, and underlying tissues may appear white; also referred to as a *third-degree burn.*

Generalized tonic clonic seizures: Seizures that affect most or all of the brain; types include petit mal and grand mal seizures.

Genitourinary system: A group of organs and other structures that eliminates waste and enables reproduction.

Gestational diabetes: A type of diabetes that occurs only during pregnancy.

Glasgow Coma Scale (GCS): A measure of LOC based on eye opening, verbal response and motor response.

Glucose: A simple sugar that is the primary source of energy for the body's tissues.

Golden Hour: A term sometimes used to describe the first hour after a life-threatening traumatic injury; providing early interventions and advanced medical care during this time frame can result in the best chance of survival.

Good Samaritan laws: Laws that apply in some circumstances to protect people who provide emergency care without accepting anything in return.

Grand mal seizures: A type of generalized seizure; involves whole body contractions with loss of consciousness.

Hallucination: Perception of an object with no reality; occurs when a person is awake and conscious; may be visual, auditory or tactile.

Hallucinogen: A substance that affects mood, sensation, thinking, emotion and self-awareness; alters perceptions of time and space; and produces hallucinations or delusions.

Hard-of-hearing: A degree of hearing loss that is mild enough to allow the person to continue to rely on hearing for communication.

Hazardous material (HAZMAT): Any chemical substance or material that can pose a threat or risk to health, safety and property if not properly handled or contained.

Hazardous materials (HAZMAT) incident: Any situation that deals with the unplanned release of hazardous materials.

Head-on collision: A collision in which a vehicle hits an object, such as a tree or other vehicle, straight on.

Head-tilt/chin-lift technique: A common method for opening the airway unless the patient is suspected of having an injury to the head, neck or spine.

Health care proxy: A person named in a health-care directive, or durable power of attorney for health care, who can make medical decisions on someone else's behalf.

Heart: A fist-sized muscular organ that pumps blood throughout the body.

Heat cramps: A form of heat-related illness; painful involuntary muscle spasms that occur during or after physical exertion in high heat, caused by loss of electrolytes and water from perspiration; may be a sign that a more serious heat-related illness is developing; usually affects the legs and abdomen.

Heat exhaustion: More severe form of heat-related illness; results when fluid and electrolytes are lost through perspiration and are not replaced by other fluids; often results from strenuous work or wearing too much clothing in a hot, humid environment.

Heat index: An index that combines the air temperature and relative humidity to determine the perceived, human-felt temperature; a measure of how hot it feels.

Heat stroke: The most serious form of heat-related illness; life threatening and develops when the body's cooling mechanisms are overwhelmed and body systems begin to fail.

Hematoma: A mass of usually clotted or partially clotted blood that forms in soft tissue space or an organ as a result of ruptured blood vessels.

Hemodialysis: A common method of treating advanced kidney failure in which blood is filtered outside the body to remove wastes and extra fluids.

Hemopneumothorax: An accumulation of blood and air between the lungs and chest wall.

Hemorrhage: The loss of a large amount of blood in a short time or when there is continuous bleeding.

Hemorrhagic shock: Shock due to excessive blood loss.

Hemostatic agent: A method of external hemorrhage control that uses a substance that absorbs or adsorbs moisture from blood and speeds the process of coagulation and clot

formation to achieve hemostasis (control of bleeding).

Hemothorax: An accumulation of blood between the lungs and chest wall; caused by bleeding that may be from the chest wall, lung tissue or major blood vessels in the thorax.

Hepatitis: An inflammation of the liver most commonly caused by viral infection; there are several types including hepatitis A, B, C, D and E.

High-order explosives (HE): Explosives such as TNT, nitroglycerin, etc., that produce a defining supersonic over-pressurization shockwave.

HIV: A virus that weakens the body's immune system, leading to life-threatening infections; causes AIDS.

Homeostasis: A constant state of balance or well-being of the body's internal systems that is continually and automatically adjusted.

Hospice care: Care provided in the final months of life to a terminally ill patient.

Hot zone: Also called the *exclusion zone*, this is the area in which the most danger exists from a HAZMAT incident.

Hyperglycemia: A condition in which too much sugar is in the bloodstream, resulting in higher than normal BGLs; also known as *high blood glucose*.

Hyperkalemia: Abnormally high levels of potassium in the blood; if extremely high, can cause cardiac arrest and death.

Hyperoxia: A condition in which an excess of oxygen reaches the body's cells.

Hypertension: Another term for high blood pressure.

Hyperthermia: Overheating of the body; includes heat cramps, heat exhaustion and heat stroke.

Hyperventilation: Rapid, deep or shallow breathing; usually caused by panic or anxiety.

Hypervolemia: A condition in which there is an abnormal increase of fluid in the blood.

Hypodermis: A deeper layer of skin, located below the epidermis and dermis, that contains fat, blood vessels and connective tissues.

Hypoglycemia: A condition in which too little sugar is in the bloodstream, resulting in lower than normal BGLs; also known as *low blood glucose*.

Hypoperfusion: A life-threatening condition in which the circulatory system fails to adequately circulate oxygenated blood to all parts of the body; also referred to as *shock*.

Hypotension: Abnormally low blood pressure.

Hypothalamus: Control center of the body's temperature; located in the brain.

Hypothermia: The state of the body being colder than the usual core temperature, caused by either excessive loss of body heat and/or the body's inability to produce heat.

Hypovolemia: A condition in which there is an abnormal decrease of fluid in the blood.

Hypovolemic shock: A type of shock caused by an abnormal decrease in blood volume.

Hypoxemia: A condition in which there are decreased levels of oxygen in the blood; can disrupt the body's functioning and harm tissues; may be life threatening.

Hypoxia: A condition in which insufficient oxygen is delivered to the body's cells.

Hypoxic: Having below-normal concentrations of oxygen in the organs and tissues of the body.

Immediate care (Red): A triage category of those involved in a MCI whose needs require urgent life-saving care.

Immobilize: To use a splint or other method to keep an injured body part from moving.

Immune system: The body's complex group of body systems that is responsible for fighting disease.

Impaled object: An object that remains embedded in an open wound; also referred to as an *embedded object*.

Implantable cardioverter-defibrillator (ICD): A miniature version of an AED, implanted under the skin, that acts to automatically recognize and help correct abnormal heart rhythms.

Implantation: The attachment of the fertilized egg to the lining of the uterus, 6 or 7 days after conception.

Implied consent: Legal concepts that assume a patient would consent to receive emergency care if he or she were physically able or old enough to do so.

In good faith: Acting in such a way that the goal is only to help the patient and that all actions are for that purpose.

Incendiary weapons: Devices designed to burn at extremely high temperatures, such as napalm and white phosphorus; mostly designed to be used against equipment, though some (e.g. napalm) are designed to be used against people.

Incident Command System (ICS): A standardized, on-scene, all-hazards incident management approach that allows for the integration of facilities, equipment, personnel, procedures and communications operating within a common organizational structure; enables a coordinated response among various jurisdictions and functional agencies, both public and private; and establishes common processes for planning and managing resources.

Indirect contact: Mode of transmission of a disease caused by touching a contaminated object.

Indirect force: A force that transmits energy through the body, causing injury at a distance from the point of impact.

Indirect medical control: A type of medical direction, also called "off-line," "retrospective" or "prospective" medical control; this type of medical direction includes education, protocol review and quality improvement for emergency care providers.

Infant: For the purpose of providing emergency medical care, anyone who appears to be younger than about 1 year of age.

Infection: A condition caused by disease-producing microorganisms, called pathogens or germs, in the body.

Infectious disease: Disease caused by the invasion of the body by a pathogen, such as a bacterium, virus, fungus or parasite.

Ingested poison: A poison that is swallowed.

Inhalant: A substance, such as a medication, that a person inhales to counteract or prevent a specific condition; also a substance inhaled to produce mood-altering effects.

Inhaled poison: A poison breathed into the lungs.

Injected poison: A poison that enters the body through a bite, sting or syringe.

In-line stabilization: A technique used to minimize movement and align the patient's head and neck with the spine.

Innate immunity: The type of protection from disease that humans are born with.

Insulin: A hormone produced by the pancreas to help glucose move into the cells; in patients with diabetes, it may not be produced at all or may not be produced in sufficient amounts.

Integumentary system: A group of organs and other structures that protects the body, retains fluids and helps to prevent infection.

Intercostal: Located between the ribs.

Internal bleeding: Bleeding inside the body.

Jaw-thrust (without head extension) maneuver: A maneuver for opening the airway in a patient suspected of having an injury to the head, neck or spine.

Joint: A structure where two or more bones are joined.

Jump kit: A bag or box containing equipment used by the EMR when responding to a medical emergency; includes items such as resuscitation masks and airway adjuncts, gloves, blood pressure cuffs and bandages.

Kinematics of trauma: The science of the forces involved in traumatic events and how they damage the body.

Labor: The birth process, beginning with the contraction of the uterus and dilation of the cervix and ending with the stabilization and recovery of the mother.

Laceration: A cut, usually from a sharp object, that can have either jagged or smooth edges.

Landing zone (LZ): A term from military jargon used to describe any area where an aircraft, such as an air medical helicopter, can land safely.

Legal obligation: Obligation to act in a particular way in accordance with the law.

Level of consciousness (LOC): A person's state of awareness, ranging from being fully alert to unconscious; also referred to as mental status.

Licensure: Required acknowledgment that the bearer has permission to practice in the licensing state; offers the highest level of public protection; may be revoked at the state level should the bearer no longer meet the required standards.

Ligament: A fibrous band that holds bones together at a joint.

Litter: A portable stretcher used to carry a patient over rough terrain.

Lividity: Purplish color in the lowest-lying parts of a recently dead body, caused by pooling of blood.

Living will: A type of advance directive that outlines the patient's wishes about certain kinds of medical treatments and procedures that prolong life.

Local credentialing: Local requirements EMRs must meet in order to maintain employment or obtain certain protocols so that they may practice.

Log roll: A method of moving a patient while keeping the patient's body aligned because of a suspected head, neck or spinal injury.

Low-order explosives (LE): Explosives such as pipe bombs, gunpowder, etc., that create a subsonic explosion.

Malpractice: A situation in which a professional fails to provide a reasonable quality of care, resulting in harm to a patient.

Mania: An aspect of bipolar disorder characterized by elation, hyperexcitability and accelerated thoughts, speech and actions.

Manual stabilization: A technique used to achieve spinal motion restriction by manually supporting the patient's head and neck in the position found *without* the use of any equipment.

Mark I™ Kit: A type of kit with pre-measured doses of antidote to counteract the effects of nerve agents.

Material Safety Data Sheet (MSDS): A sheet (provided by the manufacturer) that identifies the substance, physical properties and any associated hazards for a given material (e.g., fire, explosion and health hazards), as well as emergency first aid.

Mechanism of injury: The force or energy that causes a traumatic injury (e.g., a fall, explosion, crash or attack).

Meconium aspiration: Aspiration of the first bowel movement of the newborn; can be a sign of fetal stress and can lead to meconium aspiration syndrome.

Medical control: Direction given to EMRs by a physician when EMRs are providing care at the scene of an emergency or are en-route to the receiving facility; may be provided either directly via radio or indirectly by pre-established local medical treatment protocols.

Medical direction: The monitoring of care provided by out-of-hospital providers to injured or ill persons, usually by a medical director.

Medical director: A physician who assumes responsibility for the care of injured or ill persons provided in out-of-hospital settings.

Medical futility: A situation in which a patient has a medical or traumatic condition that is scientifically accepted to be futile should resuscitation be attempted and, therefore, the patient should be considered dead on arrival.

Meningitis: An inflammation of the meninges, the thin, protective coverings over the brain and spinal cord; caused by virus or bacteria.

Mental illness: A range of medical conditions that affect a person's mood or ability to think, feel, relate to others and function in everyday activities.

Metabolism: The physical and chemical processes of converting oxygen and food into energy within the body.

Methicillin-resistant *Staphylococcus aureus* (MRSA): A Staph bacterium that can cause infection; difficult to treat because of its resistance to many antibiotics.

Midaxillary line: An imaginary line that passes vertically down the body starting at the axilla (armpit); used to locate one of the areas for listening to breath sounds.

Midclavicular line: An imaginary line that passes through the midpoint of the clavicle (collarbone) on the ventral surface of the body; used to locate one of the areas for listening to breath sounds.

Midscapular line: An imaginary line that passes through the midpoint of the scapula (shoulder blade) on the dorsal surface of the body; used to locate one of the areas for listening to breath sounds.

Minimum data set: A standardized set of details about patients; this information is included in the *prehospital care report* (PCR).

Minute volume: The amount of air breathed in a minute; calculated by multiplying the volume of air inhaled at each breath (in mL) by the number of breaths per minute.

Miscarriage: A spontaneous end to pregnancy before the 20th week; usually because of birth defects in the fetus or placenta; also called a *spontaneous abortion*.

Moral obligation: Obligation to act in a particular way in accordance with what is considered morally right.

Morals: Principles relating to issues of right and wrong and how individual people should behave.

Morbidity: Illness; effects of a condition or disease.

Mortality: Death due to a certain condition or disease.

Mucous plug: A collection of mucus that blocks the opening into the cervix and is expelled, usually toward the end of the pregnancy, when the cervix begins to dilate.

Multidrug-resistant tuberculosis (MDR TB): A type of *tuberculosis* (TB) that is resistant to some of the most effective anti-TB drugs.

Multiple- (or mass-) casualty incident (MCI): An incident that generates more patients than available resources can manage using routine procedures.

Multiple birth: Two or more births in the same pregnancy.

Muscle: A tissue that contracts and relaxes to create movement.

Musculoskeletal system: A group of tissues and other structures that supports the body, protects internal organs, allows movement, stores minerals, manufactures blood cells and creates heat.

Myocardial infarction (MI): The death of cardiac muscle tissue due to a sudden deprivation of circulating blood; also called a heart attack.

Narcotic: A drug derived from opium or opium-like compounds; used to reduce pain and can alter mood and behavior.

Nasal (nasopharyngeal) airway (NPA): An airway adjunct inserted through the nostril and into the throat to help keep the tongue from obstructing the airway; may be used on a conscious or an unconscious patient.

Nasal cannula: A device used to administer emergency oxygen through the nostrils to a breathing person.

National Response Framework (NRF): The guiding principles that enable all response partners to prepare for and provide a unified national response to disasters and emergencies—from the smallest incident to the largest catastrophe. The *Framework* establishes a comprehensive, national, all-hazards approach to domestic incident response.

Nature of illness: The medical condition or complaint for which the person needs care (e.g., shock, difficulty breathing), based on what the patient or others report as well as clues in the environment.

Needlestick: A penetrating wound from a needle or other sharp object; may result in exposure to pathogens through contact with blood or other body fluids.

Negligence: The failure to provide the level of care a person of similar training would provide, thereby causing injury or damage to another.

Nerve agents: Toxic chemical warfare agents that interrupt the chemical function of nerves.

Nervous system: A group of organs and other structures that regulates all body functions.

Neurogenic/vasogenic shock: A type of distributive shock caused by trauma to the spinal cord or brain, where the blood vessel walls abnormally constrict and dilate, preventing relay of messages and causing blood to pool at the lowest point of the body.

Next of kin: The closest relatives, as defined by state law, of a deceased person; usually the spouse and nearest blood relatives.

Non-rebreather mask: A type of oxygen mask used to administer high concentrations of oxygen to a breathing person.

Non-swimming rescues and assists: Rescues and assists that can be performed from a pool deck, pier or shoreline by reaching, using an extremity or object, by throwing a floating object or by standing in the water to provide either of these assists; performed instead of swimming out to the person in distress.

Normal sinus rhythm (NSR): The normal, regular rhythm of the heart, set by the SA node in the right atrium of the heart.

Obstetric pack: A first aid kit containing items especially helpful in emergency delivery and initial care after birth; items can include personal protective equipment, towels, clamps, ties, sterile scissors and bulb syringes.

Obstructive shock: A type of shock caused by any obstruction to blood flow, usually within the blood vessels, such as a pulmonary embolism.

Occlusive dressing: A special type of dressing that does not allow air or fluid to pass through.

Occupational Safety and Health Administration (OSHA): Federal agency whose role is to promote the safety and health of American workers by setting and enforcing standards; providing training, outreach and education; establishing partnerships; and encouraging continual process improvement in workplace safety and health.

Ongoing assessment: The process of repeating the primary assessment and physical exam while continually monitoring the patient; performed while awaiting the arrival of more highly trained personnel or while transporting the patient.

Open fracture: A type of fracture in which there is an open wound in the skin over the fracture.

Open wound: A wound resulting in a break in the skin's surface.

Opportunistic infections: Infections that strike people whose immune systems are weakened.

OPQRST: Mnemonic to help remember the questions used to gain information about pain; the initials stand for onset, provoke, quality, region/radiate, severity and time.

Oral (oropharyngeal) airway (OPA): An airway adjunct inserted through the mouth and into the throat to help keep the tongue from obstructing the airway; used *only* with unconscious patients.

Organ: A structure of similar tissues acting together to perform specific body functions.

"O-ring" gasket: Plastic, O-shaped ring that makes the seal of the pressure regulator on an oxygen cylinder tight; can be a built-in or an attachable piece.

Overdose: The use of an excessive amount of a substance, resulting in adverse reactions ranging from mania (mental and physical hyperactivity) and hysteria, to coma and death.

Oxygen cylinder: A steel or alloy cylinder that contains 100 percent oxygen under high pressure.

Oxygenation: The addition of oxygen to the body; also, the treatment of a patient with oxygen.

Pacemaker: A device implanted under the skin, sometimes below the right collarbone, to help regulate heartbeat in someone with a weak heart, a heart that skips beats or one that beats too fast or too slow.

Packaging: The process of getting a patient ready to be transferred safely from the scene to an ambulance or a helicopter.

Pack-strap carry: A type of carry in which the patient is supported upright, across the responder's back.

Palpation: Examination performed by feeling part of the body, especially feeling for a pulse.

Pandemic influenza: A respiratory illness caused by virulent human influenza A virus; spreads easily and sustainably and can cause global outbreaks of serious illness in humans.

Panic: A symptom of an anxiety disorder, characterized by episodes of intense fear and physical symptoms such as chest pain, heart palpitations, shortness of breath and dizziness.

Paradoxical breathing: An abnormal type of breathing that can occur with chest injury; one area of the chest moves in the opposite direction to the rest of the chest.

Paramedic: Someone with more in-depth training than AEMTs and who can perform all of the former's duties plus has additional knowledge of performing physical exams; may also perform more invasive procedures than any other prehospital care provider; formerly referred to as EMT-Paramedic.

Paranoia: A condition characterized by feelings of persecution and exaggerated notions of perceived threat; may be part of many mental health disorders and is rarely seen in isolation.

Parenchyma: Tissue that is involved in the functioning of a structure or organ as opposed to its supporting structures.

Partial seizures: Seizures that affect only part of the brain; may be simple or complex.

Partial-thickness burn: A burn injury involving the epidermis and dermis, characterized by red, wet skin and blisters; also referred to as a *second-degree burn*.

Passive immunity: The type of immunity gained from external sources such as from a mother's breast milk to an infant.

Pathogen: A term used to describe a germ; a disease-causing agent (e.g., bacterium or virus).

Pathophysiology: The study of the abnormal changes in mechanical, physical and biochemical functions caused by an injury or illness.

Patient narrative: A section on the prehospital care report where the assessment and care provided to the patient are described.

Patient's best interest: A fundamental ethical principle that refers to the provision of competent care, with compassion and respect for human dignity.

Pediatric Assessment Triangle: A quick initial assessment of a child that involves observation of the child's appearance, breathing and skin.

Penetrating trauma: An injury in which a person is struck by or falls onto an object that penetrates or cuts through the skin, resulting in an open wound or wounds, the severity of which is determined by the path of the object (e.g., a bullet wound).

Percussion: A technique of tapping on the surface of the body and listening to the resulting sounds, to learn about the condition of the area beneath.

Perfusion: The circulation of blood through the body or through a particular body part for the purpose of exchanging oxygen and nutrients with carbon dioxide and other wastes.

Peritoneal dialysis: A method of treatment for kidney failure in which waste products and extra fluid are drawn into a solution which has been injected into the abdominal cavity and are withdrawn through a catheter.

Peritoneum: The membrane that lines the abdominal cavity and covers most of the abdominal organs.

Personal protective equipment (PPE): All specialized clothing, equipment and supplies that keep the user from directly contacting infected materials; includes gloves, gowns, masks, shields and protective eyewear.

Phobia: A type of anxiety disorder characterized by strong, irrational fears of objects or situations that are usually harmless; may trigger an anxiety or panic attack.

Physical exam: Exam performed after the primary assessment; used to gather additional information and identify signs and symptoms of injury and illness.

Physiology: How living organisms function (e.g., movement and reproduction).

Placenta: An organ attached to the uterus and unborn baby through which nutrients are delivered; expelled after the baby is delivered.

Placenta previa: Placental implantation that occurs lower on the uterine wall, touching or covering the cervix; can be dangerous if it is still covering part of the cervix at the time of delivery.

Pleural space: The space between the lungs and chest wall.

Pneumonia: A lung infection caused by a virus or bacterium that results in a cough, fever and difficulty breathing.

Pneumothorax: Collapse of a lung due to pressure on it caused by air in the chest cavity.

Poison: Any substance that can cause injury, illness or death when introduced into the body, especially by chemical means.

Poison Control Center (PCC): A specialized health center that provides information on poisons and suspected poisoning emergencies.

Position of comfort: The position a patient naturally assumes when feeling ill or in pain; the position depends on the mechanism of the injury or nature of the illness.

Positive pressure ventilation: An artificial means of forcing air or oxygen into the lungs of a person who has stopped breathing or has inadequate breathing.

Post-ictal phase: The final phase of a generalized seizure, during which the patient becomes extremely fatigued.

Power grip: A hand position for lifting that requires the full surface of the palms and fingers to come in contact with the object being lifted.

Power lift: A lift technique that provides a stable move for the patient and protects the person lifting from serious injury.

Pralidoxime chloride (Protopam Chloride; 2-PAM Cl): A drug contained in antidote kits used to counteract the effects of nerve agents, commonly called *2-PAM chloride*.

Preeclampsia: A type of toxemia that occurs during pregnancy; a condition characterized by high blood pressure and excess protein in the urine after the 20th week of pregnancy.

Prehospital care: Emergency medical care provided before a patient arrives at a hospital or medical facility.

Prehospital care report (PCR): A document filled out for all emergency calls; used to keep medical personnel informed so they can provide appropriate continuity of care; also serves as a record for legal and billing purposes; may be written or electronic; if electronic, it is then an E-PCR.

Premature birth: Birth that occurs before the end of the 37th week of pregnancy.

Pressure bandage: A bandage applied snugly to create pressure on a wound, to aid in controlling bleeding.

Pressure points: Sites on the body where pressure can be applied to major arteries to slow the flow of blood to a body part.

Pressure regulator: A device on an oxygen cylinder that reduces the delivery pressure of the oxygen to a safe level.

Primary (initial) assessment: A check for conditions that are an immediate threat to a patient's life.

Primary effects: In referring to explosive and incendiary devices, the effects of the impact of the over-pressurization wave from high-order explosives on body surfaces.

Prolapsed cord: A complication of childbirth in which a loop of the umbilical cord protrudes through the vagina before delivery of the baby.

Protocols: Standardized procedures to be followed when providing care to injured or ill persons.

Pulmonary embolism: Sudden blockage of an artery in the lung; can be fatal.

Pulse: The beat felt from each rhythmic contraction of the heart.

Pulse oximetry: A test to measure the percentage of oxygen saturation in the blood using a pulse oximeter.

Puncture/penetration: A type of wound that results when the skin is pierced with a pointed object.

Rabies: An infectious viral disease that affects the nervous system of humans and other mammals; has a high fatality rate if left untreated.

Radiation: One of the ways the body loses heat; heat radiates out of the body, especially from the head and neck.

Radiation burn: A burn caused by exposure to radiation, either nuclear (e.g., radiation therapy) or solar (e.g., radiation from the sun).

Rales: An abnormal breath sound; a popping, clicking, bubbling or rattling sound, also known as *crackles*.

Rape: Non-consensual sexual intercourse often performed using force, threat or violence.

Rape-trauma syndrome: The three stages a victim typically goes through following a rape: acute, outward adjustment and resolution; a common response to rape.

Rapid medical assessment: A term describing a quick, head-to-toe exam of a medical patient.

Rapid trauma assessment: A term describing a quick, head-to-toe exam of a trauma patient.

Rappelling: The act of descending (as from a cliff) by sliding down a rope passed under one thigh, across the body and over the opposite shoulder or through a special friction device.

Reaching assist: A method of rescuing someone in the water by using an object to extend the rescuer's reach or by reaching with an arm or leg.

Reactivity: The degree to which a substance may react when exposed to other substances.

Reasonable force: The minimal force necessary to keep a patient from harming him- or herself or others.

Recovery position: A posture used to help maintain a clear airway in an unresponsive, breathing patient..

Refusal of care: The declining of care by a competent patient; a patient has the right to refuse the care of anyone who responds to an emergency scene.

Respiratory arrest: A condition in which there is an absence of breathing.

Respiratory distress: A condition in which a person is having difficulty breathing or requires extra effort to breathe.

Respiratory failure: Condition in which the respiratory system fails in oxygenation and/or carbon dioxide elimination; the respiratory system is beginning to shut down; the person may alternate between being agitated and sleepy.

Respiratory rate: The number of breaths per minute; normal rates vary by age and other factors.

Respiratory shock: A type of shock caused by the failure of the lungs to transfer sufficient oxygen into the bloodstream; occurs with respiratory distress or arrest.

Respiratory system: A group of organs and other structures that brings air into the body and removes wastes through a process called breathing, or respiration.

Restraint: A method of limiting a patient's movements, usually by physical means such as a padded cloth strap; may also be achieved by chemical means, such as medication.

Resuscitation mask: A pliable, dome-shaped breathing device that fits over the mouth and nose; used to provide artificial ventilations and administer emergency oxygen.

Retraction: A visible sinking in of soft tissue between the ribs of a child or an infant.

Reye's syndrome: An illness brought on by high fever that affects the brain and other internal organs; can be caused by the use of aspirin in children and infants.

Rhonchi: An abnormal breath sound when breathing that can often be heard without a stethoscope; a snoring or coarse, dry rale sound.

Rigid splint: A splint made of rigid material such as wood, aluminum or plastic.

Risk factors: Conditions or behaviors that increase the chance that a person will develop a disease.

Roller bandage: A bandage made of gauze or gauze-like material that is wrapped around a body part, over a dressing, using overlapping turns until the dressing is covered.

Rollover: A collision in which the vehicle rolls over.

Rotational impact: A collision in which the impact occurs off center and causes the vehicle to rotate until it either loses speed or strikes another object.

Rule of Nines: A method for estimating the extent of a burn; divides the body into 11 surface areas, each of which comprises approximately 9 percent of the body, plus the genitals, which are approximately 1 percent.

"Rule of thumb": A guideline for positioning oneself far enough away from a scene involving HAZMAT: one's thumb, pointing up at arm's length, should cover the hazardous area from your view.

Run data: A section on the PCR where information about the incident is documented.

SAMPLE history: A way to gather important information about the patient, using the mnemonic SAMPLE; the initials stand for signs and symptoms, allergies, medications, pertinent past medical history, last oral intake and events leading up to the incident.

Schizophrenia: A chronic mental illness in which the person hears voices or feels that his or her thoughts are being controlled by others; can cause hallucinations, delusions, disordered thinking, movement disorders and social withdrawal.

Scope of practice: The range of duties and skills that are allowed and expected to be performed when necessary, according to the professional's level of training, while using reasonable care and skill.

Secondary assessment: A head-to-toe physical exam as well as the focused history; completed following the primary assessment and management of any life-threatening conditions.

Secondary effects: In referring to explosive and incendiary devices, the impact of flying debris and bomb fragments against any body part.

Seizure: Temporary abnormal electrical activity in the brain caused by injury, disease, fever, infection, metabolic disturbances or conditions that decrease oxygen levels.

Self-mutilation: Self-injury; deliberate harm to one's own body used as an unhealthy coping mechanism to deal with overwhelming negative emotions.

Self-splint: A splint formed by supporting one part of the body with another; also called an *anatomic splint*.

Sepsis: A life-threatening illness in which the body is overwhelmed by its response to infection; commonly referred to as *blood poisoning*.

Septic shock: A type of distributive shock that occurs when an infection has spread to the point that bacteria are releasing toxins into the bloodstream, causing blood pressure to drop when the tissues become damaged from the circulating toxins.

Service animal: A guide dog, signal dog or other animal individually trained to provide assistance to a person with a disability.

Severe acute respiratory syndrome (SARS): A viral respiratory illness caused by the *SARS-associated coronavirus* (SARS-CoV).

Sexual assault: Any form of sexualized contact with another person without consent and performed using force, coercion or threat.

Shaken baby syndrome: A type of abuse in which a young child has been shaken harshly, causing swelling of the brain and brain damage.

Shipping papers: Documents drivers must carry by law when transporting hazardous materials; list the names, possible associated dangers and four-digit identification numbers of the substances.

Shock: A life-threatening condition that occurs when the circulatory system fails to provide adequate oxygenated blood to all parts of the body; also referred to as *hypoperfusion*.

Shoulder drag: A type of emergency move that is a variation of the clothes drag.

Shunt: A surgically created passage between two natural body channels, such as an artery and a vein, to allow the flow of fluid.

Side-impact collision: A collision in which the impact is at the side of the vehicle; also known as a *broadside* or *t-bone collision*.

Signs: Term used to describe any observable evidence of injury or illness, such as bleeding or unusual skin color.

Signs of life: A term sometimes used to describe breathing and a pulse in an unresponsive patient.

Silent heart attack: A heart attack during which the patient has either no symptoms or very mild symptoms that the person does not associate with heart attacks; mild symptoms include indigestion or sweating.

Simple access: In an extrication, the process of getting to the patient without the use of equipment.

Simple partial seizures: Seizures in which a specific body part experiences muscle contractions; does not affect memory or awareness.

Simple Triage and Rapid Transport (START): A method of triage that allows quick assessment and prioritization of injured people.

Sinoatrial (SA) node: A cluster of cells in the right atrium that generates the electrical impulses that set the pace of the heart's natural rhythm.

Smooth muscles: Muscles responsible for contraction of hollow organs such as blood vessels or the gastrointestinal tract.

Soft splint: A splint made of soft material such as towels, pillows, slings, swathes and cravats.

Soft tissues: Body structures that include the layers of skin, fat and muscles.

Sphygmomanometer: A device for measuring BP; also called a BP cuff.

Spinal column: The series of vertebrae extending from the base of the skull to the tip of the tailbone (coccyx); also referred to as the *spine*.

Spinal cord: A cylindrical structure extending from the base of the skull to the lower back, consisting mainly of nerve cells and protected by the spinal column.

Spinal motion restriction: A collective term that includes all methods and techniques used to limit the movement of the spinal column of a patient with a suspected spinal injury.

Splint: A device used to immobilize body parts.

Sprain: The partial or complete tearing or stretching of ligaments and other soft tissue structures at a joint.

Squat lift: A lift technique that is useful when one of the lifter's legs or ankles is weaker than the other.

Stabilization: The final stage of labor in which the mother begins to recover and stabilize after giving birth.

Staging area: Location established where resources can be placed while awaiting tactical assignment.

Stair chair: Equipment used for patient transport in a sitting position.

Standard of care: The criterion established for the extent and quality of an EMR's care.

Standard precautions: Safety measures, including BSI and universal precautions, taken to prevent occupational-risk exposure to blood or other potentially infectious materials; assumes that all body fluids, secretions and excretions (except sweat) are potentially infective.

Standing orders: Protocols issued by the medical director allowing specific skills to be performed or specific medications to be administered in certain situations.

Status asthmaticus: A potentially fatal episode of asthma in which the patient does not respond to usual inhaled medications.

Status epilepticus: An epileptic seizure (or repeated seizures) that lasts longer than 5 minutes without any sign of slowing down; should be considered life threatening and requires prompt advanced medical care.

Stethoscope: A device for listening, especially to the lungs, heart and abdomen; may be used together with a BP cuff to measure BP.

Stillbirth: Fetal death; death of a fetus after 20 weeks gestation or of a fetus weighing more than 350 grams.

Stimulant: A substance that affects the central nervous system and speeds up physical and mental activity.

Stoma: A surgical opening in the body; a stoma may be created in the neck following surgery on the trachea to allow the patient to breathe.

Strain: The excessive stretching and tearing of muscles or tendons; a pulled or torn muscle.

Stress: The body's normal response to any situation that changes a person's existing mental, physical or emotional balance.

Stretcher: Equipment used for patient transport in a supine position.

Stridor: An abnormal, high-pitched breath sound caused by a blockage in the throat or larynx; usually heard on inhalation.

Stroke: A disruption of blood flow to a part of the brain, which may cause permanent damage to brain tissue.

Subconjunctival hemorrhage: Broken blood vessels in the eyes.

Subcutaneous emphysema: A rare condition in which air gets into tissues under the skin that covers the chest wall or neck; may occur as a result of wounds to those areas.

Substance abuse: The deliberate, persistent, excessive use of a substance without regard to health concerns or accepted medical practices.

Substance misuse: The use of a substance for unintended purposes or for intended purposes but in improper amounts or doses.

Sucking chest wound: A chest wound in which an object, such as a knife or bullet, penetrates the chest wall and lung, allowing air to pass freely in and out of the chest cavity; breathing causes a sucking sound, hence the term.

Suctioning: The process of removing foreign matter, such as blood, other liquids or food particles, by means of a mechanical or manual suctioning device.

Sudden cardiac arrest: A condition where the heart's pumping action stops abruptly, usually due to abnormal heart rhythms called arrhythmias, most commonly V-fib; unless an effective heart rhythm is restored, death follows within a matter of minutes.

Sudden death: An unexpected, natural death; usually used to describe a death from a sudden cardiac event.

Sudden infant death syndrome (SIDS): The sudden death of an infant younger than 1 year that remains unexplained after the performance of a complete postmortem investigation, including an autopsy, an examination of the scene of death and a review of the care history.

Suicide: An intentional act to end one's own life, usually as a result of feeling there are no other options available to resolve one's problems.

Sundowning: A symptom of Alzheimer's disease in which the person becomes increasingly restless or confused as late afternoon or evening approaches.

Superficial burn: A burn injury involving only the top layer of skin, characterized by red, dry skin; also referred to as a *first-degree burn*.

Supine: The body position of lying flat on the back; used when the patient has suspected head, neck or spinal injuries.

Surrogate decision maker: A third party with the legal right to make decisions for another person regarding medical and health issues through a durable power of attorney for health care.

Swathe: A cloth wrapped around a patient to securely hold the arm against the patient's chest, to add stability; also called a *binder*.

Symptoms: What the patient reports experiencing, such as pain, nausea, headache or shortness of breath.

Syncope: A term used to describe the loss of consciousness; also known as *fainting*.

Synergistic effect: The outcome created when two or more drugs are combined; the effects of each may enhance those of the other.

Systolic blood pressure: The force exerted against the arteries when the heart is contracting.

Tendon: A fibrous band that attaches muscle to bone.

Tension pneumothorax: A life-threatening injury in which the lung is completely collapsed and air is trapped in the pleural space.

Tertiary effects: The results of individuals being thrown by the blast wind caused by explosive and incendiary devices; can involve any body part.

Tetanus: An acute infectious disease caused by a bacterium that produces a powerful poison; can occur in puncture wounds, such as human and animal bites; also called *lockjaw*.

Thoracic: Relating to the *thorax*, or chest cavity.

Thready: Used to describe a pulse that is barely perceptible, often rapid and feels like a fine thread.

Thrombus: A blood clot that forms in a blood vessel and remains there, slowing the flow of blood and depriving tissues of normal blood flow and oxygen.

Throwing assist: A method of rescuing someone in the water by throwing the person a floating object, with or without a line attached.

Tidal volume: The normal amount of air breathed at rest.

Tissue: A collection of similar cells acting together to perform specific body functions.

Tolerance: A condition in which the effects of a substance on the body decrease as a result of continued use.

Tonic phase: The second phase of a generalized seizure, during which the patient becomes unconscious and muscles become rigid.

Tourniquet: A tight, wide band placed around an arm or a leg to constrict blood vessels in order to stop blood flow to a wound.

Toxemia: An abnormal condition associated with the presence of toxic substances in the blood.

Toxicity: The degree to which a substance is poisonous or toxic.

Toxicology: The study of the adverse effects of chemical, physical or biological agents on the body.

Toxin: A poisonous substance produced by microorganisms that can cause certain diseases but is also capable of inducing neutralizing antibodies or antitoxins.

Traction splint: A splint with a mechanical device that applies traction to realign the bones.

Transdermal medication patch: A patch on the skin that delivers medication; commonly contains nitroglycerin, nicotine or other medications; should be removed prior to defibrillation.

Transferring: The responsibility of transporting a patient to an ambulance, as well as transferring information about the patient and incident to more advanced medical personnel who take over care.

Transient ischemic attack (TIA): A condition that produces stroke-like symptoms but causes no permanent damage; may be a precursor to a stroke.

Trauma alert criteria: An assessment system used by EMS providers to rapidly identify those patients determined to have sustained severe injuries that warrant immediate evacuation for specialized medical treatment; based on several factors including status of airway, breathing and circulation; Glasgow Coma Scale score; certain types of injuries present; and the patient's age; separate criteria for pediatric and adult patients.

Trauma dressing: A dressing used to cover very large wounds and multiple wounds in one body area; also called a *universal dressing*.

Trauma system: A system of definitive care facilities offering services within a region or community in various areas of medical expertise in order to care for injured individuals.

Traumatic asphyxia: Severe lack of oxygen due to trauma, usually caused by a thoracic injury.

Triage: A method of sorting patients into categories based on the urgency of their need for care.

Triage tags: A system of identifying patients during a MCI; different colored tags signify different levels of urgency for care.

Triangular bandage: A triangle-shaped bandage that can be rolled or folded to hold a dressing or splint in place; can also be used as a sling to support an injured shoulder, arm or hand.

Trimester: A three-month period; there are three trimesters in a normal pregnancy.

Tripod position: A position of comfort that a person may assume automatically when breathing becomes difficult; in a sitting position, the person leans slightly forward with outstretched arms, and hands resting on knees or an adjacent surface for support to aid breathing.

Tuberculosis (TB): A bacterial infection that usually attacks the lungs.

Twisting force: A force that causes injury when one part of the body remains still while the rest of the body is twisted or turns away from it.

Two-person seat carry: A non-emergency method of carrying a patient by creating a "seat" with the arms of two responders.

Type 1 diabetes: A type of diabetes in which the pancreas does not produce insulin; formerly known as *insulin-dependent diabetes* or *juvenile diabetes*.

Type 2 diabetes: A type of diabetes in which insufficient insulin is produced or the insulin is not used efficiently; formerly known as *non-insulin-dependent diabetes* or *adult-onset diabetes*.

Umbilical cord: A flexible structure that attaches the placenta to the fetus, allowing for the passage of blood, nutrients and waste.

Universal precautions: A set of precautions designed to prevent transmission of HIV, *hepatitis B virus* (HBV) and other bloodborne pathogens when providing care; considers blood and certain body fluids of all patients potentially infectious.

Uterus: A pear-shaped organ in a woman's pelvis in which an embryo forms and develops into a baby; also called the *womb*.

Vacuum splint: A splint that can be molded to the shape of the injured area by extracting air from the splint.

Vagina: Tract leading from the uterus to the outside of the body; often referred to during labor as the *birth canal*.

Vector-borne transmission: Transmission of a pathogen that occurs when an infectious source, such as an animal or insect bite or sting, penetrates the body's skin.

Vehicle stabilization: Steps taken to stabilize a motor vehicle in place so that it cannot move and cause further harm to patients or responders.

Veins: Blood vessels that carry oxygen-poor blood from all parts of the body to the heart, except for the pulmonary veins, which carry oxygen-rich blood to the heart from the lungs.

Ventilation: The exchange of air between the lungs and the atmosphere; allows for an exchange of oxygen and carbon dioxide in the lungs.

Ventricular fibrillation (V-fib): A life-threatening heart rhythm in which the heart is in a state of totally disorganized electrical activity.

Ventricular tachycardia (V-tach): A life-threatening heart rhythm in which there is very rapid contraction of the ventricles.

Vial of Life: A community service program that provides EMS personnel and other responders with vital health and medical information (including any advance directives) when a person, who suffers a medical emergency at home, is unable to speak; consists of a label affixed to the outside of the refrigerator to alert responders and a labeled vial or container that has pertinent medical information, a list of medications, health conditions and other pertinent medical information regarding the occupant(s).

Virus: A common type of pathogen that depends on other organisms to live and reproduce; can be difficult to kill.

Visual warning devices: Warning lights in an emergency vehicle that, used together with audible warning devices, alert other drivers of the vehicle's approach.

Vital organs: Those organs whose functions are essential to life, including the brain, heart and lungs.

Vital signs: Important information about the patient's condition obtained by checking respiratory rate, pulse and blood pressure.

Voluntary muscles: Muscles that attach to bones; also called *skeletal muscles*.

Wading assist: A method of rescuing someone in the water by wading out to the person in distress.

Walking assist: A method of assisting a patient to walk by supporting one of the patient's arms over the responder's shoulder (or each of the patient's arms over the shoulder of one responder on each side).

Walking wounded (Green): A triage category of those involved in an MCI who are able to walk by themselves to a designated area to await care.

Warm zone: Also called the *contamination reduction zone*; the area immediately outside the hot zone.

Wheezing: A high-pitched whistling sound heard during inhalation but heard most loudly on exhalation; an abnormal breath sound that can often be heard without a stethoscope.

Withdrawal: The condition of mental and physical discomfort produced when a person stops using or abusing a substance to which the person is addicted.

WMDs: Weapons of mass destruction.

Work practice controls: Control measures that reduce the likelihood of exposure by changing the way a task is carried out.

Wound: An injury to the soft tissues.

Sources

Alzheimer's Association, *Alzheimer's Fact and Figures 2010*, http://www.alz.org/documents_custom/report_alzfactsfigures2010.pdf. Accessed March 8, 2011.

American Academy of Pediatrics, Changing concepts of sudden infant death syndrome: Implications for infant sleeping environment and sleep position, *Pediatrics* 2000;105:650–656 http://pediatrics.aappublications.org/cgi/content/abstract/105/3/650. Accessed March 8, 2011.

American Association of Poison Control Centers, *National Poison Data Systems*, http://www.aapcc.org/dnn/NPDSPoisonData.aspx. Accessed March 8, 2011.

American College of Obstetricians and Gynecologists, *Morning Sickness*, http://www.acog.org/publications/patient_education/bp126.cfm. Accessed March 9, 2011.

American College of Obstetricians and Gynecologists, *Repeated Miscarriage*, http://www.acog.org/publications/patient_education/bp100.cfm. Accessed March 9, 2011.

American Family Physician, *Venomous Snakebites in the United States: Management and Review Update*, http://www.aafp.org/afp/2002/0401/p1367.html. Accessed March 8, 2011.

American Foundation for Suicide Prevention, *Facts and Figures: By Gender*, http://www.afsp.org/index.cfm?fuseaction=home.viewpage&page_id=04ECB949-C3D9-5FFA-DA9C65C381BAAEC0. Accessed March 8, 2011.

American Heart Association, *Heart Disease and Stroke Statistics*, http://www.americanheart.org/presenter.jhtml?identifier=1200026. Accessed March 8, 2011.

APCO International, *9-1-1 Consumer Information: Wireless 9-1-1 Services*, http://www.apco911.org/consumer. Accessed March 7, 2011.

Arshad A., Mandava A., Kamath G., Musat D. Sudden cardiac death and the role of medical therapy. *Progressive Cardiovascular Disease* 2008;50(6):420–38.

Carnegie Mellon University Libraries, https://cameo.library.cmu.edu//uhtbin/cgisirsi/x/x/0/49/. Accessed March 8, 2011.

Centers for Disease Control and Prevention, *Asthma Fast Facts*, http://www.cdc.gov/asthma/pdfs/asthma_fast_facts_statistics.pdf. Accessed March 8, 2011.

Centers for Disease Control and Prevention, *Developmental Disabilities: Vision Impairment*, http://www.cdc.gov/ncbddd/dd/vision2.htm. Accessed March 8, 2011.

Centers for Disease Control and Prevention, *Emergency Preparedness and Response: Bioterrorism Agents/Diseases*, http://www.bt.cdc.gov/agent/agentlist-category.asp. Accessed March 8, 2011.

Centers for Disease Control and Prevention, *Foodborne Illness*, http://www.cdc.gov/women/pubs/food.htm. Accessed March 8, 2011.

Centers for Disease Control and Prevention, *Healthy Youth! Alcohol and Drug Use*, http://www.cdc.gov/HealthyYouth/alcoholdrug/index.htm. Accessed March 8, 2011.

Centers for Disease Control and Prevention, *Healthy Youth! Asthma*, http://www.cdc.gov/HealthyYouth/asthma. Accessed March 8, 2011.

Centers for Disease Control and Prevention, *How Many People Have TBI?* http://www.cdc.gov/TraumaticBrainInjury/statistics.html. Accessed March 8, 2011.

Centers for Disease Control and Prevention, *Injury Center,* http://www.cdc.gov/ncipc/factsheets/childpas.htm. Accessed March 8, 2011.

Centers for Disease Control and Prevention, Injury Prevention and Control: Traumatic Brain Injury, *Traumatic Brain Injury in the United States: Emergency Department Visits, Hospitalizations and Deaths 2002–2006* http://www.cdc.gov/traumaticbraininjury/tbi_ed.html. Accessed March 8, 2011.

Centers for Disease Control and Prevention, *National Diabetes Fact Sheet: 2005,* http://www.cdc.gov/diabetes/pubs/pdf/ndfs_2005.pdf. Accessed March 8, 2011.

Centers for Disease Control and Prevention, *Severe Acute Respiratory Synrome (SARS): Fact Sheet,* http://www.cdc.gov/ncidod/sars/factsheet.htm. Accessed March 8, 2011.

Centers for Disease Control and Prevention, *Tetanus,* http://www.cdc.gov/vaccines/pubs/pinkbook/downloads/tetanus.pdf. Accessed March 8, 2011.

Centers for Disease Control and Prevention, *Unintentional Drowning: Fact Sheet,* http://www.cdc.gov/HomeandRecreationalSafety/Water-Safety/waterinjuries-factsheet.html, Accessed March 8, 2011.

Centers for Disease Control and Prevention, *Winnable Battles: Key Data,* www.cdc.gov/WinnableBattles/ppt/WinnableBattles_CDC_KeyData.pptx. Accessed March 8, 2011.

Centers for Disease Control and Prevention, *1918 Influenza: The Mother of All Pandemics,* http://www.cdc.gov/ncidod/eid/vol12no01/05-0979.htm. Accessed March 8, 2011.

Child Help, *National Child Abuse Statistics,* http://www.childhelp.org/pages/statistics. Accessed March 8, 2011.

Epilepsy Foundation, *About Epilepsy & Seizures: Epilepsy and Seizure Statistics,* http://www.epilepsyfoundation.org/about/statistics.cfm. Accessed March 8, 2011.

Family Caregiver Alliance, *Selected Traumatic Brain Injury Statistics,* http://www.caregiver.org/caregiver/jsp/content_node.jsp?nodeid=441. Accessed March 8, 2011.

FEMA, *About the National Incident Management System,* http://www.fema.gov/emergency/nims/AboutNIMS.shtm. Accessed March 8, 2011.

FEMA, *Emergency Support Function Annexes: Introduction,* http://www.fema.gov/pdf/emergency/nrf/nrf-esf-intro.pdf. Accessed March 8, 2011.

FEMA, *National Response Framework,* http://www.fema.gov/pdf/emergency/nrf/nrf-core.pdf. Accessed March 8, 2011.

Fire Engineering, *Rescue Guidelines for Air Bag-Equipped Vehicles,* http://www.fireengineering.com/index/articles/display/60045/articles/fire-engineering/volume-150/issue-12/features/rescue-guidlines-for-air-bab-equipped-vehicles.html. Accessed March 8, 2011.

Gold B.S., Dart R.C., Barish R.A., Bites of venomous snakes, *New England Journal of Medicine* 2002;347:347–356.

Graves J.R., Austin D. Jr., Cummins R.O.: *Rapid zap: Automated defibrillation,* Englewood Cliffs, NJ, 1989, Prentice-Hall.

Hampton Roads Red Cross Chapter, *Drowning and Prevention Water Safety,* http://www.hrredcross.org/wp-content/uploads/2010/06/NewsletterSummer2010.pdf. Accessed March 8, 2011.

Maguire B. J., Hunting K. L., Smith G. S., Levick N.R. Occupational fatalities in emergency medical services: A hidden crisis, *Annals of Emergency Medicine* 2002;40: 625–632. Available at: www.paramedicduquebec.org/documents/EMS_Fatalities.pdf. Accessed March 8, 2011.

National Council on Alcoholism and Drug Dependence, *Alcoholism and Alcohol-Related Problems,* http://www.ncadd.org/facts/problems.html. Accessed March 8, 2011.

National Emergency Number Association, *9-1-1 Call Volume,* http://www.nena.org/911-statistics. Accessed March 7, 2011.

National Institute of Mental Health, *Aspergers: Introduction* http://www.nimh.nih.gov/health/publications/autism/introduction.shtml. Accessed March 8, 2011.

National Institute of Mental Health, *Older Adults: Depression and Suicide Facts (Fact Sheet),* http://www.nimh.nih.gov/health/publications/older-adults-depression-and-suicide-facts-fact-sheet/index.shtml. Accessed March 8, 2011.

National Institute of Mental Health, *The Numbers Count: Mental Disorders in America,* http://www.nimh.nih.gov/health/publications/the-numbers-count-mental-disorders-in-america/index.shtml. Accessed March 8, 2011.

National Institute of Mental Health, *Suicide in the U.S.: Statistics and Prevention,* http://www.mentalhealth.gov/health/publications/suicide-in-the-us-statistics-and-prevention/index.shtml#risk. March 8, 2011.

National Institute for Occupational Safety and Health, *Alert: Preventing Needlestick Injuries in Healthcare Settings,* http://www.cdc.gov/niosh/docs/2000-108/pdfs/2000-108.pdf. Accessed March 8, 2011.

National Survey on Drug Use and Health, https://nsduhweb.rti.org. Accessed March 8, 2011.

The Nemours Foundation, Kids Health, *Muscular Dystrophy,* http://kidshealth.org/teen/diseases_conditions/bones/muscular_dystrophy.html. Accessed March 8, 2011.

NOAA, *A Severe Weather Primer: Questions and Answers About Lightning* http://www.nssl.noaa.gov/primer/lightning/ltg_damage.html. Accessed March 8, 2011.

Psychology Today, *Elder or Dependent Adult Neglect,* http://www.psychologytoday.com/conditions/elder-or-dependent-adult-neglect. Accessed March 8, 2011.

Substance Abuse and Mental Health Services Administration (SAMHSA), *Data, Outcomes, and Quality,* http://www.samhsa.gov/dataOutcomes. Accessed March 8, 2011.

Trauma.org, *Management of the Injured Pregnant Patient,* http://www.trauma.org/archive/resus/pregnancytrauma.html. Accessed March 8, 2011.

United States Consumer Product Safety Commission, *For Kid's Sake: Think Toy Safety,* http://www.cpsc.gov/cpscpub/pubs/281.html. Accessed March 8, 2011.

United States Department of Labor, *OSHA Safety Hazard Information Bulletin on Automobile Air Bag Safety,* http://www.osha.gov/dts/hib/hib_data/hib19900830.html. Accessed March 8, 2011.

United States Food and Drug Administration, *Oxygen Units: Import Alert,* http://www.accessdata.fda.gov/cms_ia/importalert_187.html. Accessed March 8, 2011.

WebMD, *Allergy Guide: Allergies to Insect Stings,* http://www.webmd.com/allergies/guide/insect-stings. Accessed March 8, 2011.

Wellness.com, *Insect Sting Allergy,* http://www.wellness.com/reference/allergies/insect-sting-allergy. Accessed March 8, 2011.

World Health Organization, *Meningococcal Meningitis: Fact Sheet,* http://www.who.int/mediacentre/factsheets/fs141/en/. Accessed March 8, 2011.

Index

A

Abandonment, definition of, 42, 53

Abdominal injury
  assessment techniques for, 470–471
  care for, 471
  signs and symptoms of, 470

Abdominal pain, 336–337
  care for, 337
  causes of, 337
  children and, 337–338
  elderly patients and, 338
  emergencies, 338
  signs and symptoms of, 337

Abrasion
  definition of, 445
  overview of, 448

Abruptio placentae, 548
  definition of, 531
  pregnancy, trauma and, 544

Absence seizures
  definition of, 325
  signs and symptoms of, 330

Absorbed poisons
  care for, 356
  definition of, 349
  eye contact and, 356
  plant irritants and, 355–356
  signs and symptoms of, 356

Access
  complex, 608
  definition of, 602
  simple, 608
  tools, 608–609

Acetylcholine, 653

ACS. *See* Acute coronary syndrome

Activated charcoal, administration of, 367

Acute, definition of, 15

Acute abdomen, definition of, 325, 337

Acute coronary syndrome (ACS), definition of, 291, 295

Acute myocardial ischemia, definition of, 291, 295

Acute pulmonary edema, 220

ADA. *See* Americans with Disabilities Act

Adaptive immunity, definition of, 15, 19

Addiction, definition of, 349

Adult, definition of, 551

Adult respiratory distress syndrome (ARDS), definition of, 426

Advance directive
  definition of, 42, 49
  overview of, 49–52

Advanced emergency medical technician (AEMT)
  definition of, 3
  professional level of training and, 8

AEDs. *See* Automated external defibrillators

AEMT. *See* Advanced emergency medical technician

Agonal gasp
  breathing *vs.*, 144
  definition of, 136

Agricultural emergency, 501–503

AIDS
  definition of, 15, 22
  mandated reporting and, 56
  universal precautions and, 26

Air medical transport
  considerations for, 590–593
  definition of, 585

Air splint, definition of, 476, 486

Airway
  children and, 552, 556, 558–559
  definition of, 136
  foreign body obstruction in the, 223
  inadequate, 222
  lower, 68–69, 216–217
  obstruction in and clearing of, 223
  opening the, 221–223
  upper, 68–69, 216

Airway adjunct
  definition of, 252
  overview of, 254–255

All-hazards approach, definition of, 639, 645

Alphaviruses, 648

Altered mental status
  care for, 328

causes of, 327
children and, 328–329
definition of, 325
medical restraints and, 97–98
signs and symptoms of, 328

Alzheimer's disease
  definition of, 570
  overview of, 575–576

AMBER. *See* America's Missing: Broadcast Emergency Response

Ambulance, patient care in, 597–598

Ambulatory, 630

American Association of Poison Control Centers (AAPCC), 353

Americans with Disabilities Act (ADA), 578

America's Missing: Broadcast Emergency Response (AMBER), 641

Amniotic fluid, definition of, 531

Amniotic sac, definition of, 531

Amputation
  definition of, 445
  overview of, 448–449

Anabolic steroids
  abuse and misuse of, 360
  definition of, 349

Anaphylaxis
  definition of, 373
  distributive shock and, 421
  insect bites, stings and, 385
  venomous snakes and, 388

Anatomic splint, definition of, 476, 487
  See also Skill sheets

Anatomical terms, 60–64

Anatomy, definition of, 59

Aneurysm, 325, 334, 335

Angina pectoris, definition of, 291, 296

Angulation, definition of, 476, 482

Animal bites, 391

Ankle drag
  definition of, 82
  overview of, 88–89
  See also Skill sheets

Anorexia nervosa, 364

Anthrax, 648
Antibodies, definition of, 15, 18
Antidote, definition of, 349
Antihistamines
    absorbed poisons and, 356
    definition of, 349, 364
    epinephrine auto-injector and, 397
    treatment for absorbed poison, 356
Anti-inflammatory drug
    absorbed poisons and, 356
    definition of, 349
    frostbite and, 384
Antivenin
    definition of, 373
    for spider and scorpion bites, 388
Anxiety disorder
    definition of, 405
    signs and symptoms of, 407–408
APGAR (appearance, pulse, grimace, activity, respiration) score
    definition of, 151, 531
    newborns, assessment of, 539–540
Aphasia, 325, 335
Apnea
    definition of, 214
    open airway, signs of, 222
    ventilation and, 231
Apparent life-threatening event (ALTE), definition of, 551, 567
Applied ethics, definition of, 46
Aquatic creatures, 390
Arrhythmias
    definition of, 291, 296
    V-fib and, 299
Arterial bleeding, 429, 430
Arterial gas embolism
    definition of, 373, 402
    SCUBA and, 402
Arteries, definition of, 426
Arterioles, 73
Arthritis, 580
Artificial ventilation
    adequate rates of, 230
    apneic patient and, 231
    definition of, 214
    mouth-to-mask, 226–227
    mouth-to-mouth, 226

special considerations in, 228–229
ASD. See Autism spectrum disorders
Asperger syndrome, definition of, 570, 581
Aspiration, definition of, 214
Aspirin, administration of, 343–344
Assault, definition of, 42, 52
Assessment
    airway, 222
    geriatric patients and, 573–575
    pediatrics and, 554–558
    suicide, 410–411
Asthma, 218–219
    definition of, 214
    medication for, 219, 247–248
    See also Skill sheets
Asthma attack, definition of, 214
Asthma trigger, definition of, 214, 218
Asymptomatic
    definition of, 639
    discharge and, 647
Asystole, definition of, 291, 306
Atherosclerosis, definition of, 291
Atria, 72
Atrial fibrillation, definition of, 291, 296
Atrioventricular (AV) node, definition of, 291, 294
Atropine
    definition of, 639
    incapacitating agents and, 648
    nerve agent poisoning and, 654–655
Audible warning devices
    definition of, 585
    safety issues, during response and, 594
Aura phase, 325, 329
Auscultation
    blood pressure measurement and, 180
    definition of, 164
    physical exam and, 172
Autism spectrum disorders (ASD)
    definition of, 570
    overview of, 581
Automated external defibrillators (AEDs)
    children and, 307–308
    definition of, 291, 306

maintenance of, 310
operation of, 306–307
precautions for, 310
special situations, 308–310
See also Skill sheets
AVPU (alert, verbal, painful, unresponsive) scale
    definition of, 136
    overview of, 141–142
Avulsion, definition of, 445, 449

B
B NICE, definition of, 639, 646
Babesia infection, 386
Backboard, 94–95
    definition of, 82
    log rolling and, 86
Bacteria, definition of, 15
Bag-valve-mask resuscitator (BVM), 229–230
    definition of, 214
    pediatric considerations and, 229
    resuscitation mask and, 227
    See also Skill sheets
Bandage
    application of, 432–433
    definition of, 426, 431
    types of, 431–432
Bandage compress, definition of, 426, 431
Barotrauma
    definition of, 373
    SCUBA and, 402
Basket stretchers, 93
Battery, definition of, 42, 52
Behavior, definition of, 405
Behavioral emergency
    care for, 414–415
    causes, 407
    definition of, 405
    excited delirium syndrome, 407
    signs and symptoms of, 406
Bereavement care
    definition of, 570
    hospice philosophy and, 582
BGL. See Blood glucose level
Binder, definition of, 476, 486
    See also Skill sheets
Biohazard
    definition of, 15
    engineering and work practice controls and, 27

Biological disasters, response, 644–645
Biological weapons, 648–649
Bioterrorism, definition of, 639, 640
Bipolar disorder, 408
    definition of, 405
    signs and symptoms of, 408
Birth canal, definition of, 531
Bites, stings
    animal, 391
    human, 391–392
    jellyfish, stingray, sea urchin, 390–391
    snakes, 388–389
    spiders, 386–388
    ticks, 386
Blanket drag
    definition of, 82, 88
    overview of, 88
    See also Skill sheets
Blast injury, 125–126
    definition of, 115
    mechanism of, 650–651
Blast lung, definition of, 639, 651
Bleeding
    care for, 434
    controlling of, 435–436, 519
    definition of, 426
    severe, 149–150
    types of, 429–430
    See also Skill sheets
Blister agents, 647
Blocking, scene and traffic control and, 605
Blood agents, 647–648
Blood clotting, 74
Blood glucose level (BGL)
    definition of, 325
    hyperglycemia, 332
    hypoglycemia, 325, 333
    Type 2 diabetes, 325
Blood glucose monitoring
    children and, 347
    glucometer and, 346–347
Blood pressure (BP)
    definition of, 73, 164
    equipment, for measurement of, 178–179
    levels in adults, 179
    levels in children, 183
    measurement of, 179–181
    precautions, 181
    See also Skill sheets

Blood volume, definition of, 426
Bloodborne, definition of, 15
Bloodborne pathogens
    definition of, 15
    transmission of, 19–21
Bloody show, definition of, 531
Blunt trauma
    definition of, 115
    mechanism of injury, 124
Body cavities, 63–64
Body mechanics
    definition of, 82
    overview of, 84
Body substance isolation (BSI) precautions
    definition of, 15
    standard precautions and, 25
    universal precautions *vs.*, 26
Body systems
    circulatory system, 59, 71–74
    definition of, 59
    digestive system, 59, 77–78
    endocrine system, 59, 76–77
    genitourinary system, 78–79
    integumentary system, 59, 75–76
    musculoskeletal system, 59, 64–68
    nervous system, 59, 74–75
    respiratory system, 59, 68, 70–71
Body temperature, 375–376
Bone, definition of, 476
Botulism, 648
BP. *See* Blood pressure
Brachial artery, definition of, 148–149
Brain, 74–75
Braxton-Hicks contractions
    definition of, 531
    labor, assessment of, 536
Breath sounds, 244
Breathing
    adequate, signs of, 224
    inadequate, signs of, 224–227
    status of, 144–146
Breathing emergency, 216
    children and infants and, 221
    definition of, 214
    signs and symptoms of, 218
Breathing rate
    definition of, 136
    labor and, 537

normal, 144–145
    slow, 225
Breech birth
    definition of, 531
    overview of, 545–546
Brucellosis, 648
BSI. *See* Body substance isolation
Bulb syringe
    definition of, 531
    use of, 540
Bulimia, 364
Burns
    chemical, 458–459
    circumferential, 455
    classification of, 453–456
    critical, 455–456
    definition of, 445
    electrical, 445, 459
    hypothermia risk and, 458
    Lund-Browder diagram, 454
    radiation, 445, 459–460
    rule of nines and, 445, 454
    severity conditions and, 452
    thermal, 455–458
BVM. *See* Bag-valve-mask resuscitator
Bystander, communications and, 205–206
BZ. *See* 3-quinuclidinyl benzilate

C
CAMEO®, 614
CA-MRSA. *See* Community-associated MRSA
Canadian Cervical Spine (C-Spine) rule, 512
Cancer, 580
Cannabis products
    abuse and misuse of, 360
    definition of, 349
    medical use and, 362–363
Capillaries
    definition of, 426
    overview of, 72–73
Capillary bleeding, 430
Capillary refill, 150–151
    definition of, 136
    pediatric considerations and, 151
Carbon monoxide (CO) poisoning
    care for, 369
    definition of, 349, 354
    detectors of, 368
    signs and symptoms of, 368–369

Cardiac arrest
    definition of, 291
    sequence to, 298–299
Cardiac chain of survival
    definition of, 291
    overview of, 299
Cardiac emergency
    aspirin and, 298
    assessment of, 297
    care for, 298
Cardiac muscle, definition of, 476, 479
Cardiac pathophysiology
    in children, 295
    in geriatric patients, 296
Cardiogenic shock, definition of, 419, 421
Cardiopulmonary resuscitation (CPR)
    adult, child and infant, 303
    artificial ventilation and, 299–300
    breathing barriers with, 26
    cessation of, 304
    compression, breath cycles and, 303–304
    definition of, 291, 293
    external chest compressions during, 300–302
    hands-only, 304–305
    pediatric considerations and, 304
    two-rescuer, 304
    See also Skill sheets
Cardiovascular disease
    atherosclerosis and, 294–295
    children and, 295–296
    coronary heart disease and, 294–295
    definition of, 291
    diabetes and, 296
    elderly and, 296
    myocardial infarction and, 295
Carotid artery, definition of, 136
Carrying, patients, 86
Catastrophic reaction
    Alzheimer's disease and, 575–576
    definition of, 570
Cave-ins, 666
CBRNE (chemical, biological, radiological/nuclear and explosive)
    definition of, 639, 646
    incident, response to, 651–653

CDC. *See* Centers for Disease Control and Prevention
Cells, definition of, 59, 64
Cellular respiration, 70
Centers for Disease Control and Prevention (CDC), 24
Cerebral palsy, 580
Cerebrospinal fluid, definition of, 506, 508
Certification, 12
    definition of, 3
    EMTs and, 8
    maintenance of, 10
Cervical collar (C-collar)
    backboarding and, 525
    definition of, 396
    head and brain injury and, 510
Cervical spine clearing, 12
Cervix
    definition of, 531, 533
    pregnancy and, 533
Cesarean section
    definition of, 531
    limb presentation and, 546
CEUs. *See* Continuing education units
CF. *See* Cystic fibrosis
CFR. *See* Code of Federal Regulations
CG. *See* Phosgene
Chemical burns
    care of, 458–459
    definition of, 445
    signs and symptoms of, 458
Chemical digestion, 78
Chemical Transportation Emergency Center (CHEMTEC), 351, 614
Chemical weapons, 646–648
Chest compressions
    arthritis and, 301
    breathing cycles and, 302–303
    correct hand position for, 300–301
    definition of, 291
    rescuer body position during, 301–302
    xiphoid process and, 300–301
Chest injuries
    blunt trauma, 464–465
    broken ribs, 465–466
    flail chest, 466
    impaled objects, 469–470

    sucking chest wound, 467–469
    traumatic asphyxia, 462, 465
Chest tube
    definition of, 462
    pneumothorax and, 467
Chief complaint, definition of, 164, 167
Child, definition of, 551
Child abuse, 412, 564–566
    burns and, 458
    definition of, 405, 551
    documentation of, 416
    SAMPLE history and, 557
    scene size-up and, 554–555
    self-mutilation and, 411
Child development, 552–554
Child neglect, 412–413, 564–566
    definition of, 405, 551
    SAMPLE history and, 557
Children
    abdominal pain and, 337–338
    abuse, neglect, 564–566
    AEDs and, 307–308
    airway of, 552, 556, 558–559
    altered mental status and, 328–329
    anatomical differences in, 552–553
    assessment of, 554–558
    blood glucose monitoring of, 347
    and blood pressure, 183
    breathing emergencies in, 559–560
    breathing rate in, 144
    and BVMs, 229
    capillary refill in, 150–151
    cardiovascular disease, 295–296
    CPR and, 304
    emergency oxygen and, 283–284
    foreign body airway obstruction and, 258–260
    heart problems and, 295
    OPAs and, 256
    poisoning and, 562
    pulse in, 148–149, 177
    respiratory emergencies and, 221
    respiratory rates in, 176
    respiratory system and, 70
    SAMPLE history for, 557–558
    shock in, 423, 563

Full-thickness burn
    definition of, 445
    overview of, 453–454

G

GA. *See* Tabun
Gastrointestinal bleeding, 472–473
Generalized tonic clonic seizures
    definition of, 325
    signs and symptoms of, 329
    stages of, 329
Genital injuries
    care for, 473–474
    signs and symptoms of, 473
Genitourinary system
    definition of, 59
    reproductive, 79
    urinary, 78–79
Geriatric patients, 569–573
    abdominal pain in, 338
    cardiac pathophysiology in, 296
    common problems in, 575–577
    patient assessment of, 141,
        573–574
    patient care for, 574–575
    physical and mental differences
        in, 571–573
    respiratory emergency in, 221
    substance abuse and, 364
Glanders, 648
Glasgow Coma Scale (GCS)
    definition of, 136
    overview of, 161–162
Glucose, 325, 333
Golden Hour, 426, 428
Good Samaritan laws
    definition of, 42
    overview of, 45
Grand mal seizures, 325
    See also Generalized tonic
        clonic seizures

H

H.A.IN.E.S. *See* High arm in
    endangered spine
Hallucination
    behavioral emergencies and,
        406, 414
    definition of, 405
    schizophrenia and, 409
Hallucinogen
    abuse and misuse of, 358–361,
        365
    definition of, 349

Hand sanitizer, 27
Hand washing, 26–27
Hanta virus, 648
Hard of hearing
    definition of, 570–571
    geriatric patient and, 578
Hazardous materials (HAZMAT),
        606, 613–614
    definition of, 115
    scene safety and, 116
    scene size-up and, 127–128
Hazardous Materials
    (HAZMAT) EMS Response
    Unit, 661
Hazardous materials (HAZMAT)
        incident, 615
    contamination, routes of
        exposure and, 620–621
    decontamination of, 621–622
    definition of, 612
    determination, 621
    emergency medical treatment
        and, 622
    extrication involving, 603,
        606
    identification of, 621
    personal protective equipment
        and, 618–620
    preparation for, 615
    recognition of, 615–617, 621
    safety zones, establishment of,
        620
    scene safety and, 618–620
Hazardous scenes
    electricity, 131, 132
    fire, 131–132
    hostage situation, 131, 134
    hostile persons, 131, 134
    natural disasters, 131, 133
    suicide, 131, 134
    traffic, 131–132
    unsafe structures, 131, 133
    water, ice, 131, 133
Hazardous terrain, 665
HAZMAT. *See* Hazardous
    materials
HAZMAT EMS Response Unit.
    See Hazardous Materials
    EMS Response Unit
HAZMAT incident. *See*
    Hazardous materials
    incident
HCI. *See* Hydrochloric acid
HD. *See* Sulfur mustard

HE. *See* High-order explosives
Head injuries
    care for, 510–511
    helmet, equipment removal
        and, 522–524
    signs and symptoms of, 510
    skull fractures and, 508–509
    See also Skill sheets
Head-on collision, 121–122, 426
Head-splint technique, 395, 396
Head-tilt/chin-lift technique
    airway, opening of, 221
    definition of, 214
Health care proxy, definition of,
        42, 52
Health Insurance Portability and
    Accountability Act (HIPAA),
        13, 54
Health Resources and Services
    Administration (HRSA), 7
Healthcare Infection Control
    Practices Advisory
    Committee (HICPAC), 26
Heart
    definition of, 291
    electrical system in, 293–294
    function of, 293
Heart attacks, 293
    cause of, 295
    definition of, 291
    women and, 296
Heart failure. *See* Congestive heart
    failure
Heart problems, children and, 295
Heat cramps
    care for, 378
    definition of, 373
    signs and symptoms of, 378
Heat exhaustion
    care for, 379
    definition of, 373
    signs and symptoms of, 379
Heat index
    definition of, 373
    heat-related illnesses and, 377
Heat stroke
    care for, 380–381
    classic, 380
    definition of, 373
    exertional, 380
    signs and symptoms of, 380
Heat-related illnesses
    individuals at high risk for,
        376–377

predisposing factors for, 377
prevention of, 384
types of, 378–380
Helicopter emergency medical
system (HEMS), 591
Hematoma, definition of, 115, 124
Hemodialysis
definition of, 325
emergencies and, 339
special patient considerations,
338–339
Hemopneumothorax, definition
of, 462
Hemorrhage, 426
Hemorrhagic shock
definition of, 531
pregnancy and, 544
Hemostatic agent, 426, 435
Hemothorax
definition of, 462
overview of, 467–468
HEMS. *See* Helicopter emergency
medical system
Hepatitis, definition of, 15
Hepatitis A virus (HAV), 21
Hepatitis B virus (HBV), 21–22
Hepatitis C virus (HCV), 22
Hepatitis D virus (HDV), 22
Hepatitis E virus (HEV), 22
HICPAC. *See* Healthcare Infection
Control Practices Advisory
Committee
High arm in endangered spine
(H.A.IN.E.S) recovery
position, 95–96, 575
High blood pressure. *See*
Hypertension
High-order explosives (HE),
definition of, 639, 650
Highway access, emergency
response and, 595
HIPAA. *See* Health Insurance
Portability and
Accountability Act
HIV, 22
affect on body and, 18
bloodborne pathogen
transmission and, 19–20
definition of, 15
protective equipment against,
25
transmission, risk of, 21
universal precautions and, 26
Hold, triage category, 631–632

Homeland Security Presidential
Directive-5 (HSPD-5), 641
Homeostasis, definition of, 15, 18
Hospice care
definition of, 570
overview of, 581–582
Hot zone
definition of, 612, 620
safety zone establishment and,
650
HRSA. *See* Health Resources and
Services Administration
HSPD-5. *See* Homeland Security
Presidential Directive-5
Human bites, 391–392
Human-caused disasters, response,
644
Hydrochloric acid (HCI), 648
Hyoid bone, 216
Hyperglycemia, 325, 332
Hyperkalemia, 325
Hyperoxia, definition of, 278, 279
Hypertension, definition of, 291,
296
Hyperthermia
definition of, 373, 377
heat-related illnesses and, 377
Hyperventilation
definition of, 214
overview of, 220
Hypervolemia
definition of, 325
delayed dialysis signs of, 339
Hypodermis
definition of, 445
soft tissue injuries and, 446
Hypoglycemia, 325, 333
Hypoperfusion, definition of, 419,
420
See also Shock
Hypotension
definition of, 462
tension pneumothorax and,
468
Hypothalamus
body temperature and,
375–376
definition of, 373, 375
Hypothermia
care for, 381–383
contributing factors to, 380–
382
definition of, 373
signs and symptoms of, 382

Hypovolemia
definition of, 325
post dialysis signs of, 339
Hypovolemic shock
blunt trauma and, 465
care for, 434
definition of, 419, 421
Hypoxemia, 325
Hypoxia, definition of, 214, 217,
279
Hypoxic, definition of, 136, 145

I
Ice rescue, 664
ICS. *See* Incident command system
Immediate care (Red)
children and, 633
definition of, 624
in START system, 630
triage assessment and, 632
Immobilize
definition of, 476
muscle, bone, joint injuries,
care for, 483–484
Immune system, definition of, 15
Immunity, 19
Immunizations, 24
Impaled object
in chest, care for, 469–470
definition of, 462
Implantable cardioverter-
defibrillator (ICD)
AED use and, 308
definition of, 291
Implantation, definition of, 531,
534
Implied consent
definition of, 42
overview of, 47
In good faith, 45–46
definition of, 42
Incapacitating agents, 648
Incendiary weapons, 650–651
B NICE system and, 646
definition of, 639
Incident command system (ICS)
definition of, 624
EMS roles in, 625–626
overview of, 625
Incident management, 640–642
Indirect contact
bloodborne pathogens and,
20
definition of, 15, 20

Indirect force, definition of, 476, 479
Indirect medical control, definition of, 3, 11–12
Industrial emergency, 503–504
Infant(s)
 AED and, 319–321
 choking and, 269–270, 273–274
 CPR and, 303
 definition of, 551
 foreign body airway obstruction and, 258–260
 pulse oximetry on, 198
 recovery position for, 96
 shock in, 423
 ventilation and, 236–237
Infection
 cause of, 17–21
 definition of, 15
Infectious disease
 definition of, 15
 mandated reporting of, 56
 protection from, 24
 transmission of, 17–21
Influenza
 pandemic, 16, 24, 657
 seasonal, 23–24
Ingested poisons
 care for, 353
 definition of, 349, 353–354
 signs and symptoms of, 353
 types of, 353–354
Inhalants
 abuse and misuse of, 360
 definition of, 349
Inhaled poisons
 care for, 355
 definition of, 349
 signs and symptoms of, 355
 types of, 354–355
Injected poisons
 definition of, 349
 signs and symptoms of, 357
In-line stabilization
 cervical collars, backboarding and, 525
 definition of, 506
Innate immunity, definition of, 15, 19
Insect sting, care of, 385
Insulin, 325
Integumentary system
 definition of, 59
 overview of, 75–76

Intercostal, definition of, 462
Internal bleeding, 426
 assessment and care of, 436–437
 causes of, 436
Intubation, 245, 246

J
Jaw-thrust (without head extension) maneuver
 airway, opening using, 221–222
 definition of, 214
 geriatric patient and, 574
 head, neck or spinal injuries and, 229
 See also Skill sheets
Jellyfish stings, 390–391
Jewelry, piercings, AED, 309
Joint, definition of, 476
Jump kit
 definition of, 585
 overview of, 598–599
JumpSTART pediatric triage, 633–634

K
Kendrick Extrication Device (KED), 94–95
Kinematics of trauma
 definition of, 115
 falls and, 440–441
 motorcycle accidents and, 440
 vehicle collisions and, 120–121, 439–440

L
Labor
 assessment of, 536
 caring for mother in, 542
 crowning, 531, 535
 definition of, 531
 delivery, 538–539
 dilation, 531, 534–535
 expulsion, 535
Laceration
 definition of, 445
 overview of, 450–451
Landing zone (LZ)
 definition of, 585
 overview of, 592
LAPSS. *See* Los Angeles Prehospital Stroke Screen

LATCH system. *See* Lower anchors and tethers for children system
LE. *See* Low-order explosives
Legal obligation, definition of, 42
Level of consciousness (LOC)
 altered mental status and, 328
 definition of, 136
 START system and, 630
Licensure, definition of, 3, 12
Life-saving interventions (LSI), 632–633
Lifting. *See* Moving, lifting, of patient
Ligament, definition of, 476
Lightning storm, 400–401
Lights, vehicle, use of, 594
Liters per minute (LPM), 253
Litter
 definition of, 660
 hazardous terrain and, 665, 670
Lividity
 definition of, 15
 obvious death and, 55
 resuscitation and, 31
Living will, definition of, 42, 49
LOC. *See* Level of consciousness
Local credentialing, definition of, 3, 12
Log roll
 correct reaching for, 86
 definition of, 82
Los Angeles Prehospital Stroke Screen (LAPSS), 336
Lower anchors and tethers for children (LATCH) system, 607
Low-order explosives (LE), definition of, 639, 650
LSI. *See* Life-saving interventions
Lund-Browder diagram, 454
Lyme disease, 386
LZ. *See* Landing zone

M
MACS. *See* Multiagency coordination system
Malpractice
 definition of, 42
 standard of care and, 44
Mandatory reporting, 56
Mania, definition of, 405, 408

Nasal (nasopharyngeal) airways (NPAs), definition of, 252
See also Skill sheets
National Disaster Medical System (NDMS), 640
National Emergency X-Radiography Utilization Study (NEXUS) Low-Risk Criteria, 512
National Fire Protection Association (NFPA)
extrication, personal safety and, 604
HAZMAT incidents and, 614
National Highway Traffic Safety Administration (NHTSA), 5–7
National Incident Management System (NIMS), 202, 640–642
National Institute for Occupational Safety and Health (NIOSH), 614
National Oceanic and Atmospheric Administration (NOAA), 614, 641
National Response Framework (NRF)
definition of, 624, 640
NIMS and, 625
Natural disasters, response to, 644
Nature of illness
definition of, 115
overview of, 126–127
Nature of illness, definition of, 115
NDMS. *See* National Disaster Medical System
Neck, spine injuries
care for, 515–516
MOI of, 514–515
prevention of, 516–517
signs and symptoms of, 515
See also Skill sheets
Needlestick
definition of, 15
disease, spread of, and, 19
Needlestick Safety and Prevention Act, 30
Negligence
definition of, 42, 44
necessary proof for lawsuit of, 53
Nerve agents
chemical weapons and, 647

definition of, 639
self-care and peer care for, 653–655
Nervous system, 66
anatomy of, 74–75
definition of, 59
physiology of, 75
Neurogenic/vasogenic shock, definition of, 419, 421
Newborn care
APGAR score, 539–540
resuscitation, 541
umbilical cord, 532, 539
Next of kin, definition of, 42, 52
NFPA. *See* National Fire Protection Association
NGOs. *See* Nongovernmental organizations
NHTSA. *See* National Highway Traffic Safety Administration
NIMS. *See* National Incident Management System
NIOSH. *See* National Institute for Occupational Safety and Health
Nipah virus, 648
Nitrogen narcosis, 402
Nitroglycerin, administration of, 344–345
NOAA. *See* National Oceanic and Atmospheric Administration
Non-emergency moves
techniques for, 90–92
uses for, 90
Nongovernmental organizations (NGOs), 641
Non-rebreather mask, 282
definition of, 278
fixed-flow-rate oxygen and, 280
Non-swimming rescues and assists
definition of, 660
examples of, 663–664
Normal sinus rhythm (NSR), definition of, 291
Nosebleeds, 434, 511
NRF. *See* National Response Framework
Nuclear weapons, 649–650

O

Obstetric pack, definition of, 531, 536–537

Obstructive shock, definition of, 419, 421
Occlusive dressing
definition of, 426, 430–431
sucking chest wound and, 468–469
Occupational Safety and Health Administration (OSHA)
definition of, 15
exposure control plans and, 24
extrication, personal safety and, 604
HAZMAT incident and, 614
Office of Emergency Management (OEM), 614
Office of Response and Restoration (OR&R), 614
Ongoing assessment, definition of, 164
Onset, provoke, quality, region/radiate, severity, time (OPQRST), definition of, 164
Open fractures, definition of, 476, 480
Open wound
care of, 451–452
definition of, 445
types of, 448–451
Opportunistic infections, definition of, 15, 22
OPQRST. *See* Onset, provoke, quality, region/radiate, severity, time
Oral glucose, administration of, 345
Oral injuries, 514
Oral (oropharyngeal) airways (OPAs)
definition of, 252
insertion procedure, 255
pediatric considerations and, 256
See also Skill sheets
Organ, definition of, 59
Organ donors, 55
O-ring gasket
definition of, 278, 281
pressure regulator and flowmeter and, 281
OR&R. *See* Office of Response and Restoration
Orthopedic stretchers, 94

Preeclampsia, 543
    blood pressure and, 537
    definition of, 531
Pregnancy
    complications during,
        542–544, 548–549
    normal, 533–534
Prehospital care, definition of, 3
Prehospital care report (PCR)
    definition of, 200
    description and uses of,
        206–209
Premature birth
    definition of, 531
    overview of, 546–547
Preparedness
    disasters, terrorism, 638
    personal, 658
Pressure bandage, definition of,
        426, 431–432
Pressure points
    definition of, 426
    overview of, 436
Pressure regulator
    definition of, 278
    flowmeter and, 280–281
Primary assessment
    airway status, 142–143
    breathing status, 144–147
    BVMs, 146
    circulatory status, 147–151
    definition of, 136
    life threats, identification of,
        151
    LOC, 141
    patient general impression,
        139–140
    patient responsiveness,
        140–142
    scene size-up, 138–139
    shock, 151–152
    See also Skill sheets
Primary effects
    of blast injury, 650–651
    definition of, 639
Primary triage, 628–629
Prolapsed cord
    definition of, 532
    overview of, 545
Protected health information
    (PHI), 54
Protocols, definition of, 3, 11
PSAP. See Public safety answering
        point

Psychological emergencies
    anxiety disorder, 407–408
    bipolar disorder, 408
    clinical depression, 408
    paranoia, 409
    phobias, 408
    suicide, 409–411
Public safety answering point
    (PSAP), 587
Public Service Answering Point
    (PSAP), 200
Pulling, of object, 86
Pulmonary agents, 648
Pulmonary embolism
    definition of, 214
    overview of, 220
Pulmonary Overinflation
    Syndrome (POIS), 402
Pulmonary Overpressure
    Syndrome, 402
Pulse
    abnormal, 148
    definition of, 136
    normal rates, 148
    thready, 551
Pulse oximetry
    definition of, 164
    overview of, 197–198
Puncture/penetration
    definition of, 445
    overview of, 449–450
Purkinje fibers, 294
Pushing, of object, 86

Q
Q fever, 648
Quality improvement (QI), 13
3-quinuclidinyl benzilate, 648

R
Rabies
    definition of, 373, 391
    immunizations for, 391
Radiation, definition of, 373,
        376
Radiation burns
    definition of, 445
    overview of, 459–460
Radio communications,
        201–202
Radio frequency interference
    (RFI), 310
Radiological weapons, 649–650
Rales, definition of, 214, 224

Rape
    definition of, 405
    overview of, 412
    self-mutilation and, 411
Rape-trauma syndrome
    definition of, 405
    stages of, 412
Rapid medical assessment,
        definition of, 164, 169
Rapid trauma assessment,
        definition of, 164, 169
Rappelling
    definition of, 660
    hazardous terrain and, 665
Reach, throw, row then go, 133,
        394
Reaching, for patients and
        equipment, 86
Reaching assist
    definition of, 660
    ice rescue and, 664
    water rescue and, 663, 669
Reactivity, definition of, 612–613
Rear-end, vehicle crashes, 122
Reasonable force, definition of,
        82, 98
Receiving facility,
        communications and,
        204
Recovery positions
    definition of, 82
    indications for use, 95
    techniques, 96
Refusal of care, 47–49
    definition of, 42
    patient competence and, 45
Resources, students, 23
Respiration, 70–71, 376
Respiratory arrest
    definition of, 136
    resuscitation mask and, 146
Respiratory distress
    assisted ventilation during,
        230–231
    causes of, 218
    children in, 304, 559
    definition of, 136
    pulse oximetry and, 197
    resuscitation mask and, 146
Respiratory emergency
    asthma, 214, 218–219
    children and, 221
    COPD, 218
    elderly patients and, 221

suspected (jaw-thrust (without head extension) maneuver)—adult and child, 156–157

walking assist, 107

Skin, 75–76

dermis, 445, 446

epidermis, 445, 446

hypodermis, 445, 446

Sling, 486

broken ribs and, 466

triangular bandage and, 432

See also Skill sheets

Smallpox, 648

Smart Tag™ patient identification system, 630

Smooth muscles, definition of, 476, 479

Snake bites

care for, 389

signs and symptoms of, 388, 389

Soft splint

definition of, 476

overview of, 485–486

See also Skill sheets

Soft tissues, definition of, 445

Sort-Assess-Lifesaving Interventions-Treatment and/or Transport (SALT) Mass Casualty Triage, 632–633

Special events, 668–669

Special insertion and extrication (SPIE) lines, 593

Special needs patients

children, 567

chronic diseases, disabilities, 578–581

deafness, 578

hard of hearing, 578

intellectual disabilities, 577

mental illness, 577

physically challenged, 578

visual impairment, 578

Specialized Vehicle Response Unit, 661

Speed, emergency response and, 595

Sphygmomanometer, definition of, 164

Spider bites, 386–388

SPIE lines. *See* Special insertion and extrication lines

Spinal column, definition of, 506

Spinal cord, definition of, 506

Spinal motion restriction, definition of, 506

Spine, neck injuries

care for, 515–516

immobilizing the head, 526–527

MOI, 514–515

prevention of, 516–517

signs and symptoms of, 515

Splints, 484

definition of, 476

lower extremities, use on, 489–491

rules for, 484–485

types of, 485–487

upper extremities, use on, 487–489

See also Skill sheets

Sprain

definition of, 476

overview of, 481

Squat lift, definition of, 82, 86

Stabilization, definition of, 532, 535

Staging area

definition of, 612, 614

support equipment position and, 622

Staging officer, triage, 635

Stair chair, definition of, 82, 94

Standard of care, definition of, 42, 44

Standard precautions

definition of, 16

overview of, 24–26

personal protective equipment and, 118–119

Standing orders, definition of, 3, 11

Staphylococcal enterotoxin B, 648

START. *See* Simple triage and rapid transport

Status asthmaticus, definition of, 551

Status epilepticus, 326

Stethoscope, 164, 178–179

Stillbirth

definition of, 532, 542

mother, caring for, 542

Stimulants

abuse and misuse of, 359

definition of, 349

Stoma, definition of, 136, 144

Strain, 476, 481

Stress

definition of, 16, 32–33

at MCIs, 635–637

situations of, 30–31

warning signs of, 33

Stretchers

definition of, 82

EMR body mechanics and, 84

moving patients to, from bed, 91–92

types of, 92–94

Stridor, definition of, 215, 222

Stroke

care for patient having, 336

causes, 334–335

Cincinnati Prehospital Stroke Scale, 335

definition of, 326

FAST, 336

LAPSS, 336

sudden signs and symptoms of, 335

Subconjunctival hemorrhage, definition of, 462, 465

Subcutaneous emphysema, definition of, 462, 466

Substance abuse

adolescents and, 364

care for, 365

definition of, 349, 357

elderly and, 364

factors contributing to, 365–366

forms of, 357–358

prevention of, 365–366

signs and symptoms of, 364–365

substances, categories of, 358–364

Substance misuse, definition of, 349

See also Substance abuse

Sucking chest wound

care for, 468–469

definition of, 462

pneumothorax and, 467

Suctioning, 253

definition of, 215

equipment for, 253–254

pediatric consideration, 254

upper airway, foreign matter removal of, 223

See also Skill sheets

Sudden cardiac arrest (SCA)
   definition of, 292
   overview of, 298–299
Sudden death, definition of, 16, 32
Sudden infant death syndrome
   (SIDS)
   assessment of, 566–567
   definition of, 551
Suicide, 409–411
   bipolar and, 408
   clinical depression and, 408
   definition of, 405
   drug overdose and, 358
   scene size-up and, 134, 414
Sulfur mustard (HD), 647
Sundowning
   definition of, 570
   overview of, 575–576
Superficial burn, definition of,
   445, 453
Supine, definition of, 82
Supine position, 96–97
Surrogate decision maker,
   definition of, 42, 49–52
Swathe, definition of, 476, 485
Symptoms
   definition of, 136
   general impression, of patient,
   139
Syncope, 326, 328
Synergistic effect, definition of,
   349, 358
Systolic blood pressure
   blood pressure levels and, 179
   blood pressure measurement
   and, 178
   definition of, 164

T
Tabun (GA), 647
Tactical Emergency Medical
   Services (EMS) Unit, 661
Tear gas, 648
Tendon, definition of, 476
Tension pneumothorax
   definition of, 462
   overview of, 468
Terrorism, 638–656
Tertiary effects
   in blast injury, 651
   definition of, 639
Tetanus
   animal bites and, 391
   definition of, 373

jellyfish stings and, 391
   puncture/penetration wounds
   and, 450
Thermal burns, 456–458
Thoracic (cavity), definition of,
   462–463
Thready, definition of, 551, 556
360-degree assessment, 596–597
Thrombus, 326, 334, 335
Throwing assist
   definition of, 660
   ice rescue and, 664
   water rescue and, 663–664,
   669
TIA. *See* Transient ischemic attack
Tick bites, 386
Tick-borne viruses, 386, 648–649
Tidal volume, definition of, 215,
   225
Tissue, definition of, 59, 64
Tolerance, definition of, 349, 358
Tonic phase, 326, 329
Tourniquet
   definition of, 426
   overview of, 435
   See also Skill sheets
Toxemia
   definition of, 532, 543
   overview of, 543
Toxicity, definition of, 612, 614
Toxicology, definition of, 349, 351
Toxin, definition of, 349
Traction splint, definition of, 476,
   486
Traffic control, extrication and,
   605
Transdermal medication patch
   AED use and, 309
   definition of, 292
Transferring, patient
   to ambulance, 588
   definition of, 585
   to flight personnel, 592
   phases of response and, 586
Transient ischemic attack (TIA),
   326
   definition of, 326
   risks of, 334–335
Transport, of patient
   by air, 590–593
   positioning, packaging for,
   94–97
Transportation officer, triage,
   635

Trauma alert criteria
   definition of, 585
   overview of, 590
Trauma dressing, definition of,
   430, 431
Trauma system
   definition of, 426
   overview of, 428–429
Traumatic asphyxia
   definition of, 462
   overview of, 465
Traumatic brain injury, 578
Treatment officer, triage, 634–635
Triage
   assessment in, 632
   definition of, 624
   methods of, 632–633
   officer, 628
   pediatric considerations in,
   633–634
   primary and secondary,
   628–629
   staging, 635
   START system, 630–632
   tagging systems, 629–630
   transportation and, 635
   treatment in, 634–635
Triage officer, 628
Triage tags
   definition of, 624
   overview of, 629–630
Triangular bandage, definition of,
   426, 432
Trimester
   definition of, 532
   overview of, 533–534
Tripod position, definition of, 115,
   127
Tuberculosis (TB), 22
   definition of, 16
   HIV/AIDS and, 22
Tularemia, 648
Twisting force, definition of, 476,
   479
Two-person seat carry
   definition of, 82
   overview of, 90–91
   See also Skill sheets

U
Umbilical cord
   cutting of, 539
   definition of, 532
   delivery and, 539

first trimester and, 534
prolapsed, 545
Universal precautions, definition of, 16, 25
Unstable vehicles, 122–123
U.S. Department of Transportation (DOT), 4, 614
Uterus
definition of, 532
physiology of, 533
ruptured, 549

V

Vacuum splint, definition of, 476, 486
Vagina
bleeding, in pregnancy, 543–544
definition of, 532
pregnancy, physiology of, 533
Vector-borne transmission
bloodborne pathogens and, 20–21
definition of, 16
Vehicle
cleaning, disinfecting, 28–29
siren, lights and, use of, 594
Vehicle crashes
chocking and, 123
seat belts, airbags and, 123
types of, 121–122
whiplash injury from, 122
Vehicle stabilization
definition of, 602
overview of, 606–608
Veins, definition of, 426
Venous bleeding, 430
Ventilation
adequate, signs of, 224
apneic patient and, 231
artificial, 226–231
definition of, 215

inadequate, signs of, 224–225
normal *vs.* positive pressure, 230
structures supporting, 70–71
See also Skill sheets
Ventricles, 72
Ventricular fibrillation (V-fib)
arrhythmia and, 299
definition of, 292
Ventricular tachycardia (V-tach), definition of, 292, 305
Vial of life
definition of, 164
patient medical history, obtaining, 167
Viral hemorrhagic fevers, 648
Virus, definition of, 16
Visual impairment, 578
Visual warning devices
definition of, 585
safety issues, during response, 594–595
Vital organs, definition of, 59, 64
Vital signs
by age, 182
baseline, obtaining, 175
blood pressure, 177–182
definition of, 136, 151
pulse, 176–178
respiratory rate, 176
skin color, temperature, moisture, 150
See also Skill sheets
Vocal cords, 216
Voluntary muscles, definition of, 476, 479
VX. *See* Methylphosphonothioic acid

W

Wading assist
definition of, 660
water rescue and, 663–664

Walking assist
definition of, 82
overview of, 90
See also Skill sheets
Walking wounded (Green)
definition of, 624
in START system, 630
Warfarin (Coumadin®), 298
Warm zone, definition of, 612, 620
Warning systems, 641
Water pathogens, 648
Water rescue, 133, 394, 661–664
Weapons of mass destruction (WMDs), 646
biological weapons, 648–649
chemical weapons, 646–648
definition of, 639
EMS operations during, 645–646
explosives and incendiary weapons, 650–651
incident, response to, 651–653
radiological/nuclear weapons, 649–650
Weather, emergency response and, 595
Wheezing, definition of, 215, 217
Whiplash injury, 122
Withdrawal, definition of, 349, 358
WMDs. *See* Weapons of mass destruction
Work practice controls, 27–28
BSI precautions and, 25
definition of, 16
Wound, definition of, 445

Y

Yellow fever, 648